James J. Nora, M.D.
University of Colorado Medical Center
420___ ___ ___ Avenue
Denver, Colorado 80220

Other monographs in the series, *Major Problems in Clinical Pediatrics:*

Avery and Fletcher: *The Lung and Its Disorders in the Newborn Infant*—Third Edition to be published in early 1974

Bell and McCormick: *Increased Intracranial Pressure in Children*—published in July 1972

Cornblath and Schwartz: *Disorders of Carbohydrate Metabolism in Infancy*—published in February 1966

Oski and Naiman: *Hematologic Problems in the Newborn*—Second Edition published in March 1972

Rowe and Mehrizi: *The Neonate with Congenital Heart Disease*—published in June 1968

Brewer: *Juvenile Rheumatoid Arthritis*—published in January 1970

Smith: *Recognizable Patterns of Human Malformation*—published in February 1970

Markowitz and Gordis: *Rheumatic Fever*—Second Edition published in October 1972

Solomon and Esterly: *Neonatal Dermatology*—published in January 1973

AMINO ACID METABOLISM AND ITS DISORDERS

Charles R. Scriver, M.D., C.M., F.R.S.(C.)

Professor of Pediatrics; Associate Professor of Biology
McGill University
Montreal, Canada

Leon E. Rosenberg, M.D.

Professor and Chairman, Department of Human Genetics;
Professor of Pediatrics and Medicine
Yale University
New Haven, Connecticut

Volume X in the Series

MAJOR PROBLEMS IN CLINICAL PEDIATRICS

ALEXANDER L. SCHAFFER
Consulting Editor

1973
W. B. Saunders Company, Philadelphia, London, Toronto

W. B. Saunders Company: West Washington Square
                          Philadelphia, Pa. 19105

                          12 Dyott Street
                          London, WCIA 1DB

                          833 Oxford Street
                          Toronto 18, Ontario

Amino Acid Metabolism and Its Disorders   ISBN 0-7216-8044-5

Print No.   9   8   7   6   5   4   3   2   1

Foreword

Generalists, whether they deal with children or adults or both, have a hard time keeping themselves *au courant* on all fronts. Every decade or so one or another branch of medicine "takes off," either from scratch, like cytologic genetics, or from a semi-dormant state, like biochemical genetics, and grows with astonishing rapidity. One branch of biochemical genetics, disorders of protein metabolism, is a perfect example of this problem, for its recent headlong advance has left many of us badly outdistanced.

It is for this reason that we welcome this eighth volume in our series. Inborn errors of protein metabolism, one subdivision of biochemical genetics, is one of the best, if not the best example of such an occurrence. It is important not only because it involves, in the aggregate, so many infants, children and adults, but because diagnoses can now be made by properly directed studies without too much difficulty or delay, and because early diagnosis and appropriate therapy are now mandatory, since they can save life, intelligence and vision.

We have been extremely fortunate that the team of Drs. Charles R. Scriver and Leon E. Rosenberg agreed to undertake this task. Dr. Scriver, born and educated in Montreal, and trained there and in Boston and London, has devoted the major part of his fifteen years in Medicine and Pediatrics to problems concerning amino acid metabolism, both normal and deranged. He is now Professor of Pediatrics, Associate Professor of Genetics and Associate Member of the Department of Biochemistry of McGill University, as well as Associate Member of the Human Genetics Center of Laval University. Dr. Rosenberg is a Wisconsin native who received his medical training at Columbia, The National Institutes of Health and Yale. He is now Professor of Human Genetics, Pediatrics and Medicine at Yale.

Both authors have published extensively and lectured widely on the clinical and biochemical aspects of inborn errors of metabolism; both have made valuable original contributions to the subject; and both have been recipients of prestigious awards in recognition of their accomplishments. We believe in all honesty that the library of every practitioner of Pediatrics and of Medicine will be incomplete without this volume.

ALEXANDER J. SCHAFFER, M.D.

Preface

Asparagine and cystine, the first two amino acids to be recognized, were discovered in 1806 and 1810, respectively—the former in the juice of asparagus and the latter by chemical analysis of human urinary tract calculi which, incidentally, were subsequently treasured in the Guy's Hospital surgical museum for the edification of medical students. From the beginning, it was apparent that amino acids are relevant in our concerns for human health.

Just as the pace of discovery of new amino acids was slow until the beginning of the 20th century, so was the description of the disorders of amino acid metabolism in man. At the time of the first World War, all but threonine among the protein amino acids were known; a chemical method for analysis of α-amino nitrogen had become available; and the Mendelian laws of genetics had been "rediscovered" and were shown to pertain to amino acid metabolism. It was not until another Great War had occurred, and a quarter of a century had passed, that the acquisition of new knowledge about amino acid metabolism and its disorders in man achieved its current exponential rate. The introduction of new methods for analysis of amino acids, the abatement of other diseases which had long dominated medical interest and the interpretation of genetic theory in terms of modern molecular biology are the events largely responsible for the current great interest in human amino acid metabolism.

The book that we have written will not displace any of the classical treatises on amino acid biochemistry; in fact, we ourselves continue to learn from them. Our book is written for those who must deal with the human biology of health and disease where it impinges on amino acid metabolism. The book is divided into three sections. The first is a general discussion of amino acids and includes consideration of their biological chemistry. There is also an extensive discussion of methods which serve diagnosis and investigation of aminoacidopathies, revealing that quantitative and qualitative techniques of analysis form the bridge between theory and practice. Because mass screening has played such a large role in developing our awareness of human aminoacidopathies, we have also included some discussion of the principles and practices of screening.

The second part of the book brings together a series of discussions on membrane transport of amino acids and the disorders thereof. We both entered the field of amino acid metabolism through research on membrane transport of these compounds. It is now apparent to biologists in general that there is no cell, and therefore no life, without a membrane. Consequently, amino acid nutrition, considerations about distribution of amino acids between body fluids and tissues and the general metabolic traffic of amino acids cannot be viewed in proper perspective without consideration of transport phenomena. On the other hand, it is appropriate that discussions of a number of hereditary disorders of membrane transport accompany the exposition of general mechanisms: these, therefore, have been used as stimuli to interest in transport as an important constitutent of amino acid metabolism.

The third and longest part of the book presents systematic discussions of many amino acids which play important roles in human metabolism. We have again used hereditary disorders extensively to illuminate the metabolism of these amino acids. This section and the book end with a chapter on the vitamin-responsive disorders of amino acid metabolism, a topic whose lineage goes back to two of the great figures in human biochemistry, Garrod and Hopkins.

It is unfortunate that many of the published observations which could have been cited to document statements made in the text do not appear as bibliographic references, of which there are already more than 1500. In those papers that we have cited, we try to indicate how the reader's information base can be extended according to his wishes. The publishers have been generous in their allowance for tabular material and illustrations to amplify the text.

There are many many colleagues to whom we are grateful, most of whom will recognize themselves without being named in a long and thus impersonal list: those who trained us; those who through their own work instigated ours; those who are our daily associates and have endured our labor with "the book." We are particularly grateful to Dr. Alexander Shaffer for delivering the challenge to produce this book; and we warmly acknowledge the editors at Saunders for their assistance. We would have had trouble doing anything without those key people, our secretaries—Mrs. Huguette Ishmael, Miss Lynne Prevost, Miss Marilyn Feldman—and the artists and photographers, particularly Mrs. Nancy Todd, Miss Philippa Nelson, Louis and Denis Hebert and Mrs. Virginia Simon.

CHARLES R. SCRIVER
LEON E. ROSENBERG

Contents

PART III
Metabolism of Specific Amino Acids and
Their Disorders

General Aspects of Amino Acid Metabolism

Chapter One

PHYSICAL AND CHEMICAL PROPERTIES OF AMINO ACIDS

GENERAL PROPERTIES

Amino acids are the primary determinants of protein structure. Most amino acids in proteins have a free carboxyl group, a free unsubstituted amino group on the α-carbon and an R group, or side chain. The latter confers specific chemical characteristics to the individual amino acids. The general structural formula for free and peptide-linked amino acids is shown in Figure 1–1. The atoms common to protein amino acids which participate in peptide linkage are indicated in the figure.

Not all protein amino acids have α-amino groups. Proline and hydroxyproline, which are found in proteins, each have a substituted amino group; as a result, they are usually designated *imino acids*, a trivial name to distinguish them from *amino acids*.

Imino acid   Amino acid

There are many variations in R group configuration, including lengthening of the carbon chain (in the aliphatic series), ring formation (in the aromatic and heterocyclic series), addition of a charged group (in the acidic or basic series) and insertion of functional groups (e.g., SH or OH). Not all amino acids are found in protein. In those that are not, the position of the amino group may vary, appearing on the β- or α-carbon atom. In another variation, the carboxyl group may be substituted: for example, by SO_3H in taurine. The structural formulas of the 20 common protein amino acids are shown in Figure 1–2, and

3

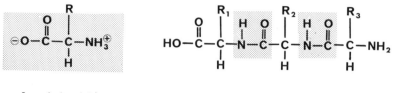

Free Amino Acid
at Isoelectric Point

Peptide—linked Amino Acid

Figure 1–1   The basic formula of a free amino acid (left). There is no net charge at the −pI, or isoelectric point.

All amino acids have carboxyl and amino groups, and all protein amino acids have an *α-amino* group. The chemical variation of amino acids resides in the R group, in the position of the amino group and in the net charge.

When amino acids are joined in peptide linkage they form peptides or proteins (right). The primary sequence of a protein is determined by variation in the sequence of R groups.

formulas of other amino acids appear in the text where they are discussed in later chapters.

CLASSIFICATION OF PROTEIN AMINO ACIDS

The amino acids can be classified in many ways, but for general purposes the most helpful division is chemical, based on R group differences and polarity. For example, many of the analytical methods take advantage of R group variation to separate one amino acid from another; and membrane transport processes are able to distinguish one amino acid from another by virtue of the side chain (Berlin, 1970; Christensen, 1967; Scriver, 1969). Moreover, about a fifth of the genetically determined variants in protein structure are recognizable by their alteration in the net charge, which results from substitution of an amino acid with different polarity for the normal residue.

The protein α-amino acids, when divided on the basis of side-chain chemistry, fall into four main classes, as indicated in Figure 1–2.

Nonpolar, Hydrophobic Amino Acids

These *neutral* amino acids, with pI values between pH 4 and pH 7*, have aliphatic or cyclic R groups. They are less soluble in water than the more polar class (solubility coefficients are given in Table 1–1), and lengthening or bulkiness of the R group further reduces solubility.

Polar, Uncharged Amino Acids

This second class of *neutral* amino acids is more soluble because hydrogen bonding with water can occur. A hydroxyl group (in serine, threonine and tyrosine), an amide group (in glutamine and asparagine) or a thiol group (in cysteine) contributes to the greater polarity of these amino acids.

Acidic Amino Acids

The dicarboxylic amino acids, glutamic and aspartic, possess a second charged carboxyl group in the side chain which confers a *net negative charge*

---

*The normal extracellular pH is about 7.34 to 7.44, whereas the normal intracellular pH is probably 6.0 to 7.0.

at physiological pH (see Table 1–1 for pK' values of the first and second carboxyl groups).

Basic Amino Acids

These amino acids possess a *net positive charge* at physiological pH. The "dibasic" compounds, lysine and ornithine, each bear a second charged amino group on the side chain, while arginine possesses a guanidinium group which dissociates (see Table 1–1). Histidine has an imidazolium function which is half-protonated (positively charged) at pH 6, but only 10 per cent charged at pH 7.

The type of amino acid side chain exposed at the active center of an enzyme and along the protein influences its catalytic and regulatory mechanisms. This topic is not dealt with here, but an appreciation of the subject can be initiated by referral to other discussions (Lehninger, 1970; Matheja and Degens, 1971).

Nonprotein and Modified Protein Amino Acids

There are over 150 nonprotein amino acids in various biological systems. Some idea of the variety and chemical properties of amino acids which occur in human tissues and which receive attention in this volume can be gained by inspection of Table 1–1. For example, β-alanine acts like a polar neutral amino acid, and taurine behaves like an acidic compound. The modified protein amino acids, hydroxylysine and hydroxyproline, are more soluble than the corresponding unhydroxylated amino acids because of the additional polar function in the R group. Some unusual amino acids may occasionally appear in human urine as artifacts or by-products of diet, medication or intestinal metabolism.

STEREOCHEMISTRY

Amino acids which possess an asymmetric carbon atom with four different substituent groups have dextrorotatory (D) and levorotatory (L) optical specificity (note the small capital letters). The L-form is the one of importance in human metabolism. A polarimeter is used to measure optical activity, which is the specific rotation (clockwise or counterclockwise) conferred on plane-polarized light of specified wave length by a solution of amino acid in water at a specified temperature and pH. The number of stereoisomers for an amino acid is 2^n, where n refers to the number of asymmetric carbon atoms. Thus, *alanine*

$$\left(\mathrm{CH_2 - \overset{\overset{\displaystyle H}{|}}{\underset{\underset{\displaystyle NH}{|}}{C}} - COOH} \right) \text{ has two stereoisomers, and } \textit{threonine} \left(\mathrm{H - \overset{\overset{\displaystyle OH}{|}}{\underset{\underset{\displaystyle CH_3}{|}}{C}} - \overset{\overset{\displaystyle H}{|}}{\underset{\underset{\displaystyle NH_2}{|}}{C}} - COOH} \right)$$

has four stereoisomers. *Glycine* (NH_2CH_2COOH) and β-alanine ($NH_2CH_2CH_2$-COOH) have no asymmetric carbon atoms; therefore, they have no stereospecificity.

Those protein amino acids which are dextrorotatory are designated by the symbol (+); for those that are levorotatory, the symbol (−) is used. We know that all protein amino acids in human amino acid metabolism are of the L-configuration; however, the specific rotation value has nothing to tell us about the stereospecificity of the amino acid. The specific rotation of L-leucine at 25°C in water ($[\alpha]_D^{25}$) is −11.0, while that for L-isoleucine is +12.4. The D- and L-stereoisomers of lysine have specific rotations of −13.5 and +13.5 respectively.

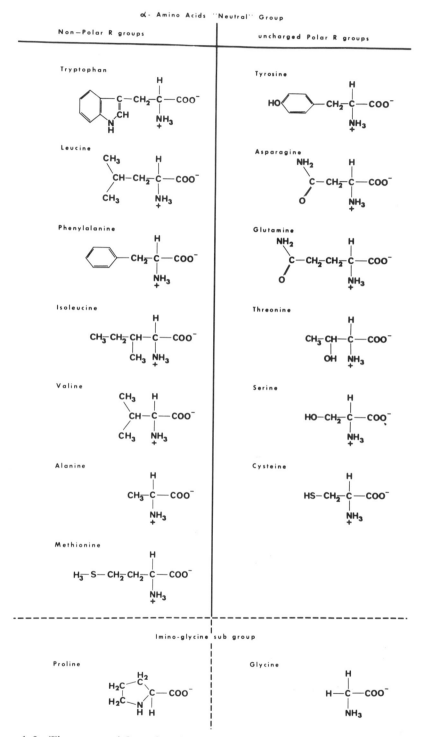

Figure 1-2 The structural formulas of the 20 protein amino acids. The amino acids are arranged into four groups: neutral, nonpolar; neutral, polar; charged, acidic; charged, basic. The amino acids have been arranged in descending order of increasing solubility. Note that proline and glycine each appear at the bottom of their respective neutral groups. Together they form a substrate group which is recognized by the "iminoglycine" membrane transport system.

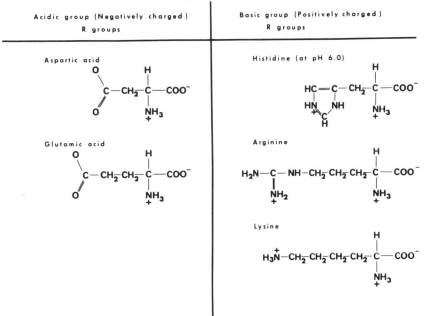

Figure 1-2   Continued

TABLE 1-1   Biological Data for Some Common Amino Acids and Peptides*

Amino Acid, Peptide, or Amine	MW	pK$_1'$ (α—COOH)	pK$_2'$ (α—NH$_3$)	pK$_R'$ (R group)	Solubility at 25°C in H$_2$O (g/100 ml)
Alanine	89.1	2.34	9.69		16.65
β-Alanine	89.1	3.55	10.24		54.5
α-Aminobutyric	103.1				S.
γ-Aminobutyric	103.1	4.03	10.56		V.S.
β-Amino *iso*butyric	103.1				S.
Anserine	240.3	2.64	9.5	7.04 (imidazole)	V.S.
Arginine	174.2	2.17	9.04	12.48	15
Asparagine	132.1	2.1	8.84		2.16
Aspartic	133.1	2.09	9.82	3.86	0.82
Citrulline	175.2	2.43	9.41		S.
Cystathionine	222.3				S.
Cysteic	169.2	1.9	8.70	1.3 (SO$_3$H)	V.S.
Cysteine	121.2	1.92	8.35	10.46 (SH)	V.S.
Cystine	240.3	<1 (1st COOH) 2.1 (2nd COOH)	8.02 (1st NH$_3^+$) 8.71 (2nd NH$_3^+$)		0.011; S in alkalis and mineral acids
Ethanolamine	61.1		~9.55		∞
Glutamic	147.1	2.1 (1st COOH) 4.07 (2nd COOH)	9.47		2.05
Glutamine	146.2	2.17	9.13		4.25
Glutathione (SH)	307.3	2.13 (1st COOH) 3.59 (2nd COOH)	8.75	9.65 (SH)	S.
Glycine	75.1	2.35	9.78		25
Histidine	155.2	1.80	9.33	6.04 (imidazole)	S.
Homocysteine	135.2	2.22	8.87	10.86	S.
Homocystine	268.4	1.59 (1st COOH) 2.54 (2nd COOH)	8.52 (1st NH$_3$) 9.44 (2nd NH$_3$)		0.02
Hydroxylysine	162.2	2.13	8.62	9.67	S.
Hydroxyproline	131.1	1.82	9.66		36.1
Isoleucine	131.2	2.32	9.76		4.12
*Allo*isoleucine	131.2	2.27	9.62		2.90 (20C)
Leucine	131.2	2.33	9.74		2.19
Lysine	146.2	2.16	9.18	10.79 (ϵ—NH$_2$)	V.S.
Methionine	149.2	2.13	9.28		S.
1-Methyl-histidine	169.2	1.69	8.85	6.48 (imidazole)	20

*Adapted from Gray and Weitzman, 1969. S. = soluble; V.S. = very soluble; (20C) = at 20°C.

TABLE 1–1 Biological Data for Some Common Amino Acids and Peptides*
(Continued)

Amino Acid, Peptide, or Amine	MW	pK' at 25°C			Solubility at 25°C in H₂O (g/100 ml)
		pK'₁ (α−COOH)	pK'₂ (α−NH₃)	pK'ᴿ (R group)	
Ornithine	132.2	1.71	8.69	10.76 (ε−NH₂)	V.S.
Phenylalanine	165.2	2.16	9.18		2.96
Pipecolic	129.2				V.S.
Proline	115.1	1.95	10.64		162.3
Putrescine	88.2		9.35 10.80 (20°C)		V.S.
Pyroglutamic	129.1	3.32			S.
Sarcosine	89.1	2.21	10.20		4.81 (20C)
Serine	105.1	2.19	9.21		25 (20C)
Taurine	125.2		9.06	−0.3 (SO₃H)	10.48
Threonine	119.1	2.09	9.10		20
Tryptophan	204.2	2.43	9.44		1.14
Tyrosine	181.2	2.20	9.11	10.13 (OH)	0.045
Valine	117.1	2.29	9.74		8.85

The stereospecificity of an amino acid is a property of the absolute configuration of the substituents around the asymmetric carbon, regardless of the direction of rotation of plane-polarized light. The reference molecule for D- and L-configurations is glyceraldehyde, a three-carbon sugar with an asymmetric carbon atom. By convention, D- and L-stereoisomers of amino acids place the amino group to the right and the left, respectively, of the plane of the molecule.

The two stereoisomers of α-alanine are mirror images of each other, as shown in Figure 1–3. The natural stereoisomer of α alanine, which is dextro

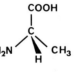

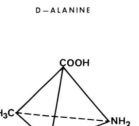

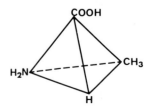

D−ALANINE

L−ALANINE

Figure 1–3 The stereoisomers of alanine. D- and L-isomers are mirror images of each other. (Adapted from Lehninger, A. L.: Biochemistry. Worth Publishers, New York, p. 74, 1970.)

rotatory, would therefore be designated L-(+)-α-alanine. Amino acids with four possible stereoisomers, such as threonine and isoleucine, have two sets of mirror-image isomers, one pair about the α-carbon atom and another pair of *allo*isomers about the second asymmetric carbon atom. For example:

L-threonine   L-allothreonine

When an equimolar mixture of the D- and L-stereoisomers exists, the mixture is said to be *racemic*. The mixture is optically inactive and is symbolized with the prefix DL-. Racemic mixtures are not normally encountered in biological systems, but awareness of their existence is important. The interpretation of physiological studies in vivo, when racemic mixtures are used, can be difficult, since only the L-stereoisomer enters catabolic pathways or incorporation reactions. The D-isomer will be rapidly excreted by the kidney or will be poorly absorbed from the intestine and into cells. A discrepancy in the distribution of D- and L-isomers will then emerge. Since most analytical methods for amino acids do not discriminate D- from L-forms, the interpretation of amino acid distributions in studies done with racemic mixtures may be fraught with error. It is for this reason that in vivo studies of amino acid metabolism should be performed with the pure L-stereoisomer.

ACID-BASE PROPERTIES OF AMINO ACIDS

Amino acids are more soluble in water than in other less polar solvents, and in the crystalline state their melting point is usually above 200°C. These properties indicate strong electrostatic forces, and it is their *dipolar* or *zwitterion* state which distinguishes amino acids from other metabolites.

undissociated form   zwitterion form

An amino acid can donate protons during titration with a base, and the proximity of electrical charges on the molecule repels H^+ from the carboxyl group, enhancing dissociation.
Recall that

$$K' = \frac{[H^+]\,[A^-]}{[HA]} \tag{1}$$

where K' is the apparent dissociation constant, and the brackets indicate concentration (moles/L) of dissociated and undissociated forms of the acid; that pK′ is the logarithmic transformation of K′, analogous to pH as a transformation of [H⁺], so that

$$pK' = \log_{10} 1/K' = -\log_{10} K' \tag{2}$$

Then, if Equation (1) is solved for [H⁺] in the customary way, the Henderson-Hasselbalch equation is obtained:

$$pH = pK' + \log\frac{[A^-]}{[HA]} \tag{3a}$$

or

$$pH = pK' + \log\frac{[\text{proton acceptor}]}{[\text{proton donor}]} \tag{3b}$$

Amino acids are characterized by two or more pK′ values during complete titration with a base—one value for the carboxyl group pK_1' and a second for the amino group pK_2'. In some cases there is a reaction function in the R group, and there will be a third value (pK_R') for this group.

The titration curve for alanine, shown in Figure 1–4, shows different ion species predominating at the various pH values. It is evident that as the carboxyl group undergoes increasingly complete dissociation with rising pH, this negatively charged group then influences dissociation of the amino group,

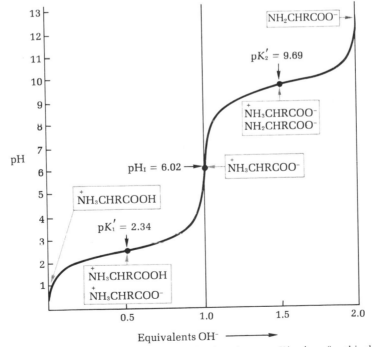

Figure 1–4 The titration curve of alanine, showing the two pK′ values for this dipolar zwitterion. The ionic species predominating at important points of the titration curve are indicated in the boxes. (From Lehninger, A. L.: Biochemistry. Worth Publishers, New York, p. 77, 1970.)

which in turn undergoes dissociation at the high pH range. There is one point in the titration when the amino acid bears no net electrical charge. This is the *isoelectric* pH (pH$_I$), which is the arithmetic mean of pK$_1'$ and pK$_2'$. Amino acids at their isoelectric point do not move in an electrical field, and this property can be used to separate uncharged amino acids from charged compounds by electrophoresis (see Chapter 5).

The zwitterion nature of amino acids yields several important results with regard to their acid-base properties. First, the carboxyl group of monoamino monocarboxylic acids is a stronger acid than the carboxyl group of the equivalent aliphatic acid; by a similar token, the α-amino group of the amino acid is a stronger acid (proton donor) than the equivalent aliphatic amine.

Second, monoamino monocarboxylic amino acids without uncharged R groups have similar pK$_1'$ and pK$_2'$ values.

Third, amino acids, with the exception of histidine which has a dissociable R group (imidazolium pK$_R'$ = 6.0), are poor buffers in the physiological range of pH.

Fourth, the "acidic" amino acids (glutamic and aspartic) have higher pK$'$ values for the second carboxyl group than for the first; the basic amino acids behave as bases, having a net positive charge at physiological pH and losing their proton only at very high pH.

The properties of "charged" amino acids will yield more negatively charged dicarboxylic amino acids inside the cell, where pH is lower, than outside, and more positively charged "dibasic" amino acids outside at the normal extracellular pH. The relationship between strong charge and impediment to membrane transport (see Chapter 6) may account for the high concentration of dicarboxylic amino acids inside cells relative to their concentration in plasma and extracellular fluid in the body.

PREBIOLOGICAL ORIGINS OF AMINO ACIDS

Long before present-day organisms synthesized their own amino acids and proteins, or came to depend on other organisms for a supply of essential amino acids, this class of organic molecules was being formed abiotically. An appreciation of the prebiological origin of amino acids and other organic molecules has been a subject of intense interest for the past 20 years (Oparin, 1965).

The Earth was formed about 4.6 billion years ago. Its earliest atmosphere probably contained water, ammonia, methane, carbon dioxide, hydrogen sulfide, nitrogen and hydrogen. The temperature was also very high. With time, some of the reducing components (hydrogen, ammonia and methane) were lost and cooling occurred. Organic compounds are believed to have appeared during this period of *chemical evolution* from the impact of energy sources (UV light, electrical discharges and heat) upon the inorganic mixtures in the atmosphere. Under appropriate conditions, the organic compounds dissolved in the sea and condensed to form polypeptides, protenoids and other species of macromolecules. These large compounds may then have been able to catalyze conversion reactions. These events presumably lasted at least one billion years.

The first organic residues in geological history were recorded about 3 to 3.5 billion years ago (Calvin, 1969). The process of chemical evolution culminated when polymeric experimentation was sufficiently stabilized for unicellular self-replicating systems to emerge. This process required a billion years and probably yielded anaerobic heterotrophs as the first living cells. The next 2.5 billion years were consumed in the process of *biological evolution*. Vertebrates did not emerge until 300 million years ago, when the oxygen content of the atmosphere had risen to 10 per cent due to the activity of photosynthetic cells. Man is so recent that his two million years of existence in a high-oxygen environment are barely discernible on the time scale of total evolution. The phenomenon of Man encompasses, among other things, polymers of amino acids (proteins) and polymers of bases, sugars and phosphates (nucleic acids). The regulation of amino acid metabolism, which is a recurring theme of this book, depends on interrelations between the two.

The apparent phenomenon of evolutionary continuity (Wald, 1964) requires that the initial origin of amino acids and other organic molecules happened with reasonable probability within the boundaries of the laws of physics and chemistry. There is considerable experimental evidence to support this assumption. Free amino acids will appear after exposure of mixtures of methane, water and ammonia at 80°C to prolonged electrical discharge (Miller, 1955; Oro, 1963). In the presence of radiant energy, HCN can be the precursor of cyanamide (NH_2—$C{\equiv}N$); and with subsequent dimerization of cyanamide to yield a series of condensing reagents, the formation of peptides from amino acids can be promoted in UV-irradiated aqueous solutions (Ponnamperuma and Peterson, 1965). Therefore, an abiotic origin for the building blocks, such as amino acids, of living cells seems likely even under primitive Earth conditions. If one accepts this, it should not be surprising then to learn that amino acids have been found in modern meteorites (Lawless et al., 1972). In this context, amino acids have true universal interest, as well as the particular perspectives discussed in this book.

REFERENCES

Specific

Berlin, R. D.: Specificities of transport systems and enzymes. Science *168*:1539–1545, 1970.

Calvin, M.: Chemical Evolution: Molecular Evolution Towards the Origin of Living Systems on the Earth and Elsewhere. Oxford University Press, London, 1969.

Christensen, H. N.: Some transport lessons taught by the organic solute. Perspect. Biol. Med. *10*: 471–494, 1967.

Lawless, J. G., Kvenvolden, K. A., Peterson, E., Ponnamperuma, C., and Jarosewich, E.: Evidence for amino-acids of extra-terrestrial origin in the Orgueil meteorite. Nature (London) *236*:66–67, 1972.

Miller, S. L.: Production of some organic compounds under possible primitive earth conditions. J. Amer. Chem. Soc. 77:2351–2361, 1955.

Oparin, A. I.: The origin of life and the origin of enzymes. Advances Enzym. *27*:347–380, 1965.

Oro, J.: Synthesis of organic compounds by electric discharge. Nature (London) *197*:862–867, 1963.

Ponnamperuma, C., and Peterson, E.: Peptide synthesis from amino acids in aqueous solution. Science *147*:1572–1574, 1965.

Scriver, C. R.: The human biochemical genetics of amino acid transport. Pediatrics *44*:348–357, 1969.

Wald, G.: The origins of life. Proc. Nat. Acad. Sci. U.S.A. *52*:595–611, 1964.

General

Edsall, J. T., and Wyman, J.: Biophysical Chemistry, Vol. 1. Academic Press, New York, 1969.

Gray, D. O., and Weitzman, P. D. J.: 1. Amino acids, amines, amides, peptides and their derivatives. *In* Dawson, R. M. C., Elliott, D. C., Elliott, W. H., and Jones, K. M., eds., Data for Biochemical Research, 2nd edition. Clarendon Press, Oxford, 1969.

Lehninger, A. L.: Biochemistry. The Molecular Basis of Cell Structure and Function. Worth Publishers, Inc., New York, 1970.

Matheja, J., and Degens, E. T.: Function of amino acid side chains. Advances Enzym. *34*:1–39, 1971.

Meister, A.: Biochemistry of the Amino Acids, 2nd edition. Academic Press, New York, 1965.

Chapter Two

NUTRITIONAL ASPECTS OF AMINO ACID METABOLISM

GENERAL CONSIDERATIONS

Amino acids enter the intracellular and extracellular pools of intermediary metabolism through endogenous routes, such as biosynthesis and tissue breakdown, or from exogenous sources, such as dietary protein and nonprotein nitrogen. Amino acids which are not synthesized by man at rates sufficient to support normal growth are considered "essential" (Rose, 1938). Consequently, a source of *nitrogen* and of *essential amino acids* is required to meet the demands for growth, protein synthesis and biosynthesis of important nitrogenous metabolites.

Protein as such is not absorbed by the intestine in any significant amount, but its nutritional requirement can be met provided the amount of dietary protein is sufficient, its amino acid composition is appropriate, it is adequately hydrolyzed in the intestine and the residues of hydrolysis are efficiently absorbed from the intestine into the portal blood. A caloric requirement must also be met by other nutrients to prevent utilization of essential amino acids as a source of energy. The average diet which satisfies these needs usually contains about 8 to 10 per cent protein.

These considerations assume special relevance during the treatment of the aminoacidopathies, because patients with inborn errors of amino acid metabolism often require special diets, strictly regulated in amino acid composition (Efron, 1967; Lowe et al., 1967; Waisman and Kerr, 1967; Scriver, 1969; Dancis, 1970). Protein and amino acid requirements must also be scrupulously considered if the patient is receiving total intravenous alimentation (Dudrick and Rhoads, 1972).

QUANTITATIVE FACTORS IN PROTEIN NUTRITION

The rate of gain in the protein component of body composition by the reference male infant is about 3.5 g/day during the first four months after birth (Fomon, 1967a). The rate falls to about 3.1 g/day between four and twelve months of age. At one year the human male infant is 14.6 per cent protein, representing a net gain of about three per cent from the time of birth. There are sex-related differences in growth, the male being larger than the female during early growth and in adulthood (Fomon, 1967b), but how this difference is reflected in the body composition of the female infant is not well known.

Nitrogen accounts for about 16 per cent of protein weight. Therefore, if the nitrogen content of the diet is multiplied by 6.25, the fraction which is protein can be calculated. The conversion factor is lower for proteins whose composition comprises less of the essential amino acids and relatively more of those with low molecular weights. Thus, in a collagenous protein like gelatin, the nitrogen fraction is proportionately greater, and the conversion factor is correspondingly lower; for example, it is 5.5 for gelatin (McCance and Widdowson, 1960). Estimates of protein requirements are most often made in one of two ways (McLaughlan and Campbell, 1969).

The Factorial Method

This method is most useful if somatic growth is not occurring. The loss of nitrogenous compounds from the body is measured under basal conditions. If the requirement for dietary protein is due to these losses, then feeding the correct amount of protein to offset the losses will indicate the requirement. The factorial method is applicable only when a plateau has been reached in nitrogen loss while on a protein-free diet. About 7 to 10 days are required to reach these basal conditions.

The obligatory losses can be represented by the equation (Dietary Standard for Canada, 1968):

$$R = (U + F + S + G) \times 1.3 \times 1.43 \times \text{body weight (kg)}$$

where U = g protein compensating for nitrogen loss in the urine/kg/day; F = g protein compensating for nitrogen loss in feces/kg/day; S = g protein compensating for nitrogen loss in skin and integument/kg/day; and G = protein growth increment/kg/day.

The calculation of the losses in urine, feces, and sweat is based on the following values expressed as a coefficient of body weight to the power 0.75:

$$
\begin{aligned}
\text{obligatory daily urinary nitrogen loss} &= 125 \text{ mg N/kg}^{0.75} \\
\text{obligatory daily fecal nitrogen loss} &= 25 \text{ mg N/kg}^{0.75} \\
\text{obligatory daily skin nitrogen loss} &= \underline{15 \text{ mg N/kg}^{0.75}} \\
\text{Total} &= 165 \text{ mg N/kg}^{0.75}
\end{aligned}
$$

or, 1.03 g protein/kg$^{0.75}$/day. The protein requirement/day is derived by dividing this value, expressed as a function of body weight to the power 0.75, by the equivalent weight in kg.

The factor 1.3 in the equation accounts for the interindividual coefficient of variation in protein requirements, which is equivalent to 2×14 per cent of the relevant mean values. The factor 1.43 accounts for the net protein utilization (NPU) value of the dietary protein (National Academy of Sciences, 1968). The reference protein (e.g., human milk or hen's egg protein) has a value of 100. The "average" protein of a typical North American diet for the adult has an NPU value of about 70 (Ballantyne and McLaughlan, 1968). Thus, the conversion factor is $\frac{100}{70}$ or 1.43.

The Direct Method

The minimum protein requirement can also be estimated by determining the nitrogen intake necessary to maintain either the grown subject in nitrogen balance or equilibrium under basal conditions or the growing subject within the normal rate of growth. If the study is carried out at several levels of dietary protein, a regression of intake upon nitrogen balance (or growth) is observed (Fig. 2–1) from which the protein requirement can be calculated. The nutritional quality of the protein relative to egg protein or breast milk must also be accounted for, since proteins of low biological value, in principle, will have to be fed at higher levels than the reference protein. Proteins seriously deficient in an essential amino acid can never satisfy requirements for nitrogen balance or growth.

Quantitative Requirements

Protein requirements have been estimated for man under a variety of conditions (WHO/FAO, 1965; National Academy of Sciences [NRC], 1968;

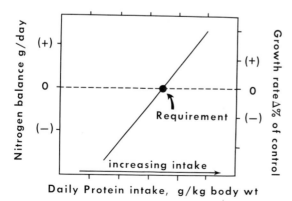

Figure 2–1 Idealized relationship between the level of protein intake and nitrogen balance or growth rate. The point at which the diagonal line, representing the regression of protein intake upon nitrogen balance or growth rate, intersects the ordinate value for nitrogen equilibrium or normal growth rate is the minimum protein requirement for the individual.

Dietary Standard for Canada, 1968). The requirements during the periods of growth are quite different from those when chemical and physical maturity has been attained and only turnover of body proteins must be met.

The requirements for dietary protein are summarized in Table 2-1. The values as presented reveal a difference between the recommendations derived by two nations for their populations living at nearly equal standards. These values, while they reveal the imprecisions in the art and science of determining protein requirements in man, nonetheless serve as a useful working guide in planning the strategy of protein nutrition for individual patients. Table 2-1 clearly shows the changing requirement for protein at different ages, and between the sexes, and conveys the idea that growth imposes special needs.

Table 2-1   Estimated Dietary Protein Requirement
(g protein/kg body weight/day)

Canadian Values[a]		United States Values[b]	
Age (years)	Protein Requirement	Age (years)	Protein Requirement
0–2 mos.	2.2[c]	0–2 mos.	2.2[c]
2–6 mos.	2.0[c]	2–6 mos.	2.0[c]
6–12 mos.	1.4[c]	6–12 mos.	1.8[c]
1–2	1.30	1–2	2.1
2–3	1.20	2–3	1.8
3–5	1.10	3–4	1.9
5–7	0.97	4–6	1.6
7–9	0.93	6–8	1.5
		8–10	1.4
9–12 Male	0.86	10–12	1.3
12–15 "	0.82	12–14	1.2
15–19 "	0.73	14–18	1.0
Adult "	0.67	18–22	0.9
		22–35	0.9
		35–55	0.9
		55–75+	0.9
9–12 Female	0.86	10–12	1.4
12–15 "	0.80	12–14	1.1
15–19 "	0.74	14–16	1.1
Adult "	0.70	16–18	1.0
		18–22	0.95
		22–35	0.95
		35–55	0.95
		55–75	0.95
Old age Male			0.78[d]

[a]Canadian values (Dietary Standard for Canada, 1968) calculated by the factorial method from the formula

$$R = (U + F + S + G) \times 1.30 \times 1.43$$

[b]U.S. values (National Academy of Sciences [NRC], 1968) calculated by a factorial method.
[c]These are direct estimates, and they indicate achievement of normal growth by subjects fed human milk of known protein content.
[d]Estimated by method employing regression of nitrogen balance vs. intake (Kountz et al., 1951) and corrected for interindividual variation (= requirement × 1.3).

Infancy

The best estimates of protein requirement in infancy (Fomon and May, 1955) were determined from subjects who were fed on pasteurized human milk, of which the average protein content is 1.1 g per cent (Macy and Kelly, 1961), and who achieved normal growth rates.

Childhood and Adolescence

The gain of body weight after one year comprises about 3 per cent nitrogen, or 18 per cent protein (Holt et al., 1960). Protein accretion can be calculated by multiplying the daily body-weight gain by 0.18. The daily protein requirement is the accretion amount plus the obligatory loss.

Old Age

Watkin (1964) suggests that old age may impose special requirements for protein. Careful studies by Kountz et al. (1957) by the staged balance method with regression analysis suggest that requirements are about 50 per cent greater than for young adults.

Special Circumstances

The stresses of ordinary life do not alter the protein requirements indicated in Table 2–1. However, serious *infection* or *illness*, and *convalescence*, will temporarily increase the requirement as tissue catabolism and nitrogen loss increase. *Heavy muscular activity* does not alter the protein needs, unless muscular hypertrophy is in progress or heavy, sustained sweat losses are encountered. *Pregnancy*, *lactation* and *menstruation* increase protein requirements. During pregnancy there is a net gain in protein of both maternal and fetal tissues. The average gain is about 900 g of protein per pregnancy (Dietary Standard for Canada, 1968). Allowing for individual variation, the estimated dietary protein supplement is about 1200 g of reference protein (NPU = 100) per pregnancy. This is equivalent to an additional protein intake of 0.5 g/day in the first trimester and 5.4 g/day in the last. *Lactation* increases the protein requirement. The supplementary allowance is about 16 g/day of reference protein. *Menstruation* causes a small loss of nitrogen. This loss (about 2 mg $N/kg^{0.75}/day$) is accounted for in the computation of the final figure for the adult and for girls in Table 2–1.

QUALITATIVE FACTORS IN PROTEIN NUTRITION

The obligatory requirement for protein of good nutritional quality in the diet of nonruminant mammals such as man is a function of their need for *essential amino acids*.* Ruminants can synthesize the carbon skeleton of all amino acids in their alimentary tract, and nitrogen is fixed by intestinal bacteria. In fact, it is even possible to raise well-nourished, fertile cattle on synthetic sources of carbon, nitrogen and sulfur, without recourse to natural foods (Virtanen,

---

*The essential amino acids for human nutrition are isoleucine, leucine, lysine, methionine, phenylalanine, threonine, tryptophan and valine (Rose, 1938). During early infancy, histidine has the characteristics of an essential amino acid (Snyderman et al., 1963).

1966). Man is unable to do this, and consequently he is dependent on an exogenous source of the essential amino acids.

The nutritional adequacy of dietary protein for man is ultimately determined by its amino acid composition (Block and Mitchell, 1946/47; Mitchell, 1954). The *biological value* (BV) or *net protein utilization* (NPU) of a protein describes its nutritional adequacy. *Reference proteins* have values of 100, and are totally utilizable for anabolic processes. Human milk whey and hen's egg protein are the most commonly used reference proteins. A protein which cannot support anabolism because it is devoid of one or more essential amino acids has a biological value of zero. When 10 per cent of the caloric intake is supplied by protein, the NPU value of the average North American dietary protein is slightly below 70 (Ballantyne and McLaughlan, 1968).

The NPU values of most dietary proteins are less than 100 because they contain essential amino acids in concentrations lower than that of the reference protein. If the concentration of each essential amino acid is taken as a percentage of its concentration in the reference protein (Table 2–2), then the essential amino acid which occurs with the lowest percentage score is designated as *the limiting amino acid* (McLaughlan and Campbell, 1969). This score is the NPU for the dietary protein. In order to sustain normal growth and anabolism, a sufficient amount of dietary protein must be supplied to make up the amount of the limiting amino acid that would be obtained from the reference protein. For example, the dietary requirement for a protein whose NPU is 66 would be $\frac{100}{66} = 1.52$ times that of the reference protein, whose NPU is 100.

It is apparent that the nutritional attributes of a protein can be evaluated in many ways. The plasma amino acid pattern as a monitor of adequacy of protein nutrition has received some attention (McLaughlan et al., 1967; Graham et al., 1970; Weller et al., 1970) since changes in plasma amino acid composition can be attributed to the nitrogen composition of the diet (Holt et al., 1960; Snyderman et al., 1968; Young and Scrimshaw, 1968). However, it is also appar-

Table 2–2   Nutritional Value of Dietary Protein

Amino Acid	*A* Human Milk[1] Amino Acids mg/g N	*B* Hen's Egg Protein[2] Amino Acids mg/g N	*C* Average[2] Dietary Protein mg/g N	Score of C, relative to A	Score of C, relative to B
Isoleucine	440	415	292	67	70
Leucine	820	553	495	60[3]	90
Lysine	403	403	385	96	96
Methionine	118	163	118	100	72
Total sulfur-containing amino acids	272	322	213	79	66[3]
Phenylalanine	326	365	289	89	79
Threonine	316	317	240	76	76
Tryptophan	112	100	77	69	77
Valine	460	454	360	78	79

[1] Data of Macy and Kelly (1961) for available amino acids in liquid milk, protein content of 1.21 g/100 ml (Fomon, 1967b). Amino acid content in milk includes free and peptide-bound forms.
[2] Data from McLaughlan and Knipfel, 1968.
[3] Lowest chemical score = limiting amino acid = NPU.

ent that the carbohydrate and fat contents of isonitrogenous diets are deter-minants of protein and amino acid requirements (Swendseid et al., 1967a, 1967b), and for this reason and because of the known effects of other nutrients upon amino acid metabolism through hormone-dependent events, plasma amino acid responses cannot be recommended in general as indices of pro-tein nutrition.

AMINO ACID REQUIREMENTS

Two types of amino acid requirements must be considered. There is the need for essential amino acids; but there is also a need for nonessential amino nitrogen. Absolute nutritional requirements for essential and nonessential ni-trogen can be spared to some extent if caloric intake is sufficient to prevent utilization of amino acids as substrates for fuel metabolism. It matters whether growth, nitrogen equilibrium or plasma aminogram is taken as the end point to evaluate specific amino acid requirements, and it matters very much whether comparative studies are done under different caloric conditions. Because of differences in methodologies and conditions of study used by various investi-gators, the reader will find an instability in the quoted values for amino acid requirements (Tables 2–3 and 2–4) similar to that which characterized the recommendations for protein requirements. The difficult subject of amino acid requirements in man has recently been well reviewed by Irwin and Hegsted (1971) and Munro (1972). A quotation from the final paragraphs of Irwin and Hegsted captures the dilemma effectively:

> The reliability of the estimates of the requirements of young children . . . cannot be de-termined. This is not stated as a criticism [of this work]. It is a general criticism of nearly all data upon nutritional requirements of man. It indicates not only the need for more data, but for continual thought toward the development of new experimental designs, more sensitive and easier criteria, and for critical statistical evaluation.
>
> The cause of the wide variations observed in the requirements of individuals or the scatter of the data obtained is also unexplained. Inspection of the data from specific in-dividuals strongly suggests that there are large inherent differences in individual require-ments. The data, however, are insufficient to provide an estimate of the error in the apparent requirement of an individual subject and thus to prove that his requirement is truly different from that of another. In any event, an average requirement is an inadequate base from which to establish safe "allowances" or dietary recommendations. These must be established enough above average need to provide for most subjects and thus an estimate of the range of require-ments (apart from errors in the determinations of such requirements) is important.
>
> In the final analysis, these data will not be of practical importance unless the data on amino acid requirements, protein requirements, and the nutritional quality of proteins provide a consistent understandable pattern. At present they do not do so.*

Holt and coauthors (1960) and Fomon and Filer (1967) have also voiced similar feelings in their earlier discussions of the topic. For these reasons some investigators have begun to re-evaluate amino acid requirements, using new approaches.

Methods for Estimating Requirements in the Adult

When growth cannot be used to evaluate the requirement of an essential nutrient, other methods of estimation must be used. Young et al. (1971) turned

---

*Irwin, M. I., and Hegsted, D. M.: A conspectus of research on amino acid requirements of man. J. Nutr. *101*:539–566, 1971.

Table 2-3 Amino Acid Requirements (Per Day) in Healthy Subjects of Both Sexes*

Amino Acid	Infant	School Child	Young Adult	Elderly	Comment
Arginine	nonessential	nonessential	probably nonessential (A₁)		A₁ = for spermato-genesis
Histidine	16–34 mg/kg	nonessential	probably nonessential (H₁)		H₁ = In disease states (e.g., uremia)
Isoleucine	17–126 mg/kg	1 g/day	250–450 mg/day		
Leucine	76–226 mg/kg	1.0–1.5 g/day	170–1100 mg/day		
Lysine	90–200 mg/kg	1.2–1.6 g/day	50–1200 mg/day	1.4–2.8 g/day	
Methionine + Cystine	20–85 mg met/kg + 15–50 mg cys/kg	0.4–0.8 g/day	0.8–1.1 g met/day (no cystine); + 75–350 mg met/day + 100–200 mg cys/day	0.29–3.0 g/day	
Phenylalanine	47–94 mg/kg (with adequate tyrosine)	0.4–0.8 g/day	0.8–1.18 g/day (no tyrosine) 120–600 mg/day with tyrosine		
Threonine	45–87 mg/kg	0.8–1.0 g/day	103–1500 mg/day		
Tryptophan	13–40 mg/kg	60–120 mg/day	2–9 mg/kg 50–250 mg/day }(T₁) 3 mg/kg (T₂)		T₁ = Nitrogen balance and equilibrium data T₂ = Plasma response data
Valine	65–115 mg/kg	0.5–0.9 g/day	230–800 mg/day		

*Condensed from Irwin, M. I., and Hegsted, D. M.: J. Nutr. *101*, 1971. The age ranges were, for infants, 6 days to 11 mos.; for children, Japanese boys, 11 to 12 years; for adults, young men and women of college age primarily; for the elderly, men 52 to 84 years.

Table 2–4   Estimated Requirements for Essential Amino Acids in
the Healthy Human Infant (mg/kg/day)

L-*Amino Acid*	Calculated from Volume of Human Milk Intake <1 mo.[a]	2–3 mos.[b]	4–5 mos.[c]	Method of Holt et al.[d] Mean	Range	Method of Fomon and Filer[e] Range
Histidine	39	33	30	34	(16–34)	19–28
Isoleucine	147	125	115	126	(80–126)	48–70
Leucine	277	234	212	150	(76–229)	111–161
Lysine	136	215	104	103	(88–103)	111–161
Methionine + Cystine[f]	39	33	30	45	(33–45)	23–29
Phenylalanine + Tyrosine[f]	110	93	85	90	(47–90)	42–61
Threonine	106	90	82	87	(45–87)	80–116
Tryptophan	38	32	29	22	(15–22)	11–17
Valine	156	130	119	105	(85–105)	64–93

[a]Fomon, 1967b; 10th percentile value for volume intake = 172 ml/kg/day.
[b]Fomon, 1967b; 10th percentile value for volume intake = 145 ml/kg/day.
[c]Fomon, 1967b; 10th percentile value for volume intake = 132 ml/kg/day.
[d]Holt et al., (1960); supplied defined L-amino acid mixture to small number of infants between two and six months of age.
[e]The diet of Fomon and Filer (1967) contained cow's milk of known amino acid composition; 22 infants evaluated over period from 8 to 112 days of age.
[f]Approximately one third of the relevant essential amino acid requirements as listed are contributed by cystine and tyrosine. Removal of the latter from the diet increases methionine and phenylalanine needs by 50 per cent.

to the specific plasma amino acid response to evaluate the tryptophan requirement. An L-amino acid mixture mimicking the amino acid pattern of egg protein was fed at a constant rate, and the tryptophan component was varied. The minimum need was judged by nitrogen equilibrium measurements and by the plasma tryptophan response. As shown in Figure 2–2, there was an abrupt rise in plasma tryptophan at daily intakes of the amino acid above 3 mg/kg. The point of demarcation was similar whether fasting or postprandial tryptophan levels were used. The point of upward deflection in Figure 2–2 was taken as the index of the minimum requirement for tryptophan in the young healthy adult subject. The estimate for tryptophan requirement achieved by the nitrogen equilibrium method in a parallel study was 15 to 30 per cent lower (2.0 to 2.6 mg/kg), but some underestimation of need by this method was assumed, since small losses of skin and sweat nitrogen were not included in the nitrogen balance data. The study of Young and colleagues reveals the plasma amino acid response curves to be of value in estimating amino acid requirements in man.

Methods for Estimating Requirements in the Infant and the Growing Child

The technique used by the New York group (Holt et al., 1960; Holt and Snyderman, 1961) to calculate the amino acid requirements of the infant employed synthetic diets which contained free L-amino acids of precisely defined composition. Growth rate and nitrogen balance were used as indices of the requirement for the single amino acid whose amount in the diet was titrated to limiting amounts. The method provided a useful estimate of the requirements

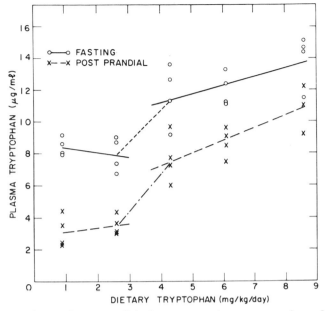

Figure 2–2 Fasting and postprandial plasma tryptophan concentrations of four adult male subjects fed a diet with various levels of tryptophan intake. The experimental protocol progressed stepwise from highest levels of tryptophan intake (8.7 mg/kg body weight) to the lowest intake (0.9 mg/kg body weight). The deflection point on the x-axis of the graph (at approximately 3 mg/kg/day), relating plasma tryptophan to intake, represents the tryptophan requirement as measured by the plasma amino acid response method. The value is the same in fasting and postprandial samples; the higher fasting value is typical of the tryptophan circadian rhythm in plasma. (From Young, V. R., et al., J. Nutr. *101*:45–60, 1971.)

for the eight essential amino acids and for histidine, *under the conditions of the study* in early infancy (Table 2–4). However, it was not determined whether these data also represent the requirements for the same amino acids when supplied as an intact dietary protein which undergoes a specified sequence of digestion and absorption of the residues.

Fomon and Filer (1967) fed a prepared diet containing cow's milk protein of known amino acid composition to male and female infants between 8 and 112 days of age. The criteria for nutritional adequacy of the diet were: normal growth in length and weight; normal retention of nitrogen relevant to intake when compared with retention on human milk diets; normal concentration of albumin in serum at 112 days. *Under the conditions of their investigation*, the amino acid requirements were even lower than those determined by the New York group (Table 2–4).

Empirical data obtained in recent years from infants with hereditary impairment of the catabolism of various essential amino acids indicate that the requirements for essential amino acids must be individualized, even though the range of requirements may resemble the data shown in Tables 2–3 and 2–4. Thus, *no precise single estimate of an amino acid requirement for the individual patient apparently exists for this most critical period in postnatal life.*

Estimates of Amino Acid Requirements

The best current estimates of the essential amino acid requirements of man have been summarized in Tables 2–3 and 2–4. Particular attention is given to the young infant, because it is in this age group that amino acid nutrition is of critical importance. The potential for treatment of certain hereditary amino-acidopathies with semisynthetic diets or by total intravenous alimentation in this age group (Ghadimi et al., 1971) imposes special demands on our knowledge of amino acid requirements for the infant.

Whether *histidine* is an essential amino acid in human metabolism has been a matter of controversy for many years (Stifel and Herman, 1972). Holt's group (Snyderman et al., 1963; Holt and Synderman, 1961) showed that the amino acid is necessary for normal growth in the young infant. This may not be true for the older child and adult subject (Nakagawa et al., 1963). However, a requirement for histidine may emerge in later life in disease states—particularly in uremia (Bergstrom et al., 1970). Endogenous synthesis of histidine has not been demonstrated in man, but if it is *not* an essential dietary amino acid in the healthy adult it must then be available from some source, perhaps the intestinal bacteria. To our knowledge this possibility has not yet been investigated. Fortunately, histidine is not a limiting amino acid in the protein of the average human diet.

An additional point emerges concerning the effect of growth on total amino acid requirements. During the period of high somatic growth rate, the proportional requirement for essential amino acids relative to nonessential nitrogen is high (Fig. 2–3), whereas it is much lower in the mature subject. This is to be expected, since protein synthesis—and hence the demand for essential amino acids in relation to total nitrogen intake—is greatest when tissue growth is greatest.

Significance of Amino Acid Requirements

The qualitative factors of nitrogen nutrition reflect variation in the amino composition of dietary proteins. McLaughlan and colleagues (1967) determined that cereal proteins (wheat, oatmeal, rye, corn and rice) and sesame are limited in lysine for human needs. Soy flour protein is limited in methionine, as are many legumes (chick pea, lentil and lima bean, for example), while peanut flour scores poorly in threonine. *Milk protein* seems to be limited in methionine when assessed by the blood amino acid response method of McLaughlan and coworkers. If the amino acid score of human milk is assessed, as indicated in Table 2–2, by comparison with a hen egg protein, then the former is indeed low in methionine. However, if human milk protein is considered the reference protein for human nutrition (and it does support an accepted standard of

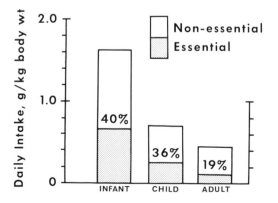

Figure 2–3   The relationship of total essential amino acids to the nonessential amino acids in the diet needed to meet requirements for growth or nitrogen equilibrium at various ages. Note that relative requirement for essential amino acids is higher during the period of rapid growth. (Redrawn from Munro, 1972.)

growth in infancy), then it can be argued that *hen egg protein* is a "superprotein" with respect to methionine and phenylalanine, while it is suboptimal in its leucine content. Considering the potential hazards of methionine toxicity (see following text) and the risks some infants face with regard to phenylalanine metabolism (see Chapter 15), one might question the use of hen egg protein as a reference standard for human nutrition. Whether human milk protein or hen egg protein should be the reference protein for human nutrition is not idle speculation. Many decisions will soon have to be made concerning the composition of amino acid mixtures for total intravenous feedings, and the decisions will require agreement concerning a reference standard for evaluation.

The reader will realize that the amino acid requirement for the *individual* human subject cannot be predicted very accurately from the data given in Tables 2–3 and 2–4 because there is likely to be considerable interindividual variation in these requirements. In a particular clinical situation, where it may be important to know the precise requirement for an essential amino acid, this information can be obtained only by the empirical approach. When minimal requirements for an amino acid are met, it is predominantly the anabolic needs which have been served. Catabolic utilization of the essential amino acid is reduced to insignificant amounts under such conditions of nutritional constraint. The corollary of this situation—namely, when catabolism is blocked, as it might be in a hereditary aminoacidopathy—can be informative about amino acid requirements. For example, in phenylketonuria, the amino acid *tolerance* is 250 to 500 mg/day. During the first year of life, this corresponds to a phenylalanine *requirement* of about 25 to 125 mg/kg; the latter values straddle the requirements listed in Table 2–4.

Certain generalizations should be reiterated concerning factors which may influence amino acid requirements in human nutrition. The amount of non-essential nitrogen in the diet is important, and it must be adequate to conserve essential amino acids from degradation for purposes of nitrogen metabolism. There is a similar need for calories derived from fat and carbohydrate sources to spare amino acids from diversion into fuel metabolism. The vitamin intake must also be sufficient, particularly the B vitamins (National Academy of Sciences [NRC], 1959; Lowe et al., 1966). The time sequence of amino acid feeding is also important, since Cannon et al. (1954) have shown that feeding of the amino acids at separate times, instead of together in a mixture, can impair growth.

Nutrition with Keto Acids

The traditional view of the *essential amino acid* has undergone further revision in recent years. Under certain conditions, indispensable nitrogen requirements can be met instead by the corresponding *keto acid* (Anonymous, 1972). An essential amino acid is one which cannot be synthesized endogenously because of an irreversible step in the normal degradative pathway. For example, in phenylalanine catabolism, it is the first hydroxylating step (which forms tyrosine) which is effectively irreversible; and in the catabolism of branched-chain amino acids (leucine, isoleucine and valine), it is the second step, involving oxidative decarboxylation of the equivalent keto acids. However, in both cases, the keto acids are in reversible equilibrium with their corresponding amino acids; in the presence of a nitrogen source, it should be possible to meet amino acid needs by feeding the keto acid. Rose (1938) questioned whether it was the aminated analogue or the carbon skeleton which was essential. Later experiments in the rat (Wood and Cooley, 1954) demonstrated that the carbon skeleton analogue, when fed in appropriate amounts, could meet the needs for growth, presumably because nitrogen fixation could occur to form the amino acids.

There are several observations which suggest that *man can utilize keto acid analogues and urea nitrogen for endogenous synthesis of essential amino acids*. Richards and coauthors (1971) showed that replacement of valine and phenylalanine by the keto acid analogues (α-keto isovaleric acid and phenylpyruvic acid respectively) in the diets of five healthy and four uremic subjects resulted in more positive (or less negative) nitrogen balances than in the absence of keto acid or amino acid replacement in all but one subject. Rudman (1971) confirmed these findings in adult subjects, but concluded that conversion efficiency for keto acids was far below 100 per cent. Neither of these studies actually proved de novo synthesis of the amino acids from the keto acids. Giardano and colleagues (1972) have come close to proving this point by demonstrating accelerated incorporation of ^{15}N into the corresponding essential amino acids of plasma albumin, when α-keto isovaleric acid and β-phenylpyruvic acid were added to a diet devoid of the corresponding amino acids, and containing ^{15}N-labeled ammonium chloride. Nitrogen balances also became less negative. The greatest rate of ^{15}N incorporation into the essential amino acids was found in a uremic patient.

The source of the amino group in such studies is of interest, particularly since uremic patients seem to be able to capitalize on their urea retention to sustain synthesis of essential amino acids. Urea can be hydrolyzed in the colonic lumen, but little of the ammonia thus formed is lost in fecal fluid (Wilson et al., 1968). Richards et al. (1967) showed that some of this ammonia is reabsorbed and utilized for protein synthesis. However, it cannot be said at present whether essential amino acid synthesis which is keto acid-dependent takes place in the liver and tissues after independent absorption of keto acid and ammonia or whether it takes place in the lower bowel lumen in the presence of bacteria with subsequent absorption of the amino acid. Questions of this nature, as well as the cost, instability and unpalatability of keto acids, relegate these nutritional studies to the class of experimentation rather than that of a practical solution to the feeding of patients. On the other hand, the very existence of potential endogenous synthesis of so-called indispensable nutrients in man illustrates one possible cause for the interindividual variation in amino acid requirements.

Complications of Amino Acid Nutrition

Several complications of amino acid nutrition may arise which may compromise that nutrition. They represent topics of broad general interest, and the reader will find more extensive discussion of them elsewhere (National Academy of Sciences [NRC], 1959; Harper, 1964). These problems are particularly relevant to the patient undergoing total intravenous alimentation or dietary management of a disturbance of amino acid metabolism.

Amino Acid Deficiency

In man, this is usually a function of protein malnutrition. However, the use of semisynthetic or modified diets restricted in particular amino acids to nourish patients has introduced the hazard of deficiency states involving essential amino acids. When therapeutic diets are used which are limited, for example, in phenylalanine (as in phenylketonuria), phenylalanine and tyrosine (as in hereditary tyrosinemia), methionine (as in homocystinuria), branched-chain amino acids (as in maple syrup urine disease and valinemia) or histidine (as in histidinemia), there is a danger that requirements for the offending amino acid may not be met. The specific manifestations of the nutritional deficiency states for tryptophan, lysine, isoleucine, threonine, methionine and valine have been described in the rat (Follis, 1948; National Academy of Sciences [NRC], 1959; Sidransky and Verney, 1964). The corresponding effects of the deficiency state in man, which may follow depletion of any of these individual amino acids, are not generally known (Follis, 1948), except where they have been evaluated under experimental conditions in relatively few infants (Table 2–5). On the other hand, the effects of phenylalanine deficiency in man have now been widely observed in the treatment of phenylketonuria (Lowe et al., 1967; Rouse, 1966).

An interesting and special example of "conditioned" amino acid deficiency in man has been described recently. Subjects with homocystinemia due to cystathionine synthase deficiency (see Chapter 11) have a block in the outflow pathway of methionine metabolism responsible for the endogenous synthesis of cyst(e)ine. Under these conditions, the patient becomes dependent on exogenous or dietary cyst(e)ine to meet his needs for protein synthesis. This need is met when the patient is consuming a normal diet; unfortunately, this will also sustain the homocystinemia. If a low-methionine diet is introduced for therapeutic reasons, it is very likely that cyst(e)ine intake will also be curtailed by such a diet. Under this new regime the patient will become deficient in a limiting amino acid, and protein synthesis will be impaired. Brenton et al. (1966) showed, by means of careful nitrogen balance studies (Fig. 2–4), that cyst(e)ine is indeed a limiting amino acid in homocystinuria. To overcome a deficiency state under these conditions, and to restore positive nitrogen balance, it is necessary to supplement the usual therapeutic diet with cyst(e)ine. This phenomenon

Table 2–5 General and Specific Manifestations of Amino Acid Deficiencies

	Human Infant[a]		Rat[b]	
	Growth Failure	Other[c]	Growth Failure	Other
Histidine	+	Dermatitis	+	
Isoleucine	+	Convulsions?	+	Muscle necrosis
Leucine	+		+	
Lysine	+		+	Achromatotrichia Fatty liver
Methionine	+		+	Anemia and hypoproteinemia[d]
Phenylalanine[c]	+	Dermatitis Osteopathy Aminoaciduria Anemia	+	
Threonine	+	Aminoaciduria	+	Periportal fat in the liver
Tryptophan	+	Niacin deficiency	+	Niacin deficiency Fatty liver
Valine	+		+	Convulsions

[a]From Holt et al., 1950; and Follis, 1948.
[b]From National Academy of Sciences (NRC), 1959, and Follis, 1948.
[c]All studies except those involving phenylalanine were short-term.
[d]These findings occur in the presence of choline and cystine supplements. Omission of former causes fatty liver; omission of latter causes liver necrosis and hair changes.

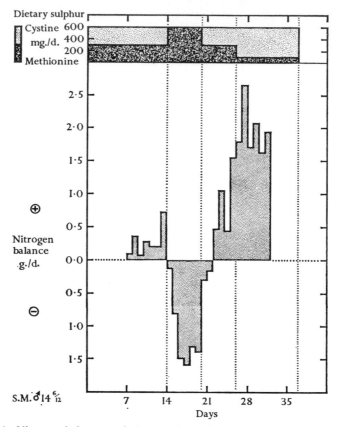

Figure 2–4   Nitrogen balance study in a patient with homocystinemia due to cystathionine synthase deficiency. The amount of sulfur in the diet derived from methionine and from cystine is indicated in the top section of the graph; nitrogen balance is shown in the lower portion. When methionine is the sole source of sulfur, cystine becomes a limiting amino acid. Positive nitrogen balance is restored only when a cystine supplement is added to sulfur intake provided by a low methionine diet, as might be done for therapeutic purposes in this disease. (From Brenton, D. P., et al., Quart. J. Med. *35*:325–346, 1966.)

of a "conditioned" deficiency (that is, conditional upon a metabolic aberration) is subtly different from amino acid unbalance and imbalance as described in the following paragraph.

Amino Acid Unbalance and Imbalance

A state of nutritional *unbalance* is said to exist when the relative proportions of amino acids in a protein deviate appreciably from the reference protein. To restore nutritional balance, the intake of the protein must be adjusted in accordance with the proportion of the limiting amino acid.

Harper (1964) introduced the concept of *imbalance* to describe that situation where the need for the limiting amino acid is actually increased because the diet contains an excess of another amino acid. Thus, by the administration of one amino acid in a marginal nutritional situation, it is possible to induce relative deficiency of a second limiting amino acid with associated effects on growth and function. The probable mechanism of the imbalance effect and its consequences have been discussed at length elsewhere (Harper, 1964; Anonymous, 1968a).

Amino Acid Antagonism

"An antagonist is considered to compete with the analogous dietary essential for a site of metabolic activity, thus preventing the normal reaction from going to completion" (National Academy of Sciences [NRC], 1959). The problem of antagonism is a more discrete event than that in imbalance. Two types of antagonism have been well documented (Harper, 1964; Anonymous, 1968b): one involving branched-chain amino acid interaction, and another involving lysine-arginine interaction. The antagonistic condition can be alleviated by supplementation with the structurally related amino acid. The condition is not prevented by supplementation with the most limiting amino acid in the diet, as it would be in the condition of imbalance.

Amino Acid Toxicity

An amino acid can be present in such excess as to cause a deleterious effect on growth and function (Anonymous, 1968a). Toxicity cannot be counteracted by administration of a structurally related amino acid or of the most limiting amino acid. The condition can only be offset by reducing the concentration of the toxic amino acid itself. Toxicity is the nutritional equivalent of the inherited aminoacidopathic phenotype and, although it is unlikely to occur as a common nutritional event, the phenomenon has often been used in attempts to develop model phenotypes in animals of human aminoacidopathies (Daniel and Waisman, 1968). (see also the discussion of animal models of phenylketonuria in Chapter 15.)

Toxicity is enhanced if the diet is low in protein. Sometimes it is alleviated by specific supplementations—for example, by threonine in tyrosine toxicity (Anonymous, 1968b), and by glycine, arginine and serine in methionine toxicity (Benevenga and Harper, 1967). The cause of toxicity is believed to be a particular chemical function of the individual amino acid involved, as illustrated, for example, by the studies of methionine and sulfur amino acid toxicity (Klavins, 1963a, 1963b, 1964, 1965) and tyrosine toxicity (Boctor and Harper, 1968). Salmon (1958) suggested that amino acids with diverse metabolic interrelations (e.g., methionine, tyrosine, tryptophan and histidine) have greater toxicity than those which have restricted catabolic pathways (e.g., branched-chain amino acids).

INTESTINAL PHASE OF AMINO ACID NUTRITION

The alimentary tract of man accommodates both the ingestion and digestion of protein nutrients and the absorption of the products of intraluminal protein and peptide hydrolysis. The preceding discussion of protein and amino acid nutrition assumed that the amino acids of protein were freely available to the subject through the processes of digestion and absorption. However, a failure of either would compromise the nutritional status of the subject (Orten, 1963).

Digestion

Intact protein and large peptides provide no nourishment because they are poorly absorbed into portal blood (Gitler, 1964). The most dramatic demonstration of human protein malnutrition due to *maldigestion* is seen in trypsinogen deficiency (Townes, 1965). Infants affected with this autosomal recessive disease fail to grow when fed a normal diet containing milk as the protein source because of their inability to digest dietary protein. The phenotypic effects of the trait can be offset by one of two methods. Nourishment with milk protein hydrolysate is immediately followed by restoration of normal growth (Townes, 1965). A similar response follows the direct approach to therapy by means of trypsinogen replacement. The ability to nourish the patient with trypsinogen deficiency by the oral feeding of free amino acids indicates the segregation of digestive and absorptive functions from each other.

Absorption

Although proteins are not absorbed, small peptides and free amino acids are absorbed, and with great efficiency, by the normal small intestine.

Amino Acids

After their release by enzymatic hydrolysis from dietary protein, free L-amino acids are absorbed from the small intestinal lumen into the intestinal absorptive cells and then, via transcellular transport, into the portal circulation (Wilson, 1962; Christensen, 1964). The small intestine is well adapted morphologically for its important absorptive role (Laster and Ingelfinger, 1961). The concentrative uptake and transcellular transport of free amino acids which occurs in intestinal absorptive cells is a mediated process (Quastel, 1960; Wilson, 1962; Scriver, 1968; Thier, 1968; Spencer, 1968) with defined chemical and physical characteristics which are under genetic control (see additional discussions in Chapters 6 through 10). Amino acid uptake from the human small intestinal lumen in vivo involves more than one mode of mediated transport for a given amino acid (Schedl et al., 1968), and many substrate-specific systems are involved in the absorption of all amino acids in a mixture (Scriver, 1969). Studies in vitro suggest that this is true of mammalian intestine generally (Spencer, 1967).

Intestinal transport of amino acids is genetically controlled. The expression of this control is apparent in various mutant phenotypes such as Hartnup disease and cystinuria. These genetic probes confirm the impressions gained by other types of analysis that several different transport systems are used for amino acid absorption by the bowel.

Ontogenetic studies (Deren et al., 1965; Spencer, 1968) indicate that maturation of intestinal transport systems occurs in the fetus in a manner analogous to that which occurs in kidney (see also Chapter 3). Specificity and capacity for absorption appear to increase with fetal development in keeping with the environmental demands and modes of nutrition which appear in postnatal life and which are not evident during intrauterine development.

During the process of absorption, it is assumed that equilibration of the free amino acid develops between the intestinal lumen and the *portal circulation* (Christensen, 1964). The *systemic circulation* and the intestinal lumen can also achieve an equilibrium (Christensen et al., 1963), so that an amino acid may move not only from intestinal lumen to plasma via the portal circulation but also from systemic plasma across the mucosal epithelium to the intestinal lumen (Fig. 2–5). Therefore, the establishment of high concentrations of amino acid in the systemic circulation will cause the same amino acid to accumulate in the intestinal lumen, and it can then influence absorption of other amino acids. A disease which causes hyperaminoacidemia may thus affect the absorption

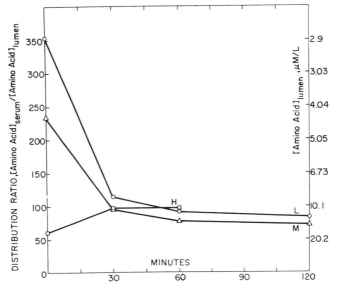

Figure 2–5 Distribution of the nonmetabolizable compound 1-aminocyclopentane carboxylic acid between serum and ileal lumen of the rat. The steady-state distribution ratio achieved after about 30 minutes was the same whether the amino acid was instilled first in the lumen (squares) or infused first into plasma (triangles and circles). H, M and L refer to high (proximal), medium and low (distal) positions of sampling along the length of the ileum. (From Christensen et al., 1963.)

of other structurally related amino acids. An acquired defect of tryptophan absorption in the presence of hyperphenylalaninemia in phenylketonuria (Yarbro and Anderson, 1965; Drummond et al., 1966) is described in Chapter 15).

Peptides

There has been renewed interest in the transport of low molecular weight peptides (oligopeptides*) as a process which is distinct from the uptake of free amino acids not only in microorganisms, where the subject has been widely studied (Payne and Gilvarg, 1971), but also in the mammalian intestine, where until recently its physiological significance had somewhat escaped the attention it deserves.

Oligopeptides (mainly di- and tripeptides) account for much of the nitrogenous material in the intestinal lumen during the digestive phase of protein nutrition (Chen et al., 1962; Mawer and Nixon, 1969). The peptides are absorbed intact across the luminal membrane, are then hydrolyzed in the mucosal cell and finally emerge into the portal circulation as free amino acids (Newey and Smith, 1960, 1962). Since several hundred combinations of amino acids in dipeptide and tripeptide linkage could result from hydrolysis of dietary proteins, the mechanisms of oligopeptide absorption are of great physiological interest and significance.

---

*Peptides are named for their constituent amino acids from the N-terminal end. Thus in glycyl-leucine, glycine has the amino group free and leucine has the carboxyl group free, while the two are attached in peptide linkage. (See Figure 1–1.)

In general, amino acids are more rapidly absorbed from human intestine when they are in the form of oligopeptides than when they are in the equivalent free state (Craft et al., 1968). This seems to be true also for nonhuman mammalian intestine (Lis et al., 1971). However, not all peptide combinations or all peptides will yield free amino acids in portal or systemic blood more rapidly than absorption from intestine of their free constituents. Asatoor et al. (1970a) demonstrated that the absorption rates for free β-alanine and L-histidine into systemic venous plasma are each slightly more rapid than when they are peptide-linked in the form of carnosine (β-alanyl-L-histidine). This finding suggests that hydrolysis is the point of delay in the assimilation of this particular dipeptide for amino acid nutrition. It is known that intracellular aminopeptidase activity is not equivalent for all peptide combinations, and hydrolysis is the limiting step in nutrition for several species of oligopeptide.

Asatoor et al. (1970a, 1970b) and Navab and Asatoor (1970) went on to show that the absorption of dipeptides is an important compensatory mechanism for delivery of amino acids into the portal circulation in the patient with Hartnup disease, an inborn error of membrane transport involving the neutral α-amino acid group (but excluding proline and glycine) and affecting intestinal and renal tubular epithelium (Scriver, 1965). The British group suggested that adequate amino acid nutrition was maintained in Hartnup disease because peptide absorption could offset the deficiency of free amino acid absorption under conditions of adequate protein nutrition.

Investigation of oligopeptide absorption has revealed the following points of general interest.

(1) Rates of amino acid absorption from peptides are generally faster than from *mixtures* of the equivalent free constituents, at all levels of the small bowel (duodenum, jejunum and ileum) in man (Adibi and Morse, 1971) (Fig. 2–6).

(2) Intracellular peptide hydrolysis is greater in the ileum than in the jejunum (Adibi and Morse, 1971).

(3) Kinetic analysis of "neutral" peptide transport (in rabbit ileum) indicates that more than one type of uptake mechanism is available for the dipeptide glycyl-L-proline (Fig. 2–7). One type of uptake has high affinity but low capacity, while the other has low affinity but high capacity (Rubino et al., 1971).

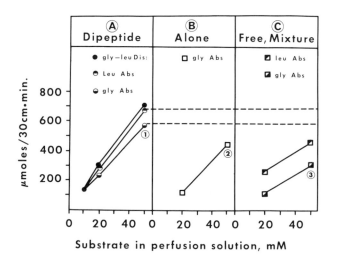

Figure 2–6 The rates of absorption and disappearance from the small jejunal lumen (in man) of free amino acids (glycine or leucine) and the dipeptide glycyl-L-leucine when either the dipeptide alone, the amino acid alone or an equimolar mixture of the constituent free amino acids is perfused through the jejunum in vivo. Note that the absorption rate of the dipeptide is faster than that of the constituent free amino acids. Note also that absorption from the mixture of free amino acids is associated with partial inhibition of free amino acid uptake. (Redrawn from data of Adibi and Morse, 1971.)

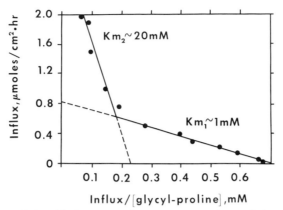

Figure 2-7 The relationship between substrate concentration and the uptake of the dipeptide glycyl-L-proline by segments of rabbit intestine in vitro. The graph indicates biphasic uptake kinetics, with more than one rate constant and more than one apparent affinity constant for 1 minute uptake of the intact dipeptide. The two observed types of dipeptide transport are independently saturable. Glycylproline is transported intact, but intracellular hydrolysis occurs very rapidly after uptake. The net transepithelial flux of constituent free amino acids from luminal peptide into portal blood therefore involves transport of the intact dipeptide by more than one peptide-specific site of entry (as is the case also for free glycine and free proline [Mohyuddin and Scriver, 1970]), followed by a process of peptide hydrolysis and efflux on the opposite border of the cell. (Redrawn from data of Rubino et al., 1971.)

These characteristics resemble those which have also been identified for transport of free amino acids (Spencer, 1967; Schedl, 1968; Scriver, 1969).

(4) The absorptive mechanism for a neutral dipeptide such as glycyl-L-proline is mediated and is enhanced by Na^+. The reactive site specifically excludes inhibition by the free constituent amino acids (L-proline and glycine) but allows interaction with other α-amino dipeptides with different N-terminal or C-terminal constituents* (Rubino et al., 1971).

These characteristics of peptide transport reveal that mammalian intestine absorbs the intraluminal products of protein digestion more efficiently when they are in the form of oligopeptides. However, net absorption of dipeptides and tripeptides into portal blood requires both peptide-specific membrane transport sites and intracellular amino peptidases. For this reason, it is likely that *protein-calorie malnutrition (kwashiorkor)* will produce more profound effects on protein nutrition than will the inborn errors of membrane transport which affect only free amino acid absorption in the intestine. Usually, only one type of amino acid transport (the high-capacity, low-affinity mode of uptake) is lost in the inborn error (Scriver, 1969), while the auxiliary transport systems remain intact throughout the intestine. Transport is also supplemented by the various peptide transport systems, and under these conditions one would not anticipate a serious impairment of protein nutrition. On the other hand, in mammalian protein-calorie malnutrition, there are extensive cellular changes in the intestinal mucosa accompanied by atrophy of the absorptive area (Burman, 1965) and loss of intracellular peptide hydrolases (Kumar and Chase, 1971). Under these conditions, not only will the capacity of all transport sites for

*Kidney transports the free amino acids proline and glycine by low-affinity and high-affinity systems (Mohyuddin and Scriver, 1970). Glycylproline does not interact with these systems (Scriver, 1965).

amino acids and peptides be diminished, but intraluminal digestion and intra-cellular peptide hydrolysis will also be compromised. This extensive disruption of absorptive mucosal activity may explain the difficulties encountered with initial re-alimentation of patients severely affected with protein-calorie malnu-trition. Initial intravenous feeding with solutions containing suitable free amino acid mixtures would seem to be preferable to oral alimentation under these conditions.

Interactions Between Substrates During Absorption

The composition of the diet can apparently modify the effectiveness of protein nutrition by directly influencing free amino acid absorption. Animal studies show that when dietary fructose and sucrose are replaced by corn-starch, the uptake of essential amino acids by intestinal tissue in vitro is im-proved, with the exception of threonine (Human Nutrition Research Division, USDA, 1971). This interesting observation merits careful additional docu-mentation because of the implication, from yet another vantage point, that nonprotein nutrients can affect the efficiency of protein amino acid nutrition in vivo. Studies performed by Cook (1971) showed that glucose or galactose, when present at twice the concentration of the amino acid, can inhibit the absorption of isosmotic glycine (100 mM) from the perfused upper jejunal lumen in man. This finding has practical relevance for the non-Caucasian populations of the world, among whom protein malnutrition is most prevalent. The latter populations have a high prevalence of inherited intestinal lactase deficiency. The intraluminal concentration of milk-derived free glucose and lactose in lactase-deficient individuals is likely to be lower than in subjects with higher intestinal lactase activity. Under conditions of marginal protein nutrition, lactase-deficient subjects have a mechanism which provides them with a selective advantage for amino acid absorption from milk (Cook, 1971).

The mechanism by which monosaccharides impair amino acid transport in vivo and in vitro has been the subject of much discussion (Alvarado, 1970). It is likely that the effect is *not* due to interaction between carbohydrate and amino acid at a common membrane carrier site; it is more probable that the inhibition represents some form of noncompetitive interaction arising during the transport of the sugar and which indirectly affects the amino acid during its intracellular and transcellular transport (Genel et al., 1971).

FECAL AMINO ACIDS

Fecal amino acids may be informative about the intestinal handling of protein and amino acids, as, for example, in Hartnup disease, where an im-pairment of amino acid transport is reflected in the fecal amino acid pattern (Scriver, 1965). Sheffner, et al. (1948) and Ross (1965) concluded that the fecal pattern is a reflection of the dietary protein. Seakins and colleagues (1970) and Ersser et al. (1971) concluded from more recent investigations that fecal amino acids were derived primarily from bacterial hydrolysis of dietary protein reaching the large bowel. Any effect of diet upon the pattern, as, for example, in early postnatal life, appears to reflect the response of gut flora to a changing dietary pattern. Thus, when there is maldigestion and malabsorption of nitro-genous material, as in cystic fibrosis, fecal amino acids are likely to be increased; under such conditions, the pattern of fecal amino acids will change according to the amino acid sequence in the predominant dietary protein (Seakins et al., 1970).

Fecal bacteria acting further upon liberated amino acids may yield by-products and nonprotein amino acids. The literature (discussed by Seakins et al., 1970) describes many unusual compounds in feces, including β-alanine (decarboxylated aspartate), γ-aminobutyric acid (decarboxylated glutamate), γ-amino-n-valeric acid (a degradation product of lysine and proline), the diamines cadaverine (from lysine) and putrescine (from ornithine) and related compounds. The diamines can be absorbed and re-excreted in urine, where they may serve as markers of an intestinal transport defect, as, for example, in some forms of cystinuria (Bremer and Kohne, 1971). (See also the specific discussion of cystinuria, Chapter 7). Phenylacetylglutamine is usually considered to be of endogenous origin (see Chapter 15). However, it may also be formed by intestinal bacteria acting upon phenylalanine released from fecal protein, to yield the decarboxylation product phenylethylamine. When the latter is absorbed, it can be converted, conjugated and then excreted as phenylacetylglutamine (Seakins, 1971). Urinary tyramine can also arise from intracolonic decarboxylation of tyrosine (Seakins et al., 1970). Direct contamination of urine by feces is a hazard of urine collection in young infants. This artifact should be considered, particularly when interpreting unusual urine amino acid patterns in the newborn (Levy et al., 1969).

In summary, fecal amino acid loss is likely to be increased with any condition which enhances protein transit to the large bowel (e.g., diarrhea in infancy and cystic fibrosis). When the free amino acid content of the large bowel is augmented by bacterial hydrolysis of protein or when delivery of free amino acids to the colon is enhanced, because of aberrant peptide or amino acid absorption in the small bowel, unusual decarboxylation products of amino acids are likely to be found not only in the feces but also in the urine.

REFERENCES

Adibi, S. A., and Morse, E. L.: Intestinal transport of dipeptides in man: Relative importance of hydrolysis and intact absorption. J. Clin. Invest. 50:2266–2275, 1971.

Alvarado, F.: Intestinal transport of sugars and amino acids: Independence or federalism. Amer. J. Clin. Nutr. 23:824–828, 1970.

Anonymous: The mechanism of lysine-arginine antagonism in the chick. Nutr. Rev. 26:89–92, 1968a.

Anonymous: Imbalance and toxicity of amino acids. Nutr. Rev. 26:115–118, 1968b.

Anonymous: Annotation. Synthesis of essential amino acids. Lancet (i), 191, 1972.

Asatoor, A. M., Bandoh, J. K., Lant, A. F., Milne, M. D., and Navab, F.: Intestinal absorption of carnosine and its constituent amino acids in man. Gut 11:250–254, 1970a.

Asatoor, A. M., Cheng, B., Edwards, D. G., Lant, A. F., Matthews, D. M., Milne, M. D., Navab, F., and Richards, A. J.: Intestinal absorption of two dipeptides in Hartnup disease. Gut 11:380–387, 1970b.

Ballantyne, R. M., and McLaughlan, J. M.: The quality of the "protein" of the Canadian diet. Canad. Nutr. Notes 24:79–80, 1968.

Benevenga, N. J., and Harper, A. E.: Alleviation of methionine and homocystine toxicity in the rat. J. Nutr. 93:44–51, 1967.

Bergstrom, J., Fürst, P., Josephson, B., and Noree, L. O.: Improvement of nitrogen balance in a uremic patient by the addition of histidine to essential amino acid solutions given intravenously. Life Sci. 9:787–791, 1970.

Block, R. J., and Mitchell, H. H.: Correlation of amino acid composition of proteins with their nutritive value. Nutr. Abstr. Rev. 16:249–278, 1946/47.

Boctor, A. M., and Harper, A. E.: Tyrosine toxicity in the rat: Effect of high intake of p-hydroxyphenylpyruvic acid and of force-feeding high tyrosine diet. J. Nutr. 95:535–540, 1968.

Bremer, H. J., and Kohne, E.: The excretion of diamines in human urine. II. Cadaverine, putrescine 1,3-diamino propane, 2,2'-dithiobis-(ethylamine) and spermidine in urine of patients with cystinuria and cystinlysinuria. Clin. Chim. Acta 32:407–418, 1971.

Brenton, D. P., Cusworth, D. C., Dent, C. E., and Jones, E. E.: Homocystinuria. Clinical and dietary studies. Quart. J. Med. 35:325–346, 1966.

Burman, D.: The jejunal mucosa in kwashiorkor. Arch. Dis. Child. *40*:526–531, 1965.

Cannon, P. R., Steffee, C. H., Frazier, L. J., Rowley, D. A., and Stepto, R. C.: The influence of time of ingestion of essential amino acids upon utilization in tissue synthesis. Fed Proc. *6*:390, 1947.

Chen, M. L., Rogers, Q. R., and Harper, A. E.: Observations on protein digestion in vitro. IV. Further observations on the gastrointestinal contents of rats fed different dietary proteins. J. Nutr. *76*:235–241, 1962.

Christensen, H. N.: Free amino acids and peptides in tissues. *In* Munro, H. N., and Allison, J. B., eds., Mammalian Protein Metabolism, Vol. I. Academic Press, New York, pp. 105–124, 1964.

Christensen, H. N., Feldman, B. H., and Hastings, A. B.: Concentrative and reversible character of intestinal amino acid transport. Amer. J. Physiol. *205*:255–260, 1963.

Cook, G. C.: Impairment of glycine absorption by glucose and galactose in man. J. Physiol. (London) *217*:61–70, 1971.

Craft, I. L., Geddes, D., Hyde, C. W., Wise, I. J., and Matthews, D. M.: Absorption and malabsorption of glycine and glycine peptides in man. Gut *9*:425–437, 1968.

Dancis, J.: Nutritional management of hereditary disorders. Med. Clin. N. Amer. *54*:1431–1448, 1970.

Daniel, R. G., and Waisman, H. A.: The effects of excess amino acids on the growth of the young rat. Growth *32*:255–265, 1968.

Dietary Standard for Canada. Protein requirements. *In* Canadian Bulletin on Nutrition, Dec. 1968, (1964, revised.)

Dudrick, S. J., and Rhoads, J. E.: Total intravenous feeding. Sci. Amer. *226*(5):73–81, 1972.

Efron, M. L.: Dietary management of patients with inborn errors of amino acid metabolism. J. Amer. Diet. Ass. *51*:40–45, 1967.

Ersser, R. S., Seakins, J. W. T., and Gibbons, I. S. E.: Effect of diet and bacteria on the faecal amino acid pattern in the newborn. Z. Kinderheilk, *110*:276–285, 1971.

Follis, R. M., Jr.: The Pathology of Nutritional Disease. III. The essential amino acids. Charles C Thomas, Springfield, Ill., pp. 73–88, 1948.

Fomon, S. J.: Body composition of the male reference infant during the first year of life. Pediatrics *40*:863–870, 1967a.

Fomon, S. J.: Infant Nutrition. W. B. Saunders Company, Philadelphia, 1967b.

Fomon, S. J., and Filer, L. J., Jr.: Amino acid requirements for normal growth. *In* Nyhan, W. L., ed., Amino Acid Metabolism and Genetic Variation. McGraw-Hill, New York, pp. 391–401, 1967.

Fomon, S. J., and May, C. D.: Metabolic studies of normal full-term infants fed pasteurized human milk. Pediatrics *22*:101–115, 1958.

Genel, M., Rea, C. F., and Segal, S.: Transport interaction of sugars and amino acids in mammalian kidney. Biochim. Biophys. Acta *241*:779–788, 1971.

Ghadimi, H., Abaci, F., Kumar, S., and Rathi, M.: Biochemical aspects of intravenous alimentation. Pediatrics *48*:955–965, 1971.

Giardano, C., Phillips, M. E., DePascale, C., De Santo, N. G., Fürst, P., Brown, C. L., Houghton, B. J., and Richards, P.: Utilization of keto acid analogues of valine and phenylalanine in health and uraemia. Lancet (i), 178–182, 1972.

Graham, G. C., Placko, R. P., Morales, E., Acevedo, G., and Cordano, A.: Dietary protein quality in infants and children. VI. Isolated soy protein milk. Amer. J. Dis. Child. *120*:419–423, 1970.

Harper, A. E.: Amino acid toxicities and imblances. *In* Munro, H. N., and Allison, J. B., eds., Mammalian Protein Metabolism, Vol. II. Academic Press, New York, pp. 87–134, 1964.

Holt, L. E., Jr., Gyorgy, P., Pratt, E. L., Snyderman, S. E., and Wallace, W. M.: Protein and Amino Acid Requirements in Early Life. New York University Press, New York, 1960.

Holt, L. E., Jr., and Snyderman, S. E.: The amino acid requirement of infants. Report to the Council on Food and Nutrition. J.A.M.A. *175*:100–103, 1961.

Human Nutrition Research Division, Agricultural Research Service, U.S. Department of Agriculture: Amino Acid Absorption Progress Report, U.S. Govt. Printing Office, Washington, D.C., p. 29, 1971.

Irwin, M. I., and Hegsted, D. M.: A conspectus of research on amino acid requirements of man. J. Nutr. *101*:539–566, 1971.

Klavins, J. V.: Pathology of amino acid excess. II. Effects of administration of excess amounts of sulphur containing amino acids: L-cystine. Brit. J. Exp. Path. *44*:516–519, 1963b.

Klavins, J. V.: Pathology of amino acid excess. V. Effects of methionine on free amino acids in serum. Biochim. Biophys. Acta *104*:554–565, 1965.

Klavins, J. V., and Peacocke, I. L.: Pathology of amino acid excess. III. Effects of administration of excessive amounts of sulphur-containing amino acids: methionine with equimolar amounts of glycine and arginine. Brit. J. Exp. Path. *45*:533–547, 1964.

Kountz, W. B., Hofslatter, L., and Ackermann, P. G.: Nitrogen balance studies in 4 elderly men. J. Geront. *6*:20–33, 1951.

Kumar, V., and Chase, H. P.: Progressive protein undernutrition and intestinal enzyme activities in monkeys. Amer. J. Clin. Nutr. *25*:485–489, 1972.

Levy, H. L., Madigan, P. M., and Lum, A.: Fecal contamination in urine amino acid screening. Amer. J. Clin. Path. 57:765–768, 1969.

Lis, M. T., Crampton, R. F., and Matthews, D. M.: Rates of absorption of a dipeptide and the equivalent free amino acid in various mammalian species. Biochim. Biophys. Acta 233: 453–455, 1971.

Lowe, C. U., et al., Committee on Nutrition, American Academy of Pediatrics: Vitamin B6 requirements in man. Pediatrics 38:1068–1076, 1966.

Lowe, C. U., et al., Committee on Nutrition, American Academy of Pediatrics: Nutritional management in hereditary metabolic disease. Pediatrics 40:289–304, 1967.

Macy, I. G., and Kelly, H. J.: Human milk and cow's milk in infant nutrition. In Kon, S. K., and Cowie, A. T., eds. Milk: The Mammary Gland and Its Secretion, Vol. II. Academic Press, New York, pp. 265–304, 1961.

Mawer, G. E., and Nixon, E.: The net absorption of the amino acid constituents of a protein meal in normal and cystinuric subjects. Clin. Sci. 36:463–477, 1969.

McCance, R. A., and Widdowson, E. M.: The Composition of Foods, 3rd edition. Great Britain Medical Research Council, Special Report Series, No. 297, 1960.

McLaughlan, J. M., and Campbell, J. A.: Methodology of protein evaluation. In Munro, H. N., and Allison, J. B., eds., Mammalian Protein Metabolism, Vol. III. Academic Press, New York, pp. 391–423, 1969.

McLaughlan, J. M., Venkat Rao, S., Noel, F. J., and Morrison, A. B.: Blood amino acid studies. VI. Use of plasma amino acid score for predicting limiting amino acid(s) in dietary proteins. Canad. J. Biochem. 45:31–37, 1967.

Mitchell, H. H.: The dependence of the biological value of food proteins upon their content of essential amino acids. In Nehring, K., ed., Die Bewertung der Futterstoffe und andere Probleme der Tiererriahrung. Wiss Abhandl dent., Akad. Landwirtsch 5(Vol. 2):279–325, 1954.

Mohyuddin, F., and Scriver, C. R.: Amino acid transport in mammalian kidney: Multiple systems for imino acids and glycine in rat kidney. Amer. J. Physiol. 219:1–8, 1970.

Munro, H. N.: Basic concepts in the use of amino acids and protein hydrolysates for parenteral nutrition. In Symposium on Total Parenteral Nutrition, Food Science Committee, Council on Foods and Nutrition, American Medical Association, Nashville, pp. 7–35, 1972.

Nakagawa, I. I., Takahashi, T., Suzuki, T., and Kobayashi, K.: Amino acid requirements of children: Minimal needs of tryptophan, arginine, and histidine based on nitrogen balance method. J. Nutr. 80:305–310, 1963.

National Academy of Sciences (National Research Council), Food and Nutrition Board, Division of Biology and Agriculture, Committee on Amino Acids: Evaluation of protein nutrition. The Academy—The Council, Washington, D.C., Publ. 711, 1959.

National Academy of Sciences (National Research Council): Recommended Dietary Allowances. The Academy—The Council, Washington, D.C. Publ. 1694, 1968.

Navab, F., and Asatoor, A. M.: Studies on intestinal absorption of amino acids and a dipeptide in a case of Hartnup disease. Gut 11:373–379, 1970.

Newey, H., and Smith, D. H.: Intracellular hydrolysis of dipeptides during intestinal absorption. J. Physiol. (London) 152:367–380, 1960.

Newey, H., and Smith, D. H.: Cellular mechanisms in intestinal transfer of amino acids. J. Physiol. (London) 164:527–551, 1962.

Payne, J. W., and Gilvarg, C.: Peptide transport. Advances Enzym. 35:188–244, 1971.

Richards, P., Brown, C. L., Houghton, B. J., and Thompson, E.: Synthesis of phenylalanine and value by healthy and uremic men. Lancet (ii), 128–134, 1971.

Richards, P., Metcalfe-Gibson, A., Ward, E. E., Wrong, O. M., and Houghton, B. J.: Utilization of ammonia nitrogen for protein synthesis in man and the effect of protein restriction on uraemia. Lancet (ii), 845–849, 1967.

Rose, W. C.: The nutritive significance of the amino acids. Physiol. Rev. 18:109–136, 1938.

Ross, C. A. C.: Faecal excretion of amino acids in infants. Lancet (ii), 190–194, 1951.

Rouse, B. M.: Phenylalanine deficiency syndrome. J. Pediat. 69:246–249, 1966.

Rubino, A., Field, M., and Schwackman, H.: Intestinal transport of amino acid residues of dipeptides. I. Influx of the glycine residue of glycyl-L-proline across mucosal border. J. Biol. Chem. 246:3542–3548, 1971.

Rudman, D.: Capacity of human subjects to utilize keto acid analogues of valine and phenylalanine. J. Clin. Invest. 50:90–96, 1971.

Salmon, W. D.: The significance of amino acid imbalance in nutrition. Am. J. Clin. Nutr. 6:487–494, 1958.

Schedl, H. P., Pierce, C. E., Rider, A., and Clifton, J. A. (with technical assistance of Nokes, G.): Absorption of L-methionine from the human small intestine. J. Clin. Invest. 47:417–425, 1968.

Scriver, C. R.: Glycyl-proline in urine of humans with bone disease. Canad. J. Physiol. Pharmacol. 42:357–364, 1964.

Scriver, C. R.: Hartnup disease. A genetic modification of intestinal and renal transport of certain neutral α-amino acids. New Eng. J. Med. *273*:530–532, 1965.

Scriver, C. R.: Treatment of inherited disease: Realized and potential. Med. Clin. N. Amer. *53*: 941–963, 1969.

Scriver, C. R.: The human biochemical genetics of amino acid transport. Pediatrics *44*:348–357, 1969.

Seakins, J. W. T.: The determination of urinary phenylacetylglutamine as phenylacetic acid. Studies on its origin in normal subjects and children with cystic fibrosis. Clin. Chim. Acta *35*:121–131, 1971.

Seakins, J. W. T., Ersser, R. S., and Gibbons, I. S. E.: Studies on the origin of faecal amino acids in cystic fibrosis. Gut *11*:600–609, 1970.

Sheffner, A. L., Kirsner, J. B., and Palmer, W. L.: Studies on amino acid excretion in man. 2. Amino acids in feces. J. Biol. Chem. *176*:89–93, 1948.

Sidransky, H., and Verney, E.: Chemical pathology of acute amino acid deficiencies. VII. Morphological and biochemical changes in young rats force-fed arginine-, leucine-, isoleucine-, and phenylalanine-devoid diets. Arch. Path. *78*:134–148, 1964.

Snyderman, S. E., Boyer, A., Roitman, E., Holt, L. E., Jr., and Prose, P. H.: The histidine requirement of the infant. Pediatrics *31*:786–801, 1963.

Snyderman, S. E., Holt, L. E., Jr., Norton, P. M., Roitman, E., and Phansalkar, S. V.: The plasma aminogram. I. Influence of the level of protein intake and a comparison of whole protein and amino acid diets. Pediat. Res. *2*:131–144, 1968.

Stifel, F. B., and Herman, R. H.: Is histidine an essential amino acid in Man? Amer. J. Clin. Nutr. *25*:182–185, 1972.

Swendseid, M. E., Tuttle, S. G., Drenick, E. J., Joven, C. B., and Massey, F. J.: Plasma amino acid response to glucose administration in various nutritive states. Amer. J. Clin. Nutr. *20*:243–249, 1967.

Swendseid, M. E., Yamada, C., Vinyard, E., Figueroa, W. G., and Drenick, E. J.: Plasma amino acid levels in subjects fed isonitrogenous diets containing different proportions of fat and carbohydrate. Amer. J. Clin. Nutr. *20*:52–55, 1967.

Virtanen, A. I.: Milk production of cows on protein free feed. Science *153*:1603–1614, 1966.

Waisman, H. A., and Kerr, G. R.: Advantages and disadvantages in the use of restricted diets in the treatment of inborn errors of metabolism. *In* Nyhan, W. L., ed., Amino Acid Metabolism and Genetic Variation. McGraw-Hill, New York, pp. 365–378, 1967.

Watkin, D.: Protein metabolism and requirements in the elderly. *In* Munro, H. N., and Allison, J. B., eds., Mammalian Protein Metabolism, Vol. II. Academic Press, New York, Chap. 17, 1964.

Weller, L. A., Calloway, D. H., and Margen, S.: Plasma amino acids in subjects on three diets. J. Amer. Diet. Ass. *57*:234–238, 1970.

Wilson, D. R., Ing, T. S., Metcalfe-Gibson, A., and Wrong, O. M.: In vivo dialysis of faeces as a method of stool analysis. 3. The effect of intestinal antibiotics. Clin. Sci. *34*:211–221, 1968.

Wilson, T. H.: Intestinal Absorption. Chapter 5. Amino acids. W. B. Saunders Company, Philadelphia, pp. 110–133, 1962.

Wood, J. L., and Cooley, S. L.: Substitution of α-keto acids for 5 amino acids essential for growth of rat. Proc. Soc. Exp. Biol. Med. *85*:409–411, 1954.

World Health Organization/Food and Agriculture Organization: Protein Requirements. U.N. Technical Report Series #301, 1965.

Young, V. R., and Scrimshaw, N. S.: Endogenous nitrogen metabolism and plasma free amino acids in young adults given a "protein-free" diet. Brit. J. Nutr. *22*:9–20, 1968.

Young, V. R., Hussein, M. A., Murray, E., and Scrimshaw, M. S.: Plasma tryptophan response curve and its relation to tryptophan requirements in young adult men. J. Nutr. *101*:45–60, 1971.

Chapter Three

DISTRIBUTIONS OF AMINO ACIDS IN BODY FLUIDS

GENERAL CONSIDERATIONS

The amino acids of plasma and other compartments of extracellular fluid comprise not only those absorbed from the intestinal pool but also those derived from the endogenous tissue pools, both free and peptide-bound (Holden, 1962). The total concentration of free amino acids in mammalian plasma is about 2 mM, while the corresponding amount of amino acids in the form of plasma proteins is 300 times greater. The concentration of free amino acids in the intracellular space is about 10 times greater than in plasma water, and the amount present as protein in tissues is 30 to 60 times greater than the corresponding free amount (Christensen, 1964). One must conclude from these data that the randomly sampled plasma pattern of free amino acids merely reflects a moment of their traffic during a diurnal round of commerce in cellular metabolism.

Van Slyke and Meyer (1913) first drew attention to the important role played by membrane transport in the internal ecology of the free amino acids, and it is the process of mediated transport across cell membranes in which some aspects of regulation of amino acid metabolism can take place. Specific discussion of transport is taken up in Chapter 6, and other aspects of its role in regulation have been mentioned in Chapter 2. In the present chapter, we are primarily concerned with so-called steady-state distribution patterns of free amino acids in the various body fluids.

Quantitative analysis of amino acids has been advanced greatly in recent years: it is now possible to define accurately for healthy human subjects many aspects of interindividual and intraindividual variations in amino acid distribution provided pitfalls of analysis are avoided (Perry and Hansen, 1969; Scriver et al., 1971). Some of the distributions which are more readily accessible to analysis, and thus are likely to be of particular clinical interest, include the age-dependent plasma concentrations of amino acids, circadian variation in plasma concentration, urine excretion and renal conservation of free amino acids, erythrocyte:plasma distribution ratios, fetal:maternal distribution ratios and the pattern and concentration in amniotic fluid, cerebrospinal fluid, sweat and saliva. Knowledge of normal amino acid levels is essential before normal physiological or disease perturbation of these levels can be recognized.

AMINO ACIDS IN PLASMA

Concentration

There have been many studies of plasma amino acids in infants, children and adults. The subjects of these investigations come primarily from the Caucasian and Negro races and from the North American, Arctic, European and African regions; although these subjects may have had widely different types of diets, there has been found a relative constancy of age-specific amino acid levels in these samplings of human plasma, bearing out the concept that storage and flux through intracellular pools is probably a more important regulation of plasma patterns than variation in the composition of the normal diet (Christensen, 1964; Scriver, 1969). The regulatory components which allow such stability must be impressive. One component of what is obviously a multi-factorial system is genetic regulation. This is clearly illustrated by the elegant data of Nance and Nance (1971), which showed the striking concordance for plasma amino acids in newborn monozygotic twins and the relative discordance in dizygotic twins (Fig. 3–1). To our knowledge, these are the first data revealing the genetic component in plasma amino acid homeostasis in normal human subjects.

The mean plasma concentration of some amino acids (such as the branched-chain group) is lower during infancy than in later life (Table 3–1), even though the amount of amino acids ingested per kg body weight is greater during early life than in adulthood (see Chapter 2). The lower concentration of certain plasma amino acids during the period of rapid somatic growth presumably reflects greater uptake into tissues from plasma at this time of life (Christensen and Streicher, 1948). Noall and colleagues (1957) showed that even the non-metabolizable amino acid α-aminoisobutyric acid, which cannot be incorporated into protein, is concentrated more avidly from plasma in the animal during rapid somatic growth than during maturity. Recognition of such age-dependent phenomena is important if the normal limits of amino acid concentrations in plasma are to be used precisely for recognition of aberrations in amino acid levels.

Physiological Variation in Steady-State Plasma Amino Acid Levels

There are some important time-dependent changes in plasma amino acids during the first few hours and days of life. Dickenson, Rosenblum and Hamilton (1970) showed that the levels of most plasma amino acids fall during the first *days* of life. Reisner et al. (1973) have confirmed this finding (Fig. 3–2); they believe that it probably reflects redistribution of amino acid pools in early life under normal hormonal and dietary influences. Lindblad and Baldesten (1969) examined the change in plasma amino acids during the first few *hours* after birth. The change between the levels in cord blood and in the cubital vein plasma of

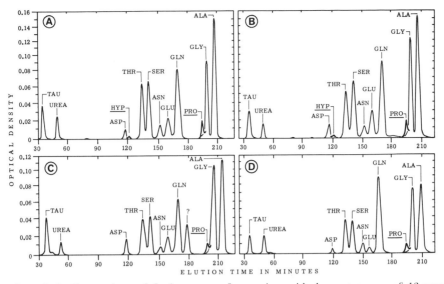

Figure 3–1 Comparison of fasting serum free amino acid chromatograms of 13-year-old monozygotic male twins (*A* and *B*) and 12-year-old dizygotic male twins (*C* and *D*). Both twins in the pairs were studied in identical fashion. After processing of the plasma, the amino acids in equivalent volumes were examined by elution chromatography using a lithium buffer system on ion-exchange resin columns in a pair of consecutive runs.

Note the striking concordance of plasma amino acid levels in the monozygotic twins and the relative discordance in the dizygotic twins: these indicate genetic components among the multi-factorial regulators of plasma amino acid levels in man. Small peaks take on biological significance when they are present in both members of the monozygotic twin pair. Note, for example, the unusual occurrence of a small hydroxyproline peak in both monozygotic twins. In contrast, the dizygotic twins show both qualitative and quantitative intra-pair differences (e.g., discordance for the small phosphoethanolamine peak [appearing as a shoulder on taurine in *C*] and for the unknown peak following glutamine [also in *C*]; the relative sizes of the taurine, aspartic acid, glutamic acid, glutamine, glycine and alanine peaks). (Data of Nance and Nance, 1971.)

full-term infants obtained two to six hours after birth (Table 3–2) was different from the pattern of change between the first day of extrauterine life and the third day (Fig. 3–2). The change between extrauterine cord blood and venous blood patterns probably reflects the emergence of infant tissues as important modulators of amino acid levels in plasma, since cord-blood amino acids have been delivered by the placenta but have not yet equilibrated with the tissues of the infant.

Placental insufficiency affects plasma amino acid levels in the newborn, causing the concentration to be generally lower in the infant who is born small for his gestational age (Table 3–2). The changes resemble those of starvation and protein depletion (Mestyán et al., 1969; Lindblad, 1970; Reisner et al., 1973) and are therefore appropriate for the physiological effects of placental malnutrition.

Pregnancy affects maternal plasma amino acid levels (Armstrong and Yates, 1964). Maternal plasma amino acid levels are generally significantly lower in the first half of pregnancy than in nonpregnant control females, and urea cycle intermediates (citrulline, ornithine and arginine) are particularly low. Blood levels tend to rise toward normal at term (Reid et al., 1971). The causes of the relative hypoaminoacidemia in early pregnancy are probably numerous and complex. It is a point of interest that tyrosine falls relative to phenylalanine

Table 3-1   Amino Acid Concentration in Plasma or Serum[a] (μmole/L)

Amino Acid	"Prematures"[1] Mean	± SD	Neonates[2] Mean	± SD	Infants[3] Mean	± SD	Children[4] Mean	± SD	Children[5] Mean	Range	Children[6] Mean	Range	Adults[7] Mean	Adults[8] Range	Adults[9] Mean	± SD	Range
Taurine	180	75	141	40					80	57–115	49	19–91	66	27–168	59	12	41–78
Hydroxyproline	40	40		32						25			16	0–24			tr–5
Aspartic acid	10	10	8	4	19	2	16	3	10	4–20	2	0–9					
Threonine	215	60	217	21	177	36	145	16	76	42–95	60	33–128	162	79–246	138	31	75–189
Serine	270[c]	75	163	34	131	27[c]	121	14[c]	94	79–112	92	24–172	112	67–193	99	19	67–129
Asp (NH₂) + Glu (NH₂)[b]	905[c]	250	759	136	193	52	176	33	295	57–467	135	46–290	603	413–690	696[d]	73[d]	554–824[d]
Proline	230	75	183	32					106	68–148	115	51–185	233	100–442	185	48	90–270
Glutamic acid	65	35	52	25					110	23–250			58	14–192	24	12	10–67
Glycine	460	275	343	69	213	35	219	33	166	117–223	170	56–308	231	120–553	284	44	162–335
Alanine	375	50	329	55	292	53	271	36	234	137–305	219	99–313	344	209–659	360	71	205–496
Valine	130	50	136	39	161	38	181	20	162	128–283	127	57–262	169	116–315	225	40	151–302
Half Cystine	65	10	62	13	42	9	44	7	60	45–77			74	48–141	49	9	34–67
Methionine	35	5	29	8	18	3	16	3	14	11–16	21	3–29	21	6–39	21	4	13–32
Isoleucine	40	20	39	8	39	8	44	6	43	28–84	44	26–94	54	35–97	60	12	38–83
Leucine	70	25	72	17	77	21	90	13	85	56–178	75	45–155	100	71–175	115	23	77–162
Tyrosine	120	100	69	16	54	21	45	8	43	31–71	45	11–122	50	21–87	54	11	40–80
Phenylalanine	90	20	78	14	55	10	47	5	42	26–61	40	23–69	57	37–115	48	7	37–61
Ornithine	90	20	91	25	50	11	46	8	33	27–86	40	10–107	69	29–125	58	14	32–88
Lysine	190	60	200	46	135	28	130	20	111	71–151	87	45–144	173	82–236	186	36	99–249
Histidine	50	20	77	16	78	14	80	13	55	24–85	64	24–112	79	31–106	88	16	65–119
Arginine	50	20	54	17	62	9	85	16	53	23–86	31	11–65	81	21–137	82	17	53–115
Tryptophan	30	15	32	17										25–73	31	6	19–45
β-alanine			14.5														

[a] All data obtained by elution chromatography on ion exchange resin columns.

[b] Asparagine and glutamine, as combined amounts.

[c] Includes asparagine.

[d] Signifies pooled glutamine and asparagine. The individual values for the mean ± SD (and range) are glu (NH₂) 640 ± 58, (520–742); asp (NH₂) 56 ± 15, (34–82).

[e] Signifies glutamine alone.

[1] Adapted from Dickinson, Rosenblum, and Hamilton, 1970. Data for the first day of life from 10 premature infants with birth weights less than 2500 grams. Some of these infants may have been small-for-gestational-age rather than prematurely born.

[2] Recalculated from Dickinson et al., 1965; 25 infants (more than 2500 grams) studied before first feeding.

[3] Recalculated from Brodehl and Gellisen, 1968; 12 infants, 16 days to 4 months of age, studied after 6- to 8-hour fast.

[4] Recalculated from Brodehl and Gellisen, 1968; 12 children, 2 to 12 years of age, studied after overnight fast.

[5] Scriver and Davies, 1965; 9 children, 3 to 10 years of age, studied after overnight fast.

[6] Soupart, 1962; 20 children, 9 months to 2 years of age, studied after overnight fast.

[7] Recalculated from Dickinson et al., 1965; 8 adults.

[8] Data on 76 adults compiled from nine sources by Dickinson et al., 1965; includes variation recorded by Soupart, 1962.

[9] Data on 10 men and 10 women (age range 33 to 56 years), from Perry and Hansen, 1969.

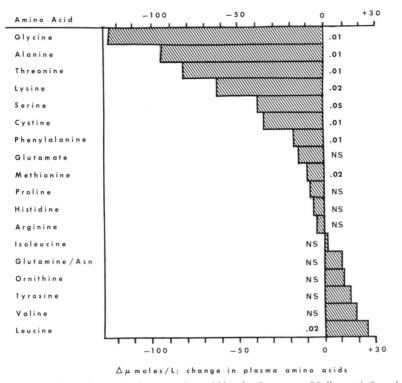

Figure 3–2   Relative change in plasma amino acid levels of a group of full-term infants between the day of birth (mean age 12½ hours) and the third day of extrauterine life (mean age 80 hours). The change is expressed as Δ μmoles per liter plasma; −Δ indicates a fall by the third day; +Δ indicates a rise in the plasma concentration of the amino acid. (Data of Reisner et al., 1973.)

in early pregnancy; the phenylalanine:tyrosine ratio consequently rises and vitiates the use of the phe/tyr ratio for diagnosis of phenylketonuria heterozygosity under these conditions. Churchill et al. (1969) observed a positive correlation between total maternal plasma amino acid levels in the last trimester and birth weight and cranial volume of the offspring at birth. The authors suggested that fetal development was influenced by maternal plasma amino acids. Dawson and McGanity (1970) showed that adolescent pregnancy, when *maternal and fetal* growth rates could be great enough to compromise protein and amino acid nutrition, affects plasma amino acid patterns in accordance with a marginal nutritional hypothesis. The situation with regard to pregnancy is likely to be complicated by physiological stimuli which clearly affect amino acid distributions (Noall et al., 1957), and it is not surprising that even the normal menstrual cycle and oral contraceptive administration affect plasma amino acids so that levels oscillate downward by as much as 50 per cent during the latter half of the normal or contraceptive-regulated cycle (Craft and Peters, 1971).

Circadian Rhythms in Plasma Amino Acid Levels

The measurement of plasma amino acid levels is usually made only at one point in time, and it is often upon such data that decisions must be made as to whether a subject manifests normal or aberrant amino acid metabolism. Under such conditions, there is no evaluation of the *variation from moment*

Table 3–2   Plasma Amino Acid Levels (μmoles/L) in the First Hours of Life in Normal Full-Term and "Small-for-Gestation" Infants

| | Full-Term Systemic Venous Blood | | "Small-for-Gestation" Systemic Venous Blood | |
	$\Delta\%$[a]	Mean $\pm$ SD[b]	Mean $\pm$ SD[c]	p
Isoleucine	−52	33	11	21	7	<.05
Leucine	−49	62	19	57	28	NS
Ornithine	−46	64	18	53	36	NS
Tyrosine	−43	55	14	51	24	NS
Valine	−42	116	35	85	46	NS
Glutamate	−41	81	34	97	32	NS
Lysine	−40	193	58	155	81	NS
Arginine	−35	51	14	41	21	NS
Taurine	−33	124	42	135	38	NS
Phenylalanine	−27	64	12	53	26	NS
Methionine	−22	30	8	19	7	<.02
Alanine	−20	355	75	296	92	NS
Proline	−12	181	46	155	35	NS
Histidine	−9	86	26	57	25	<.05
Glutamine	+15	710	154	421	05	<.001
Glycine	+25	340	94	205	56	<.005
Serine	−	177	65	107	49	<.05

[a]Percentage difference between cord-blood level and fasting systemic venous plasma level at 2 to 6 hours after birth (from Lindblad and Baldesten, 1969).

[b]Data from 13 infants at $12\frac{1}{2}$ hours mean age after birth (data of Reisner et al., 1973).

[c]Data from 6 infants at 9 hours mean age after birth (same source as for footnote b); p value from Student's t test for difference between full-term and low birth-weight infants.

to moment in the apparent steady-state level or of the *flux of amino acids through the pool being measured.* The latter problem is discussed further in Chapter 4; the former is a function of *circadian variation,* among other regulatory events.

Physiological rhythms throughout the biological realm have been identified and studied in recent years (Hastings, 1970), and the term "circadian" (Halberg, 1959, 1969) is commonly used to describe these phenomena, referring as it does to periodicity around *(circa)* the day *(diem).*

The "normal" interindividual variation in plasma concentration of amino acids is usually defined either in terms of the *fasting* mean value ±1 SD, or as the mean value and range of data under these conditions. The data in Table 3–1 are of this nature. Feigin and colleagues (1967) were the first to report circadian periodicity of blood amino acid levels in the adult. The observation was subsequently confirmed (Wurtman et al., 1967, 1968) and extended to the infant, even as early as the first day of life (Feigin and Haymond, 1970), where the rhythm is similar, but not identical, to that of adults and older children. The concentration of total amino acids is normally lowest in the pre-dawn hours, and the apogee of the rhythm occurs in midafternoon or early evening (Fig. 3–3). The periodicity for individual amino acids resembles that for total amino acids, but the former is less consistent. The amplitude of the circadian variation for total amino acids is about ±30 per cent around the diurnal mean, which occurs at about 12 noon (Feigin et al., 1967, 1970), and it is rarely more than ±50 per cent for individual amino acids (Wurtman et al., 1968).

The source of the periodicity and its phasing has been investigated, but no simple explanation has been found. For example, enzymes which catabolize amino acids themselves exhibit cyclic activity (Rapaport et al., 1966; Wurtman and Axelrod, 1967). The latter type of periodicity may reflect intermittent sub-

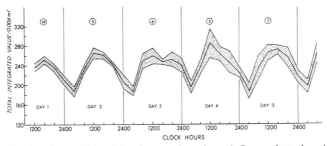

Figure 3–3 Total amino acid level in plasma of newborn infants, plotted against time of day. A circadian periodicity is apparent, with the peak level occurring in the afternoon-evening period and the nadir occurring in the predawn period. The phase of periodicity is similar to that of the adult (Feigin et al., 1967), but absolute levels and duration of phases in the cycle are different in the two age groups. The mean values ± SEM are shown by the shaded area in the graph; the number of infants examined on each day is also indicated. (From Feigin, R., and Haymond, M.: Pediatrics 45:782–791, 1970.)

strate induction or hormonal induction linked to circadian variation in steroid secretion (Rivlin, 1965). Moreover, the oscillations in plasma tyrosine and its hepatic transaminase are mutually linked to the availability of tryptophan in the liver (Wurtman et al., 1968), indicating that the periodicity of catabolic enzyme activity and the amino acid level in plasma may be interacting. However, enzyme activity is not the major cause of periodicity, since tyrosine oscillations are not extinguished even in the hypertyrosinemic newborn infant in whom tyrosine oxidation is impaired (Feigin and Haymond, 1971). It has also been shown that tryptophan availability does not determine periodicity, since a zero-tryptophan diet does not extinguish the plasma amino acid rhythms in adult men (Hussein et al., 1971).

The relationships which impinge on plasma amino acid periodicity are clearly multifactorial. Feigin and coauthors (1971) could not assign the responsibility for the phenomenon to any one regulatory event. In Feigin's own study of the problem (Feigin et al., 1968), it was surmised that although exogenous synchronizers influenced the *amplitude* of the rhythm, both *phase* and amplitude were generated by unknown endogenous signals. Normal or exaggerated protein intake is not responsible for initiation or maintenance of the rhythm, although absolute levels of amino acids in the blood can be modulated by diet. Endogenous hormones such as insulin, steroid and growth hormones probably exert a permissive effect on periodicity but are not essential for its presence. Changes in cellular uptake rates correlate with periodicity, and fluxes through plasma from one tissue pool to another (e.g., muscle to liver), which are dependent on release of amino acid in the tissue of origin and uptake at the destination, undoubtedly play a role in the oscillation of plasma amino acid levels. Regulatory events of this nature are more likely to affect individual amino acids less systematically than total amino acid levels, this assumption being supported by experimental observations in man.

The phase of circadian rhythm can be reversed or extinguished with certain stimuli. A 12-hour shift of the waking-sleep cycle reverses the phase, so that nadir and apogee now appear in the afternoon and predawn periods, respectively (Feigin et al., 1968). The plasma phenylalanine rhythm is reversed from normal phenylketonuria by the autosomal recessive trait (the lowest phenylalanine level occurs in the afternoon), whereas the plasma tyrosine rhythm remains normal (Güttler et al., 1969). Chloramphenicol not only raises the absolute level of total amino acids in plasma, but it also extinguishes the circadian rhythm (Burghen et al., 1970).

In summary, circadian periodicity is an important cause of intraindividual variation in plasma amino acid levels, but it is only a modest determinant of the interindividual variation in absolute values. The cause of periodicity and its phasing is clearly heterogeneous, and it includes normal endogenous and exogenous stimuli plus perturbations of these stimuli. Awareness of circadian variation in plasma amino acid levels is important if one is to interpret accurately the significance of minor differences in the absolute concentration of an amino acid between individuals at any moment in time. For example, such small differences become very important in the classification of phenylketonuric heterozygotes. Rosenblatt and Scriver (1968) found that circadian variation should be taken into account in the identification of heterozygotes by means of plasma amino acid levels. Periodicity will also influence the interpretation of plasma amino acid variation under nutritional and hormonal stimuli or during prolonged investigative protocols where repeated sampling of blood amino acids may be necessary.

RENAL EXCRETION AND REABSORPTION OF AMINO ACIDS

One fifth of the systemic blood supply reaches the kidneys each minute, and in the adult about 120 ml of plasma is filtered by the glomeruli in that time. The filtrate in Bowman's space contains free amino acids which are topologically "outside" the body until tubular absorption occurs. In the normal adult, only about 2 or 3 per cent of the total urinary nitrogen in bladder urine is accounted for by amino acids, and this fraction represents less than 5 per cent of the filtered amino acid load. These calculations indicate that the majority of the filtered amino acid load has disappeared from urine by the process of tubular absorption (Cushny, 1917). In man and other mammals, net tubular reabsorption occurs against a concentration gradient (Christensen and Jones, 1962; Christensen and Clifford, 1962). The tubular absorptive process is both mediated and energy-dependent (Scriver, 1962, 1967; Young and Freedman, 1971).

The pattern and concentration of amino acids present initially in the glomerular filtrate and the efficiency of the absorptive process each modulate the composition of the final aminoaciduria. The normal pattern of aminoaciduria in man is quite variable (Scriver, 1962). Diet, age, sex and physiological status of the subject, as well as disease processes, each account for some of the variation; and circadian variation is again apparent in aminoaciduria (Tewksbury and Lohrenz, 1970).

Qualitative analysis of urine amino acids by partition chromatography on filter paper (see Chapter 5) is often the simplest way to recognize the normal and abnormal patterns of *aminoaciduria*. Westall (1962) published a valuable compendium of the many abnormal chromatographic patterns of urine amino acids. Recognition and interpretation of such abnormal patterns may be more difficult if the investigator relies on quantitative data, unless the corresponding normal values for amino acid excretion can be compared. However, the data for amino acid excretion are expressed in so many different coefficients (e.g., mg or μmole amino acid/day; mg or μmole amino acid/mg total creatinine or /mg nitrogen) that it is difficult to give a survey of the quantitative data for normal amino aciduria (Scriver, 1962). Soupart (1962) constructed a useful diagram (Fig. 3–4) which reveals the essential features of normal aminoaciduria in adult and young human subjects.

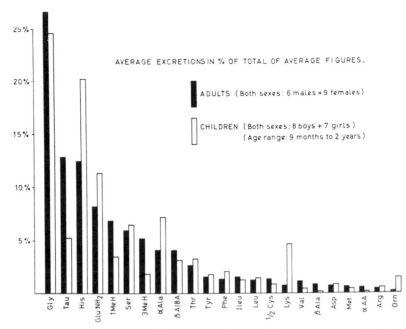

Figure 3–4 Urinary excretion of free amino acids by children and adults of both sexes. The principal feature is a diminishing rate of excretion when there is a lengthened or charged side-chain in the amino acid. The plasma concentrations of the individual amino acids are rather comparable, and therefore excretion rates inversely reflect reabsorption to a considerable extent. (From Soupart, P.: *In* Holden, J. T., ed., Amino Acid Pools. Elsevier, New York, 1962.)

Since a quantitative description of the amino acid content of urine may not indicate the cause of an abnormality, the *endogenous renal clearance* of amino acids should be evaluated wherever possible. In this way, a more precise description of abnormal excretion rates can be obtained to indicate whether it is of pre-renal or renal origin (see Chapter 6). Renal clearance rates reveal some of the characteristics of tubular transport for the particular amino acid, as shown in Figure 3–5; deviation from the normal clearance rate may indicate disease. Recognition of the abnormal requires definition of the normal clearance rate, and normal data are available for children and adults (Table 3–3).

Renal clearance rates of amino acids are age-dependent, clearance rates being higher in the young infant than in the more mature subject (Table 3–3). The higher clearance rates in infancy reflect lower tubular reabsorption rates in this age group (Fig. 3–6).

The ontogeny of amino acid reabsorption by kidney has been studied in considerable detail. For example, Baerlocher and colleagues (1970) showed that exaggerated excretion of proline, hydroxyproline and glycine was characteristic of the immature mammalian kidney in many species (Fig. 3–7). They noted that the excessive excretion of imino acids in the rat pup disappeared at an earlier age after birth than did the accompanying postnatal hyperglycinuria. This feature has also been demonstrated in the human infant by Woolf and Norman (1957) and by Baerlocher et al. (1971a). Baerlocher et al. (1971b, 1971c) showed that the developing mammalian nephron was deficient in high-affinity, low-capacity proline-specific and glycine-specific sites at birth. Maturation of

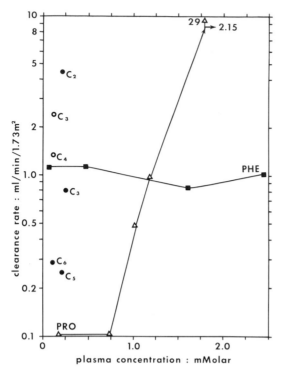

Figure 3–5 Endogenous renal clearance is an indirect measure of the net tubular absorption of amino acids under endogenous conditions. Note the diminished renal clearance (increased tubular absorption) of amino acids with long, apolar side chains compared to those with short carbon chains (left hand side of graph). Proline and phenylalanine clearance rates illustrate the saturable characteristics of tubular transport mechanisms. The proline system saturates at relatively low plasma concentrations. Phenylalanine is absorbed with equal efficiency at high and at normal concentrations of phenylalanine in the plasma of a patient with phenylketonuria, off and on treatment, respectively. (From Scriver, C. R.: Pediatrics *44*:348–357, 1969.)

tubular function involved the early appearance of the proline-specific site and a later emergence of the glycine-specific site. The in vitro demonstration of transport site ontogeny coincided with the in vivo disappearance of the specific hyperexcretion of amino acid. Baerlocher and his colleagues also showed that tubular maturation involved an increase in the total functional capacity for transport. The change in function coincides with a change in structure.

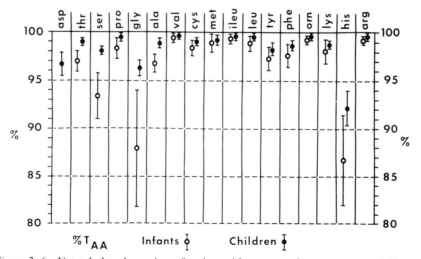

Figure 3–6 Net tubular absorption of amino acids, expressed as percentage of filtered load, in infants and children. Efficiency of absorption improves with age. (Redrawn from Brodehl, J., and Gellissen, K.: Pediatrics *42*:395–404, 1968.)

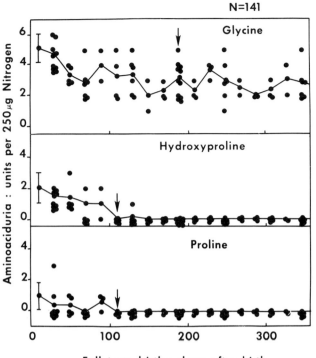

Figure 3-7   Urinary excretion of proline, hydroxyproline and glycine by 141 full-term human infants. Proline and hydroxyproline are excreted in excess for about the first three months after birth; hyperexcretion of glycine continues until about six months. The prior disappearance of the imino acids reflects earlier emergence of the imino acid-specific transport system in mammalian kidney, as documented in vitro by Baerlocher et al. (1970, 1971b, 1971c). An independent change in the specific activities of various transport sites during ontogeny is one explanation for the changing, age-dependent composition of aminoaciduria. The other important determinant is a change in morphology, with an increase in the absorptive area during maturation (see also Figure 3–8). (Data of Baerlocher, Clow, Mackenzie and Scriver, 1971a.)

ONTOGENY OF "SPECIFIC ACTIVITY" AND OF "TOTAL ACTIVITY" FOR AMINO ACID TRANSPORT IN KIDNEY TUBULE

Figure 3-8   A model depicting the change in specific activity and total activity of renal tubular absorptive mechanisms during postnatal development, to account for the changing, age-dependent pattern of amino acid excretion and reabsorption. Data for model obtained in the rat (Baerlocher et al., 1971c).

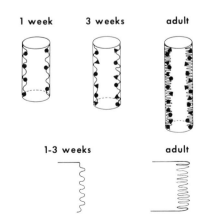

Table 3-3   Endogenous Renal Clearance of Amino Acids[a]
(ml/min/1.73 M²)

Amino Acid	Infants			Children				Adults
	Range[1]	Mean	± SD[2]	Mean	± SD[3]	Mean[4]	Range[4]	Range[5]
Taurine	0.1–3.8	–	–	–	–	13.7	9.9–26.2	1.7–14
Hydroxyproline	tr–34	–	–	–	–	–	0–tr	0
Aspartic acid	tr–16	–	–	3.6	0.9	2.8	tr–8.8	0–2.4
Threonine	3.0–8.2	2.0	1.4[b]	1.0	0.2[b]	1.4	0.5–2.5	0.8–1.5
Serine	4.5–13.0	4.1	1.9	2.4	0.5	2.4	1.2–3.4	1.9–3.0
Asp + Glu (amides)	1.2–3.6	–	–	–	–	1.3	0.1–2.3	0.7–1.8
Proline	1.7–14.0	1.0	0.7	0.3	0.2	–	0–0.3	0
Glutamic acid	0.1–3.0	–	–	–	–	0.8	0.1–2.4	0.3–0.7
Glycine	12–44	7.4	3.2	4.2	1.4	4.4	1.2–8.6	2.7–5.8
Alanine	1.5–4.2	1.6	0.7	0.8	0.4	0.8	0.2–1.3	0.3–0.9
Valine	0.2–0.6	0.3	0.1	0.2	0.1	0.2	0.18–0.3	0.1–0.3
Half Cystine	2.5–8.8	1.1	0.3	0.8	0.2	–	1.0–1.4	0.7–2.9
Methionine	2.3–5.8	0.8	0.5	0.8	0.3	1.9	1.0–3.4	1.1
Isoleucine	0.4–1.7	0.3	0.2	0.3	0.1	0.5	0.2–1.0	0.2–1.0
Leucine	0.4–1.3	0.8	0.5	0.5	0.1	0.5	0.2–0.9	0.2–0.9
Tyrosine	0.5–2.6	1.8	0.4	2.0	0.8	2.0	0.8–3.3	1.0–1.7
Phenylalanine	1.0–2.2	1.7	0.9	1.5	0.3	1.2	0.3–2.3	0.7–1.4
Ornithine	0.6–1.1	0.4	0.1	0.4	0.1	0.5	0.2–0.8	tr
Lysine	1.6–6.3	1.3	0.4	1.2	0.4	1.1	0.3–2.4	0.2–1.9
Histidine	12–29	8.5	4.4	9.5	2.6	9.2	1.9–21.8	4.7–9.1
Arginine	tr–1.0	0.4	0.1	0.3	0.1	0.5	0.15–1.2	0.2–0.8

[a]Determined by elution chromatography on ion exchange resins.
[b]Includes asparagine.
[1]O'Brien and Butterfield, 1963; 4 premature and 3 full-term infants, 30 to 60 days old; short-term clearance after 4-hour fast.
[2]Brodehl and Gellissen, 1968; 12 infants, 16 days to 4 months of age; short-term clearance after fasting.
[3]Brodehl and Gellissen, 1968; 12 children, 2 to 13 years of age; short-term clearance after overnight fast.
[4]Scriver and Davies, 1965; 9 children, 3 to 12 years of age; short-term clearance after overnight fast.
[5]Cusworth and Dent, 1960; 4 adults; short-term clearance after overnight fast.

Nephron development involves lengthening of the absorptive segment of the nephron (Fetterman et al., 1965) and augmentation of brush border density (Suzuki, 1958). The concept that specific activity and total activity of epithelial transport are both changing during maturation of the nephron is summarized graphically in Figure 3–8.

The normal variation of free amino acid excretion in the neonatal period should not be confused with artifacts arising from fecal contamination of urine. The latter is a common hazard in the newborn and must be considered when interpreting urine patterns in screening programs (Levy et al., 1969).

FREE AMINO ACIDS IN BLOOD CELLS

The intracellular amino acid concentration may be used as an index of abnormal amino acid metabolism under certain conditions. For example, cystinosis can be identified in its infantile (Schneider et al., 1967), adult (Schneider et al., 1968) and adolescent forms (Goldman et al., 1971) through analysis of the cystine concentration in isolated blood leukocytes. Shih (1973) reports that erythrocyte arginase deficiency causes arginine to accumulate in erythrocytes while the plasma arginine level remains normal. McMenamy and colleagues (1960) were among the first to study erythrocyte and leukocyte amino acid levels relative to plasma in man. Erythrocytes do not concentrate the less polar neutral amino acids against a gradient relative to plasma, whereas the more polar neutral amino acids and the charged amino acids are usually present in erythrocyte water at more than 1.5 times their level in plasma. These findings were confirmed in general by Levy and Barkin (1971). McMenamy et al. (1960) also showed that leukocytes accumulate neutral and charged amino acids very well as compared to erythrocytes, and leukocytes can achieve cell:plasma distribution ratios exceeding 5.0. The concentration of arginine in both blood cell types is low relative to other amino acids and relative to its plasma concentration. This finding presumably reflects the high arginase activity of blood cells. The level of the important tripeptide glutathione is particularly high in erythrocytes (Levy and Barkin, 1971). Human reticulocytes concentrate amino acids more avidly than mature erythrocytes (Allen, 1960). This may reflect the presence in mammalian reticulocyte membranes of efficient auxiliary transport systems which are lost during maturation to the erythrocyte stage (Winter and Christensen, 1965).

Levy and Barkin (1971) studied erythrocyte amino acid levels in several disease states. The usual erythrocyte:plasma distribution ratio was unperturbed for the branched-chain amino acids in maple syrup urine disease, for glycine in hyperglycinemia and for tyrosine, phenylalanine, ornithine and histidine in the four different traits which cause plasma accumulation of each of these amino acids. Homocystinemia was associated with a reduced distribution ratio for methionine and homocystine, implying that these amino acids are excluded from the red cell despite abnormal accumulation in plasma. The findings of Levy and Barkin indicate that blood cell analysis offers no advantage over plasma analysis except in cystinosis and perhaps in erythrocyte arginase deficiency.

TRANSPLACENTAL AMINO ACID GRADIENT
(FETAL:MATERNAL RATIO)

A transplacental gradient of free amino acids exists in favor of the fetus (Table 3–4) (Christensen and Streicher, 1948; Crumpler and Dent, 1950;

Table 3–4   Human Transplacental Gradient of Amino Acids*

Amino Acid	Maternal Venous Plasma ($\mu moles/L$)		Fetal:Maternal Ratio	
	Mean	± SD	Mean	± SD
Taurine	62	16	3.1	0.6
Aspartic acid	8.1	4.6	2.8	2.3
Threonine	159	51	1.7	0.3
Serine	77	6	1.9	0.5
Proline	89	26	1.7	0.4
Glutamic acid	91	18	1.7	0.6
Glycine	144	22	2.1	0.3
Alanine	286	66	1.7	0.3
Valine	118	13	1.7	0.8
Half Cystine	43	12	1.6	0.5
Methionine	15	5.5	1.6	0.6
Isoleucine	37	73	1.9	0.4
Leucine	67	10	1.7	0.3
Tyrosine	30	7	2.2	0.5
Phenylalanine	39	6	1.8	0.3
Ornithine	28	7	2.9	0.9
Lysine	97	16	3.1	0.4
Histidine	34	10	2.3	0.4

*Data of Butterfield and O'Brien, 1963; obtained from seven normal deliveries at term.

Clemetson and Churchman, 1954; Butterfield and O'Brien, 1963; Ghadimi and Pecora, 1964). The same is true of other primates (Kerr, 1968) and of the rat (Lines and Waisman, 1971). The placenta apparently has the ability to act as a "pump" to deliver amino acids to the fetus, and disorders of placental function tend to reduce the transplacental amino acid gradient (Clemetson and Churchman, 1954; Butterfield and O'Brien, 1963; Lindblad and Zetterström, 1968). It is also possible that the fetus acts as a holding place for amino acids relative to the nonfetal (maternal) pool and that the process of fetal growth accounts in part for the transplacental gradient (Christensen and Streicher, 1948). This interpretation finds support from the fact that concentrations of amino acids in maternal plasma tend to be lower in pregnancy than in the nonpregnant state (Reid et al., 1971). Because of the apparent importance of the transplacental gradient which provides the fetus with optimal amino acid nutrition, it is surprising that more is not known about the normal gradient and its significance for the fetus.

Transplacental delivery of amino acids is a benefit only under normal conditions of maternal metabolism, and the fetal:maternal gradient can achieve a threatening significance when the fetus is carried by a mother with hyperaminoacidemia. In this case, the placenta becomes a mechanism to produce marked intrauterine fetal hyperaminoacidemia. The infant could thus be exposed to extreme amino acid imbalance throughout fetal development. Kerr and coworkers (1968) studied the phenomenon in the rhesus monkey with artificially induced maternal hyperphenylalaninemia and examined its effect on fetal aminoacidemia. When the maternal plasma phenylalanine concentration was 1.65 mM, the fetal cord blood concentration was 2.62 mM. The usual fetal:maternal gradient for phenylalanine of about 1.5 was retained. The finding indicates that the ability to maintain a fetal:maternal gradient for phenylalanine is presumably not saturated even at high substrate concentrations. The comparable situation in man has now been documented by Howell and Stevenson (1971). The normal transplacental gradient for phenylalanine permitted marked hyperphenylalaninemia to develop in the offspring of a mother with hyperphenylalaninemia. The fetus was irrevocably damaged. (See Chapter 15.)

AMINO ACIDS IN AMNIOTIC FLUID

Evaluation of the amino acids in human amniotic fluid reveals a consistent pattern throughout the course of pregnancy. Levy and Montag (1969) showed that individual amino acids, with the exception of taurine, are present at lower concentrations in amniotic fluid at term than in maternal or fetal plasma. Emery et al. (1970), Thomas and colleagues (1971) and Reid and associates (1971) confirmed this finding while examining the amniotic fluid pattern at various stages of pregnancy. On the other hand, these investigators also observed that the concentration of amino acids in the amniotic fluid of early pregnancy exceeds that of fetal or maternal blood. The amino acid pattern during pregnancy followed three trends. Emery et al. (1970) and Rosenblatt et al. (1971) observed that some amino acids do not change their concentration through pregnancy (cysteic acid, phosphoethanolamine, proline and ethanolamine); other amino acids achieve higher concentrations in the early midtrimester and decline thereafter to term levels (the majority of amino acids); the concentrations of a few amino acids fall steadily during the course of pregnancy (serine, glycine, phenylalanine, lysine and arginine). Rather similar trends are characteristic of pregnancy and amniotic fluid amino acids in other primates also (Kerr and Kennan, 1969). Several unusual ninhydrin-positive substances, which are not readily evident in newborn or maternal urine or blood, have also been detected in the amniotic fluid.

Thomas et al. (1971) have carried out an unusual study on amniotic fluid amino acids. They monitored two successive pregnancies of a homozygous phenylketonuric patient. Phenylalanine was present at very high levels (about 2 mM; normal is <0.1 mM) in first-trimester amniotic fluid. The concentration fell to about 0.5 mM at term (normal is <0.02 mM), while tyrosine and other amino acids were present at normal concentrations in the amniotic fluid of this patient. These findings concerning maternal disease, which confirm an early similar report by Woolf et al. (1961), harbinger the other possibility that amniotic supernatant fluid could be used to monitor aminoacidopathies in the fetus. This likelihood has not escaped the notice of numerous investigators, but it has been given little attention so far (Nadler, 1969).

The source of amino acid homeostasis in amniotic fluid is not known. Maternal blood and the blood, urine and skin cells of the fetus probably contribute amino acids in varying degrees, and the overall decline of amniotic fluid amino acids in the later stages of pregnancy may reflect improved retention and incorporation by the fetus during rapid growth. Maternal tissues may also contribute to amino acid homeostasis in amniotic fluid.

Human uterine muscle is of interest because it exhibits a phasic distribution of free amino acids during pregnancy (Lorincz and Kuttner, 1969). Several amino acids are retained by uterine muscle at high concentrations relative to maternal serum during late pregnancy. When compared to the nonpregnant uterus, the concentration of essential free amino acids and of glycine is lower in the pregnant uterus at term. These findings are compatible with uterine growth, muscle hypertrophy and protein incorporation. Rather oddly, the threonine content of uterus rises during pregnancy, as it does in maternal plasma. The significance of this finding in the physiology of pregnancy is not known.

AMINO ACIDS IN HUMAN SPINAL FLUID

Metabolites in cerebrospinal fluid (CSF) originate from neural and extraneural tissue as well as by filtration from the choroid plexus (Rall, 1964). Simple diffusion of amino acids into CSF via choroid plexus or through brain from plasma should yield a uniform plasma:CSF ratio approaching unity. However, the concentrations of most amino acids in CSF (Table 3–5) are usually lower than their equivalent concentrations in plasma (Knauff et al., 1961; Perry and Jones, 1961; Dickenson and Hamilton, 1966). Moreover, the plasma:CSF ratio is not uniform for the individual amino acids, suggesting that CSF composition is controlled by efflux from, and uptake into, nervous and ependymal tissue, as well as by diffusion across the choroid plexus.

Cerebral tissue is capable of concentrative uptake of amino acids, both in vitro (Neame, 1961; Abadom and Scholefield, 1962; Blasberg and Lajtha, 1965) and in vivo (Gruemer et al., 1971). This mediated process may constitute the so-called blood-brain barrier (Rall, 1964), since there is little extracellular fluid interposed between the blood space and brain cells. Subsequent efflux of amino acids from brain is likely to be the principal source of CSF amino acids (Levi et al., 1965). Amino acid clearance from CSF has been studied in the living cat (Snodgrass et al., 1969; Murray and Cutter, 1970), and these studies probably describe the comparable events in man. Amino acids are removed from CSF by mediated transport systems which resemble those found, for example, in kidney (see Chapter 6). After loss into the CSF, amino acids are removed into

Table 3–5 Concentration of Amino Acids in Cerebrospinal Fluid
(μmoles/L)

Amino Acid	Pooled Data[a] (Range)	Dickinson and Hamilton (1966)[b] Mean	± SD[b]	Normal Plasma:CSF ratio[b]
Taurine	1.9–13.9	6.3	1.8	11
Aspartic acid	1.6–7.6*	0.9	0.5	18
Threonine	9.9–51.3	25	10	7
Serine	13.1–70	38	23	4
Glutamine	161–533	509	144	1
Proline	0–4.2	0.6	—	392
Glutamic acid	0–117[c]	7.0	4.9	8
Glycine	1.6–19.5	6.6	1.8	35
Alanine	12.6–36.6	23	9.4	15
Valine	3.2–26	14	5.5	5
Half Cystine	—	0.2	—	368
Methionine	1–4.3	2.6	1.6	8
Isoleucine	2.4–14.8	4.4	1.3	12
Leucine	5.6–17.7	11	3.6	9
Tyrosine	1.2–11	9.1	5.0	6
Phenylalanine	2.4–10	9.2	5.8	6
Ornithine	3–8.2	5.7	1.8	12
Lysine	13.4–42	19	6.6	9
Histidine	2.4–31.4	13	4.4	6
Arginine	5.8–29.3	20	5.8	4

[a]Pooled data of Perry and Jones, 1961; Efron, 1965; Fisher et al., 1968; from healthy adults.
[b]The data of Dickinson and Hamilton, 1966, obtained from 18 patients, aged 4 months to 42 years.
[c]Possible artifact of sample processing may explain high values.

the periventricular brain tissue, choroid plexus and extrachoroidal sites in the subarachnoid compartment in the spinal cord and over the brain. Therefore, we deduce that active transport out of CSF maintains the normal low concentration of amino acids in that fluid relative to plasma and brain. A change in CSF amino acid content should reflect either primary changes in plasma or brain tissue or a change in the transport mechanisms which evacuate CSF. Less efficient exit transport is likely to alter the distribution of amino acids in CSF in a manner analogous to the change in urine amino acids which accompanies impaired tubular reabsorption. In this context, it is surprising to find few published abnormalities of CSF amino acids in the inborn errors of amino acid transport. This may reflect a dearth of such studies, but in those which have been published (for example, in Lowe's syndrome [Perry and Jones, 1961; Hambraeus et al., 1970], in familial iminoglycinuria [Joseph et al., 1958] and in Hartnup disease [Baron et al., 1956]) no abnormality is described. This may indicate that the mutant genes do not affect amino acid reabsorption from the CSF.

One would expect the aminoacidopathies which are accompanied by hyperaminoacidemia, and which retain intact cellular transport because they are caused by an extracerebral enzyme deficiency, to show accumulation of the relevant amino acid in CSF but little or no lowering of the plasma:CSF ratio. Diseases such as phenylketonuria, maple syrup urine disease and hyperprolinemia show little alteration of the plasma:CSF ratio of the relevant amino acid (Table 3–6). But if the mutant enzyme is present in brain, and amino acid accumulation can be initiated in brain itself and independent of plasma changes, one would anticipate that significant lowering of the plasma:CSF ratio could occur. For example, the urea cycle is present in brain (Sporn et al., 1959) and in its hereditary disorders, the relevant plasma:CSF amino acid ratios are markedly depressed, even below unity (Table 3–6).

AMINO ACIDS IN OTHER BODY FLUIDS

In 1962, Westall described the amino acid composition of saliva, tears and sweat. Saliva secreted by the parotid and submaxillary glands contains phosphoethanolamine. However, saliva collected without cannulation of the ducts will show little phosphoethanolamine because it is cleaved by the alkaline phosphatase normally found in this fluid. The phosphoethanolamine content of saliva should be elevated in hypophosphatasia. Saliva is also said to contain γ-aminobutyric acid, which, if present, is probably an artifact of bacterial decarboxylation of salivary glutamic acid. Others (Dreyfus et al., 1968) believe that the substance identified as γ-aminobutyrate is in fact γ-aminovaleric acid, another putrefactive product. The amino acid content of saliva has been quantitated by Dreyfus and colleagues (1968).

Tears contain amino acids in pattern comparable to that of sweat. Sweat and tears resemble an ultrafiltrate of plasma, with the addition of citrulline. There are differences in the amino acid composition of sweat collected from various regions of the body (Hadorn et al., 1967), and contamination of glassware by hand sweat is an important potential artifact to be avoided in the microanalysis of amino acids (Hamilton, 1965). Baron et al. (1956) showed that the amino acid content of sweat, saliva and tears is normal in Hartnup disease, an inborn error of amino acid transport which affects kidney and gut.

Fecal amino acids are discussed in Chapter 2.

Table 3-6   Plasma:CSF Ratios in Aminoacidopathies

Disorder	Amino Acid	Plasma conc. μmoles/L	CSF conc. μmoles/L	P:CSF Ratio in Disease	Normal P:CSF Ratio[a]	References
Phenylketonuria	Phenylalanine	2000	323	6	6	Perry and Jones, 1961
		2600	585	4.5		McKean and Boggs, 1966
Maple syrup urine disease	Leucine	2570	443	5.8	12	
	Isoleucine	1090	223	4.9	9	
	Valine	1920	325	5.9	5	
Citrullinemia	Citrulline			4.2	15	McMurray et al., 1963
Argininosuccinicaciduria	ASA	133	363	0.3	0	Moser et al., 1967
	Citrulline	334	44	8	15	
Hyperprolinemia	Proline	750	tr	750	392	Schafer et al., 1962
Hyper-β-alaninemia	β-alanine	33	45	0.7	1	Scriver et al., 1966
	GABA	4	2	2.0	0	
Cystathioninemia	Cystathionine	25	11	2.3	1	Berlow, 1966
	Cystathionine	11	0.5	22		Perry et al., 1968

[a]From Dickinson and Hamilton, 1966.

REFERENCES

Abadom, P. N., and Scholefield, P. G.: Amino acid transport in brain cortex slices. Canad. J. Biochem. *40*:1591–1602, 1962.

Allen, D. W.: Amino acid accumulation by human reticulocytes. Blood *16*:1564–1571, 1960.

Baerlocher, K., Clow, C., Mackenzie, S., and Scriver, C.: Ontogeny of amino acid transport sites in kidney; specific and total activity. (Abstract.) Pediat. Res. 5:382–383, 1971a.

Baerlocher, K., Scriver, C. R., and Mohyuddin, F.: Ontogeny of iminoglycine transport in mammalian kidney. Proc. Nat. Acad. Sci. U.S.A. *65*:1009–1016, 1970.

Baerlocher, K. E., Scriver, C. R., and Mohyuddin, F.: The ontogeny of amino acid transport in rat kidney. I. Effect on distribution ratios and intracellular metabolism of proline and glycine. Biochim. Biophys. Acta *249*:353–363, 1971b.

Baerlocher, K. E., Scriver, C. R., and Mohyuddin, F.: The ontogeny of amino acid transport in rat kidney. II. Kinetics of uptake and effect of anoxia. Biochim. Biophys. Acta *249*:364–372, 1971c.

Baron, D. N., Dent, C. E., Harris, H., Hart, E. W., and Jepson, J. B.: Hereditary pellagra-like skin rash with temporary cerebellar ataxia, constant renal amino aciduria and other bizarre biochemical features. Lancet (ii), 421–428, 1956.

Berlow, S.: Studies in cystathioninuria. Amer. J. Dis. Child. *112*:135–142, 1966.

Blasberg, R., and Lajtha, A.: Substrate specificity of steady-state amino acid transport in mouse brain slices. Arch. Biochem. *112*:361–377, 1965.

Brodehl, J., and Gellissen, K.: Endogenous renal transport of free amino acids in infancy and childhood. Pediatrics *42*:395–404, 1968.

Burghen, G. A., Beisel, W. R., and Bartelloni, P. J.: Influences of chloramphenicol administration on whole blood amino acids in man. Clin. Med. *77*:26–29, 1970.

Butterfield, L. J., and O'Brien, D.: The effect of maternal toxaemia and diabetes on transplacental gradients of free amino acids. Arch. Dis. Child *38*:326–327, 1963.

Christensen, H. N.: Free amino acids and peptides in tissues. In Munro, H. N., and Allison, J. B., eds., Mammalian Protein Metabolism, Vol. I. Academic Press, New York, pp. 105–124, 1964.

Christensen, H. N., and Clifford, J. A.: Excretion of 1-amino-cyclopentane-carboxylic acid in man and the rat. Biochim. Biophys. Acta *62*:160–162, 1962.

Christensen, H. N., and Jones, J. C.: Amino acid transport models: Renal resorption and resistance to metabolic attack. J. Biol. Chem. *237*:1203–1206, 1962.

Christensen, H. N., and Streicher, J. A.: Association between rapid growth and elevated cell concentrations of amino acids. J. Biol. Chem. *175*:95–100, 1948.

Churchill, J. A., Moghissi, K. S., Evans, T. N., and Frohman, C.: Relationships of maternal amino acid levels to fetal development. Obstet. Gynec. *33*:492–495, 1969.

Clemetson, C. A. B., and Churchman, J.: The placental transfer of amino acids in normal and toxaemic pregnancy. J. Obstet. Gynaec. Brit. Comm. *61*:364–371, 1954.

Craft, I. L., and Peters, T. J.: Quantitative changes in plasma amino acids induced by oral contraceptives. Clin. Sci. *41*:301–307, 1971.

Crumpler, H. R., Dent, C. E., and Lindan, O.: The amino acid pattern in faetal and maternal plasma at delivery. Biochem. J. *47*:223–227, 1950.

Cushny, A. R.: The Secretion of the Urine. Longmans, Green and Co., London, 1917.

Cusworth, D. C., and Dent, C. E.: Renal clearances of amino acids in normal adults and in patients with aminoaciduria. Biochem. J. *74*:550–561, 1960.

Dawson, E. B., and McGanity, W. J.: Plasma amino acid alteration during teen-age pregnancy. Amer. J. Obstet. Gynec. *107*:585–594, 1970.

Dickinson, J. C., and Hamilton, P. B.: The free amino acids of human spinal fluid determined by ion exchange chromatography. J. Neurochem. *13*:1179–1187, 1966.

Dickinson, J. C., Rosenblum, H., and Hamilton, P. B.: Ion exchange chromatography of the free amino acids in the plasma of the newborn infant. Pediatrics *36*:2–13, 1965.

Dickinson, J. C., Rosenblum, H., and Hamilton, P. B.: Ion exchange chromatography of the free amino acids in the plasma of infants under 2500 grams at birth. Pediatrics *45*:606–613, 1970.

Dreyfus, P. M., Levy, H. L., and Efron, M. L.: Concerning amino acids in human saliva. Experientia *24*:447–448, 1968.

Emery, A. E. H., Burt, D., Nelson, M. M., and Scrimgeour, J. B.: Antenatal diagnosis and amino acid composition of amniotic fluid. Lancet (i), 1307–1308, 1970.

Feigin, R. D., Beisel, W. R., and Wannemacher, R. W.: Rhythmicity of plasma amino acids and relation to dietary intake. Amer. J. Clin. Nutr. *24*:329–341, 1971.

Feigin, R. D., Klainer, A. S., and Beisel, W. R.: Circadian periodicity of blood amino-acids in adult men. Nature (London) *215*:512–514, 1967.

Feigin, R. D., and Haymond, M. W.: Circadian periodicity of blood amino acids in the neonate. Pediatrics *45*:782–791, 1970.

Fetterman, G. H., Shuplock, N. A., Philipp, F. J., and Gregg, H. S.: The growth and maturation of human glomeruli and proximal convolutions from term to adulthood: Studies by microdissection. Pediatrics 35:601–619, 1965.

Fisher, R. G., Pomeroy, J., and Henry, J. P.: The free amino acids in adult human cerebrospinal fluid. Acta Neurol. Scand. 44:619–630, 1968.

Ghadimi, H., and Pecora, P.: Plasma amino acids after birth. Pediatrics 34:182, 1964.

Goldman, H., Scriver, C. R., Aaron, K., Delvin, E., and Canlas, Z.: Adolescent cystinosis: Comparisons with infantile and adult forms. Pediatrics 47:979–988, 1971.

Gruemer, H. D., Grannis, G. F., Hetland, L. B., and Constantini, M. L.: Amino acid transport and mental retardation. Clin. Chem. 17:1129–1131, 1971.

Güttler, F., Olesen, E. S., and Warnberg, E.: Diurnal variations of serum phenylalanine in phenylketonuric children on low-phenylalanine diet. Amer. J. Clin. Nutr. 22:1568–1570, 1969.

Hadorn, B., Hanimann, F., Anders, P., Curtius, H.-Ch., and Halverson, R.: Free amino acids in human sweat from different parts of the body. Nature (London) 215:416–417, 1967.

Halberg, F.: Physiologic 24-hour periodicity; general and procedural considerations with reference to the adrenal cycle. Z. Vitamin Hormon Fermentforsch. 10:225–296, 1959.

Halberg, F.: Chronobiology. Ann. Rev. Physiol. 31:675–725, 1969.

Hambraeus, L., Pallisgaard, G., and Kildeberg, P.: The Lowe syndrome: Observations on the amino acid metabolism in a 2-year-old affected boy. Acta Paediat. Scand. 59:631–636, 1970.

Hamilton, P. B.: Amino acids on hands. Nature (London) 205:284–285, 1965.

Hastings, J. W.: The biology of circadian rhythms from man to micro-organism. New Eng. J. Med. 282:435–441, 1970.

Holden, J. T., ed.: Amino Acid Pools. Distribution, Formation and Function of Free Amino Acids. Elsevier, New York, 1962.

Howell, R. R., and Stevenson, R. E.: The offspring of phenylketonuric women. Soc. Biol. 18: S19–S29, 1971.

Hussein, M. A., Young, V. R., Murray, E., and Scrimshaw, N. S.: Daily fluctuation of plasma amino acid levels in adult men: Effect of dietary tryptophan intake and distribution of meals. J. Nutr. 101:61–70, 1971.

Joseph, R., Ribierre, M., Job, J.-C., and Girault, M.: Maladie familiale associante des convulsions à début très précoce, une hyperalbuminorachie et une hyperaminoacidurie. Arch. Franc. Pediat. 15:374–387, 1958.

Kerr, G. R.: The free amino acids of serum during development of macaca mulatta. II. During pregnancy and fetal life. Pediat. Res. 2:493–500, 1968.

Kerr, G. R., and Kennan, A. L.: The free amino acids of amniotic fluid during pregnancy of the rhesus monkey. Amer. J. Obstet. Gynec. 105:363–367, 1969.

Knauff, H. G., Schabert, P., and Zickgraf, H.: Die Konzentration der freien Amino-säuren im Liquor cerebrospinalis und ihre Beziehungen zu Konzentration der freien plasma Amino-säuren. Klin. Wschr. 39:778–784, 1961.

Levi, G., Cherayil, A., and Lajtha, A.: Cerebral amino acid transport in vitro. 3. Heterogeneity of exit. J. Neurochem. 12:757–770, 1965.

Levy, H. L., and Barkin, E.: Comparison of amino acid concentrations between plasma and erythrocytes. Studies in normal human subjects and those with metabolic disorders. J. Lab. Clin. Med. 78:517–523, 1971.

Levy, H. L., Madigan, P. M., and Lum, A.: Fecal contamination in urine amino acid screening. Amer. J. Clin. Path. 51:765–768, 1969.

Levy, H. L., and Montag, P. P.: Free amino acids in human amniotic fluid. A quantitative study by ion exchange chromatography. Pediat. Res. 3:113–120, 1969.

Lindblad, B. S.: The venous plasma free amino acid levels during the first hours of life. I. After normal and short gestation complicated by hypertension with special reference to the 'small for dates' syndrome. Acta Paediat. Scand. 59:13–20, 1970.

Lindblad, B. S., and Baldesten, A.: Time studies on free amino levels of venous plasma during the neonatal period. Acta Paediat. Scand. 58:252–260, 1969.

Lindblad, B. S., and Zetterström, R.: The venous plasma free amino acid levels of mother and child during delivery. II. After short gestation and gestation complicated by hypertension with special reference to the 'small-for-dates' syndrome. Acta Paediat. Scand. 57:195–204, 1968.

Lines, D. R., and Waisman, H. A.: Placental transport of phenylalanine in the rat: maternal and fetal metabolism. Proc. Soc. Exp. Biol. Med. 136:790–793, 1971.

Lorincz, A. B., and Kuttier, R. E.: Free amino acids in the pregnant uterus. Amer. J. Obstet. Gynec. 105:925–932, 1969.

McKean, C. M., and Boggs, D. E.: Influence of high concentrations of phenylalanine on the amino acids of cerebrospinal fluid and blood. Proc. Soc. Exp. Biol. Med. 122:987–991, 1966.

McMenamy, R. H., Lund, C. C., Neville, G. J., and Wallach, D. F. M.: Studies of unbound amino acid distributions in plasma, erythrocytes, leukocytes and urine of normal human subjects. J. Clin. Invest. *39*:1675–1687, 1960.

McMurray, W. C., Rathbun, J. C., Mohyuddin, F., and Keegler, S. J.: Citrullinuria. Pediatrics *32*: 347–357, 1963.

Mestyán, J., Fekete, M., Járai, I., Sulyok, E., Imkof, S., and Soltész, G. Y.: The postnatal changes in the circulating free amino acid pool in the newborn infant. II. The plasma amino acid ratio in intrauterine malnutrition ('small for dates,' full-term, pre-term and twin infants). Biol. Neonat. *14*:164–177, 1969.

Moser, H. W., Efron, M. L., Brown, H., Diamond, R., and Neumann, C. G.: Argininosuccinic aciduria. Report of two new cases and demonstration of intermittent elevation of blood ammonia. Amer. J. Med. *42*:9–26, 1967.

Murray, J. E., and Cutler, R. W. P.: Transport of glycine from the cerebrospinal fluid. Arch. Neurol. *23*:23–31, 1970.

Nadler, H. L.: Prenatal detection of genetic defects. J. Pediat. *74*:132–143, 1969.

Nance, W. E., and Nance, C.: Personal communication, 1971.

Neame, K. D.: Uptake of amino acids by mouse brain slices. J. Neurochem. *6*:358–366, 1961.

Noall, M. W., Riggs, T. R., Walker, L. M., and Christensen, H. N.: Endocrine control of amino acid transfer. Distribution of an unmetabolized amino acid. Science *126*:1002–1005, 1957.

O'Brien, D., and Butterfield, L. J.: Further studies on renal tubular conservation of free amino acids in early infancy. Arch. Dis. Child. *38*:437–442, 1963.

Perry, T. L., and Hansen, S.: Technical pitfalls leading to errors in the quantitation of plasma amino acids. Clin. Chim. Acta *25*:53–58, 1969.

Perry, T. L., Hardwick, D. F., Hansen, S., Love, D. L., and Israels, S.: Cystathioninuria in two healthy siblings. New Eng. J. Med. *278*:590–592, 1968.

Perry, T. L., and Jones, R. T.: The amino acid content of human cerebrospinal fluid in normal individuals and in mental defectives. J. Clin. Invest. *40*:1363–1372, 1961.

Rall, D. P.: The structure and function of the cerebrospinal fluid. *In* Hoffman, J. F., ed., The Cellular Functions of Membrane Transport. Prentice-Hall, Englewood Cliffs, N.J., pp. 269–282, 1964.

Rapoport, M. I., Feigin, R. D., Burton, J., and Beisel, W. R.: Circadian rhythm for tryptophan pyrrolase activity and its circulating substrate. Science *153*:1642–1644, 1966.

Reid, D. W. J., Campbell, D. J., and Yakymyshyn, L. Y.: Quantitative amino acids in amniotic fluid and maternal plasma in early and late pregnancy. Amer. J. Obstet. Gynec. *111*:251–258, 1971.

Reisner, S. H., Aranda, J. V., Colle, E., Papageorgiou, A., Schiff, D., Scriver, C. R., and Stern, L.: An effect of intravenous glucagon on plasma amino acids in the newborn. Pediat. Res. *7*:184–191, 1973.

Rivlin, R. S., and Melmon, K. L.: Cortisone-provoked depression of plasma tyrosine concentration: Relation to enzyme induction in man. J. Clin. Invest. *44*:1690–1698, 1965.

Rosenblatt, D. S., Kinch, R. A. H., and Scriver, C. R.: Metabolites in amniotic fluid as a function of gestational age. (Abstract.) Clin. Res. *18*:727, 1970.

Rosenblatt, D., and Scriver, C. R.: Heterogeneity in genetic control of phenylalanine metabolism in man. Nature (London) *218*:677–678, 1968.

Schafer, I. A., Scriver, C. R., and Efron, M. L.: Familial hyperprolinemia, cerebral dysfunction and renal anomalies occurring in a family with hereditary nephritis and deafness. New Eng. J. Med. *267*:51–60, 1962.

Schneider, J. A., Bradley, K., and Seegmiller, J. E.: Increased cystine in leucocytes from individuals homozygous and heterozygous for cystinosis. Science *157*:1321–1322, 1967.

Schneider, J. A., Wong, V., Bradley, K., and Seegmiller, J. E.: Biochemical comparisons of the adult and childhood forms of cystinosis. New Eng. J. Med. *279*:1253–1257, 1968.

Scriver, C. R.: Hereditary amino aciduria. *In* Bearn, A., and Steinberg, A. G., Progress in Medical Genetics, Vol. 2. Grune & Stratton, New York, pp. 83–186, 1962.

Scriver, C. R.: Amino acid transport in mammalian kidney. *In* Nyhan, W. L. ed., Amino Acid Metabolism and Genetic Variation. McGraw-Hill, New York, pp. 327–340, 1967.

Scriver, C. R.: The human biochemical genetics of amino acid transport. Pediatrics *44*:348–357, 1969.

Scriver, C. R., Clow, C. L., and Lamm, P.: Plasma amino acids: Screening quantitation and interpretation. Amer. J. Clin. Nutr. *24*:876–890, 1971.

Scriver, C. R., and Davies, E.: Endogenous renal clearance rates of free amino acids in pre-pubertal children. Pediatrics *32*:592–598, 1965.

Scriver, C. R., Pueschel, S., and Davies, E.: Hyper-β-alaninemia associated with β-aminoaciduria and γ-aminobutyricaciduria, somnolence and seizures. New Eng. J. Med. *274*:636–643, 1966.

Shih, V. E.: Personal communication, 1973.

Snodgrass, S. R., Cutler, R. W. P., Kang, E. S., and Lorenzo, A. V.: Transport of neutral amino acids from feline cerebrospinal fluid. Amer. J. Physiol. *217*:974–980, 1969.

Soupart, P.: Free amino acids of blood and urine in the human. *In* Holden, J. T., ed., Amino Acid Pools. Elsevier, pp. 220–262, 1962.

Sporn, M. B., Dingman, W., Defalco, A., and Davies, R. K.: The synthesis of urea in the living rat brain. J. Neurochem. *5*:62–67, 1959.

Suzuki, Y.: Electron microscopy of the renal differentiation. I. Proximal tubule cells. J. Electron Micr. (Tokyo) *6*:52–65, 1958.

Tewksbury, D. A., and Lohrenz, F. N.: Circadian rhythm of human urinary amino acid excretion in fed and fasted states. Metabolism *19*:363–371, 1970.

Thomas, G. H., Parmley, T. H., Stevenson, R. E., and Howell, R. R.: Developmental changes in amino acid concentrations in human amniotic fluid: Abnormal findings in maternal phenylketonuria. Amer. J. Obstet. Gynec. *111*:38–42, 1971.

Van Slyke, D. D., and Meyer, G. M.: The absorption of amino acids from the blood by the tissues. J. Biol. Chem. *16*:197–212, 1913.

Westall, R. G.: The free amino acids of body fluids and some hereditary disorders of amino acid metabolism. *In* Holden, J. T., ed., Amino Acid Pools. Elsevier, New York, pp. 195–219, 1962.

Winter, C. G., and Christensen, H. N.: Contrasts in neutral amino acid transport by rabbit erythrocytes and reticulocytes. J. Biol. Chem. *240*:3594–3600, 1965.

Woolf, L. I., and Norman, A. P.: The urinary excretion of amino acids and sugars in early infancy. J. Pediat. *50*:271–295, 1957.

Woolf, L. I., Ounsted, C., Lee, D., Humphrey, M., Chesire, N. M., and Steed, G. R.: Atypical phenylketonuria in sisters with normal offspring. Lancet (ii), 564–565, 1961.

Wurtman, R. J., and Axelrod, J.: Daily rhythmic changes in tyrosine transaminase activity of the rat liver. Proc. Nat. Acad. Sci. U.S.A. *57*:1594–1599, 1967.

Wurtman, R. J., Chou, C., and Rose, C. M.: Daily rhythm in tyrosine concentration in plasma: Persistence in subjects fed low-protein diet. Science *158*:660–663, 1967.

Wurtman, R. J., Rose, C. M., Chou, C., and Larin, F. F.: Daily rhythms in the concentrations of various amino acids in human plasma. New Eng. J. Med., *279*:171–175, 1968.

Wurtman, R. J., Shoemaker, W. J., and Larin, F.: Mechanism of daily rhythm in hepatic tyrosine transaminase activity: Role of dietary tryptophan. Proc. Nat. Acad. Sci. U.S.A. *59*:800–807, 1968.

Young, J. A., and Freedman, B. S.: Renal tubular transport of amino acids. Clin. Chem. *17*:245–266, 1971.

Chapter Four

BIOCHEMISTRY AND PHYSIOLOGICAL CHEMISTRY OF AMINO ACIDS

61

INTRODUCTION

Knowledge of the biochemistry and physiological chemistry (metabolism) of amino acids is important in the interpretation of steady-state amino acid levels in body fluids and tissues. The nutritional components of amino acid metabolism were discussed in Chapter 2. However, it will be made apparent in this chapter that *biosynthesis* of the "nonessential" amino acids occurs endogenously in man. Amino acid steady states in body fluids were the subject of Chapter 3, but the flow of amino acids through the pools in question has not yet been discussed; some aspects of *amino acid pools and fluxes*, and the factors which modulate them, are examined in this chapter.

Amino acids participate in chemical *conversion reactions*, many of which are described in detail in Part III of the book. However, most interconversions are initiated by a series of typical reactions which involve the amino group, the carboxyl group or the side chain. The chemical reactions which initiate *catabolic* or *anabolic* interconversions of amino acids are described in this chapter. Finally, some comment about *regulation* of catalytic steps is in order, because the boundary between health and disease is often drawn at the level of regulatory events. The general relationships between amino acid conversion reactions and nitrogen intake, retention and loss are summarized in Scheme 4–1.

BIOSYNTHESIS OF AMINO ACIDS IN MAN

Biosynthesis involves those amino acids which are nonessential (except under unusual circumstances which affect the essential amino acids; see Chapter 2). Twelve of the amino acids which participate in protein biosynthesis can be synthesized by man. They are alanine, arginine, asparagine, aspartic acid, cysteine, glutamic acid, glutamine, glycine, histidine, proline, serine and tyrosine. Biosynthesis requires the utilization of a reduced form of nitrogen and a carbon skeleton to which the nitrogen moiety will be attached. Since nitrogen economy is the important limiting factor, one anticipates that stringent mechanisms of reduced nitrogen salvage and recycling are involved in the biosynthetic reactions. These reactions usually involve short pathways, or a single step, and are conservative, being relatively invariant among mammalian species. The sources of the carbon atoms and the non-amino nitrogen atoms of the nonessential amino acids are listed in Table 4–1. Three important routes of entry for carbon chains are evident in the biosynthesis of nonessential amino acids.

SCHEME 4–1

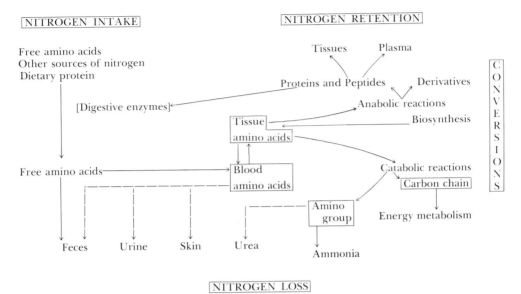

Table 4–1 Origins of Carbon and Non-Amino Nitrogen Atoms in the Non-Essential Amino Acids Synthesized by Man

Amino Acid	Source of Carbon Atoms	Source of Non-Amino Nitrogen Atoms
Alanine	Pyruvate	
Arginine	Glutamate, (C–1 to C–5) CO_2, (in guanidino C—N)	NH_3 (in guanidino C—N) Aspartate (in guanidino N)
Aspartic Acid	Oxaloacetate	
Asparagine	Oxaloacetate	NH_3
Cysteine*	Serine	
Glutamic Acid	α-Ketoglutarate	
Glutamine	α-Ketoglutarate	NH_3
Glycine	Pyruvate, via serine	
Histidine	Unknown; probably from ribose and adenylic acid	Unknown; probably from adenylic acid (imidazole N–1) and amide of glutamine (imidazole N–3)
Proline	Glutamate	
Serine	Pyruvate, via P-glycerate	
Tyrosine	Phenylalanine	

*S atom from methionine.

Biosynthesis Originating in α-Ketoglutarate

Glutamic Acid

Synthesis of glutamate involves α-ketoglutarate, as the source of the carbon chain, in either of two reactions. The reaction shown in Equation 1 is catalyzed by *glutamic acid dehydrogenase* (L-glutamate:NAD oxido-reductase [deaminating]). Direct amination of the keto acid occurs in the presence of ammonia.

$$NH_3 + \alpha\text{-ketoglutarate} + NADPH + H^+ \rightleftarrows \boxed{\text{L-glutamate}} + NADP^+ \qquad \textbf{(1)}$$

This reaction is the major route by which α-amino groups are formed directly from ammonia.

The other reaction which involves α-ketoglutarate directly is catalyzed by a transaminase for which the keto acid is the acceptor; another amino acid is the donor of the amino group. Pyridoxal phosphate is the coenzyme for this and all other transamination reactions (see subsequent text).

Glutamine

Glutamine is formed indirectly from α-ketoglutarate, via glutamate. *Glutamine synthetase* catalyzes the ATP-dependent amination of glutamate in the presence of ammonia (Equation 2). The reaction is complex and involves intermediate steps.

$$\text{L-(or D-) Glutamic acid} + ATP \rightleftarrows ADP + [\gamma\text{-glutamyl phosphate}] \qquad \textbf{(2.a)}$$

$$[\gamma\text{-glutamyl phosphate}] + NH_3 \rightleftarrows \boxed{\text{L-glutamine}} + Pi \qquad \textbf{(2.b)}$$

$$\text{Glutamic acid} + ATP + NH_3 \rightleftarrows \boxed{\text{L-glutamine}} + ADP + Pi \qquad \textbf{(2.c)}$$

Glutamine synthesis is not mandatory to generate a tissue level of glutamine. For example, it is believed that man generates glutamine in kidney predominantly by extraction from renal arterial blood (Lyon and Pitts, 1969; Marliss et al., 1971).

The enzymes which regulate glutamate and glutamine synthesis are two of the most important and interesting of the multienzyme complexes. Their presence is ubiquitous in nearly all organisms, and they have been widely studied because of their susceptibility to allosteric regulation.

Proline

Proline is synthesized from glutamate via the intermediate, glutamic acid-γ-semialdehyde (Equation 3); the pathway is a reversal of the degradation sequence for proline.

$$\text{Glutamic acid} + NADH + ATP \rightleftarrows \text{glutamic-}\gamma\text{-semialdehyde} + NAD + ADP + Pi \qquad \textbf{(3.a)}$$

$$\text{Glutamic-}\gamma\text{-semialdehyde} + NADPH \rightleftarrows \boxed{\text{Proline}} + NADP \qquad \textbf{(3.b)}$$

$$\rightarrow \text{(nonenzymatic)} \rightarrow \Delta'\text{-Pyrroline-5'-carboxylic acid}$$

In microorganisms, proline is an allosteric inhibitor of the initial step committing the carbon chain of glutamate to proline synthesis. Less is known about the regulation of proline synthesis in human tissues.

Arginine

Glutamate can also contribute to arginine biosynthesis through its conversion first to *ornithine* via glutamic-γ-semialdehyde (see Equation 23). Ornithine is then condensed with carbamyl phosphate, $\boxed{H_2N}$—C—O~P, to form *citrulline*;

$$\underset{O}{\overset{\|}{C}}$$

the latter, in the presence of aspartate, yields *argininosuccinate*, which is split to form *arginine* and fumarate. In this way, the amino group of aspartate and ammonia, carried as carbamyl phosphate, is lost as *urea*, and ornithine is re-formed. The carbon chain of glutamate continues to recycle in the urea cycle, and the carbon chain of oxaloacetate exits as fumarate after appearing transiently as aspartate.

Summary

The above-mentioned biosynthetic interrelations are summarized in Scheme 4–2.

$$SCHEME\ 4\text{--}2$$

Proline

↑

$\boxed{NH_3}$ + $\boxed{\alpha\text{-ketoglutarate}}$ → glutamate → glutamic-γ-semialdehyde

↓   ↓

glutamine   ornithine

↓

arginine

Biosynthesis Originating in Pyruvate

Alanine

Alanine arises in human tissues by the transfer of NH_3 (transamination) to pyruvic acid (Equation 4).

$$\text{Glutamate} + \text{pyruvic acid} \rightleftarrows \alpha\text{-ketoglutarate} + \boxed{\text{alanine}} \qquad (4)$$

Serine

Pyruvic acid contributes indirectly to serine synthesis when it is cycled anaplerotically via the pyruvate carboxylase and phosphoenol pyruvate carboxykinase reactions to reappear in the gluconeogenic pathway as 3-phosphoglyceric acid; the latter is, of course, also formed as an intermediate of glycolysis. Serine is then synthesized via the intermediates 3-phosphohydroxypyruvate and 3-phosphoserine (Equation 5).

$$3\text{-phospho-D-glycerate} + NAD^+ \rightarrow 3\text{-phosphohydroxypyruvate} + NADH \quad \textbf{(5.a)}$$

$$3\text{-phosphohydroxypyruvate} + \text{glutamate} \rightarrow 3\text{-phosphoserine} + \alpha\text{-ketoglutarate}$$
$$\textbf{(5.b)}$$

$$3\text{-phosphoserine} \rightarrow \boxed{\text{serine}} + Pi \qquad \textbf{(5.c)}$$

Two coenzymes, NAD^+ in reaction 5a and pyridoxal phosphate in reaction 5b, are required in the catalysis of serine synthesis.

Cysteine

The biosynthesis of cysteine involves *degradation of methionine* (see Chapter 11) and *serine incorporation* at the stage of cystathionine formation. The sulfur atom from methionine and the carbon chain and amino group of serine come together, with loss of the hydroxyl group of serine, to form cysteine. The overall reaction is accomplished by a series of complex steps (Equation 6) which can be summarized as follows:

$$\boxed{\text{Methionine}} + ATP + \text{methyl acceptor} + H_2O + \boxed{\text{serine}} \rightarrow$$
$$\text{methylated acceptor} + \text{adenosine} + \alpha\text{-ketobutyrate} + NH_3 +$$
$$\boxed{\text{cysteine}} + PPi + Pi \qquad \textbf{(6)}$$

Glycine

Glycine synthesis is complex by one route and is catalyzed by serine transhydroxymethylase. The β-carbon of serine is lost, and tetrahydrofolate (FH_4) is the acceptor of the methyl group (Equation 7). The overall reaction requires 2 cosubstrates and the coenzyme pyridoxal phosphate.

$$\text{Serine} + FH_4 \rightarrow \boxed{\text{glycine}} + N^5,N^{10}\text{-methylene } FH_4 \qquad \textbf{(7)}$$

The β-carbon of serine is a precursor of the ureido carbon atoms of uric acid.

Summary

The biosynthetic relationships involving *pyruvate* are summarized in Scheme 4–3.

SCHEME 4–3

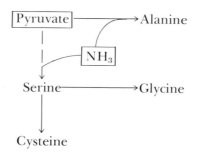

Biosynthesis Originating in Oxaloacetate

Aspartic Acid

The third major route of entry of carbon chains into nonessential amino acid metabolism is through oxaloacetic acid (Equation 8). Transamination of oxaloacetate yields aspartic acid.

$$\text{Glutamic acid} + \text{oxaloacetate} \rightleftarrows \alpha\text{-ketoglutarate} + \boxed{\text{aspartic acid}} \qquad \textbf{(8)}$$

Asparagine

Aspartic acid is believed to be the direct precursor of aspargine (Equation 9), the synthesis being served presumably by a reaction analogous to glutamine synthesis and catalyzed by an asparagine synthetase.

$$\text{Aspartic acid} + NH_3 + \text{ATP} \rightleftarrows \boxed{\text{asparagine}} + \text{ADP} + \text{Pi} \qquad \textbf{(9)}$$

The reaction has not been well characterized in mammalian tissues.

Summary

The oxaloacetate-derived relationships are summarized in Scheme 4–4.

SCHEME 4–4

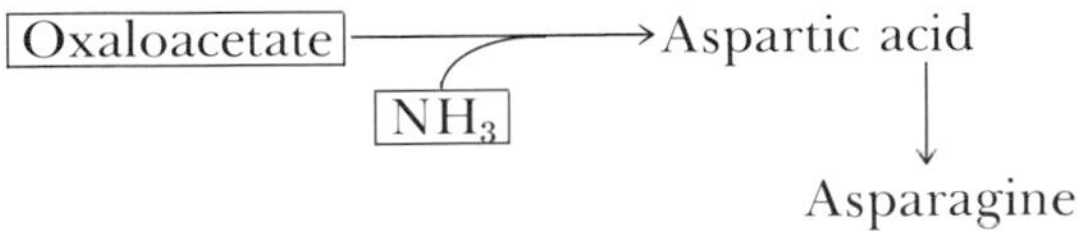

$$\boxed{\text{Oxaloacetate}} \xrightarrow[\boxed{NH_3}]{} \text{Aspartic acid}$$
$$\downarrow$$
$$\text{Asparagine}$$

Keto Acid–Independent Biosynthesis

The synthesis of tyrosine and histidine in human tissues is not comparable to the above-mentioned reactions. *Tyrosine* synthesis requires hydroxylation of the essential amino acid *phenylalanine*. Tyrosine may also be formed from its keto acid (*p*-hydroxyphenylpyruvic acid) by transamination when the latter is present in large amounts (see discussion of neonatal tyrosinemia, Chapter 16).

The biosynthesis of *histidine* is a tour de force in microorganisms, nine enzymes being under the control of one operon which is subject to coordinate repression by the end product, histidine. The mechanism of histidine synthesis in man is not known, and in fact, this amino acid has some features of an essential amino acid (Stifel and Herman, 1972).

Precursor Functions of Some Amino Acids

Amino acids participate as precursors in the synthesis of other compounds. We have seen that serine participates in the synthesis of *cysteine* and *cystathionine*. Tyrosine is the precursor of *thyroxine* and *catecholamines*, and glycine is required for the synthesis of *porphyrins*. Glycine, cysteine and glutamate can be joined in peptide linkage to form the important tripeptide *glutathione* (Equation 10).

$$\text{glutamate} + \text{cysteine} + \text{ATP} \xrightarrow{\text{Mg}^{++}} \gamma\text{-glutamyl cysteine} + \text{ADP} + \text{Pi} \qquad \textbf{(10.a)}$$

$$\gamma\text{-glutamyl cysteine} + \text{glycine} + \text{ATP} \xrightarrow{\text{Mg}^{++}} \text{glutathione} + \text{ADP} + \text{Pi} \textbf{ (10.b)}$$

Some of the products derived from amino acid precursors mentioned elsewhere in this book or otherwise of interest are listed in Table 4–2.

AMINO ACID FLUXES AND METABOLIC POOLS

Plasma proteins are vehicles of limited capacity for the transfer of amino acids from one tissue or organ to another, and peptides do not play a significant part in such fluxes. It follows that any major flux of amino acids must occur while they are in their free forms. Unfortunately, steady-state measurements of free amino acid levels in body fluids tell us nothing about flux through the pool under scrutiny; nor do they tell us anything about episodic variation in the pool size. Circadian variation hints at the ebb and flow of plasma amino acids, but why does it occur? As we shall see, it is the oscillation in relative rates of deposit and demand, with reference to the intracellular stores of protein and free amino acids, that underlies these fluxes. In this section, we describe briefly the flow of amino acids between blood and tissues and how it may be carried out. Later in this chapter, we will discuss some of the events which regulate it.

Where Amino Acids Go

Amino acids enter metabolic traffic at many points, such as from the intestine during protein digestion or from the muscle or liver after proteolysis and release of free amino acids. Thereafter, the amino acids may be carried to another tissue, where they leave the interorgan traffic in the vascular space to enter intracellular protein synthesis or anabolic and catabolic pathways. Some amino acids will also be lost from the body, and they will constitute a portion of the daily nitrogen loss. Figure 4–1 depicts the flow of amino acids in broad terms.

Table 4–2   Derivatives of Amino Acid Precursors

Precursor	Derivative	Mechanism of Formation
Arginine	Putrescine	Decarboxylation
Aspartate	Pyrimidine	Incorporation
Cysteine	Glutathione	Peptide Linkage
Glutamate	γ-Aminobutyrate	Decarboxylation
	Glutathione	Peptide linkage
Glycine	Purines	Incorporation
	Porphyrins	Incorporation
	Creatine	Incorporation
	Glutathione	Peptide linkage
Histidine	Histamine	Decarboxylation
Lysine	Cadaverine	Decarboxylation
Serine	Ethanolamine	Conversion
	Choline	Conversion
Tyrosine	Catecholamine	Conversion and decarboxylation
	Thyroxine	Conversion
	Melanin	Conversion
Tryptophan	Serotonin	Conversion and decarboxylation
	Nicotinic acid	Conversion

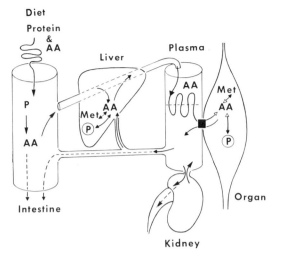

Figure 4-1 The flow of free (un-bound) amino acids from the nutritional phase (*Intestine*), through metabolic pools (*Met*) in organs such as liver and muscle, into bound pools (*P*). Plasma and erythrocytes mediate the interorgan fluxes with oscillations in the plasma steady state. Regulators, such as hormones, influence supply and chemical demand at various sites (viz., muscle-plasma interface).

We see that three tissues, besides the intestine, play a large role in the regulation of free amino acid traffic in blood: skeletal muscle, liver and kidney.

Relative Pool Sizes

If we return, for a moment, to the early work of Van Slyke and Meyer (1913; cited in Chapter 3), we find that uptake (influx) into tissues accounts for the rapid disappearance of α-amino nitrogen from dog plasma after intravenous infusion of an amino acid. The amino acid has moved into the animal's skeletal muscle, where it resides in the free form until it is incorporated or oxidized or until it effluxes to reach another destination. Many years after these early experiments, Boorsook et al. (1950) confirmed that less than three per cent of the amino acid dose is found in the blood stream of the mouse 10 minutes after the injection; these investigators found the amino acid first in muscle and then, after recirculation, in the liver, where it entered pathways of protein synthesis or intermediary metabolism.

Skeletal muscle has the largest pool of free amino acids in the body of the rat (Munro, 1970), and presumably the same is true of man. At least 35 per cent and sometimes as much as 80 per cent of the total body pool of any free, essential amino acid resides in muscle; and muscle holds at least 50 per cent of the total body pool for any of the nonessential amino acids. By comparison, the liver pool of any amino acid rarely holds more than 10 per cent of the total body pool; the kidney pool is uniformly less than four per cent, and the plasma pool is estimated to be between about one and six per cent of the total. It is not surprising that there is considerable variation in the relative interorgan pool sizes among the various amino acids, but the details are not pertinent here.

Subcellular Pools

It is not likely that the intracellular pools are any more uniform than the various organ pools, since compartmentalization is evident at the subcellular level. Isolated nuclei and mitochondria will accumulate free amino acids readily, and lysosomes can retain a pool of some amino acids after proteolysis has occurred. For example, there is tentative evidence that cystine storage in cystinosis occurs because its efflux from lysosomes is abnormal in some way (see

Chapter 11). Nevertheless, the subcellular compartmentalization of amino acid pools and metabolism has received relatively little attention up to now despite an awareness that different organelles contain different isozymes for the regulation of amino acid metabolism—for example, tyrosine transaminase in cytosol and mitochondria (see Chapter 16).

The recent studies of valine metabolism in perfused rat liver by Mortimer, Mondon and colleagues (1970, 1972) reveal that one pool of valine which equilibrates readily with the extracellular pool is presumably cytoplasmic in location and serves protein synthesis or oxidative metabolism; another pool, which does not equilibrate readily with the extracellular pool, may be a transient intralysosomal pool formed during proteolysis prior to the efflux of amino acids from lysosome to cytoplasm.

Relative Changes in Tissue Pools

The intracellular amino acid pools which are available for protein synthesis ("nitrogen retention" in Scheme 4–1) and catabolism or biosynthesis ("nitrogen conversion" in Scheme 4–1) are in dynamic equilibrium. Gan and Jeffay (1967) showed that the intracellular amino acid pools of liver and muscle undergo constant dilution, apparently by the release from intracellular protein of amino acids which then enter the intracellular pool. In the fed animal, up to 50 per cent of the intracellular amino acid pool of liver is derived from protein turnover; the corresponding figure in muscle is 30 per cent. In the fasted state, the contribution from proteolysis rises to 90 per cent in liver and to 65 per cent in muscle, at which time amino acids efflux from the intracellular pools and are transported to other tissues. There appears to be a hierarchy to the order in which labile proteins are degraded to provide free amino acids to the body, liver giving up its amino acids first and muscle thereafter.

Mechanisms of Interorgan Flux

The gut delivers free amino acids to the liver in the plasma fraction of the splanchnic portal circulation. Muscle and peripheral tissues also provide amino acids to the splanchnic tissues for metabolic functions such as gluconeogenesis, urea synthesis, protein synthesis and catabolism to yield energy. On the other hand, the liver is also asked to deliver free amino acids to the peripheral tissues, particularly in the postabsorptive state. Does this bidirectional interorgan flux occur exclusively in plasma? Elwyn and colleagues (1972) suggest that it may not. These investigators, and others before them, examined amino acid flux rates between blood and tissues and found that transit across the plasma membranes of tissue cells does not impede the rate at which amino acids equilibrate between tissues and whole blood in vivo. In fact, cell membrane transport (discussed in Chapter 2 and in the chapters of Part II) facilitates flux under normal circumstances, although it is likely to be one of the places at which amino acid metabolism is regulated.* It follows then that pool size in a tissue is a function of amino acid concentration on either side of the membrane and blood flow past the mem-

---

*Christensen and Cullen (1968) showed that interaction between amino acids at membrane transport sites was itself a determinant of intracellular pool size. An excess of one amino acid in blood could lead to the depletion of another amino acid in tissue. The detrimental effects of amino acid imbalance probably can be attributed in part to this type of interaction.

brane. The relative size of intracellular and extracellular pools must then be a function of the net flux across the membrane, which is, in turn, determined by two unidirectional fluxes ("in" or "out") and the concentration of amino acids at the origins of the fluxes. Elwyn and colleagues showed that the half-life of amino acids in plasma is extremely short—on the order of a minute—and that the rate of flux into tissue is very high. They estimated that the liver in the dog cleared the circulating plasma of 50 to 90 per cent of its total free amino content each minute.

During the course of their study of tissue-plasma fluxes of amino acids in vivo, Elwyn's group also discovered anomalous behavior with regard to the erythrocyte pool of amino acids in the blood. The velocity of change in erythrocyte amino acid content in vivo was found to be 100-fold greater than would occur in vitro when erythrocytes and plasma were mixed together under comparable conditions of substrate concentration. They also observed that the change in the erythrocyte pool is independent of the change in plasma amino acid flux rates, and they concluded that liver must contribute something to the amino acid content of erythrocytes during the passage of these cells through the liver sinusoids. It was suggested that anatomically distinct hepatic cells which line the sinusoids might participate in an erythrocyte-tissue exchange which was distinct from the plasma-tissue exchange. Such a hypothesis and an elaboration from it (Fig. 4–2) await confirmation. Nonetheless, it is attractive because it offers a mechanism for bidirectional flux between splanchnic and peripheral tissues whereby plasma and erythrocytes play independent and even opposing roles in the interorgan transport of amino acids. Plasma is predominantly responsible for interorgan flux toward liver; erythrocytes accommodate flux away from liver. Since transmembrane tissue blood flux is very rapid and not limiting, interorgan flux is achieved without great changes in amino acid concentration in blood.

This hypothesis has recently gained unexpected support from a study reported by Cahill's group (Aoki et al., 1972). These investigators found a discrepancy between the data for *plasma* arterio-deep venous glutamate difference and the *whole blood* arterio-deep venous glutamate difference in human forearm vessels. The plasma data revealed no increase in glutamate uptake by muscle in the presence of insulin, whereas the whole-blood data showed a striking effect of insulin on glutamate uptake. One must conclude from analysis of the data that the cellular fraction of whole blood plays a dynamic role in glutamate transport to peripheral striated muscle, and the data are compatible with the Elwyn hypothesis.

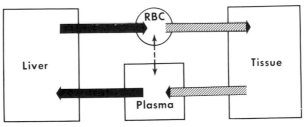

Figure 4–2 A hypothesis based on the studies of Elwyn et al. (1972) for the mechanism of amino acid flux between a peripheral tissue, such as muscle, and a central tissue, such as liver. Erythrocytes take up amino acids in liver sinusoids and deliver them to a peripheral capillary bed and tissue. Blood plasma extracts amino acids from peripheral tissue and delivers them to liver. The latter tissue can clear plasma of 50 to 90 per cent of its free amino acid load each minute. There is relatively little exchange of amino acids between the plasma and erythrocytes.

CATABOLISM (DEGRADATION) OF AMINO ACIDS

Catalytic Options

About 400 g of protein (amino acids) turn over daily in the normal adult; about one quarter is oxidized to CO_2 and water. The amino groups either are transferred into other pools and utilized for biosynthetic processes or are lost from the body as ammonia or urea; the carbon chains are ultimately oxidized in the tricarboxylic acid cycle.

The initial catalytic attack upon the amino acid most often occurs around the α-carbon atom. The result is either decarboxylation, removal of the α-amino group or cleavage and modification of the side chain. These enzyme-catalyzed reactions usually require pyridoxal-phosphate as coenzyme. The proposed relationship between the substrate and coenzyme, which facilitates electron mobilization and transfer around the α-carbon atom, is depicted in Figure 4–3.

The following discussion of amino acid degradation is organized to make clear the ultimate fate of the carbon chain and its contribution to energy metabolism, the general outcome of decarboxylation (a reaction which usually diverts the amine residue toward a special anabolic function) and the mechanisms of amino group transfer generating the α-keto acid that enters the pathways of carbon chain oxidation.

Fate of the Carbon Skeleton

The catabolic pathways which direct the stepwise oxidation of each of the specific amino acids are complex; these are the subject of more detailed examination in the various chapters of Part III. Each amino acid has a final destination in the tricarboxylic acid cycle, where the carbon chain can be oxidized; the entry points are illustrated in Figure 4–4. The carbon skeletons of amino acids need not be oxidized completely, and under some circumstances they are reutilized for the synthesis of glucose and glycogen or they recirculate from tissue to tissue as ketone bodies. Most amino acids are glucogenic and can promote net synthesis of glucose via phosphoenol pyruvate; one is solely ketogenic; and a few (those which yield acetoacetyl-CoA) can be both ketogenic and glucogenic (Table 4–3).

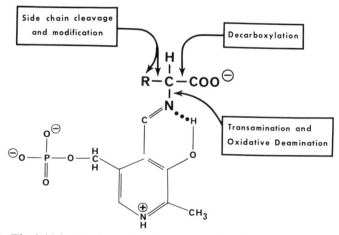

Figure 4–3   The initial catalytic reactions in amino acid catabolism. Pyridoxal-5′-phosphate is required as a coenzyme by most amino acids during their decarboxylation, transamination, deamination or modification of their side chain.

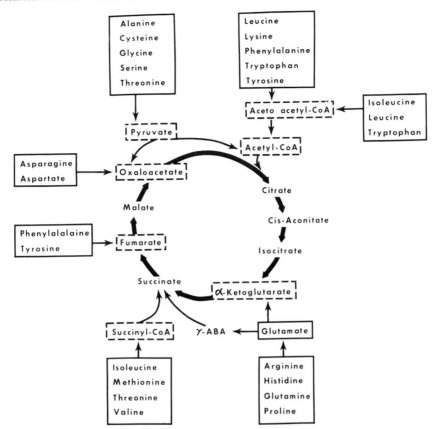

Figure 4–4 Catabolic fates of amino acids; final destinations for oxidation of carbon chains in the tricarboxylic acid cycle.

Table 4–3 Fate of Amino Acid Carbon Skeleton

Glucogenic	Glucogenic and ketogenic	Ketogenic
Alanine	Isoleucine	Leucine
Arginine	Lysine	
Aspartic acid	Phenylalanine	
Asparagine	Tyrosine	
Cyst(e)ine		
Glutamic acid		
Glutamine		
Glycine		
Histidine		
Methionine		
Proline		
Serine		
Threonine		
Tryptophan		
Valine		

Catabolism of amino acids may share some of the same steps in reverse that serve their biosynthesis, but reversibility at every step in the modification of the carbon chain obviously does not exist. An irreversible step in catabolism confers essentiality upon an amino acid (see Chapter 2).

Not all tissues and cells have identical capacities to oxidize or utilize amino acids anaplerotically. For example, skin fibroblasts do not oxidize tyrosine or convert sarcosine to serine; and neither leukocytes nor fibroblasts can support glucogenesis via the pyruvate carboxylase reaction with amino acids which generate pyruvate. The major organs for amino acid catabolism are the liver and, to a lesser extent, the kidney. However, these tissues oxidize branched-chain amino acids relatively poorly, and the latter are degraded more efficiently in such peripheral tissues as muscle (Miller, 1962).

Threonine possesses two types of oxidative conversion, one demanding R-group cleavage, the other initiated by removal of the amino group (Fig. 4–5). The bidirectional oxidative option for threonine may explain why it alone among the essential amino acids has not yet been associated with an inborn error of its catabolism and excessive accumulation in body fluids.

There are six types of ATP-generating mechanisms in human tissues: two in the anaerobic glycolysis of carbohydrate; three in the electron transport of molecular oxygen; and one in the oxidative decarboxylation of α-keto acids to carboxylic acids (Krebs, 1964). Oxidation of the deaminated carbon chains yields ATP, and the estimates for ATP yield per amino acid are given in Table 4–4. Certain assumptions are made to derive these data—namely, that all steps of oxidative phosphorylation are coupled with phosphorylation; that each atom of amino acid nitrogen consumes two molecules of ATP during ureogenesis (with the exception of one arginine nitrogen which enters urea without ATP consumption); and that the carbon skeletons of glycine, cyst(e)ine and tryptophan as well as 12 per cent of the carbon chain of all other amino acids are not oxidized (Krebs, 1964).

Decarboxylation and Oxidative Decarboxylation

Initial decarboxylation is not important, in quantitative terms, for the disposal of amino acids in human metabolism. However, the amine products of initial decarboxylation often possess potent pharmacologic activity, and it is for this reason that decarboxylation is a focus of interest not only for the interpretation of disease (phenotype) in the aminoacidopathies but also for an appreciation of the therapeutic approach which may modulate decarboxylase activity.

Amino acid decarboxylation in human tissues is catalyzed by an L-amino acid decarboxylase activity. The decarboxylase may serve many substrates (as for the decarboxylation of phenylalanine, tyrosine, tryptophan, histidine, 5-hydroxytryptophan and 3,4-dihydroxyphenylalanine), or it may possess considerable substrate specificity (as for L-glutamic acid). The general reaction is most active at neutral or slightly alkaline pH, and it yields an amine plus CO_2. The more important endogenous decarboxylation reactions of human tissues are listed in Table 4–5. Not every amino acid can participate in decarboxylation reactions, in human tissues, and those that do not include alanine, asparagine, cyst(e)ine, glutamine, glycine, hydroxyproline, methionine, proline, free serine and threonine. Decarboxylation products which do not originate from endogenous decarboxylation reactions are also found in human tissues and body fluids, and it should be remembered that microorganisms can be an important source of decarboxylase activity. For example, the putrescine and cadaverine found in the urine in some forms of cystinuria arise in the intestinal lumen

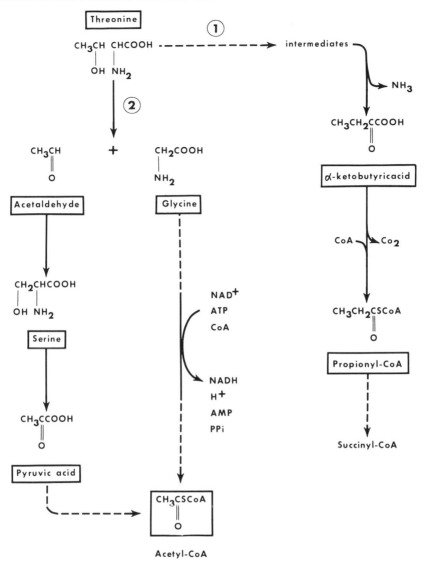

Figure 4–5 Pathways of threonine oxidation. Two major pathways for degradation are available. The initial attack in one is deamination, and in the other it is against the side chain.

as the result of bacterial action on nonabsorbed amino acid substrates. This consideration is relevant to the interpretation of the phenotype in several of the aminoacidopathies described in Parts II and III of this book.

Oxidative decarboxylation of the branched-chain keto acids pyruvate and α-ketoglutarate is an essential step in the conversion of the respective corresponding amino acid. These reactions are complex, and they are discussed in more detail under the section on branched-chain amino acids.

Transfer and Fate of the Amino Group

Liberation of ammonia from the carbon skeleton yields an amino group which can be either salvaged or excreted. Transfer of the nitrogen moiety

Table 4-4   Maximum ATP Yields From Amino Acids[a]

Substrate	Net ATP Yield (moles/mole amino acid)
Alanine	16
Arginine	29
Aspartic acid	16
Glutamic acid	25
Histidine[b]	21
Isoleucine	41
Leucine	40
Lysine	35
Methionine[c]	18
Phenylalanine	39
Proline	30
Serine	13
Threonine[d]	21
Tyrosine	42
Valine	20

[a]From Krebs (1964), based on assumptions listed in text.
[b]No net change in ATP in the metabolism of formyltetrahydrofolate.
[c]Methyl group inert in ATP balance.
[d]Oxidation via α-ketobutyrate.

Table 4-5   Enzymatic Decarboxylation of L-Amino Acids

Amino Acid[a]	Amine Product and Function	Location of Enzyme
Cysteic acid[b]	Taurine; bile salt formation	Liver
Cysteine sulfinic acid[b]	Hypotaurine; neural activity	Liver, brain
3,4-Dihydroxyphenylalanine	3,4-dihydroxyphenylethanolamine; neuroendocrine function	Adrenal medulla
Glutamic acid	γ-amino butyric acid; neural activity; renal ammoniagenesis	Brain, kidney
Histidine	Histamine; neurovascular activity	Mast cells (specific enzyme); liver, kidney, etc. (nonspecific enzyme)
5-Hydroxytryptophan	Serotonin; neuroendocrine role	Brain, other tissues
Serine (as phosphatidyl-serine)	Ethanolamine; cephalin synthesis	Brain, other tissues

[a]Other amino acids for which endogenous decarboxylative reactions may be of significance in certain diseases include phenylalanine ($\rightarrow$ phenylethylamine, in phenylketonuria) and tyrosine ($\rightarrow$ tyramine, in tyrosine disorders).
[b]Decarboxylation in man in doubt.

during catabolism of amino acids ultimately involves either transamination or deamination whose activity can be summarized by the general reactions:

Transamination:
$$\text{Amino acid} + \alpha\text{-ketoglutarate} \rightleftarrows \alpha\text{-keto acid} + \text{glutamate} \qquad \textbf{(11.a)}$$

Deamination:
$$\text{Glutamate} - 2H + H_2O \rightleftarrows \alpha\text{-ketoglutarate} + NH_3 \qquad \textbf{(11.b)}$$

Combined:
$$\text{Amino acid} - 2H + H_2O \rightleftarrows \alpha\text{-keto acid} + NH_3 \qquad \textbf{(11.c)}$$

Transamination and deamination reactions serve different metabolic functions, and they will be discussed separately. It should be remembered that mammals are unable to fix nitrogen (as $N\equiv N$), a capacity available to only a few bacteria and algae. Nor can man assimilate reduced nitrogen (as NH_3) in his search for a nitrogen source; ruminants, among the mammals, can do so in symbiosis with their ruminant bacteria. Man must obtain nitrogen in a form which is nontoxic and which is readily transferable. Protein is his major source of nitrogen, and therein is found the source of essential amino acids and nitrogen for other anabolic reactions. The constraints on nitrogen metabolism apparent in its assimilation are also evident in its disposal. Man is *ureotelic*. Free ammonia is toxic to all his tissues and particularly to the brain. Elaborate disposal mechanisms are available to facilitate the safe transfer of free ammonia from amino acids to receptors or to carriers which direct it into the pathway of urea synthesis.

Small amounts of tissue nitrogen are excreted as free NH_3 by man, but he is not *ammonotelic* like the teleost fish or the tadpole. When NH_3 excretion occurs, it is a mechanism peculiar to kidney for purposes of acid titration and excretion (Pitts, 1971). The ammonia for compensation of metabolic acidosis in man is derived from plasma glutamine (Lyon and Pitts, 1970). When formed under the action of renal glutaminase-I, it is excreted preferentially into an acid urine by the process of nonionic diffusion (Milne et al., 1958), where it combines with H^+ to yield NH_4^+, a new ionic species which cannot diffuse back into tubular cells and must be excreted in the urine. Man also excretes a small fraction of his nitrogen waste products in the form of uric acid, but he is not *uricotelic* like the avian and reptilian phyla. Thus our attention should focus on the mechanisms of ammonia transfer and urea synthesis, which serve amino acid catabolism in man.

Transamination

Removal of the α-amino (or ω-amino) group either initiates or continues the catabolism of most amino acids. The amino group is usually transferred to one of three α-keto acids: pyruvate, oxaloacetate or α-ketoglutarate, as indicated in reactions 11a and 12. A new amino acid is formed during the generation of the α-keto acid analogue, and under these conditions there is no net loss of nitrogen, only transfer and collection of nitrogen in a different metabolic pool. Transamination reactions are freely reversible, their equilibrium being the same from either direction.

The general constraints on acceptance of amino groups result in their collection in the form of only a few new amino acids. The relevant transaminases are named after the product formed by the transfer-acceptance reaction. Thus, when pyruvate is the acceptor, the catalyst is *alanine transaminase*; alternatively the enzyme may have a specific *aminotransferase* designation which recognizes the substrate and the acceptor, e.g., *glutamate:pyruvate* aminotransferase. Both terms just mentioned could be used to describe Equation 12:

$$\text{glutamate} + \text{pyruvate} \rightleftarrows \alpha\text{-ketoglutarate} + \text{alanine} \qquad (12)$$

The other important catalysts are *glutamate transaminase* and *aspartate transaminase*; they also are "specific" for the keto acid analogue (amino group receptor) and "nonspecific" for the substrate (amino group donor). The amino groups are ultimately transferred to one major common acceptor, α-ketoglutarate.

Evaluation of the kinetics of transamination reactions indicates that they proceed by a complex sequence of events whereby cosubstrates — amino acid donor and keto acid acceptor — are bound by the apoenzyme sequentially and in the presence of coenzyme (Cleland, 1964; La Du, 1967). This type of reaction, depicted in Figure 4–6, is said to observe "ping-pong" kinetics. Transaminases are also complex in that they occur as isozymes and are inducible in eukaryotic (nucleated) diploid cells (see following material). These characteristics are anticipated, since transaminases command important positions for regulating metabolism. The isozymic nature of transaminases may determine their differential distribution in the cell, one form of a transaminase usually being found in the cytoplasm and another in the mitochondria, for example. The differences in physical and chemical properties of mitochondrial and extramitochondrial transaminases allow interplay between the compartments during catabolism and biosynthesis of amino acids. The main thrust of this interplay seems to be to accumulate the amino groups in glutamate in the cytoplasm so that glutamate can be transported into the mitochondria via an inward-directed amino acid carrier. Conversion of glutamate to α-ketoglutarate in the mitochondrial compartment then occurs, and the keto acid can be oxidized by the intramitochondrial tricarboxylic acid cycle (Fig. 4–7).

Oxidative Deamination

Two types of oxidative deamination occur in mammalian cells. Both yield free ammonia and an α-keto acid analogue; the more important deaminative mechanism is intramitochondrial and is catalyzed by a powerful amino acid dehydrogenase. The other mechanism is cytoplasmic and requires many different oxidases.

Glutamate Dehydrogenase.   Animal tissues and microorganisms possess

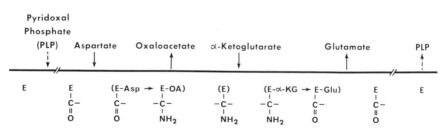

Figure 4–6   The kinetics of a transamination reaction. The enzyme *(E)* binds first the pyridoxal form of coenzyme *(E—C═O)*. Next it reacts with the first substrate (aspartate) to form the first product *(OA)*. The enzyme then reacts with the second substrate (α—KG), transferring the amino group from coenzyme transformed to the pyridoxamine form in the first reaction, to form the second product, glutamate. Free enzyme is regenerated at the end of this "ping-pong" sequence of reactions.

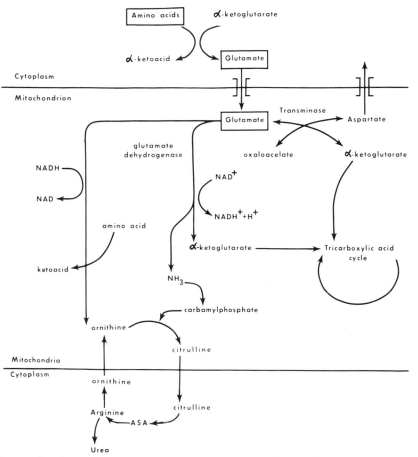

Figure 4–7 Glutamate shuttle from cytosol to mitochondria and formation of urea under conditions favoring the collection of cellular ammonia in glutamate. The aspartate shuttle is a rapid export system (vs. oxaloacetate movement) which provides carbon chain and reducing equivalent for gluconeogenesis in the cytosol. A bidirectional shuttle for movement of α-ketoglutarate across the membrane also exists but is not shown.

a dehydrogenase which is specific for glutamic acid, the relative importance of which is greatest in ammonotelic organisms. The intramitochondrial enzyme catalyzes the reaction shown in Equation 11b. It is *pyridine-linked* and, unlike many other dehydrogenases, the enzyme will react with either NAD^+ or $NADP^+$ coenzymes. In the oxidized form, the apoenzyme transfers one hydrogen to the coenzyme, while the other becomes a proton; reduction of the coenzyme occurs during the process which involves the formation of two binary complexes — E-NAD^+ and E-NADH — and two tertiary complexes — substrate$_{(oxid)}$-E-NADH and substrate$_{(reduc)}$-E-NAD^+. Substrate conversion is summarized in Equation 13.

$$
\begin{array}{ccccccccc}
R & & & & R & & & R & \\
| & & & & | & & & | & \\
CHNH_2 & - & 2H & \rightarrow & C{:}NH & + & H_2O & \rightarrow & C{=}O & + & NH_3 \\
| & & & & | & & & | & \\
COOH & & +\ NAD^+ & & COOH & & & COOH & & +\ NADH \\
& & (or\ NADP^+) & & & & & & (or\ NADPH)
\end{array}
$$

$$(13)$$

Glutamate dehydrogenase is an allosteric enzyme which has a molecular weight in beef liver of about 280,000, the enzyme containing subunits of about 40,000 molecular weight. It aggregates into a rod-shaped complex of about 2.2 million particle weight under appropriate conditions. Amino acids activate the enzyme, while reduced coenzyme is an inhibitor.

Amino Acid Oxidases.   Amino acid deamination may also proceed in the presence of *oxidases*, of which there are two different types: L-*amino acid oxidase* and D-*amino acid oxidase*. These enzymes require flavin coenzymes, and they are active in the cytoplasm (Neims and Hellerman, 1970). The L-amino acid oxidase catalyzes a reaction in the endoplasmic reticulum in the presence of a flavin mononucleotide coenzyme (Equation 14):

$$\text{L-amino acid} + \text{E-FMN} \rightarrow \alpha\text{-keto acid} + NH_3 + \text{E-FMNH}_2 \qquad (14)$$

The D-amino acid oxidase activity of mammalian cells is situated in the microbodies (peroxisomes), and it requires a flavin adenine dinucleotide coenzyme to catalyze the reaction summarized in Equation 15.

$$\text{D-amino acid} + \text{E-FAD} \rightarrow \alpha\text{-keto acid} + NH_3 + \text{E-FADH}_2 \qquad (15)$$

The function of D-amino oxidase in animal cells is not known with certainty. However, Neims and Hellerman (1962) suggest that this curious activity may be an incidental property of glycine oxidase.

Both types of amino acid oxidase result in the formation of reduced flavin nucleotides which react with molecular oxygen to form H_2O_2. The hydrogen peroxide is subsequently converted in peroxisomes to $H_2O + \frac{1}{2}O_2$ in the presence of catalase. The relative activities of L- and D-amino acid oxidases, in reference to different amino acid substrates, can be compared in mammalian kidney, as shown in Table 4–6. D-amino acid oxidase has very much lower activity toward the L-substrate, and the corresponding degree of stereospecificity is observed toward D-amino acids by the L-amino acid oxidase.

Table 4–6   Relative Specificity of Amino Acid Oxidases
in Mammalian Kidney[a]

Substrate	L-*Oxidase* (Rat Kidney)	D-*Oxidase* (Sheep Kidney)
Leucine	[100]	7
Methionine	81	42
Proline	77	78
Isoleucine	71	12
Phenylalanine	45	14
Tryptophan	40	19
Valine	28	18
Tyrosine	20	[100]
Cystine	15	1
Histidine	9	3
Aspartate	0	0.5
Glutamate	0	0
Lysine	0	0.3
Ornithine	0	2
Serine	0	22
Threonine	0	1

[a]Relative activities expressed as per cent of maximum activity observed (=100). Adapted from Krebs (1964) and Meister (1965).

Removal of Ammonia

The body has recourse to one of three alternatives for the removal of ammonia:

(i) It may be salvaged by reversal of the glutamate dehydrogenase reaction (Equation 16):

$$\alpha\text{-ketoglutarate} + NH_3 + NADH + H^+ \rightarrow \text{glutamate} + NAD^+ \qquad (16)$$

(ii) It may be incorporated as the amide nitrogen of glutamine, in the presence of glutamine synthetase (or in the analogous form as asparagine), by the reaction shown in Equation 17.

$$\text{glutamate} + NH_3 + ATP \xrightarrow{Mg^{++}} \text{glutamine} + ADP + Pi \qquad (17)$$

(iii) It may be used for the synthesis of urea, the principle excretion product of nitrogen metabolism in man. Urea synthesis is described in detail in Chapter 12, but the overall reaction (Equation 18) is of interest in the present context.

$$\boxed{NH_3} + CO_2 + 3ATP + \text{Aspartate} \rightarrow$$

$$\boxed{\text{Urea}} + \text{fumarate} + 2ADP + AMP + P{\sim}Pi + 2Pi \qquad (18)$$

Four high-energy phosphate bonds are consumed in the process, corresponding to an energy expenditure of 35 to 40 kcal. Two moles of ATP are consumed during the incorporation of NH_3 and CO_2 to form carbamyl phosphate, $\boxed{H_2N}{-}C{-}O{-}PO_3{-}H$. The latter is condensed with ornithine to form citrul-
line. The synthesis of argininosuccinic acid from citrulline and aspartate requires the third mole of ATP; the ejected $P{\sim}Pi$ is then cleaved immediately by pyrophosphatase, causing a net consumption to two high-energy phosphate bonds at this step. Argininosuccinate, when cleaved, yields arginine and fumarate. The synthesis of arginine in this fashion is found throughout the animal kingdom; however, it is the cleavage of arginine to ornithine and urea in the presence of large amounts of arginase that is unique in ureotelic organisms. The major organ of urea production is the liver, but brain and kidney can also synthesize urea on a small scale.

Urea synthesis is a mitochondrial activity in the liver; its objective is to prevent NH_3 accumulation. The latter is toxic to organisms unable to excrete ammonia to the environment immediately after its formation.

The toxicity of ammonia is related in part to its ability to reaminate α-ketoglutarate in the presence of glutamate dehydrogenase whose equilibrium is shifted to the right in the presence of NADH (Equation 19).

$$NH_3 + H^+ + \alpha\text{-ketoglutarate} + NADH \rightarrow \text{glutamate} + NAD^+ \qquad (19)$$

Depletion of α-ketoglutarate will occur in the presence of ammonia excess, and respiration will be inhibited.

Synthesis of ornithine from glutamate consumes NADH while priming the urea cycle as shown in Equation 20.

$$\text{glutamate} + \text{NADH} \rightarrow \text{glutamine-}\gamma\text{-semialdehyde} + \text{NAD}^+ \qquad \textbf{(20a)}$$

$$\text{glutamic-}\gamma\text{-semialdehyde} + \text{amino acid} \rightleftarrows \text{ornithine} + \alpha\text{-keto acid} \quad \textbf{(20b)}$$

Once ornithine enters the urea cycle, nitrogen incorporation via carbamyl phosphate is irreversible and the organism is protected from ammonia intoxication.

Glutamine synthesis (Equation 17) is another important protective mechanism against hyperammonemia. Glutamine is the most prevalent amino acid in human blood plasma and cerebrospinal fluid (see Chapter 3), and this amino acid can be considered an important vehicle for the transport of ammonia from peripheral to splanchnic tissues (Marliss et al., 1971). Its synthesis is dependent on the allosteric enzyme glutamine synthetase, which is present in muscle and other tissues. Glutamine cleavage is carried out predominantly in splanchnic tissues by glutaminase to yield glutamate and free ammonia.

METABOLIC INTERFACES IN AMINO ACID METABOLISM

The preceding section has described a number of reactions which link the metabolism of keto acids and ammonia with amino acids. The mechanisms of amino acid flux between the organs have also been discussed. In the present section we will describe the events which link amino acid metabolism with other phases of metabolism in tissues such as liver, kidney and skeletal muscle. Each of these organs plays a major role in the final stages of amino acid metabolism (Elwyn, 1970; Cahill and Owen, 1970; Young, 1970).

Gluconeogenic Functions

If muscle is a major holding place for amino acids, liver and kidney are important furnaces where they are burned for energy metabolism; and the latter are also the forges where amino acids are converted to glucose and glycogen. Amino acids account for about half of the glucose formed by isolated rat liver when it is perfused with a plasma-like mixture of substrates (Exton and Park, 1967). Hepatic conversion of amino acids to glucose was first documented by Bach and Holmes in 1937, and in the same year Benoy and Elliott noted that kidney was also capable of gluconeogenesis. However, not until three decades later was it shown that renal extraction of amino acids plays an important quantitative role in gluconeogenesis (Goodman et al., 1966; Goorno et al., 1967).

The release of amino acids from skeletal muscle provides gluconeogenic precursors for use by splanchnic tissues to maintain blood glucose during starvation. Increased net amino acid release from skeletal muscle follows modulation of either the rate of protein synthesis (decreased), the rate of peripheral oxidation of amino acids (decreased) or the rate of protein degradation and release of free amino acids (increased). The rate of release from peripheral tissues (muscle) and delivery to central (splanchnic) tissues will directly influence gluconeogenesis in the latter area, because amino acids are the most potent modulator of gluconeogenic rates in liver (Exton et al., 1970).

Among the individual amino acids, alanine is one of the most important precursors of glucose in liver (Mallette et al., 1969; Felig et al., 1970). Glutamine is also extracted in large amounts by the splanchnic tissues of man (Marliss et al., 1971), also for purposes of gluconeogenesis. There is reason to believe that kidney is another important tissue for glutamine extraction, since this amino acid supports ammoniagenesis as well in man. Other amino acids are also extracted in significant amounts from systemic plasma by the mammalian splanchnic circulation—notably, glycine and proline.

Two "cycles" have been proposed whereby carbon chains and ammonia are shuttled from peripheral to central tissues under conditions of metabolic stress, such as starvation. One is called the "alanine cycle" (Mallette et al., 1969; Felig et al., 1970), the other the "glutamine cycle" (Marliss et al., 1971) (Fig. 4–8). In the alanine cycle, pyruvate is the acceptor of amino groups in peripheral tissues; the donor amino acids are taken up by the tissues or released from protein stores, and the pyruvate is derived from blood glucose or tissue glycogen. The alanine thus formed in muscle is delivered into plasma; it is then carried

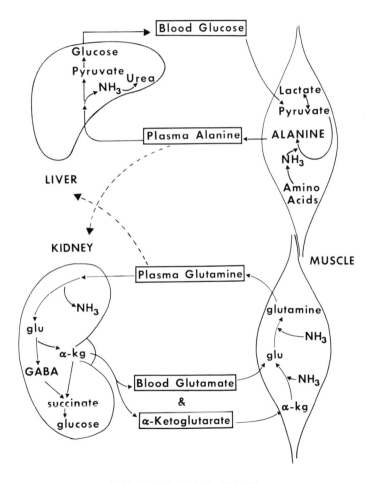

THE "ALANINE CYCLE"

THE "GLUTAMINE CYCLE"

Figure 4–8 So-called "alanine cycle" and "glutamine cycle" in which carbon chains and ammonia are shuttled back and forth between peripheral and central tissues. Not all steps of either cycle have been demonstrated unequivocally, but current evidence suggests that alanine and glutamine move as shown. Muscle has adequate glutamine synthetase to form glutamine; liver and kidney both extract alanine and glutamine. Since glutamine enters special pathways of interest in the kidney, the latter organ is shown participating in the "glutamine cycle," whereas the liver is shown for the "alanine cycle."

and extracted by the splanchnic tissue (in particular, the liver). Ammonia is removed and excreted as urea; the pyruvate moiety is converted back to glucose, released from liver and recirculated to the peripheral tissue. This process provides an effective means of maintaining blood glucose at the expense of protein catabolism while preventing the accumulation and release of NH_3.

The glutamine shuttle is analogous to the alanine cycle on its centripetal journey. The "carrier" is glutamate, which can be extracted by skeletal muscle from blood or synthesized peripherally from α-ketoglutarate. Glutamine is presumably formed from glutamate in skeletal muscle under the influence of glutamine synthetase which is present in this tissue (Iqbal and Ottaway, 1970). The glutamine "carrier" is then transferred in plasma to the central tissues, where it is extracted by liver and kidney; gluconeogenesis will be supported in both tissues by the glutamate carbon chain. Urea metabolism and ammoniagenesis will then transpire in the two organs respectively through the normal course of events described earlier.

Ketogenic Functions

Another important metabolic interface concerns those amino acids which are pyruvigenic or ketogenic (see Table 4–3 and Figure 4–4). Conversion of pyruvate to acetyl-CoA via the pyruvate dehydrogenase-catalyzed reaction, or oxidation of ketogenic amino acids under certain conditions, generates an excess of acetyl-CoA. The subsequent utilization of acetyl-CoA proceeds in the following manner:

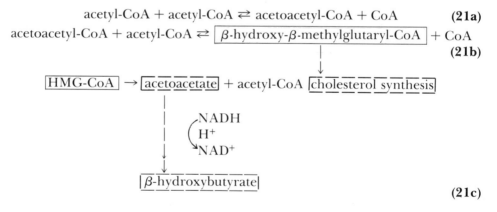

$$\text{acetyl-CoA} + \text{acetyl-CoA} \rightleftarrows \text{acetoacetyl-CoA} + \text{CoA} \qquad \textbf{(21a)}$$

$$\text{acetoacetyl-CoA} + \text{acetyl-CoA} \rightleftarrows \boxed{\beta\text{-hydroxy-}\beta\text{-methylglutaryl-CoA}} + \text{CoA}$$
$$\textbf{(21b)}$$

$$\boxed{\text{HMG-CoA}} \rightarrow \boxed{\text{acetoacetate}} + \text{acetyl-CoA} \boxed{\text{cholesterol synthesis}}$$

$$\boxed{\beta\text{-hydroxybutyrate}}$$
$$\textbf{(21c)}$$

β-hydroxy-β-methylglutaryl-CoA (HMG-CoA) is an intermediate in the genesis of ketone bodies (acetoacetate and β-hydroxybutyrate) and in cholesterol biosynthesis. Therefore, metabolic states such as fasting and starvation, or insulinopenia, will promote amino acid export from peripheral pools such as muscle to splanchnic tissues where, in the absence of insulin, their oxidation to CO_2 will be impaired. Conversion to ketone bodies provides a substrate which can still fuel metabolism in vital tissues such as brain and heart (Cahill, 1971).

REGULATION OF AMINO ACID METABOLISM

This complex subject cannot receive due recognition in the space available, and the reader who wishes to know more should read the discussions, among many possible selections, by Munro (1970a), Manchester (1970), Schimke (1970) and Kaplan and Pitot (1970).

Regulation of amino acid metabolism can take place with respect to the determination of pool size, the flux of amino acids, the rate of amino acid incorporation and the rate of amino acid degradation. Regulation thus seems to be focused on three different types of events: mechanisms of protein synthesis; transfer across membranes; and activity of enzymes in catabolic or anabolic interconversions. The *regulators* of these events also fall into three classes — namely, hormones, coenzymes and metabolites. The last of these are either amino acid substrates (usually "inducers" of enzymes), products of conversion reactions (usually acting as inhibitors) or non-amino acid metabolites.

Hormonal Effects

At Membranes

Insulin and *glucagon* can be cited as examples of hormones apparently active at the membrane level of amino acid metabolism. Administration of *insulin* causes amino acids to be retained by skeletal muscle and their plasma levels to be depressed (Pozefsky et al., 1969). This response is particularly evident with the branched-chain amino acids. Conversely, a rise in plasma insulin follows protein feeding; this response is mediated particularly through the branched-chain amino acids and phenylalanine by mechanisms which are not yet clear. The principal metabolic interrelation between amino acids and insulin appears to be in peripheral tissue pools and appears to hinge around branched-chain amino acids which are feedback regulators of insulin release (Munro, 1969). Insulin, like growth hormone and testosterone, is an anabolic hormone with respect to amino acid metabolism, capable of stimulating free amino acid retention in peripheral pools and permitting synthesis of protein.

Glucagon infusion also causes plasma amino acids to fall; this response is the result of a central or splanchnic effect of the hormone which allows amino acids to serve gluconeogenesis in liver and other central tissues. Glucagon is thus anabolic and catabolic in its actions on amino acids. Certain amino acids infused at rates of 1mM/kg body weight have a profound glucagon-stimulating effect, particularly those which enter the gluconeogenic pathway in the form of pyruvate (Rocha et al., 1972). Other amino acids fail to stimulate glucagon release effectively; among these are the branched-chain amino acids.

A balancing effect of glucagon and insulin upon nitrogen metabolism emerges. In periods of nitrogen abundance (postprandial), certain nitrogenous precursors of glucose can be removed centrally for gluconeogenesis and glycogen synthesis. In late starvation, when glucagon release is minimal, nitrogen is conserved for its own essential needs or is available for release from peripheral pools in the absence of insulin for use as glucogenic precursors in central tissues. In the presence of glucose or branched-chain amino acid excess, amino acids are retained in peripheral pools until they are called upon. These seemingly effective regulatory mechanisms can, however, work against the host, as we shall see later in discussions of the effects of malnutrition and obesity upon aminoacidemia.

Two other hormones exhibit general translocational actions on amino acids. Both are catabolic in this action. *Corticosteroids* and *thyroxine* each cause the loss of protein and amino acids from skeletal muscle and other peripheral tissues; at the same time, splanchnic tissues are encouraged to gain protein and amino acids. However, the two hormones have quite different effects at the finer levels of intracellular control. For instance, corticosteroid hormones lower tyrosine in plasma by the induction of hepatic tyrosine transaminase despite accelerated tyrosine transfer to the liver (Betheil et al., 1965), whereas thyroxine raises plasma tyrosine because catabolism in liver does not increase to compensate for the increased transfer (Rivlin and Melmon, 1965).

A transport-oriented interpretation of hormonal effects on amino acids originated in the seminal work of Christensen's group (Noall et al., 1957), who showed that several hormones could stimulate the net uptake of a metabolically inert amino acid (α-aminoisobutyric acid) by different tissues. Responsiveness to the particular hormone was, in general, tissue-specific. The mechanism by which hormone responsiveness is translated into a membrane event is still largely unknown—that is, whether it is through synthesis of new membrane transport protein(s), improved coupling of cumulative transport with energy metabolism, change in efflux barrier or enhancement of membrane affinity for substrate binding uptake (Akedo and Christensen, 1962; Elsas et al., 1968).

At Enzymes

Hormones also regulate amino acid metabolism by modulating intracellular enzyme activity. Amino acid outflow or inflow into metabolic pools can be retarded or accelerated by hormonal control of enzymes which are situated at key entry or exit points and which have a high turnover number (short half-life). The effect of hormones is again target-specific: for example, corticosteroids augment hepatic tyrosine transaminase activity, the first step in tyrosine oxidation, whereas thyroxine does not affect this step.

The mechanisms by which steroids regulate amino acid catabolism have been extensively examined, particularly through the study of tryptophan pyrrolase and tyrosine transaminase and their induction (increase in specific activity of the enzyme) by hydrocortisone (Civen and Knox, 1959; Knox, 1963; Wicks, 1968). The inductive effect of the hormone is inhibited by puromycin and actinomycin, both being agents which block protein synthesis. The hormone does not affect the interaction between the relevant apoenzyme and its *coenzyme* (or cofactor), yet it causes both *apoenzyme* and *holoenzyme* (apoenzyme plus coenzyme) to accumulate in the cell. This could occur either by an increase in the number of RNA templates upon which the enzyme is synthesized, or by a blockade of enzyme degradation, in the face of a constant rate of RNA-dependent protein synthesis. The latter mechanism accounts for the induction of tryptophan pyrrolase by cortisone (Schimke, 1970). Hormonal "induction" of this type may reflect a conformational change in the enzyme brought about by the hormone so that the affinity of the enzyme for degradative processes is lessened; or the hormone may affect the activity of the degradative process itself. Induction of enzyme activity and thus regulation of amino acid metabolism is, however, itself dependent on the availability of amino acids. For example, induction of hepatic tyrosine transaminase by hydrocortisone is dependent on the availability of free tryptophan to maintain enzyme synthesis (Wurtman et al., 1968). Since the same hormone also accelerates tryptophan catabolism, intracellular depletion of tryptophan by its own oxidation must be offset to allow tyrosine transaminase induction.

Conformational changes in enzymes with subunits and a defined quaternary structure can occur under the influence of hormones. The classic model for this type of regulation is mitochondrial glutamate dehydrogenase. The enzyme is a tetramer with a molecular weight of 250,000 to 300,000. The enzyme can polymerize, at higher protein concentrations, to a molecule of about four times its usual weight; or it can be dissociated into subunits. The physical state of the molecule determines its activity. In the associated state, it has potent glutamate dehydrogenase activity; the dissociated form, however, has weak activity toward glutamate and a shift in substrate preference to alanine. Dissociation in vitro is promoted by the sex steroids progesterone, stilbestrol and estradiol and by thyroxine.

Regulation by Coenzyme or Cofactor

Many of the apoenzymes which catalyze interconversion, biosynthesis and degradation of amino acids and their derivatives require a *coenzyme* (see Chapter 22). The most important coenzyme in amino acid metabolism is pyridoxal-5-phosphate (see Figure 4–4), a derivative of *vitamin B_6*. But other coenzymes are also involved. *Vitamin B_{12}* coenzymes are required in the remethylation stage of methionine metabolism and in methylmalonate conversion to succinate; *folate* plays many roles in the transfer of methyl, methylene, formyl and formimino groups. *Vitamin B_1* (thiamine) coenzyme, thiamine pyrophosphate, participates in oxidative decarboxylation reactions. *Vitamin B_2* (riboflavin) contributes the flavin mononucleotide and flavin adenine nucleotide coenzymes required for several conversion reactions involving derivatives from amino acid precursors. *Biotin* controls the carboxylation steps in amino acid catabolism, and *ascorbic acid* is the coenzyme for *p*-hydrophenylpyruvic acid oxidase, an important enzyme in tyrosine oxidation.

In addition to the coenzyme derivatives of vitamins, there are other *cofactors* which are necessary to maintain optimal activity of holoenzymes. Some of these are metal ions, while others are more complex, such as the hematin moiety of tryptophan pyrrolase. In general, the cofactors are tightly bound, as *prosthetic groups*, to the apoenzyme, whereas the coenzymes experience a complex but reversible type of binding (Mudd, 1970).

Depletion of coenzyme, or cofactor, depresses catalytic activity of enzymes. Regulation in the form of specific activation or induction of enzyme activity has been carefully examined in three different situations: pyridoxal-5-phosphate induction of certain transaminases; hematin induction of tryptophan pyrrolase; and ascorbate activation of *p*-HPPA oxidase.

Induction by Pyridoxal-5-Phosphate

Vitamin B_6 (pyridoxine, pyridoxamine or pyridoxal) is transported into the cell, where phosphorylation takes place to form the coenzyme (McCormick et al., 1961; Pal and Christensen, 1961). Administration of pyridoxine to the intact animal significantly augments the activity of certain hepatic transaminases (Lin and Knox, 1958; Greengard and Gordon, 1963). Specific activity increases, and the net concentration of apoenzyme rises. The mechanism for this effect is still unclear, but it is suspected that saturation of apoenzyme with the coenzyme retards its degradation (turnover) (Mudd, 1970; Mudd et al., 1970).

Hematin Induction

The effect of hematin upon tryptophan pyrrolase activity is apparently the best example of the retarded turnover mechanism of induction. Fiegelson and Greengard (1961) and Greengard (1963) showed that tryptophan pyrrolase requires hematin cofactor; saturation with cofactor caused induction, with an increase in the effective concentration of apoenzyme in the cell. A shift in equilibrium from dissociated enzyme complex to the cofactor saturated state occurred during cofactor induction. The evidence suggests that the enzyme concentration rises because the rate of degradation (turnover) has been attenuated by cofactor-apoenzyme interaction.

Activation by Ascorbate

This event is not a true enzyme induction, but it is a mechanism by which regulation of tyrosine oxidation can occur. The p-HPPA oxidase apoenzyme must be in the reduced form for optimal activity (see Chapter 16). The enzyme can be inhibited by its substrate in the absence of ascorbic acid; saturation with the cofactor restores activity. These relationships are of particular interest in the neonatal period, when tyrosine oxidation is in precarious balance. The intake of substrate is high, while the available amount of hepatic oxidase is low. Administration of large amounts of ascorbate (25 times the dosage required by the adult on the basis of a body weight coefficient) maintains tyrosine oxidation effectively by activating the critical enzyme.

Regulation by Substrate and Product

Amino acid metabolism in microorganisms is exquisitely regulated through substrate induction and product (feedback) inhibition. In the mammal, amino acid metabolism is less adaptive, and several of the highly adaptive steps identified in microorganisms are virtually constitutive in the mammal. However, some enzyme proteins have a relatively short half-life in mammalian cells, and it is these enzymes that are often involved in regulation. For example, the half-life of the soluble tyrosine transaminase in rat liver is two to three hours, and that of tryptophan pyrrolase is two to four hours (Schimke, 1970). Both enzymes have the capacity for substrate induction within a few hours. Protein (enzyme) synthesis must be intact for rapid induction to occur, while the mechanism of substrate induction is carried out by attenuation of the apoenzyme degradation rate. For substrate induction of tryptophan pyrrolase to occur there must already be conjugation of hematin with apoenzyme to form the activated holoenzyme; the latter does not occur effectively in the absence of substrate.

Induction of other enzymes in critical areas of amino acid metabolism may require a much longer time scale. Alanine transaminase requires 24 hours, and arginase, 48 hours, to respond with a twofold increase in activity to an inductive stimulus. As expected, the half-life of these enzymes is measured in days instead of hours. Schimke (1970) has shown that under steady-state dietary conditions, arginase activity rises in liver when the animal has a very high protein diet; the augmentation of arginase reflects a change in the rate of its synthesis while degradation rates are constant. On the other hand, acute changes from one level of protein intake to another influence degradation rates, so that adaptation to changing substrate intake occurs at this level, according to the specific environmental condition.

Isozymes

The presence of more than one form of an enzyme in the cell affords another mechanism for regulation of amino acid metabolism. Isozymes are usually formed from different combinations of subunits shared among the different forms of the enzyme. In this way, conservatism at the genetic level is compatible with diversity at the phenotypic level. Several enzymes controlling the catabolism of amino acids exist as isozymes. Several transaminases occur in more than one form, such as the amino transferases for glutamic-oxaloacetic (Wada and Morino, 1964), γ-aminobutyric-α-ketoglutarate (Waksman and Bloch, 1968) and tyrosine-α-ketoglutarate substrate pairs (Fellman et al., 1969). The various isozymes are usually located in different subcellular compartments: for example, one form in the mitochondria, another in the cytoplasm. The dispersal between segregated cellular locations must, of course, serve different metabolic needs. Thus, to find a difference in the kinetic properties of the isozymes would not be surprising. This is true of substrate binding by isozymic transaminases (Henson and Cleland, 1964) and also of coenzyme binding: for example, the affinity of the soluble glutamic-oxaloacetic transaminase for coenzyme (pyridoxal-5-phosphate) is almost 1000-fold greater than its mitochondrial form (Wada and Morino, 1964). "Direction" of metabolic flow may be possible because of isozymes in subcellular compartments, although the full significance of the phenomenon is not yet clear. One important role they may have is regulation of metabolism when cellular differentiation is in progress during ontogeny (Knox, 1972).

GENERALIZED PERTURBATIONS OF AMINO ACID METABOLISM

In addition to the specific, inherited disorders of amino acid metabolism to be described in Parts II and III of this book, there are other acquired and multifactorial conditions which broadly perturb the balance of amino acid metabolism.

Obesity

Plasma amino acid levels are altered in the euglycemic obese subject (Felig et al., 1969a). The branched-chain amino acids and tyrosine and phenylalanine are significantly elevated, while glycine is depressed. The hyperaminoacidemia apparently reflects insulin ineffectiveness in the control of amino acid uptake and release at the level of skeletal muscle. Postprandial peaking of amino acids may be the feedback signal for the exaggerated release of insulin which accounts for the high plasma content of the hormone in the presence of normal blood glucose levels in obese subjects.

Starvation

Amino acid levels in plasma experience cyclic changes in starvation (Fig. 4–9). These undulations reflect progressive changes in the amino acid pools of skeletal muscle and the splanchnic handling of amino acids (Felig et al., 1969b; Adibi et al., 1970; Cahill, 1970). In early starvation, branched-chain and other amino acids exit from muscle into plasma, and so a rise in their plasma content is seen. This stage reflects the abatement of insulin control on muscle pools; a new equilibrium follows as starvation proceeds. Plasma alanine and other glycogenic amino acids fall from the outset, probably because liver augments their extraction and utilization for gluconeogenesis in early starvation. At a later stage in the progress of starvation, substrate depletion occurs; alanine remains low, and hepatic gluconeogenesis dependent on this amino acid is ultimately attenuated, the concomitant drain on protein being diminished also. During the evolution of starvation, brain adapts to fueling from ketone bodies in place of glucose (Owen et al., 1967); at the same time, kidney assumes an increasingly large role in gluconeogenesis and ammoniagenesis. It is able to do this by extracting more glycine, alanine and proline as gluconeogenic substrates; glutamine extraction under these conditions will serve ammoniagenesis and

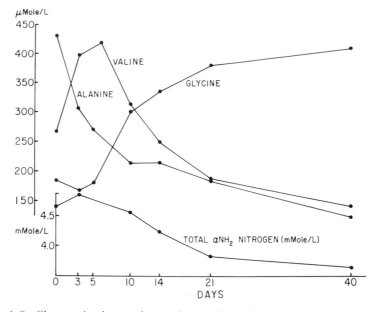

Figure 4–9 Changes in the steady-state levels of certain amino acids in plasma chosen to represent three types of response to starvation in adult human subjects. Alanine falls steadily, as it is extracted more avidly from the splanchnic circulation and is depleted in peripheral tissues. Insulinopenia in early starvation permits exaggerated branched-chain amino acid release initially; with progressive starvation, delivery is depleted and the plasma level falls. Glycine rises steadily for reasons not yet fully explained. Splanchnic tissues (kidney particularly) extract glycine avidly for gluconeogenesis during starvation. (From Cahill, G. F.: New Eng. J. Med. *282*:668, 1970.)

glucogenesis (Marliss et al., 1971). The combination of augmented supply of glycine in plasma during starvation (Fig. 4–9) and enhanced renal extraction of glucogenic substrates represents one of the most important adaptations of amino acid metabolism to a threatening pathophysiological situation.

Protein-Calorie Malnutrition (Kwashiorkor)

Typical and striking changes in the plasma amino acid pattern have been demonstrated in kwashiorkor (Holt, 1963). They are characterized by relative elevations of proline, serine, glycine and phenylalanine in plasma as well as relative deficiencies of the branched-chain amino acids tryptophan, methionine and threonine and of arginine and citrulline (Holt et al., 1963; Saunders et al., 1967) (Fig. 4–10). The pattern resembles the effect of starvation complicated by nitrogen deficiency. Marked oscillation of plasma amino acids occurs during the early stages of protein depletion in protein-calorie malnutrition, and treatment is difficult—a reflection, probably, of the depletion of tissue pools in which to store amino acids and the loss of enzymes to regulate catabolism and anabolism. Intestinal changes also compromise the availability of dietary nitrogen in these states (see Chapter 2).

Liver and Kidney Disease

Diseases of organs controlling amino acid equilibrium should perturb metabolism. Felig and colleagues (1970) showed that viral hepatitis blunts the

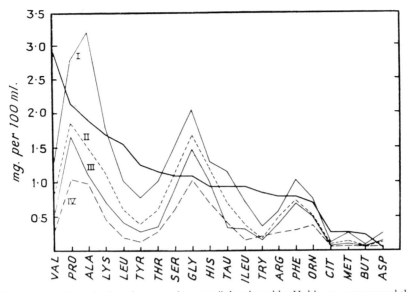

Figure 4-10 The classic "plasma aminogram" developed by Holt's group to reveal the impact of protein-calorie malnutrition at various stages of severity (*I*, mildest; *IV*, most severe). The thicker solid line is the mean plasma value for the amino acid profile in healthy control children. The distortion of the profile reflects many effects of protein calorie malnutrition. (From Holt, L. E., Jr., et al.: Lancet (ii), 1343, 1963.)

response of plasma amino acids to a glucagon stimulus, and they suggested that hepatocellular disease blocks the ability to support gluconeogenesis from amino acids. Acute hepatocellular disease causes a rise in tyrosine and methionine in plasma, whereas biliary disease does not (Feigin, 1972). Generalized hyperaminoacidemia and other amino acid changes have long been recognized in acute hepatic deterioration and other types of liver disease (Munro, 1970).

Advanced renal failure and, in particular, uremia cause changes in plasma amino acids, but these are difficult to evaluate because of the unusual dietary factors which prevail in advanced renal disease. One finding of interest—the abnormal presence of 3-methylhistidine in plasma—presumably reflects breakdown of actin and myosin, which are myofibrillar proteins in muscle and which contain this unusual amino acid (Condon and Asatoor, 1971). Other workers find that essential amino acids are lower than normal in uremia, when protein intake is drastically restricted (McGale et al., 1972). These changes are probably the effect of starvation and protein depletion more than they reflect the course of uremia.

Infection

Acute infection depresses plasma amino acids. Absolute levels fall in bacterial infection, and circadian periodicity is altered in viral infection. The changes occur very early in the host response—in fact, prior to the onset of clinical disease. The amino acid response is believed to be mediated by a leukocyte factor whose release is initiated by the infection (Feigin, 1972).

REFERENCES

Adibi, S. A., Drash, A. L., and Livi, E. D.: Hormone and amino acid levels in altered nutritional states. J. Lab. Clin. Med. *76*:722–732, 1970.

Akedo, H., and Christensen, H. N.: Nature of insulin action on amino acid uptake by the isolated diaphragm. J. Biol. Chem. *237*:118–122, 1962.

Aoki, T. T., Brennan, M. F., Muller, W. A., Moore, F. D., and Cahill, G. F., Jr.: Effect of insulin on muscle glutamate uptake; whole blood versus plasma glutamate analysis. J. Clin. Invest. *51*: 2889–2894, 1972.

Bach, S. J., and Holmes, E. G.: The effect of insulin on carbohydrate formation in the liver. Biochem. J. *31*:89–95, 1937.

Benoy, M. P., and Elliott, K. A. C.: The metabolism of lactic and pyruvic acids in normal and tumor tissues. V. Synthesis of carbohydrate. Biochem. J. *31*:1268–1274, 1937.

Betheil, J. J., Feigelson, M., and Feigelson, P.: The differential effects of glucocorticoid on tissue and plasma amino acid levels. Biochim. Biophys. Acta *104*:92–97, 1965.

Borsook, M., Deasy, C. L., Haagen-Smith, A. J., Keighley, G., and Lowy, P. H.: Metabolism of C¹⁴-labelled glycine, L-histidine, L-leucine, L-lysine. J. Biol. Chem. *187*:839–848, 1950.

Cahill, G. F., Jr.: Starvation in man. New Eng. J. Med. *282*:668–675, 1970.

Cahill, G. F., Jr., and Owen, O. E.: The role of the kidney in the regulation of protein metabolism. *In* Munro, H. N., ed., Mammalian Protein Metabolism, Vol. IV. Academic Press, New York, pp. 539–585, 1970.

Christensen, H. N.: Free amino acids and peptides in tissues. *In* Munro, H. N., and Allison, J. B., eds., Mammalian Protein Metabolism, Vol. I. Academic Press, New York, pp. 105–124, 1964.

Christensen, H. N., and Cullen, A. M.: Effects of non-metabolizable analogs on the distribution of amino acids in the rat. Biochim. Biophys. Acta *150*:237–252, 1968.

Civen, M., and Knox, W. E.: The independence of hydrocortisone and tryptophan inductions of tryptophan pyrrolase. J. Biol. Chem. *234*:1787–1790, 1959.

Cleland, W. W.: The kinetics of enzyme-catalyzed reactions with two or more substrates or products. I. Nomenclature and rate equations. Biochim. Biophys. Acta *67*:104–137, 1963.

Coleman, J. E.: Metabolic interrelationships between carbohydrates, lipids and proteins. *In* Bondy, P. K., ed., Duncan's Diseases of Metabolism, 6th edition. W. B. Saunders Company, Philadelphia, pp. 89–198, 1968.

Condon, J. R., and Asatoor, A. M.: Amino acid metabolism in uraemic patients. Clin. Chim. Acta *32*:333–337, 1971.

Elsas, L. J., Albrecht, I., and Rosenberg, L. E.: Insulin stimulation in rat diaphragm: Relationship to protein synthesis. J. Biol. Chem. *243*:1846–1853, 1968.

Elwyn, D. H.: The role of liver in regulation of amino acid and protein metabolism. *In* Munro, H. N., ed., Mammalian Protein Metabolism, Vol. IV. Academic Press, New York, pp. 523–558, 1970.

Elwyn, D. H., Launder, W. J., Parikh, H. C., and Wise, E. M., Jr.: Roles of plasma and erythrocytes in interorgan transport of amino acids in dogs. Amer. J. Physiol. *222*:1333–1342, 1972.

Exton, J. H., Mallette, L. E., Jefferson, L. S., Wong, E. H. A., Friedmann, N., Miller, T. B., Jr., and Park, C. R.: The hormonal control of hepatic gluconeogenesis. Recent Progr. Hormone Res. *126*:411–461, 1970.

Exton, J. H., and Park, C. R.: Control of gluconeogenesis in liver. I. General features of gluconeogenesis in the perfused livers of rats. J. Biol. Chem. *242*:2622–2636, 1967.

Feigin, R. D.: Personal communication, 1972.

Felig, P., Brown, W. V., Levine, R. A., and Klatskin, G.: Glucose homeostasis in viral hepatitis. New Eng. J. Med. *283*:1436–1440, 1970.

Felig, P., Marliss, E., and Cahill, G. F., Jr.: Plasma amino acid levels and insulin secretion in obesity. New Eng. J. Med. *281*:811–816, 1969a.

Felig, P., Owen, O. E., Wahren, J., and Cahill, G. F., Jr.: Amino acid metabolism during prolonged starvation. J. Clin. Invest. *48*:584–594, 1969b.

Felig, P., Pozefsky, T., Marliss, E., and Cahill, G. F., Jr.: Alanine: Key role in gluconeogenesis. Science *167*:1003–1004, 1970.

Fellman, J. H., Vanbellinghen, P. J., Jones, R. T., and Koler, R. D.: Soluble and mitochondrial forms of tyrosine aminotransferase. Relationship to human tyrosinemia. Biochemistry *8*:615–622, 1969.

Gan, J. C., and Jeffay, H.: Origins and metabolism of the intracellular amino acid pools in rat liver and muscle. Biochim. Biophys. Acta *148*:448–459, 1967.

Goodman, A. D., Fuisz, R. E., and Cahill, G. F., Jr.: Renal gluconeogenesis in acidosis, alkalosis and potassium deficiency: Its possible role in regulation of renal ammonia production. J. Clin. Invest. *45*:612–619, 1966.

Goorno, W. E., Rector, F. C., Jr., and Seldin, D. W.: Relation of renal gluconeogenesis to ammonia production in the dog and rat. Amer. J. Physiol. *213*:969–974, 1967.

Greengard, O.: The role of coenzymes, cortisone and RNA in the control of liver enzyme levels. Advances Enzym. Regulat. *1*:61–76, 1963.

Greengard, O., and Gordon, M.: The cofactor-mediated regulation of apoenzyme levels in animal tissues. I. The pyridoxine-induced rise of rat liver tyrosine transaminase level in vivo. J. Biol. Chem. *238*:3708–3710, 1963.

Henson, P., and Cleland, W.: Kinetic studies of glutamic oxaloacetic transaminase isozymes. Biochemistry *3*:338–356, 1964.

Holden, J. T., ed.: Amino Acid Pools. Distribution, Formation and Function of Free Amino Acids. Elsevier, London, 1962.

Holt, L. E., Jr., Snyderman, S. E., Norton, P. M., Roitman, E., and Finch, J.: The plasma aminogram in kwashiorkor. Lancet (ii), 1343–1348, 1963.

Iqbal, K., and Ottaway, J. H.: Glutamine synthetase in muscle and kidney. Biochem. J. *119*:145–156, 1970.

Kaplan, J. H., and Pitot, H. C.: The regulation of intermediary amino acid metabolism in animal tissues. *In* Munro, H. N., ed., Mammalian Protein Metabolism, Vol. IV, Academic Press, New York, pp. 388–444, 1970.

Knox, W. E.: The adaptive control of tryptophan and tyrosine metabolism in animals. Trans. N.Y. Acad. Sci., Series II *25*:502–512, 1963.

Knox, W. E.: The protoplasmic patterns of tissues and tumors. Amer. Sci. *60*:480–488, 1972.

Krebs, H. A.: The metabolic fate of amino acids. *In* Munro, H. N., and Allison, J. B., eds., Mammalian Protein Metabolism, Vol. I. Academic Press, New York, pp. 125–176, 1964.

La Du, B. N.: Genetic variation in metabolic disorders. *In* Nyhan, W. L., ed., Amino Acid Metabolism and Genetic Variation. McGraw-Hill, New York, pp. 121–130, 1967.

Lehninger, A. L.: Biochemistry. The Molecular Basis of Cell Structure and Function. Worth Publishers, Inc., 1970.

Lin, E. C. C., and Knox, W. E.: Effect of vitamin B_6 deficiency on the basal and adapted levels of rat liver tyrosine and tryptophan transaminases. J. Biol. Chem. *233*:1183–1185, 1958.

Lyon, M. L., and Pitts, R. F.: Species differences in renal glutamine synthesis in vivo. Amer. J. Physiol. *216*:117–122, 1969.

Mallette, L. E., Exton, J. H., and Park, C. R.: Control of gluconeogenesis from amino acids in the perfused rat liver. J. Biol. Chem. *244*:5713–5723, 1969.

Manchester, K. L.: Sites of hormonal regulation of protein metabolism. *In* Munro, H. N., ed., Mammalian Protein Metabolism, Vol. IV. Academic Press, New York, pp. 229–298, 1970.

Marliss, E. B., Aoki, T. T., Pozefsky, T., Most, A. S., and Cahill, G. F., Jr.: Muscle and splanchnic glutamine and glutamate metabolism in postabsorptive and starved man. J. Clin. Invest. *50*: 814–817, 1971.

McCormick, D. B., Gregory, M. E., and Snell, E. E.: Pyridoxal phosphokinase. I. Assay, distribution, purification and properties. J. Biol. Chem. *236*:2076–2084, 1961.

McGale, E. H. F., Pickford, J. C., and Aber, G. M.: Quantitative changes in plasma amino acids in patients with renal disease. Clin. Chim. Acta *38*:395–403, 1972.

Meister, A.: Biochemistry of the Amino Acids, 2nd edition. Academic Press, New York, 1965.

Miller, L. L.: The role of the liver and the non-hepatic tissues in the regulation of free amino acid levels in the blood. *In* Holden, J. T., ed., Amino Acid Pools. American Elsevier, New York, pp. 708–721, 1962.

Milne, M. D., Scribner, B. H., and Crawford, M. A.: Non-ionic diffusion and the excretion of weak acids and bases. Amer. J. Med. *24*:709–729, 1958.

Mortimer, G. E., and Mondon, C. E.: Inhibition by insulin of valine turnover in liver. Evidence for a general control of proteolysis. J. Biol. Chem. *245*:2375–2383, 1970.

Mortimore, G. E., Woodside, K. H., and Henry, J. E.: Compartmentation of free valine and its relation to protein turnover in perfused rat liver. J. Biol. Chem. *247*:2776–2784, 1972.

Mudd, S. H.: Pyridoxine-responsive genetic disease. Fed. Proc. *30*:970–976, 1971.

Mudd, S. H., Edwards, W. A., Loeb, P. M., Brown, M. S., and Laster, L.: Homocystinuria due to cystathionine synthase deficiency: the effect of pyridoxine. J. Clin. Invest. *49*:1762–1773, 1970.

Munro, H. N.: Amino acids as feedback regulators of insulin. New Eng. J. Med. *281*:847–848, 1969.

Munro, H. N.: Free amino acid pools and their role in regulation. *In* Munro, H. N., ed., Mammalian Protein Metabolism, Vol. IV. Academic Press, New York, pp. 299–387, 1970.

Neims, A. H., and Hellerman, L.: Specificity of the D-amino acid oxidase in relation to glycine oxidase activity. J. Biol. Chem. *237*:PC976–PC978, 1962.

Neims, A. H., and Hellerman, L.: Flavoenzyme catalysis (740) Ann. Rev. Biochem. *39*:867–888, 1970.

Noall, M. W., Riggs, T. R., Walker, L. M., and Christensen, H. N.: Endocrine control of amino acid transfer. Distribution of an unmetabolized amino acid. Science *126*:1002–1005, 1957.

Owen, O. E., Morgan, A. P., Kemp, H. G., Sullivan, J. M., Herrera, M. G., and Cahill, G. F.: Brain metabolism during fasting. J. Clin. Invest. *46*:1589–1595, 1967.

Pal, P. N., and Christensen, H. N.: Uptake of pyridoxal and pyridoxal phosphate by Ehrlick ascites tumor cells. J. Biol. Chem. *236*:894–897, 1961.

Pitts, R. F.: The role of ammonia production and excretion in regulation of acid base balance. New Eng. J. Med. *284*:32–38, 1971.

Pozefsky, T., Felig, P., Tobin, J. D., Soeldner, J. S., and Cahill, G. F., Jr.: Amino acid balance across tissues of the forearm in post absorptive man. Effects of insulin at two dose levels. J. Clin. Invest. *48*:2273–2282, 1969.

Rivlin, R. S., and Melmon, K. L.: Cortisone-provoked depression of plasma tyrosine concentration: Relation to enzyme induction in man. J. Clin. Invest. *44*:1690–1698, 1965.

Rocha, D. M., Faloona, G. R., and Unger, R. H.: Glucagon stimulating activity of 20 amino acids in dogs. J. Clin. Invest. *51*:2346–2352, 1972.

Saunders, S. J., Truswell, A. S., Barbezat, G. O., Wittman, W., and Hansen, J. D. L.: Plasma free amino acid pattern in protein-calorie malnutrition. Reappraisal of its diagnostic value. Lancet (ii), 795–797, 1967.

Schimke, R. T.: Regulation of protein degradation in mammalian tissues. *In* Munro, H. N., ed., Mammalian Protein Metabolism, Vol. IV. Academic Press, New York, pp. 178–228, 1970.

Stifel, F. B., and Herman, R. H.: Is histidine an essential amino acid in man? Amer. J. Clin. Nutr. *25*:182–185, 1972.

Van Slyke, D. D., and Meyer, G. M.: The absorption of amino acids from the blood by the tissues. J. Biol. Chem., pp. 197–212, 1913.

Wada, H., and Morino, Y.: Comparative studies on glutamic-oxaloacetic transaminases from the mitochondrial and soluble fractions of mammalian tissues. *In* Harris, R. S., Wool, I. G., Loraine, J. A., eds., Vitamins and Hormones, Vol. 22. Academic Press, New York, pp. 411–443, 1964.

Waksman, A., and Bloch, M.: Identification of multiple forms of aminobutyrate transaminase in mouse and rat brain: subcellular localization. J. Neurochem. *15*:99–105, 1968.

Wicks, W. D.: Induction of tyrosine-α-ketoglutarate transaminase in fetal rat liver. J. Biol. Chem. *243*:900–906, 1968.

Wurtman, R. J., Shoemaker, W. J., and Larin, F.: Mechanism of daily rhythm in hepatic tyrosine transaminase activity: Role of dietary tryptophan. Proc. Nat. Acad. Sci. U.S.A. *59*:800–807, 1968.

Young, V. R.: The role of skeletal and cardiac muscle in the regulation of protein metabolism. *In* Munro, H. N., ed. Mammalian Protein Metabolism, Vol. IV. Academic Press, New York, pp. 586–674, 1970.

Chapter Five

METHODS OF ANALYSIS AND DIAGNOSIS OF AMINO-ACIDOPATHIES

INTRODUCTION

Advances in the technology of amino acid analysis have been, to a great extent, responsible for the growth of our knowledge about the diseases of amino acid metabolism. Without the technology there would be less material of interest to physicians in this book, and for that reason, it is appropriate to describe the methods which have brought us so much information—and so many patients.

Analytical methods will be discussed. Some of these reach back to the beginning of the 20th century, when Garrod first introduced his concepts about the inborn errors of metabolism. At that time, there were but two inborn errors of amino acid metabolism (alcaptonuria and cystinuria) known to cause abnormal urinary excretion of detectable metabolites. They, like many later-discovered aminoacidopathies, betrayed their presence initially through the application of simple chemical tests to the patient's urine. Phenylketonuria and tyrosinosis (Medes type) were subsequently discovered with the help of such tests, some of which are discussed in this chapter and elsewhere in the book.

Garrod had died by the time partition chromatography on filter paper, coupled with the ninhydrin stain, gained recognition for its ability to detect amino acids in body fluids and became widely applied to the investigation of human disease. Two decades later, the exponential growth of knowledge fostered by this technology had spawned some 50 "ninhydrin-positive" traits (Fig. 5–1); and the list of aminoacidopathies continues to grow as further technological developments, notably gas-liquid chromatography coupled with mass spectrometry, reveal new forms of "ninhydrin-negative" metabolic disorders.

The steady improvement in diagnostic precision and the broadening of the disease spectrum of interest to health-oriented scientists promoted more concern for the role of treatment of the inborn errors of amino acid metabolism. Theoretical principles were first successfully applied to the treatment of phenylketonuria in the early 1950's (see Chapter 15). Here, an element of success awakened interest in the value of early diagnosis in those rare patients with inborn errors, among the thousands of normal births, who could benefit from specific diagnosis and treatment. Enter, the age of mass screening. Before this era, diagnosis had been episodic; prospective diagnosis was confined to pedigrees in which mutations affecting amino acid metabolism were known to be segregating. Simple, economical, semiquantitative or qualitative methods for the accurate detection of perturbed amino acid steady states in body fluids became objectives of interest to many people. We see now that screening technology yields data on the prevalence of hereditary and acquired aminoacidopathies in the world's populations while providing societies with the opportunity to establish nationwide or regional programs for the screening, diagnosis, counseling and treatment of patients with disordered amino acid metabolism.

Because of their importance, we have devoted a section of the chapter to the principles and practices of screening for aminoacidopathies. We suspect that Garrod would have appreciated this. In his Croonian lectures, he observed that the aminoacidopathies would "advertise their presence in some conspicuous way, either by some strikingly unusual appearance of surface tissues or of ex-

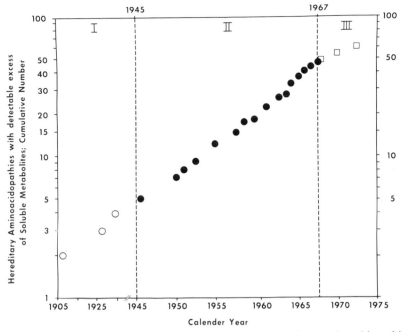

Figure 5–1   Three stages of development in our knowledge about aminoacidopathies. *I*, the pre-chromatography period (Garrod, 1908 → Dent, 1946), slow to yield up its puzzles, and only to those imaginative investigators who knew which chemical tests to use; *II*, the era of partition chromatography (Dent, 1946) in which the ninhydrin stain reigned supreme and which cast up a long series of "ninhydrin-positive" traits; *III*, the gas chromatography era, in which "new" diseases are being found through the identification of "ninhydrin-negative" compounds.

creta, *by the excretion of some substance which responds to a test habitually applied in the routine of clinical work* or by giving rise to obvious morbid symptoms" (Garrod, 1908, italics added). It is the desire of everyone today to prevent the appearance of 'obvious morbid symptoms'—hence the interest in screening. Because the options for screening and diagnosis now include prenatal diagnosis and heterozygote detection, we have also included abbreviated notes on the latter; and the chapter is rounded off with a classification of the diseases and traits known at present to reflect perturbed amino acid metabolism.

GENERAL METHODS FOR QUANTITATIVE AND QUALITATIVE ANALYSIS

Estimation of Total Amino Nitrogen

The amino acid nitrogen fraction in the urine normally represents about 3 to 4 per cent of the total nitrogen content. Analysis of amino nitrogen can therefore detect hyperexcretion of free amino acids (hyperaminoaciduria).

There are a number of methods for estimation of "α-amino nitrogen" (Scriver, 1962), and each suffers to a greater or lesser degree from the same drawbacks. First, these methods lack specificity, and as a result, substances other than free amino acids may be measured during the analysis. Second, the methods are usually cumbersome to use. But the most important objection is that biochemically significant variation in the concentration of a single amino acid may cause only a minor quantitative variation of total α-amino nitrogen;

this may not be distinguishable by a method which is designed to discriminate universal rather than particular variation.

Determination of Individual Amino Acids

Chemical, microbiological, chromatographic and electrophoretic methods are available for the measurement of specific amino acids.

Chemical Methods

Chemical methods are of most value to the investigator who wishes to study the metabolism of a particular amino acid. The investigations of hyperglycinemia, histidinemia, phenylketonuria and cystinuria, for example, were greatly assisted because specific chemical methods of analysis were available. Fluorometric methods which can be automated have been used widely in screening programs.

Microbiological Methods

Microbiological methods can be applied in several ways: amino acid auxotrophs can be used for quantitative analysis of particular amino acids, since, under the appropriate conditions, growth of the dependent organism is proportional to the amount of the amino acid in the sample. The early classic study of cystinuria by Yeh and colleagues (1947), which identified the presence of lysine and arginine in addition to cystine in the urine of affected patients, depended on microbiological methods. Specific enzymatic systems in microorganisms can be utilized to measure concentration of the relevant substrate; and the "inhibition assay," first adapted by Guthrie and colleagues (1963, 1964) for the measurement of phenylalanine, has gained widespread favor as an ingenious and effective method for quantitative analysis of some amino acids (see section on methods for screening, p. 105).

Electrophoretic Methods

Separation of amino acids in an electrical field, on a supporting medium of filter paper soaked with an appropriate buffer, has been exploited in many ways for qualitative analysis of amino acids. The zwitterion properties of amino acids offer the investigator the chance to choose buffers which allow selective analysis of different amino acids according to their pKa' values (Fig. 5–2). This aspect of electrophoretic analysis has been carefully investigated by Evered (1959), who employed low-voltage methods. High-voltage methods (Efron, 1960) offer the advantages of speed and compactness of the bands or spots, which are shown up by subsequent staining. However, monodimensional electrophoresis (Mabry and Karam, 1964) has severe limitations in its ability to separate, in a single run, all the amino acids of interest in a sample of urine or deproteinized plasma, and for this reason the two-dimensional method pioneered by Efron (1959), which employs filter-paper electrophoresis in one direction followed by partition chromatography in the second direction (Fig. 5–3), has found wide application and emulation.

Chromatography

The science of chromatography continues to develop, the literature expanding at the rate of about 4000 papers per year (Zweig et al., 1970; Juvet et al.,

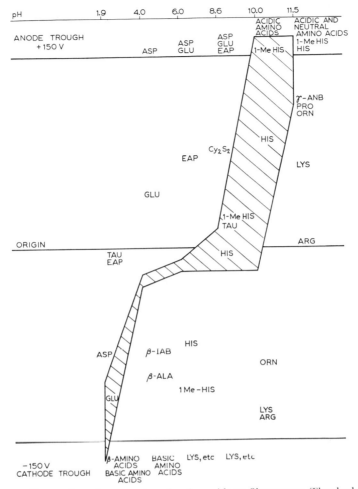

Figure 5–2　Electrophoretic separation of amino acids on filter paper. The shaded area represents neutral amino acid species; other amino acids are indicated by standard abbreviations. EAP = phosphoethanolamine; β-IAB = β-aminoisobutyrate; γ-ANB = γ-amino-n-butyrate. The effect of pH on separation is shown in this representative "map of the spots" which can be obtained by electrophoresis; the buffer pH required to obtain the desired separation is determined by placing a ruler on the vertical axis to intersect the line showing the pH values at the top. (From Evered, D. F.: Biochim. Biophys. Acta *36*:14–19, 1959.)

1970). Among the many forms of liquid column and partition chromatography, certain methods have served the analysis of amino acids in biological fluids particularly well.

Partition Chromatography.　This technique is used primarily for qualitative analysis. Development of the chromatogram in only one dimension may be effective for analysis of simple mixtures of amino acids, and this approach has been exploited for mass screening of blood and plasma amino acids. However, when the mixture is complex, the positions of different amino acids often coincide; resolution is improved if the chromatogram is developed in a different solvent in the second dimension (Consden et al., 1944; Dent, 1948). A wide repertoire of solvents for development of chromatograms and of stains for location of the amino acids and their derivatives has been developed over the

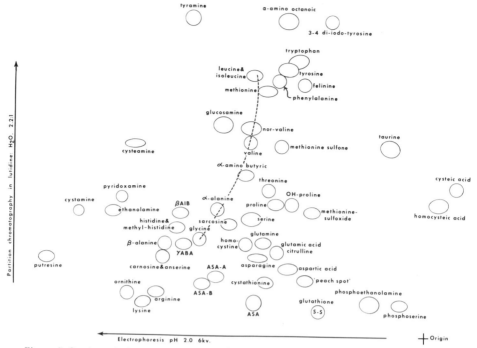

Figure 5–3   A typical "map of the spots" obtained by two-dimensional separation of amino acids and other ninhydrin-positive compounds. In this example, high-voltage electrophoresis is used in the horizontal axis, followed by partition chromatography in the vertical axis; after staining with ninhydrin, the amino acids are made visible. The map, as shown, is amplified from that published by Efron (1959), who originated this particular method. Other combinations of separation have been used to yield many different maps which aid the investigator in the study of amino acid patterns in body fluids.

years, many of which are described in books on the subject (Block et al., 1958; Hais and Macek, 1958; Smith, 1968, 1969).

Filter paper is generally used as the supporting medium in partition chromatography, particularly because many sheets (and samples) can be processed batchwise (Datta et al., 1950). In recent years, thin-layer chromatography, on preparations of silica and other inert materials spread over glass or plastic, has gained favor for its speed of solvent development (Jackson et al., 1968; Jørgensen et al., 1970). Urine may require treatment with urease and desalting in order to obtain satisfactory chromatograms on some thin-layer supporting materials. These preparative steps are usually not required for filter paper techniques.

Liquid Elution Chromatography on Ion-Exchange Resin Columns.   This method (illustrated in Figure 3–1) has become the standard for quantitative analysis of complex mixtures of amino acids in solution, particularly since semi-automation (Moore et al., 1958; Spackman et al., 1958) superseded the manual methods originally developed by Moore and Stein (1954). Data on the amino acid content of various body fluids (see Tables 3–1 through 3–6) are obtained almost exclusively by this method of analysis. Programs for step-wise elution with a sequence of buffers (Moore et al., 1958) or for gradient elution (Piez and Morris, 1960) are usually employed to obtain reproducible resolution of the amino acids. The amino acid composition of physiological fluids is often very complex, and Hamilton's study (1963) showed that urine contains in excess of 150 ninhydrin-reacting compounds, not all of which are amino acids.

The increased demand for precise quantitative methods for the investigation of amino acid metabolism in man, and for the studies of protein structure, stimulated much activity in the development of methodology, many aspects of which have been reviewed elsewhere (Peters and Berridge, 1970; Zweig et al., 1970; Berridge et al., 1971; Scriver et al., 1971). Studies of specific groups of amino acids by column methods have been assisted by the development of selective programs for accelerated analysis on short resin columns (see, for example, Shih et al., 1967; Benson et al., 1967; Scriver et al., 1968; Grimble and Whitehead, 1971). The advantages of the latter type of analysis are related to the use for which they are intended, but by way of example we can mention the short column analysis of phenylalanine and tyrosine, which requires less than an hour to obtain values for which the analytical error is $<\pm3\%$ (Shih et al., 1967; Scriver et al., 1968). Standard column methods would demand six hours of analyzer time to obtain the same result. Levy and colleagues (1971) have recently shown that blood collected on filter paper can be quantitatively transferred to short ion-exchange columns for rapid analysis of phenylalanine and tyrosine, thus providing a useful back-up procedure for mass screening programs which use blood spots collected on filter paper.

Gas Chromatography (With Mass Spectrometry). For many years there has been interest in the potential advantages of gas chromatography (GC) with gas-liquid interface for analysis of amino acids in biological fluids. The very small sample size which is required, the high sensitivity of the method (capable of detecting 10^{-10}M amino acid) and the high speed of analysis (two hours or less) are all desirable features. However, consistency in the derivatization procedure prior to analysis has been a troublesome matter met to some extent by the formation of N-trifluoroacetyl, N-butyl esters (Darbre and Islam, 1968). Zumwalt, Kuo and Gehrke (1971) were ultimately able to publish GC data on the total amino acid content (about 5 μg) in about 25 μl of plasma which compared favorably with data obtained by standard ion-exchange, resin-column, elution chromatography of much larger plasma samples. However, the preparatory work is still too cumbersome to allow GC analysis any advantage for routine analysis of urine amino acids.

GC is at present the method of choice for the identification of "ninhydrin-negative" derivatives of free amino acids. Horning and Horning (1971), Mamer et al. (1971) and Jellum et al. (1971, 1972) have published representative papers describing the potential of GC to identify metabolites in body fluids. The power of the instrumentation is further increased if the GC outflow can be coupled to the inlet of a mass spectrometer (MS), so that mass numbers of the compounds can be determined. A Norwegian group (Jellum et al., 1972) has discovered three "new" diseases (methylmalonic aciduria, β-methylcrotonyl-CoA carboxylase deficiency and pyroglutamic aciduria) since they initiated GC-MS methods to study selected patients; and a Canadian group (Daum et al., 1971) discovered a new disorder of isoleucine catabolism (Fig. 5-4) shortly after initiating a GC-MS analytic program. The use of computerized data processing to match the unknown mass spectra with a library of reference spectra (17,000 examples in the Norwegian library) will enhance the ease and reliability with which unusual compounds in biological fluids are first recognized and subsequently identified. A résumé of the known inborn errors of amino acid metabolism would include all the conditions detectable by the GC-MS system, according to the recent survey by Jellum et al. (1972). It is equally apparent that many "*unborn*" errors of metabolism merely await discovery by this approach in the future.

Mass spectrometry will distinguish compounds labeled with nonradioactive-stable isotopes from those containing no ^{15}N, ^{14}C or deuterium. Therefore, it

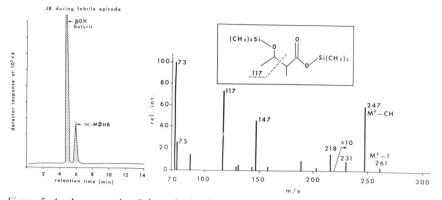

Figure 5-4   An example of data obtained by combined gas chromatography–mass spectrometry (GC-MS). The initial separation of the derivatized metabolite is achieved by GC; the outflow from the GC analytic column is then directed to the inlet of the mass spectrometer, where the compounds undergo ion bombardment and disintegration to yield a series of spectra, from which the mass number and probable structure of the molecule can be deduced. The figure shows the GC chromatogram and the corresponding MS spectra of the silylated derivative of α-methyl-β-hydroxybutyric acid, a derivative of isoleucine which was present in large excess in the urine of a patient with a recently discovered hereditary disorder of isoleucine metabolism first described by Daum et al. (1971). (See Chapter 14.)

should be possible to examine the metabolism of amino acids safely with these techniques in normal subjects and in those with inborn errors of metabolism. These methods should be applicable also to the study of mutant traits in somatic cell culture systems, where relatively little has been done, so far, to study the metabolite pools in fibroblast culture systems. The use of stable isotopes in the culture system should permit the investigator to follow metabolic conversions of amino acids in the cultured cells and in the medium, despite the small amount of available material. We anticipate developments in this area in the immediate future. In the meantime, investigators have already begun to use deuterated amino acids to re-examine the classic hereditary aminoacidopathies and their genetic variants. A recent paper by Curtius, Völlmin and Baerlocher (1972) describes the use of deuterated phenylalanine to study phenylalanine metabolism in patients with phenylketonuria and other hyperphenylalaninemic traits.

PITFALLS IN THE INTERPRETATION OF QUANTITATIVE DATA

Knowledge of the normal patterns and concentrations of amino acids in body fluids permits the investigator to recognize the abnormal finding when it is encountered. However, there is a danger that artifacts in the preparation and analysis of samples may alter their amino acid content, so that the distinction between genuine and false abnormalities will be blurred. It *is* important to pay attention to the details of sample preparation, and the following are points of interest in the handling of plasma or serum for column chromatography (Hansen and Perry, 1969; Scriver, Clow and Lamm, 1971).

The Effect of Venipuncture

The concentration of taurine and glutamic acid in plasma falls after venipuncture and returns to normal in about one hour (Rouser et al., 1962). This artifact should be recognized in studies requiring multiple, sequential venipunctures.

Plasma versus Serum, and Choice of Anticoagulant. In general, plasma is easier to prepare for application to the resin column. Plasma can be deproteinized within a few minutes after the venipuncture once the blood cells are separated by centrifugation, whereas serum may experience changes in its amino acid composition while standing at room temperature during clot retraction.

The choice of anticoagulant is also important. Most investigators use heparin; however, an excess of this anticoagulant may cause hemolysis, leading to release of ninhydrin-positive constituents from the red blood cells (see subsequent text). Impurities in some batches of ethylenediaminetetraacetic acid (EDTA), which is sometimes used as an anticoagulant, can produce ninhydrin-positive peaks in the elution chromatogram (Perry and Hansen, 1969).

Deproteinization

Many investigators prefer to deproteinize plasma with 3% sulfosalicylic acid (Gerritson et al., 1965; Dickinson et al., 1965) (plasma, 1 vol.:3% sulfosalicylic acid, 5 vol.), or with direct addition of 30 mg sulfosalicylic acid powder/ml plasma. After high-speed centrifugation (21,000 × g) for 10 minutes, the supernatant may be applied directly to the ion exchange column.

The other popular method of deproteinization (Moore and Stein, 1954) uses picric acid, which, because of its yellow color, must be removed on Dowex-1 or -2 resin before the deproteinized sample can be analyzed for taurine and urea. The sulfosalicylic acid method of deproteinization prevents substantial losses of tryptophan, citrulline and homocitrulline; the latter occur during the removal of picric acid from deproteinized samples. The arguments are numerous, both for and against sulfosalicylic acid versus picric acid as the agent of choice for deproteinization in various situations, and several discussions on the matter can be consulted: for example, Gerritson et al., 1965; Dickinson et al., 1965; DeWolfe et al., 1967; Knipfel et al., 1969.

Immediate removal of protein from the sample is important so as to avoid significant losses of disulfide amino acids that will bind to plasma proteins on standing at room temperature or in the refrigerator (Moore and Stein, 1954; Crawhall et al., 1966). Rapid deproteinization is necessary in field studies, in those situations in which shipment of samples is required or when the treatment of patients with disorders of sulfur amino acid metabolism is being monitored. This artifact explained why homocysteine was not found in plasma samples obtained from the original patients with homocystinuria (Carson et al., 1963).

Contamination

Hamilton (1965) has mentioned that contamination of glassware with sweat from a fingertip can jeopardize the reliability of analyses obtained by some high-sensitivity methods.

Platelets and leukocytes contain large amounts of taurine and dicarboxylic amino acids (Rouser et al., 1962; Soupart, 1962). Therefore, plasma or serum samples can be contaminated when these substances are released from the cellular constituents in the buffy coat. Plasma should be drawn off from the cell-plasma interface with care in order to avoid disturbing the buffy coat.

Hemolysis of Red Blood Cells

Glutathione (both reduced and oxidized) is present in red cells. Arginase from erythrocytes may diminish arginine and increase ornithine in plasma.

Plasma cystine may be lowered, either by dilution with an intracellular pool that is low in cystine, or by binding to protein in the hemolysate. The concentration of other amino acids is not significantly altered by hemolysis, since their concentration in mature red cells is similar to that of plasma (Soupart, 1962; Winter and Christensen, 1964; Levy and Barkin, 1971).

Storage

The concentration of glutamic and aspartic acids rises slowly, and glutamine and asparagine fall equivalently, in samples stored for long periods at −20°C. These changes are minimized by storage at −68°C and enhanced at −4°C or at room temperature (Dickinson et al., 1965; DeWolfe et al., 1967; Perry and Hansen, 1969). Evaporation of samples, or elution of amino acids from ion exchange columns, at temperatures above 40°C will reduce the glutamine and asparagine content of plasma samples.

Table 5–1 summarizes the artifacts related to techniques of processing the blood sample which affect its amino acid content. Many of these hazards pertain also to the handling of urine, cerebrospinal fluid and amniotic fluid. In the case of urine, the presence of enzymes released from damaged kidney tissue or contamination with bacteria may increase free amino acids by hydrolysis of peptides and proteins or remove free amino acids through degradation.

Metabolic events unrelated to any primary aminoacidopathy may also affect the amino acid steady state. Some of these (e.g., the nutritional state, circadian variation and infection) are discussed elsewhere in this book. They constitute a form of artifact which modifies the qualitative amino acid pattern and must be considered in its interpretation.

METHODS FOR MASS SCREENING

The techniques described in the previous section were developed primarily to analyze amino acids in aqueous solutions under convenient laboratory

Table 5–1   Artifacts Which Affect the Amino Acid Content of Plasma Samples

| | Effect on Particular Amino Acids | |
Procedure	Concentration in Sample Decreases	Concentration in Sample Increases
1. Repeated venipuncture (effect on serum or plasma)	Taurine, glutamic acid	
2. Clotting of serum standing at room temperature	Glutamine, asparagine	Taurine, aspartic acid, glutamic acid
3. Delay in deproteinization of sample	Cystine, homocystine, and mixed disulfides	
Picric acid method[a]	Citrulline, homocitrulline, tryptophan	
4. Contamination with platelets and WBC		Taurine, aspartic acid, glutamic acid
RBC (hemolysis)	Arginine, cystine	Glutathione, ornithine
"Fingerprints" (sweat)		Many amino acids
5. Storage of sample at temperature above −68°C	Glutamine, asparagine, tryptophan	Glutamic acid, aspartic acid
Handling and elution at temperature >4°C	Glutamine, asparagine	Glutamic acid, aspartic acid

[a]Losses occur during step when picric acid is removed on Dowex-1 or -2 resin.

conditions. Although any of these methods can be used to screen for aminoacidopathies, they are generally too cumbersome or expensive for purposes of mass screening of populations.

Effective liquid urine testing programs which employ imaginative adaptations of chemical tests and chromatographic methods have been developed (Dent, 1951, 1957; Perry et al., 1966; Tocci, 1967; Berry et al., 1968; Buist, 1968). However, the adaptation of these same methods to mass screening of newborn infants has been impractical, usually because the techniques cannot be sufficiently automated. Since the examination of liquid urine from the newborn infant is not compatible with the practical requirements of mass screening, initial collection of urine samples on filter paper has been emphasized, and many aminoacidopathies are identifiable when partition chromatography is applied to such samples (Levy et al., 1968b; Levy et al., 1972). The use of dried blood samples, collected and shipped on filter paper, was the initial and major advance in the application of screening technology to the detection of human aminoacidopathies (Guthrie and Susi, 1963). The technique effectively bridged the distance between the population in the field and the laboratory in which analysis of the sample must be performed. Heparinized capillary tubes can also be used to obtain samples of whole blood or plasma for mass screening purposes (Culley et al., 1962; Scriver, 1964), but there is not the same simplicity of handling and storage which is found in the filter paper method.

The analytical methods for mass detection of diseases of amino acid metabolism measure the free amino acid content of the sample; none measure the relevant enzyme activity directly. Three different methods of amino acid analysis have been employed.

Microbiological Methods

Guthrie and Susi (1963) adapted the "microbial inhibition assay" to screen for phenylketonuria. The principle of the method is simple. An organism (*B. subtilis* ATCC-6051) is suspended in an agar medium, into which is also incorporated the chemical β-2-thienylalanine, an inhibitor of the organism's growth. Phenylalanine in sufficient concentrations will overcome the effect of the inhibitor, and growth of the organism will occur. If a filter paper disc impregnated with blood is applied to the surface of the agar, one can determine whether the sample contains excessive amounts of phenylalanine by the size of the growth zone which appears around the disc (Fig. 5–5). Under defined conditions, the inhibition assay will distinguish phenylalanine levels in excess of about 4 mg% in whole blood. This particular test has now been used to screen over 12 million infants, and its technical adequacy has been clearly proved. When properly used, its ability to detect hyperphenylalaninemia is impressive.

The inhibition assay method has been adapted for the detection of other amino acids. In each, the unleashing of growth in the "detector" strain of microorganism around a blood-impregnated filter paper disc is used to ascertain whether the concentration of an index metabolite is present in excess in the sample. These supplementary assays will detect leucine, tyrosine, methionine, histidine, valine and argininosuccinic acid (the latter is, in fact, an auxotroph assay) (Guthrie, 1972).

Chemical Methods

Automated chemical and fluorometric analysis of amino acid content in dried blood samples, collected on filter paper, is the most sophisticated proced-

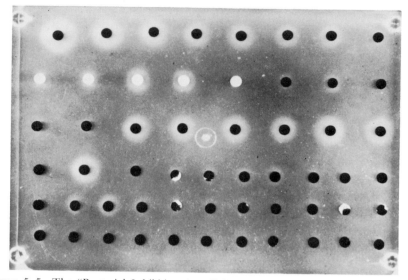

Figure 5–5   The "Bacterial Inhibition Assay" for phenylalanine applied to dried blood on filter paper discs (Guthrie and Susi, 1963). Pale areas around the dark, blood-soaked discs are the growth zones of microorganisms suspended in agar medium. Size of the zone is equivalent to amount of phenylalanine diffusing out of the blood sample on the disc. (Photograph kindly supplied by Dr. Michael Partington.)

ure now in use for mass screening. With electronic processing of the data, it is possible to obtain quantitation over a wide concentration range and total automation with precise internal and external controls. The first move to this type of screening was initiated by Hill and colleagues (1965), who automated the fluorometric method of McCaman and Robins (1962) for analysis of phenylalanine; an automated fluorometric method for determination of tyrosine in whole blood was soon added by Hochella (1967). Further diversification of completely automated, chemical analysis of selected amino acids can be anticipated in the future.

Chromatographic Methods

Partition chromatography provides a useful semiquantitative method for mass screening of amino acids in blood and urine. Chromatography in one dimension has been adapted for analysis of whole blood collected on filter paper discs (Efron et al., 1964) or of plasma from blood collected in heparinized capillary tubes (Scriver et al., 1964). Both methods, and useful modifications of them (Szeinberg et al., 1969; Adriaenssen et al., 1967), can identify many of the amino acids whose concentration in plasma will be altered in a number of the hereditary aminoacidopathies. Several large field trials (Levy et al., 1968a; Levy et al., 1972, dried blood spot method; Clow et al., 1969; Applegarth et al., 1970; Komrower et al., 1968, 1969; Raine et al., 1972, heparinized capillary tube method) have demonstrated the value of this approach to comprehensive mass screening for aminoacidopathies in the newborn population. Unfortunately, chromatographic methods resist automation, they depend on a dedicated human factor for interpretation of the amino acid patterns, and there are nagging technical variables.

One-dimensional partition chromatography of amino acids has also been successfully adapted for urine screening on a population basis (Levy et al.,

1968b; Levy, Madigan and Shih, 1972). Thus, any disease of amino acid metabolism which causes a significant change in the amino acid pattern of blood or urine can, in theory, be detected by these methods.

PRINCIPLES OF SCREENING FOR AMINOACIDOPATHIES

Over 90 per cent of North American infants are screened for metabolic disease of one form or another shortly after birth. Screening for genetic variation may serve one or more purposes. There is still a basic need for information about the frequency, natural history and inheritance of much genetic disease; some types of screening can help to supply this information. It may also be practical to establish mass screening for purposes of diagnosis, counseling and treatment of some forms of genetic disease; and in a number of situations, specialized screening procedures and prenatal diagnosis have widened the options available to persons at risk for major genetic illness.

The World Health Organization has issued two instructive technical reports (WHO, 1968, 1972) which discuss the practice and impact of screening for hereditary metabolic disease (including the disorders of amino acid metabolism). These reports recommend that pilot studies be carried out to gather information relevant to proposed mass screening programs, but mass screening on a public health basis is not recommended if there are no facilities for patient retrieval, diagnosis, counseling and treatment. Centralized facilities for the specific diagnosis, genetic counseling and subsequent management of the patient are strongly encouraged in both reports, which recognize that collaborative and interdisciplinary efforts are required if the scientific and social consequences of screening are to be realized.

A screening procedure has two primary objectives (Wilson and Jungner, 1966): it should be able to discriminate simply and accurately between those individuals who have the mutant phenotype and those who do not; and it should provide the opportunity for early detection of such individuals, so that the appropriate options for management of the problem can be undertaken. The real and potential assets of screening methods for genetic disease have been a major stimulus for widespread interest in development and use of them in the community (Fogarty International Centre, 1972). Diseases of amino acid metabolism have long been prime targets for the application of mass screening.

Targets of the Screening Test (Levels of Application)

Screening for amino acid disease may be done at four primary levels (Scriver, 1965):

(1) the genetic material, where the mutation occurs;
(2) the gene product, modified by the mutation;
(3) the cellular function, or metabolic equilibrium, which is controlled by the gene product; and
(4) the disease caused by the perturbation of cellular function.

To screen at any of these levels has its own merit and hazard. Screening at the first level (the gene) is not yet practical, although we anticipate that mapping of the human genome by cell hybridization (Ruddle et al., 1972), and pedigree analyses, will eventually yield useful information for purposes of genetic counseling under certain circumstances. However, the subsequent discussion will be confined to the last three levels of phenotypic expression, because the practical advantages are apparent.

Screening for the Gene Product (Enzyme Phenotype)

The gene product, whether it is an enzyme or other cellular protein, will usually be altered in some way when the mutation is expressed, so that either the primary structure of the protein or the amount of the protein is affected. It has been customary to think that regulator genes are responsible for the amount of protein in the cell. However, there is no firm evidence at the present time for the presence of regulator genes influencing amino acid metabolism in human cells. Nonetheless, the amount of an enzyme acting at some stage of amino acid metabolism may be altered, if the mutation affects the structure of the enzyme in such a way that its turnover number in the cell has been altered. One can visualize that the degradation rate, in the presence of a constant rate of enzyme synthesis, could be increased or decreased so that the amount of enzyme would be diminished or augmented, respectively. The amount of enzyme in the cell could also be affected if the final form of the enzyme reflects genes acting in sequence. For example, if a protein, formed under the influence of one gene, is modified by the addition of side groups through the action of a second enzyme acting on the first, then mutation at the gene locus responsible for the second enzyme could prevent synthesis of the final form of the first enzyme; this could be reflected by a diminished quantity of the first enzyme. Alternatively, if the final form of the first enzyme is composed of subunits, or if it is a multienzyme complex, then mutation affecting synthesis of structure of one of the components of a final enzyme complex could alter the amount of the intact enzyme.

Enzyme screening requires either that the enzyme be present in an active and soluble form in body fluids or that the tissue source of the enzyme be available to simple and effective biopsy. It is clear that a test requiring biopsy of fixed tissues is not compatible with the principles of mass screening. However, such an approach may be very useful in the investigation of a single patient or a pedigree. If, on the other hand, the formed elements of blood or free-floating cells in urine or amniotic fluid, for example, are a source of the enzyme, it may be possible to obtain material for purposes of diagnosis or screening. (Tissue sources of material which can be used to investigate a number of diseases of amino acid metabolism are summarized in Table 5–2.)

Screening for Metabolic Imbalance (Chemical Phenotype)

If the gene product (enzyme) regulates a metabolic pathway, or transport function, alteration in the function of the enzyme or transport site may cause imbalance between precursor and product stage of the pathway or transfer; this will declare itself either as an accumulation of the substrate or as a deficiency of the product of the reaction catalyzed by the mutant enzyme (Fig. 5–6). Furthermore, accumulation or depletion of metabolites may lead to secondary or tertiary levels of imbalance which may be identifiable by the appropriate screening test. For example, phenylalanine hydroxylase deficiency (gene product level) causes accumulation of phenylalanine and of its by-product, phenylpyruvic acid (metabolite level). Phenylalanine accumulation secondarily causes serotonin and catecholamine depletion and inhibition of melanin synthesis.

Screening methods that are to be sensitive to variation in the concentrations of metabolites in body fluids must be able to detect significant changes in those concentrations. Great efforts have been made in recent years to develop techniques with sufficient specificity and sensitivity for this purpose (see following text for definitions of specificity and sensitivity). A number of physiological factors influence how the screening test should be applied. Amino acids which are very efficiently reabsorbed by the renal tubule may experience large

Table 5–2 Use of In Vitro Techniques to Investigate Some Diseases of Amino Acid Metabolism

Phenotype	Tissue Source of Phenotype[a]		
	White Blood Cells[b]	Cultured Skin Cells	Amniotic Fluid or Cultured Amniotic Cells[c]
hyperAlaninemia (Pyr. carboxylase deficiency)	O	O	
(Pyr. dehydrogenase deficiency)	+	+	
hyperAmmonemia (OCT deficiency)	O	O	
Argininosuccinicaciduria	+	+	⊕
Branched-chain ketoaciduria (and variants)	+	+	+ (cells)
Citrullinemia	O	+	⊕
Cystathioninuria	O	O	⊕
Cystinosis (and variants)	+	+	⊕
Homocystinuria(s) (cystathionine synthase deficiency)	+[d]	+	+ (cells)
Hypophosphatasia	+		
Isovalericacidemia	+	+	
hyperLeucinemia	+	⊕	
hyperLysinemia		+	⊕
Methylmalonicaciduria(s)	+	+	+ (fluid)
Ornithine, α-ketoglutaric acid transaminase deficiency		⊕	
Propionic acidemia(s)	+	+	+ (cells)
Sarcosinemia	O	O	
hyperValinemia	+	⊕	

Symbols: + = trait detected by either enzyme defect or metabolite accumulation.
⊕ = detection of trait feasible but no documented experience.
O = not expressed in these tissues because enzyme is normally absent.

[a]Phenotype expressed as deficiency of enzyme (e.g., branched-chain keto acid decarboxylase) or accumulation of a metabolite (e.g., cystine in cystinosis).
[b]Mixed leukocyte population from peripheral blood (adapted and extended from Nadler and Hsia, 1968).
[c]Adapted and extended from paper by Milunsky, A., et al. (New Eng. J. Med. *283*:1370*ff*.; 1498*ff*.; 1504*ff*., 1970).
[d]Phytohemagglutinin stimulated cultured lymphocytes

quantitative changes in the plasma and relatively small changes, by comparison, in their urine concentration. An amino acid with this type of renal excretion is more readily screened by plasma methods. Amino acids which are rapidly cleared from plasma by the kidney experience large changes in their urinary excretion and relatively small changes, by comparison, in their plasma concentration. Dent and Walshe (1954) described these as high-threshold (prerenal) and low-threshold (renal) aminoacidopathies, respectively. Thus, conditions which affect only the membrane transport of an amino acid are most appropriately detected by urine screening, where large changes in concentration will occur; any small decrease in the plasma concentration which may be caused by the transport defect is unlikely to be detectable by even the best of screening methods.

It has been argued (Dent, 1951, 1957) that, for general purposes of diagnosis, urine is the ideal fluid to mirror the state of amino acid metabolism. The physiological events which control the formation of urine and its amino acid content, beyond the period of infancy (see Chapter 3), render it a very sensitive "biological amplifier" of any signal indicating a change in prerenal metabolism

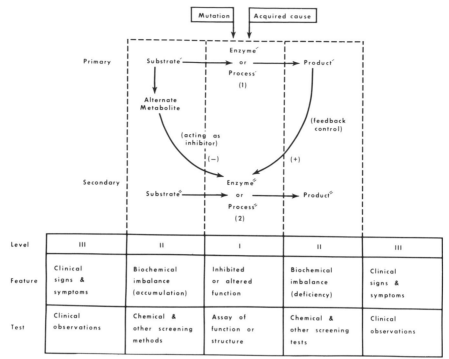

Figure 5–6 Scheme showing the effect of mutation at various phenotypic levels. Level I (enzyme phenotype) is the most specific for screening purposes. Level II (metabolic or biochemical phenotype) may be less precise but technically more accessible for purposes of screening. Level III (clinical phenotype) is not preferred, since prevention of disease is the primary objective of screening. Note that mutation may affect one biochemical sequence which, when perturbed, may affect a second and unrelated reaction or metabolic sequence. Appropriate interpretation of the screening test requires recognition of this possibility.

or renal transport of amino acids (Table 5–3). However, as indicated earlier, logistical problems make mass screening of liquid urine samples in the newborn less appealing than the screening of blood samples for amino acid content.

Clinical Disease (Disease Phenotype)

Screening for diagnosis in the presence of disease is not desirable, since it may be too late to help the patient. The objective of screening is to prevent pathological change or at least to recognize the disease at its incipient stage. Unfortunately, our knowledge of amino acid metabolism has not yet developed to the extent that the appearance of clinical disease can be prevented in all disorders of amino acid metabolism. A patient may be irrevocably affected before a family can be counseled to avoid further risk. However, it may be possible to recognize these phenotypes in utero by means of prenatal diagnostic techniques. Those disorders of amino acid metabolism in which the phenotype is expressed in cultured amniotic fluid cells are indicated in Table 5–2 and are discussed in more detail below.

Specificity and Sensitivity of Screening Tests (Signal and Noise)

Screening methods are effective in direct proportion to the ratio of "signal-to-noise." The term implies a relationship between the test signal and the back-

Table 5-3 Urine as a "Biological Amplifier" and Screen for the Inborn Error of Amino Acid Metabolism

	Normal Phenotype[a]	Prerenal[b] Aminoacidopathy	Renal[c] Aminoacidopathy
Filtered load of amino acid	100	400	100
Reabsorbed load	99	396	90
Excreted load	*1*	*4*	*10*

[a]Physiological data (filtered, reabsorbed and excreted load of the amino acid) are standardized for simplicity.

[b]"Prerenal" phenotype is the term used by Dent and Walshe (1954) to indicate a defect in amino acid catabolism which causes an increase in metabolite concentration in blood first and in urine second.

[c]"Renal" phenotype is the term (Dent and Walshe, 1954) used to indicate a disorder of membrane transport which causes an increase in metabolite concentration of urine first (and either no change or a decrease in blood second).

ground against which it is used. A positive test carries with it a certain amount of noise generated by false-positive tests, misdiagnosis and various other perturbations of screening efficiency. To be precise with the analogy, the signal is the index phenotype to be identified by the screening method, while noise is nondisease, genetic heterogeneity in the phenotype and other sources of a faulty signal. A high noise level makes the screening test "costly." The value of any screening method lies in its ability to yield an acceptable signal-to-noise ratio. The signal must be amplified so that it can be detected as efficiently as possible; and the noise must be damped to keep extraneous signals to a minimum. There are many ways in which the signal-to-noise ratio may be improved (Scriver, 1972).

A statistical definition of a "positive" signal (test) may be the only alternative when a single test for metabolite concentration or enzyme activity is used to discriminate between the abnormal phenotype (signal) and the normal phenotype (silence). The investigator may have to establish a value for metabolite concentration or enzyme activity which is two or three standard deviations from the mean of a normal distribution, and accept this as the cut-off point which is indicative of an abnormal test result. However, depending on the rarity of the index phenotype and the size of the population to be screened, a large number of repeat tests may be required to find the patient with the disease (Table 5-4).

Table 5-4 Screening "Noise" and the Relative Strength of the "Signal" (Positive Test) The Statistical Approach

	Size of Population Screened:100,000 Signal:Noise Ratio When Disease Frequency[b] Is	
Criteria for "Positive Test"	*10^{-5}*	*10^{-4}*
>2 SD from mean[a]	1:2250	1:225
>3 SD from mean	1:160	1:16

[a]Assuming normal (Gaussian) distribution of normal values. SD = standard deviation.

[b]"Disease frequency" refers to frequency of index problem in population at which preventive screening is directed. Noise is the number of positive tests in the range of values >2 SD, or >3 SD, from the mean which are *not* caused by the index problem; in other words, "false positive" results.

In these terms, the follow-up noise is appreciable. Only when the discriminant test is fortunate enough to yield a clear signal such as visualization of an abnormal protein (gene product) band on an electrophoretic strip (as for example hemoglobin S in the sickle cell trait), can the noise problem be avoided.

The choice of test and the criteria by which the abnormal is distinguished from the normal are usually arrived at by compromise between an acceptable signal-to-noise ratio and the overall benefits which accrue from application of the screening method to a population. Figure 5–7 summarizes in graphic terms how considerations of specificity and sensitivity of the screening test influence the relative costs of screening. The *specificity* of a screening test is defined as the fraction of healthy subjects, a, with a negative screening test in the population $a + b$ (see matrix in Figure 5–7). The *sensitivity* of a screening test is defined as the fraction of diseased patients, d, who are identified by means of a positive screening test in the population $c + d$. The "cost" of the screening test can then be defined in terms of the number of errors $(b + c)$, i.e., normal subjects with positive tests (b) and diseased subjects with negative tests (c), encountered when the test is applied to the total population of healthy and diseased subjects. The cost (according to the matrix of Figure 5–7) is defined as the fraction $\dfrac{b+c}{a+b+c+d}$. Screening costs vary according to the efficiency of the test and the criteria used for discrimination between normal and abnormal test results. Relative cost functions for "good" and "poor" tests are shown in Figure 5–7.

Appropriate signal amplification can improve the efficiency of screening and reduce its costs. Sometimes this can be achieved by biological methods — for example, by picking the appropriate body fluid to screen, as shown in Table 5–3.

Appropriate choice of screening method can broaden the receiving band so that many signals can be received from a signal test. Partition chromatography applied to urine or blood, and location of amino acids with a ninhydrin stain, provides a high signal-to-noise ratio with a broad-band reception pattern. Partition chromatography, in fact, provides the opportunity to screen for over 50 abnormalities of amino acid metabolism.

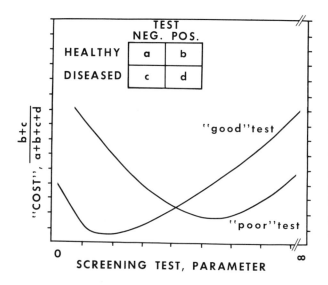

Figure 5–7 A graph depicting the "cost" of a screening test in relation to its application and interpretation. The proportion of negative and positive tests in relation to healthy and diseased phenotypes, respectively, is indicated in the matrix at the top of the figure. A decrease in specificity $\left(\dfrac{a}{a+b}\right)$ or in sensitivity $\left(\dfrac{d}{c+d}\right)$ leads to a rise in the noise or cost of the testing procedure, which is expressed as the fraction $\dfrac{b+c}{a+b+c+d}$. (Adapted from Partington, 1968.)

Resources for Screening

The numerous and various aspects of these important issues are discussed in many writings on the subject, and the interested reader is referred to them: Clow et al., 1971; Clow, 1972; Raine, 1972; Levy, 1972; WHO, 1968, 1972.

Laws

There is controversy concerning legislation for mass screening. The American Academy of Pediatrics (1965) recommends that legislation neither enforce screening nor specify the technology to be used. Legislation can enable screening by recommending the extent of the resources and by making provision for funding.

Centralized Facilities

Quality control of the screening procedure is important if the costs and "noise" components of screening are to be kept to a minimum. This can be achieved best at a centralized facility, such as the public health laboratory for the region, preferably working in liaison with a university (WHO, 1972). Experience with interpretation of the test, recognition of the diagnostic alternatives in the positive test, resources for confirmatory tests and a mechanism to record data and to reach the subjects who require follow-up study must all be available through the central laboratory.

Satellite centers for confirmatory diagnosis, counseling and treatment of patients will usually be required if a large geographic area is covered by the screening program. Management of the patient on an in-home basis is desirable, and the cost of such management is substantially lower than in traditional hospital-oriented programs (Clow et al., 1971).

Communications

Delivery of blood samples of neonates to the laboratory from the region, reporting of results and retrieval of patients for follow-up require an efficient communication network. It is desirable to operate the screening network so that the first test in newborn programs is complete by the third week of the infant's life (Clow et al., 1972). If a positive test is found, then follow-up work and initiation of treatment, if indicated, can usually be accomplished before clinical disease has appeared in most aminoacidopathies. (A patient with classical maple syrup urine disease will probably not benefit from this pacing of newborn screening, but the rarity of the trait — at least 10 times less common than such other diseases as phenylketonuria — precludes changing the logistics of newborn screening programs, for economic reasons.)

Education of the community about the existence and objectives of screening is an important factor in running successful programs. The physicians and the "consumers" are equally important targets for the educational material.

Economics and Industrial Resources

The major costs of screening programs are in personnel, hardware and overhead. The tests themselves are invariably inexpensive to perform, or they would not be screening tests. The cost per patient, when cost is accounted over the whole program, should not be greater than the cost for care of the unscreened patient who develops disease and requires medical care. A distinct cost-benefit from screening is desirable.

Treatment options are taken up in most situations where mass screening identifies the patient. Most treatment procedures involve some process of "environmental engineering" (Scriver, 1969) which neutralizes the mutant allele or prevents expression of disease. Dietary and pharmacological modes of treatment are the mainstay of intervention, but at present food engineering and drug design have lagged behind what is required for mutants, who are "consumers with special needs" (Scriver, 1971).

DIAGNOSIS OF AMINOACIDOPATHIES

Classification of Hereditary Phenotypes and Acquired Disorders

Diagnosis may be arrived at rationally by the application of the investigative methods alluded to earlier in this chapter; or it may be revealed by serendipity, through the routine use of screening methods. The differential diagnosis of the disorders of amino acid metabolism is extensive. The classification presented in Table 5–5 divides them into acquired and inherited types, and it includes disturbances related to perinatal adaptive phenomena having various causes. The classification also recognizes physiological factors affecting amino acid distribution between plasma and urine and whether the disorder primarily affects catabolism or membrane transport of an amino acid. Conditions listed in the table are discussed in more detail in Parts II and III under the appropriate sections dealing with transport and catabolism of individual amino acids.

Frequencies of Amino Acid Phenotypes

Too little is known about the real frequencies of the hereditary aminoacidopathies. Uneven segregation of mutant genes occurs among the populations of the world, often showing remarkable variation in frequency between geographic regions and ethnic groups and demes. For this reason, it is difficult to give true frequency data for amino acid traits that are meaningful to everyone. Nonetheless, the available data (Table 5–6) illuminate some of the quantitative aspects of the inborn errors of amino acid metabolism, such as the number of potential patients involved and the demand they will make upon services for diagnosis, counseling and treatment. The effect of relaxed selection (i.e., the effect of treatment on genetic fitness) on the frequency of the mutant gene in the future is also of concern (WHO, 1972). If complete ascertainment of the trait is achieved now, it will be possible to monitor its frequency over future generations. In this way, we may also be able to detect changes in frequency which reflect variation in the mutation rate at the relevant gene locus; from these data we may detect environmental factors which are influencing the mutation rate. The obvious and immediately pertinent applications, as well as these long-range perspectives, suggest why screening and surveillance of amino acid disorders in populations has grown in relevance.

How to Investigate the Patient with a Suspected Aminoacidopathy

The problem of diagnosis may present itself at any moment in the patient's lifetime; it may appear as an emergency or incidentally, during the course of other investigations. Once the possibility has arisen that the patient may have a disorder of amino acid metabolism, one must attempt to arrive at a reasonable diagnosis. Certain parts of the investigation can be done simply and effectively

Table 5-5 Hereditary and Acquired Aminoacidopathies[a], Classified According to Mechanism and Preferred Fluid for Detection

Group I. A: Primary Defect in Catabolism
Low Renal Clearance of Amino Acid
Hyperaminoaciduria by Saturation of Transport System
Detection Preferable in Plasma

Condition or Disease	Amino Acids Affected	Abnormal Enzyme	Comment
Common Perinatal (Adaptive) Traits			
Neonatal hyper-phenylalaninemia[a]	Phenylalanine	Phenylalanine hydroxylating system (?)	Benign; may respond to folic acid; often occurs with tyrosinemia
Neonatal tyrosinemia[b]	Tyrosine	*p*-Hydroxyphenyl-pyruvate hydroxylase (E.C. 1.14.2.2)	Benign; responds to ascorbic acid and reduced protein intake
Hypermethioninemia[b]	Methionine	ATP: 1-methionine S-adenosyl transferase (?) (E.C. 2.5.1.6)	Benign; usually found with high protein intake
Hyperhistidinemia[b]	Histidine	L-Histidine ammonia-lyase (?) (E.C. 4.3.1.3)	Benign; related to high protein intake
Inherited Aminoacidopathies			
The hyperphenylalaninemias Classical phenylketonuria[b]	Phenylalanine	L-Phenylalanine, tetrahydropteridine: oxygen oxidoreductase (4-hydroxylating) (E.C. 1.14.3.1)	Plasma phenylalanine >16 mg/100 ml; causes mental retardation. When treated, L-phenylalanine tolerance in diet is 250–500 mg phe/day
Atypical phenylketonuria[b]	Phenylalanine	L-Phenylalanine, tetrahydropteridine: oxygen oxidoreductase (4-hydroxylating) (E.C. 1.14.3.1)	Plasma phenylalanine >16 mg/100 ml; similar to classical form but dietary tolerance for L-phenyl alanine is >500 mg/day
Transient phenylketonuria[b]	Phenylalanine	L-Phenylalanine, tetrahydropteridine: oxygen oxidoreductase (4-hydroxylating) (E.C. 1.14.3.1)	Plasma phenylalanine >16 mg/100 ml; change in status to benign form, or normal, several months or years after birth
Benign hyper-phenylalaninemia[b]	Phenylalanine	L-Phenylalanine, tetrahydropteridine: oxygen oxidoreductase (4-hydroxylating) (E.C. 1.14.3.1)	Plasma phenylalanine <16 mg/100 ml on normal diet; benign trait
The hypertyrosinemias Tyrosinosis (Medes)	Tyrosine	L-tyrosine:pyruvate aminotransferase (?) (E.C. 2.6.1.20)	One case known; myasthenia gravis, probably incidental finding
Hypertyrosinemia[b]	Tyrosine	Soluble (cytosol) tyrosine aminotransferase	One case; associated developmental retardation
Hereditary tyrosinemia[b]	Tyrosine (and methionine)	*p*-Hydroxyphenyl-pyruvate hydroxylase (E.C. 1.14.2.2) (Primary or secondary defect?)	Hepatic cirrhosis, and renal tubular failure, eventually fatal; responds to tyrosine restriction.

Table 5–5   Hereditary and Acquired Aminoacidopathies[a], Classified
According to Mechanism and Preferred Fluid for Detection (*Continued*)

| Group I. | A: | Primary Defect in Catabolism
Low Renal Clearance of Amino Acid
Hyperaminoaciduria by Saturation of Transport System
Detection Preferable in Plasma | | |

Condition or Disease	Amino Acids Affected	Abnormal Enzyme	Comment
The hyperhistidinemias Classical form[b]	Histidine (alanine in some cases)	L-Histidine ammonia-lyase (E.C. 4.3.1.3) (liver and skin)	Usually associated with mental retardation and speech defect.
Variant form	Histidine	L-Histidine ammonia-lyase (E.C. 4.3.1.3) (liver only)	As above
The branched-chain hyperaminoacidemias Classical maple syrup urine disease[b]	Leucine, isoleucine, valine	BCKA: Lipoate oxidoreductase (acceptor acylating) (E.C. 1.2.4.–)	Postnatal collapse, mental retardation in survivors; diet therapy can be effective
Intermittent form	Leucine, isoleucine, valine	Same	Intermittent symptoms; development may be otherwise normal
Mild form	Same	Same	Unremittent; milder than classical form
Thiamine-responsive	Same	Same	Mild form; B_1-responsive
Hypervalinemia	Valine	Valine aminotransferase (E.C. 2.6.1.–)	Retarded development and vomiting; responds to diet
Hyperleucinemia	Leucine/isoleucine	Leucine/isoleucine aminotransferase (E.C. 2.6.1.–)	Retarded development
Others[d]			
Sulfuraminoacidemias Homocystinuria[b]	Methionine and homocystine	L-Serine hydrolyase (deaminating); ("cystathionine synthetase") (E.C. 4.2.1.13)	Usually associated with thromboembolic disease, mental retardation, and Marfan phenotype
Cystathioninuria[c]	Cystathionine	L-Homoserine hydrolyase (deaminating) (E.C. 4.2.1.15)	Probably benign trait; vitamin B_6 corrects biochemical trait in most patients
The hyperglycinemias Ketotic form[b]	Glycine and other glucogenic acids	Propionyl-CoA: carbon-dioxide ligase (ADP) (E.C. 6.4.1.3)	Ketosis, neutropenia, mental retardation; often fatal
Nonketotic form[b]	Glycine	Same or "glycine decarboxylase" (?)	Milder form of trait
Sarcosinemia[c]	Sarcosine (ethanolamine)	Sarcosine: oxygen oxidoreductase (demethylating) (E.C. 1.5.3.1)	Benign trait (probably)
The hyperprolinemias Type I[b]	Proline	L-Proline: NAD(P) 5-oxidoreductase ("proline oxidase") (E.C. 1.5.1.2)	Benign trait, which is sometimes associated with hereditary nephritis

Table 5–5 Hereditary and Acquired Aminoacidopathies[a], Classified According to Mechanism and Preferred Fluid for Detection (*Continued*)

Group I. A: **Primary Defect in Catabolism**
Low Renal Clearance of Amino Acid
Hyperaminoaciduria by Saturation of Transport System
Detection Preferable in Plasma

Condition or Disease	Amino Acids Affected	Abnormal Enzyme	Comment
Type II	Proline	"Δ'-pyrroline-5-carboxylate dehydrogenase"	Possibly benign trait, sometimes associated with CNS disease; ΔPC excreted in urine; proline concentration greater than Type I.
Hydroxyprolinemia	Hydroxyproline	"Hydroxyproline oxidase"	Two cases, associated with CNS disease; others normal
The hyperlysinemias Type I	Lysine (and glutamine)	Lysine:α-ketoglutarate: triphosphopyridine nucleotide (TPNH), oxidoreductase (ϵ-N-[L-glutaryl-2]-L-lysine forming)	Associated with mental retardation and hypotonia
Type II	Lysine, arginine (NH_3)	Partial defect of type I, or different enzyme?	Hyperammonemia symptoms, related to protein intake
Saccharopinuria[c]	Lysine, saccharopine, citrulline	"Saccharopinase" (?)	One case; associated with mental retardation and short stature
Pipecolicacidemia[c]	Pipecolic acid	"Pipecolate oxidase" (?)	Hepatomegaly and mental retardation
The hyperammonemias Type I	Glycine, glutamine	ATP: carbamate phosphotransferase (E.C. 2.7.2.2)	A group of diseases that show ammonia intoxication, protein intolerance, hepatomegaly, vomiting etc. ASAuria also has trichorrhexis nodosa
Type II[b]	Glutamine	Carbamoylphosphate: L-ornithine carbamoyltransferase (E.C. 2.1.3.3)	
Hyperornithinemia	Ornithine	Ornithine-keto-acid amino-transferase (E.C. 2.6.1.13)	
Citrullinemia[b]	Citrulline	L-Citrulline: L-aspartate ligase (AMP) (E.C. 6.3.4.5)	
Argininosuccinicaciduria[c]	ASA	L-Argininosuccinate arginine-lyase (E.C. 4.3.2.1)	
Argininemia	Arginine	L-Arginineamidino hydrolase (E.C. 3.5.3.1)	
Glutamicacidemia	Glutamate	Unknown	X-linked mental retardation
The hyperalaninemias	Alanine	Pyruvate decarboxylase (E.C. 4.1.1.1) (dehydrogenase, E.C. 1.2.4.1) deficiency	Lactic acidosis, intermittent ataxia, mental retardation
		Pyruvate carboxylase deficiency (E.C. 6.4.1.1)	Intermittent lactic acidosis, intermittent hypoglycemia

Table 5–5   Hereditary and Acquired Aminoacidopathies[a], Classified According to Mechanism and Preferred Fluid for Detection (*Continued*)

Group I.   A: **Primary Defect in Catabolism**
Low Renal Clearance of Amino Acid
Hyperaminoaciduria by Saturation of Transport System
Detection Preferable in Plasma

Condition or Disease	*Amino Acids Affected*	*Abnormal Enzyme*	*Comment*
Aspartylglycosaminuria	Glycoasparagines	2-acetamido-1-(β^1-L-aspartamido)-1,2-dideoxyglucoseamido hydrolase	Lysosomal disease? Mental retardation
"Glutathionemia"	Glutathione or related peptide	γ-glutamyltranspeptidase deficiency	Mental retardation associated with finding

Nutritional and Other Diseases Which May Affect Amino Acids in Plasma

Protein-calorie malnutrition	Tryptophan/leucine/isoleucine/valine ↓ ; tyrosine/glycine/proline ↑		Severity of change related to severity of malnutrition
Prolonged fasting	Alanine ↓ ; threonine/glycine ↑		Early fasting does not show same pattern
Obesity	Leucine/isoleucine/valine/phenylalanine/tyrosine ↑ ; glycine ↓		Reflects insulin insensitivity
Hepatitis	Methionine/tyrosine ↑		Reflects severity of liver disease

Group I.   B: **Primary Defect in Catabolism**
High Renal Clearance of Amino Acid
Hyperaminoaciduria by Saturation
Detection Preferable in Urine

Condition or Disease	*Amino Acids Affected*	*Abnormal Enzyme*	*Comment*
Hypophosphatasia	Phosphoethanolamine	? Deficiency of *o*-phosphorylethanolamine phospho-lyase (E.C. 4.2.99.–)	"Rickets"-unresponsive to vitamin D; carniosynostosis; hypercalcemia
Pseudohypophosphatasia	Phosphoethanolamine	"Alkaline phosphatase" activity present but altered (K_m mutant)	
β-Aminoisobutyricaciduria	βAIB	?	Benign polymorphic trait
Hyper-β-alaninemia	β-Alanine	β-Alanine transaminase?	Seizures; somnolence; mental retardation
Carnosinemia	Carnosine	Carnosinase	Seizures and mental retardation

(See also homocystinuria, cystathioninuria and argininosuccinicaciduria under Group I.A, Inherited Aminoacidopathies)

Pyroglutamic-aciduria	5-oxo-L-proline (pyrrolidone-2-carboxylic acid)	5-oxo-pro conversion to CO_2 (L-pyroglu. hydrolase system?)	One patient known, 5-O-P in urine; origin in kidney?

Table 5–5 Hereditary and Acquired Aminoacidopathies[a], Classified According to Mechanism and Preferred Fluid for Detection (*Continued*)

Group II: **Primary Defect in Catabolism; Secondary Defect in Transport Hyperaminoaciduria of Combined Origin (Saturation and Competition) Detection Possible in Plasma and Urine**

Disease	*Amino Acids Affected in Plasma*	*Amino Acids Present in Urine*	*Comment*
Hyperprolinemia Types I and II	Proline	Proline plus hydroxy-proline and glycine	(See hyperproline-mias) Competition occurs on iminoglycine transport system (See iminoglycinuria)
Hyper-β-alaninemia	β-Alanine	β-alanine plus βAIB	(See hyper-β-alaninemia.) Competition occurs on β-amino transport system
Hyperlysinemia	Lysine	Lysine plus ornithine and arginine	(See hyperlysinemias). Competition occurs on "dibasic" transport system (See cystinuria) (See Argininemia)
Argininemia	Arginine	Arginine plus lysine and ornithine	

Group III: **Primary Defect in Membrane Transport Site High Renal Clearance of Amino Acid Detection Possible Only in Urine**

Disease or Trait	*Amino Acids Affected*	*Abnormal Transport System*	*Comment*
Common Perinatal (Adaptive) Traits			
Neonatal iminoglycinuria	Proline, hydroxy-proline, and glycine	Low-capacity system for proline; same for glycine	Iminoaciduria persists about 3 mos.; glycinuria persists 5–6 mos.
Hereditary Traits Cystinuria[b]	Dibasics and cystine	High-capacity, diamino-monocarboxylic (involving cysteine during efflux only)	
Type I Type II Type III		Kidney plus gut Kidney plus gut Kidney plus gut (partial)	Cystine stone formation in urinary tract is major hazard.
Hypercystinuria	Cystine only	Substrate-specific system for cystine	Renal calculi
Renal iminoglycinuria[b]	Proline, hydroxypro-line, and glycine	High-capacity system for imino acids and glycine	
Type I Type II		Kidney and gut Kidney alone	Benign trait

Table 5–5   Hereditary and Acquired Aminoacidopathies,[a] Classified According to Mechanism and Preferred Fluid for Detection (*Continued*)

Group III: Primary Defect in Membrane Transport Site
High Renal Clearance of Amino Acid
Detection Possible Only in Urine

Disease or Trait	Amino Acids Affected	Abnormal Transport System	Comment
Hartnup disease[b]	Neutral monoamino-monocarboxylic acids (except imino acids and glycine)	High-capacity system shared by neutral amino acids	Pellagra-like symptoms under condition of marginal protein nutrition
Type I Type II		Kidney and gut Kidney only	
Blue-diaper syndrome	Tryptophan	Low-capacity system for specific amino acid (in the intestine)	Hypercalcemia
Methionine malabsorption	Methionine		Mental retardation

Group IV: Generalized Inhibition of Transport Processes
High Renal Clearance of Substrates
Detection Best in Urine

Condition or Disease	Amino Acids Affected	Comment
Fanconi syndrome[b] (multiple causes; see Chapter 10)	Generalized amino-aciduria plus other solutes	Symptoms related to proximal tubular dysfunction, plus primary trait
Oculocerebrorenal syndrome	Generalized	X-linked; glaucoma, hypotonia and mental retardation
Busby syndrome	Generalized	Severe growth failure and pulmonary disease

[a] Table refers only to those conditions associated with perturbation of the normal content of ninhydrin-reactive metabolites in plasma or urine.
[b] These conditions have been detected by screening methods applied in the neonatal period of life.
[c] Urine screening is probably preferable in these conditions.
[d] A number of disorders of branched-chain amino acid catabolism cause accumulation of substances which are ninhydrin-negative. These compounds can usually be detected by gas-liquid chromatographic methods.

in the clinic or the doctor's office; other stages require special techniques and referral of the patient to a center where the work-up can be performed. The investigative protocol currently in use in the public health urine screening program of Massachusetts, organized by Levy and colleagues (1972), indicates to what limits "preliminary diagnosis" can be carried; in practice, however, most work-ups are only simpler modifications of this complete and elegant program. A description of the use and interpretation of several clinical tests which can be applied in an office or clinic setting is given in the Appendix to this chapter.

Clinical Aids

The investigation begins always with a careful *history*, which includes details about the *environment*, including toxins, drugs and foods which may cause the

Table 5–6 Approximate Frequency of Some Hereditary Aminoacidopathies

Phenotype	Apparent Frequency per 100,000 Live Births	Region or Population
Argininosuccinicaciduria	0.4	N.E. N. Amer.
Branched-chain ketoaciduria(s)	0.3	General
Cystinuria	7	General
Fanconi syndrome	0.4	N.E. N. Amer.
Hartnup disease	4	General
Histidinemia	4	General
Iminoglycinuria	5	General
*hyper*Lysinemia	0.4	N.E. N. Amer.
*hyper*Methioninemia (with homocystinuria)	0.4	General
*hyper*Prolinemia	2	General
Phenylketonuria	8	General (PKU rare in Ashkenazic Jews)
*hyper*Phenylalaninemia	3	General
Tyrosinemia (persistent)	<0.1	General
	30	Isolate of French Canadians in Quebec

excretion or accumulation of amino acids or their by-products, and about the *family*, with details about consanguinity, origins of the parents and health in sibs, parents and collateral branches of the pedigree.

The proband may provide helpful *clinical signs*. News from the nose should not be ignored; *odors* can be diagnostic of aminoacidopathies (Cone, 1968; Anonymous, 1967; Anonymous, 1968; Buist, 1968; Snyderman, 1970; Raine, 1972):

—Phenylacetic acid (phenylketonuria) causes a musty or mousy odor.

—Branched-chain amino acid derivatives produce the maple-syrup odor characteristic of diseases associated with branched-chain keto acid decarboxylase deficiency.

—α-Hydroxybutyric acid (and perhaps other substances) produce an "oast-house" odor in the oast-house syndrome (Smith and Strang, 1958).

—α-Ketobutyrate or α-keto-γ-methiolbutyrate excreted in urine in hyper-methioninemic states causes a fishy or cabbage-like odor.

—Trimethylaminuria is associated with a powerful fishy odor.

—Isovaleric acid yields a characteristic cheesy odor likened to sweaty feet by those who are less enthusiastic about cheese.

Urine color should be noted. It darkens from the surface down on exposure to air, light and alkali in alcaptonuria, and it is indigo blue in the blue-diaper syndrome (Cone, 1968).

Hair color can be diagnostic of some aminoacidopathies (Rook, 1969). The pigmentation is diluted in phenylketonuria and in the Chediak-Higashi syndrome; and it is completely or almost completely deficient in various forms of albinism. Patients with oasthouse urine disease, methionine malabsorption or homocystinuria have unusually fair hair. In cystinosis the hair is straw-like, and the pigment is yellowed.

Chemical Tests for Screening

A series of simple chemical tests can be used to yield considerable information during the preliminary stages of investigation (Scheme 5–1). For example,

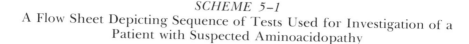

SCHEME 5–1

A Flow Sheet Depicting Sequence of Tests Used for Investigation of a
Patient with Suspected Aminoacidopathy

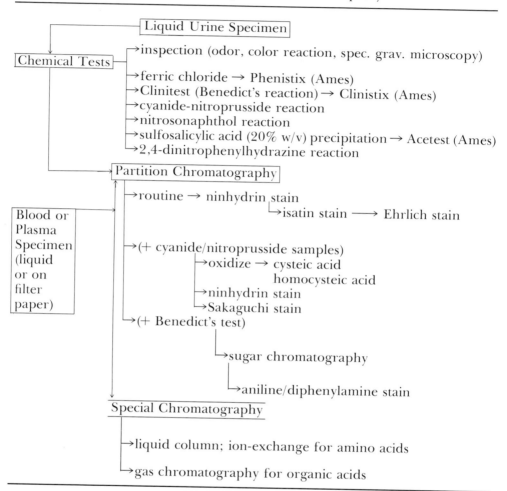

an infant in the second half of his first year of life with pale hair, polyuria and recent history of weight loss can be given a tentative diagnosis of the Fanconi syndrome if the urine contains glucose, a cyanide-nitroprusside-positive substance and a heat-soluble low-molecular-weight protein. Should inspection of the patient's eyes with the +40-diopter lens of the ophthalmoscope under lateral illumination reveal crystals in the cornea, the diagnosis of cystinosis would be highly probable. The preliminary work-up would have taken 10 minutes!

Several descriptions of the office or "side-room" tests which can be applied to screen liquid urine have been published (O'Brien, 1965; Perry et al., 1966; Berry et al., 1968; Buist, 1968). Some of the tests are summarized in the Appendix to this chapter; we recommend them to the house officer, the clinician and health workers everywhere whose job it is to recognize disease at incipient or established stages.

There are, of course, pitfalls in the use of chemical screening tests, and they require careful interpretation. For example, the Benedict's test identifies reducing substances, but a positive (confirmatory) glucose oxidase reaction (on a dip stick) does not eliminate the presence of substances other than glucose; sugar chromatography should *always* be done on the urine sample that yields a positive Benedict's test to identify the substance(s) (see Appendix). A positive ferric chloride test is not specific for phenylpyruvic acid; many other substances produce the classic green color with the ferric chloride reagent (see Appendix). A negative ferric chloride reaction does *not* exclude hyperphenylalaninemia in the neonatal period, because the conversion of phenylalanine to phenylpyruvic acid may be impaired at this age. A positive 2,4-dinitrophenylhydrazine test may only indicate ketonuria, and the test for acetone will also be positive in this circumstance. But ketosis may occur in several diseases of amino acid metabolism, and if the 2,4-DNPH test remains positive after heating the urine to rid it of acetone, then the possibility of an aminoacidopathy should be investigated. In this situation, gas chromatography of the urine may reveal one of the unusual organic acids. However, presence of the latter may also reflect bacterial contamination of urine (Hansen et al., 1972), and this artifact should not be interpreted as an index of disease. The intestinal lumen may be the origin of metabolites in urine, another artifact which must not be forgotten. In other words, chemical tests can be used successfully, provided precautions are taken with their interpretation.

Special Studies

The detailed investigation with specific chromatographic and chemical methods applied to the identification and measurement of metabolites in body fluids usually lies in the realm of a research laboratory experienced in the investigation of amino acid disorders. However, physiological studies to identify whether the aberration is one of catabolism (prerenal) or transport (renal) can be carried out quite simply (Scriver and Davies, 1965). Tissue studies using blood leukocytes, cultured skin fibroblasts or amniotic fluid cells can provide a definitive diagnosis in many instances (Table 5–2).

Special Problems of Diagnosis

On occasion there is no option for treatment of an inherited aminoacidopathy, and postnatal diagnosis therefore has nothing to offer to proband or family. Identification of the heterozygote and the opportunity for intrauterine diagnosis are valuable options when they are available under such circumstances.

Identification of Heterozygotes

Most inborn errors of amino acid metabolism are autosomal recessive, and inheritance of a pair of rare mutant alleles, one from each heterozygous parent, is required for the phenotype to be expressed under normal environmental conditions. When the two mutant alleles are identical, the proband is *homozygous* for the mutation. However, the two alleles can be different (*heteroallelism*), as we know to be the case in cystinuria and hereditary iminoglycinuria and probably also in many forms of hyperphenylalaninemia and maple syrup urine disease. If the two different alleles occur at the *same* genetic locus, the affected proband is said to be a *genetic compound*; when they occur at two *different* genetic loci (no example being known yet among the aminoacidopathies), the proband is said to be *doubly heterozygous* for the mutant genotype. The hereditary amino-acidopathies which are not autosomal recessive are X-linked in their mode of inheritance. At present, ornithine carbamyl transferase deficiency with hyper-ammonemia and the oculocerebrorenal syndrome are the only known examples of X-linked disorders of amino acid metabolism. At least one dominantly inherited form of the Fanconi syndrome has been identified, and this requires the appropriate genetic counseling.

The frequency of the "homozygote" for any given inborn error of amino acid metabolism is not great in the population, the range being in the order of 4 per million births (as in the case of maple syrup urine disease in the general population) to 400 per million births (for example, with hereditary tyrosinemia in French Canadians). Consequently, vast numbers of screening tests are usually performed to find one patient with a particular hereditary aminoacidopathy. However, if it were possible to screen for carriers of the mutant allele (heterozygotes), the efficiency with which at-risk couples could be identified might be much higher. When the carrier is known, it may often be possible to introduce preventive genetic counseling and to anticipate the appearance of an affected offspring. Carrier detection, as a general form of applied genetics, is a much debated issue (Hsia, 1969; Danks, 1966). However, when the inheritance of a trait is under investigation, or when there are high-risk circumstances to be counseled, or when the sibs of affected probands seek counseling with respect to prospective marriage partners, there is need for effective methods to identify the pertinent heterozygous genotype. It is for this reason that there is concern for heterozygote identification in the field of hereditary aminoacidopathies.

Homozygotes are often recognized by some expression of biochemical imbalance in physiological fluids. Heterozygotes rarely exhibit significant deviation from the normal. This is so because they have one normal allele, and about half of the normal amount of an enzyme is sufficient to maintain metabolic equilibrium. The performance of a loading test, which stresses the capacity of the relevant metabolic pathway, may demonstrate reduced catalytic capacity in the heterozygote. Table 5–7 lists traits in which this form of discrimination has been of use. However, such tests require the administration of a chemical, either by mouth or intravenously, followed by numerous samplings of blood or urine, to document its subsequent metabolism. Tests of this nature are inconvenient and usually cannot be used for general screening purposes, although they can be of value for specific investigative or counseling purposes.

Assay of the enzyme affected by the mutation can also be adapted for ascertainment of the heterozygote (Table 5–7). In this case, however, there is the problem of sampling. A "biopsy," be it blood cells or otherwise, is usually required, because the enzyme used for assay is rarely available in plasma or serum.

The major difficulty in heterozygote screening nearly always lies in the segregation of heterozygotes from the normal homozygotes; rarely is the heterozygote mistaken for the mutant homozygote. If more than one mutant allele accounts for the trait, and different heterozygous genotypes exist, discrimination between the different mutant genotypes may further complicate the issue.

Segregation of the heterozygous from the normal genotype, by a single unequivocal test, is difficult in all hereditary aminoacidopathies and may even be impossible within the limits of statistical confidence. Because people are rarely satisfied with the news that "they have less than 5 per cent chance of being a carrier" (and particularly if an elaborate procedure was required to arrive at this unenthusiastic statement), heterozygote ascertainment has to be unequivocal if the information is to be of any use at the level of human behavior.

High reliability in the classification of heterozygotes is particularly im-

Table 5–7 Hereditary Aminoacidopathies in Which Mutant Phenotype Is Detectable in the Heterozygote*

| Phenotype[a] | Metabolite level[b] | | Enzyme level in[c] | | |
	No Load	After Load Test	WBC[d]	Fibroblast[e]	Other
hyperAmmonemia (X-linked OCT deficiency)		↑ NH₃ (B)			
Argininosuccinic aciduria					↓ (RBC)
Branched-chain keto-amino aciduria(s)		↑ BCKA (B)	[↓]	[↓]	
Cystathioninuria		↑ (U)			
Cystinosis (+ variants)	↑ Cys (in WBC fibroblasts)				
Cystinuria (types II and III)	↑ Cys, lys (U)				
hyperDibasic amino-aciduria (type II)	↑ (U)				
Histidinemia(s)	↓ urocanic (in sweat)				↓ (epidermis)
Homocystinuria (cystathionine synthase deficiency)				[↓]	
Hypophosphatasia	↑ EAP (U)				↓ (serum)
Hydroxykynureninuria		↑ Xanthurenic (U)			
Iminoglycinuria (type III)	↑ gly (U)				
hyperLysinemia(s)		↑ lys (B)			
Methylmalonicaciduria (mutase deficiency)			[↓]	[↓]	
hyperPhenylalaninemia(s)	↑ P/T ratio (B)	↑ Phe (B)			
hyperProlinemia (type I)	↑ Pro (B)				
Propionicacidemia (propionate carboxylase deficiency)			↓	↓	
Sarcosinemia		[↑] (B)			

*Adapted and expanded from Hsia, 1969.

[a] Genetic heterogeneity exists for some conditions; not all conditions cause disease.

[b] Metabolite is usually the *substrate* of the mutant enzyme or membrane transport system. However, it may be a by-product, or the *product.* ↑ = increased amount. ↓ = decreased amount.

[c] Enzyme means "mutant gene product." ↓ = decreased activity by assay.

[d] WBC = mixed blood leukocytes.

[e] Fibroblast = cultured skin fibroblasts.

Symbols: (U) = urine, (B) = blood, [ ] = needs confirmation.

portant in the difficult situation faced by *consultand sibs* of affected probands. Yet, when the mutant phenotype is autosomal recessive, the unaffected sib has an *a priori* probability of 0.66 that he or she is a carrier. Unfortunately, most aminoacidopathies do *not* permit unequivocal classification of the carrier, and Gold and coauthors (1972) have reminded us that, in this circumstance, it is usually impossible to counsel the consultand sib that he is homozygous normal with any statistical confidence, regardless of the test result. That being the case, it is wiser to designate the sib as heterozygous. *Counseling of the sib's intended spouse then becomes the focus of attention.* The spouse, who presumably will come from a random population, has an a priori probability of about 0.02 for heterozygosity if the aminoacidopathy in question has a typical homozygous frequency of about 10^{-4} at birth. Classification of the intended spouse can be achieved with much greater confidence, particularly if a two-test solution is adopted (Rosenblatt and Scriver, 1968) and Bayesian statistical methods are applied (Gold et al., 1972; Murphy and Mutalik, 1969), a factor ignored by Farriaux and Delabre (1972) in their unsuccessful attempt to identify the heterozygote in phenylketonuria. The two-test solution for heterozygote classification is illustrated in Figure 15–9 in the discussion of phenylketonuric heterozygote classification. Rational counseling for the inheritance risks with the inborn errors of amino acid metabolism will be a greater problem in the future and will demand the use of sophisticated methods for heterozygote discrimination.

Prenatal Diagnosis of Aminoacidopathies

The principles and practice of prenatal diagnosis (Milunsky et al., 1970) are well established, and it is evident that in utero diagnosis of the homozygous phenotype is feasible for some aminoacidopathies (Table 5–2) and is warranted in the appropriate clinical circumstance. Prenatal diagnosis in the last trimester could alert the physician to the need for dietary or intravenous therapy immediately after birth of the infant in some of the life-threatening aminoacidopathies. If the disorder, on the other hand, cannot be treated successfully and it will inevitably maim the child, a midtrimester diagnosis allows the parents to take up the option of induced abortion. Moreover, some families already committed to the care of a proband, and unable or unwilling to undertake the treatment regimen for an additional affected offspring, would welcome the option of prenatal diagnosis and selective abortion of an affected fetus. Because work in prenatal diagnosis of aminoacidopathies is still in the experimental stage, counseling should not be entered upon without the support of a genetics center skilled in the methodology, and then only if the interested parties accept the limitations and commitments of the exercise.

Diagnosis of Hereditary Aminoacidopathies in the Acutely Ill Newborn

Several aminoacidopathies (Table 5–8) can cause acute, life-threatening illness in the first month of life (O'Brien and Goodman, 1970; Rosenberg, 1972). None of these diseases was known before 1958, and over half have been described in the past half-decade; the list will continue to grow.

Despite differences in their enzymatic and biochemical phenotypes, each aminoacidopathy listed in the table is strikingly similar to the others in the manner of its clinical presentation in the newborn period. Failure to feed, vomiting, seizures, lethargy and coma occur, and if the clinical course progresses, death is to be expected in the absence of aggressive intervention. When faced with a clinical problem of this nature, the physician can resort to a matrix of diagnostic procedures which should rapidly yield a reasonably specific diagnosis (Scheme 5–2). The best indication to proceed with this investigative protocol is a high index of clinical suspicion, perhaps triggered by clinical signs such as odor, eye signs and neurological findings (Raine, 1972). Metabolic acidosis or respiratory alkalosis, hypoglycemia, ketosis and hyperammonemia, alone or in combination with each other, can signal this type of disease in the newborn.

The underlying inborn error of metabolism is all too frequently mistakenly diagnosed as neonatal sepsis, transient hypoglycemia or tetany of the

Table 5–8 Inherited Aminoacidopathies Causing Severe Disease in the Newborn

Amino Acid Classification	Disorder	Clinical Findings	Laboratory Findings	Available Leukocyte Assay	Enzymatic Defect
Branched-Chain	Branched-chain ketoaciduria (maple syrup urine disease)	Feeding difficulty, lethargy, coma, maple syrup-like odor	Metabolic acidosis; hypoglycemia; elevated blood and urine leucine, isoleucine and valine; branched-chain ketoaciduria	Yes	Branched-chain ketoacid decarboxylase
	Valinemia	Feeding difficulty, vomiting, lethargy	Elevated blood and urine valine	Yes	Valine: α-ketoglutarate transaminase
	Isovalericacidemia	Progressive neurologic dysfunction, odor of "sweaty feet"	Metabolic acidosis; elevated blood and urine isovaleric acid	Yes	Isovaleryl-CoA dehydrogenase
	β-Hydroxyisovalericaciduria	Feeding difficulty, acrid urine odor	Urinary excretion of β-hydroxyisovaleric acid and β-methylcrotonylglycine	No	β-Methylcrotonyl-CoA carboxylase (?)
	Propionicacidemia (ketotic hyperglycinemia)	Feeding difficulty, vomiting, lethargy, seizures	Metabolic ketoacidosis; hypoglycemia; hyperammonemia; hyperglycinemia and -uria; long-chain ketonuria; elevated blood and urine propionate	Yes	Propionyl-CoA carboxylase
	Methylmalonicaciduria (B_{12}-unresponsive)	Feeding difficulty, vomiting, lethargy	Metabolic ketoacidosis; hypoglycemia; hyperammonemia; hyperglycinemia and -uria; long-chain ketonuria; methylmalonicacidemia and -uria	Yes	Methylmalonyl-CoA mutase
	Methylmaloricaciduria (B_{12}-responsive)	Feeding difficulty, vomiting, lethargy	(See B_{12}-unresponsive form)	Yes	Defective conversion of vitamin B_{12} to deoxyadenosyl-B_{12}
	Methylmalonicaciduria and homocystinuria	Feeding difficulty, lethargy, coma	Methylmalonicaciduria; cystathioninemia; homocystinuria; hypomethioninemia	Yes	Defective conversion of vitamin B_{12} to deoxyadenosyl-B_{12} and methyl-B_{12}

Table 5-8   Inherited Aminoacidopathies Causing Severe Disease in the Newborn (*Continued*)

Amino Acid Classification	Disorder	Clinical Findings	Laboratory Findings	Available Leukocyte Assay	Enzymatic Defect
Urea Cycle	Hyperammonemia	Feeding difficulty, vomiting, lethargy, coma	Respiratory alkalosis; hyperammonemia	No	Ornithine transcarbamylase
	Citrullinemia	Feeding difficulty, vomiting, coma	Respiratory alkalosis; hyperammonemia; elevated blood and urine citrulline	No	Argininosuccinate synthetase
	Argininosuccinicaciduria	Ataxia, seizures	Hyperammonemia; argininosuccinicacidemia and -uria	Yes	Argininosuccinate lyase
	Argininemia	Spastic diplegia, seizures	Hyperammonemia; elevated blood and urine arginine	No	Arginase
Sulfur-Containing	Methionine malabsorption (oast-house syndrome)	Hypotonia, seizures, musty urine odor	α-Hydroxybutyricaciduria; elevated urine methionine (?)	No	Gut transport of methionine
	Sulfituria and thiosulfaturia	Pyramidal tract signs, blindness, dislocated lenses	Elevated urine sulfite, thiosulfate and S-sulfo-cysteine	No	Sulfite oxidase
Glycine	Hyperglycinemia (nonketotic)	Developmental failure, seizures	Elevated blood and urine glycine	No	Glycine decarboxylase (?)
Aromatic	Tyrosinemia	Cirrhosis, rickets, Fanconi syndrome	Hypophosphatemia; tyrosinemia and tyrosyluria; generalized aminoaciduria	No	p-Hydroxyphenylpyruvic acid oxidase (?)
β-Amino	β-Alaninemia	Lethargy, seizures	Elevated blood and urine β-alanine; γ-aminobutyricaciduria	No	β-Alanine: α-ketoglutarate transaminase (?)
Dipeptide	Carnosinemia	Seizures	Elevated blood and urine carnosine	No	Carnosinase

SCHEME 5–2

Flow Sheet Depicting Sequence of Investigation for the Acutely Ill Neonate with Suspected Aminoacidopathy

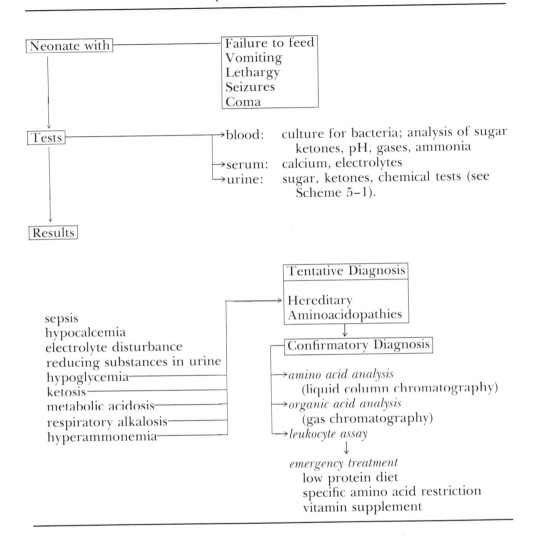

newborn. Failure to recognize the presence of life-threatening aminoacidopathy is less likely to occur if the family history reveals a previous sibling with similar manifestations; if there is no obvious cause for severe metabolic acidosis (found in branched-chain amino acid diseases) or alkalosis (found in diseases of the urea cycle); if symptoms follow the onset of protein feeding or a catabolic insult such as infection or reduced food intake; or if the blood ammonia is elevated.

The work-up of the patient may begin with the identification of ninhydrin-positive or ninhydrin-negative metabolites in blood and urine. Blood leukocytes can then be used to assay the activity of the enzyme relevant to the metabolite in excess (see Table 5–8). Unfortunately, diagnosis is dependent on special methodology which may be available only at certain referral centers. If the fetus is suspected of being at high risk because of the family history and if prenatal diagnosis is not feasible, leukocytes from cord blood may be useful to identify the enzyme phenotype; if the infant is affected, treatment could be initiated before symptoms appear. The appropriate arrangements should be made, taking this option into account, when counseling families in which there is an increased risk that offspring will be affected with a life-threatening aminoacidopathy.

A feeding regimen which restricts nitrogen intake to the absolute minimum for anabolic needs (i.e., no more than 2 g protein per kg body weight per day) and provides sufficient calories to prevent tissue catabolism should be started immediately and continued until the results of investigation are obtained. Appropriate measures to offset acidosis or alkalosis and to prevent hyperammonemia or hypoglycemia are also recommended where relevant; the appropriate specific treatment can be initiated when the diagnosis is known.

REFERENCES

Adriaenssens, K., Vanheule, R., and Van Belle, M.: A new simple screening method for detecting pathological aminoacidemias with collection of blood on paper. Clin. Chim. Acta *15*:362–364, 1967.

American Academy of Pediatrics: Committee statement on screening of newborn infants for metabolic disease. Pediatrics *35*:499–501, 1965.

Anonymous: Perception of isovalericacidemia. New Eng. J. Med. *277*:371, 1967.

Anonymous: Body odor and metabolic defects. Nutr. Rev. *26*:107–111, 1968.

Applegarth, D. A., Hardwick, D. F., Israels, S., and Ross, P. M.: Results of a screening program for aminoacidopathies in British Columbia. B. C. Med. J. *12*:129–132, 1970.

Benson, J. V., Jr., Cormick, J., and Patterson, J. A.: Accelerated chromatography of amino acids associated with phenylketonuria, leucinosis (maple syrup urine disease) and other inborn errors of metabolism. Anal. Biochem. *18*:481–492, 1967.

Berridge, B. J., Chao, W. R., and Peters, J. H.: Analysis of plasma and urinary amino acids by ion-exchange column chromatography. Amer. J. Clin. Nutr. *24*:934–939, 1971.

Berry, H. K., Leonard, C., Peters, H., Granger, M., and Chunekanrai, N.: Detection of metabolic disorders. Chromatographic procedures and interpretation of results. Clin. Chem. *14*:1033–1065, 1968.

Block, R. J., Durrum, E. L., and Zweig, G.: A Manual of Paper Chromatography and Paper Electrophoresis, 2nd edition. Academic Press, New York, 1958.

Buist, N. R. M.: Set of simple side-room urine tests for detection of inborn errors of metabolism. Brit. Med. J. *2*:745–749, 1968.

Carson, N. A. J., Cusworth, D. C., Dent, C. E., Field, C. M. B., Neill, D. W., and Westall, R. G.: Homocystinuria: A new inborn error of metabolism associated with mental deficiency. Arch. Dis. Child *38*:425–436, 1963.

Clow, C. L., Fraser, F. C., Laberge, C., and Scriver, C. R.: On the application of knowledge to the patient with genetic disease. Progr. Med. Genet. *9*:162–213, 1973.

Clow, C., Reade, T., and Scriver, C. R.: Management of hereditary metabolic disease. The role of allied health personnel. New Eng. J. Med. *284*:1292–1298, 1971.

Clow, C. L., Scriver, C. R., and Davies, E.: Results of mass screening for hyperaminoacidemias in the newborn infant. Amer. J. Dis. Child. *117*:48–53, 1969.

Cone, T. E., Jr.: Diagnosis and treatment: Some syndromes, diseases and conditions associated with abnormal coloration of the urine or diaper. Pediatrics *41*:645–658, 1968.

Cone, T. E., Jr.: Diagnosis and treatment: Some diseases, syndromes and conditions associated with an unusual odor. Pediatrics *41*:993–995, 1968.

Consden, R., Gorden, A. H., and Martin, A. J. P.: Qualitative analysis of proteins: A partition chromatographic method using paper. Biochem. J. *38*:224–232, 1944.

Crawhall, J. C., Thompson, C. J., and Bradley, K. H.: Separation of cystine, penicillamine, disulfide and cysteine-penicillamine mixed disulfide by automatic amino acid analysis. Anal. Biochem. *14*:405–413, 1966.

Culley, W. J., Mertz, E. T., Luce, M. W., Calandro, J. M., and Jolly, D. H.: Paper chromatographic estimation of phenylalanine and tyrosine using finger-tip blood. Clin. Chem. *8*:266–269, 1962.

Curtius, H.–Ch., Vollmin, J. A., and Baerlocher, K.: The use of deuterated phenylalanine for the elucidation of the phenylalanine-tyrosine metabolism. Clin. Chim. Acta *37*:277–285, 1972.

Danks, D. M.: Detection of heterozygotes. *In* Crow, J. F., and Neel, J. V., eds., Proceedings of the

Third International Congress of Human Genetics (Chicago, 1966). Johns Hopkins Press, Baltimore, pp. 61–67, 1967.

Darbre, A., and Islam, A.: Gas-liquid chromatography of trifluoroacetylated amino acid methyl esters. Biochem. J. *106*:923–925, 1968.

Datta, S. P., Dent, C. E., and Harris, H.: An apparatus for the simultaneous production of many two-dimensional paper chromatograms. Science *112*:621–622, 1950.

Daum, R. S., Lamm, P. H., Mamer, O. A., and Scriver, C. R.: A "new" disorder of isoleucine catabolism. Lancet (ii), 1289–1290, 1971.

Dent, C. E.: Detection of amino acids in urine and other fluids. Lancet (ii), 637–639, 1946.

Dent, C. E.: A study of the behaviour of some sixty amino acids and other ninhydrin reacting substances on phenol-"collidine" filter paper chromatograms with notes as to the occurrence of some of them in biological fluids. Biochem. J. *43*:169–180, 1948.

Dent, C. E.: Paper chromatography and medicine. In Dyke, S. C., ed., Recent Advances in Clinical Pathology, 2nd edition. Blakiston, Philadelphia, pp. 238–258, 1951.

Dent, C. E.: Clinical applications of amino acid chromatography. Scand. J. Clin. Lab. Invest. Supplement 31 *10*:122–127, 1957.

Dent, C. E., and Walshe, J. M.: Amino acid metabolism. Brit. Med. Bull. *10*:247–250, 1954.

DeWolfe, M. S., Baskurt, S., and Cochrane, W. A.: Automatic amino acid analysis of blood serum and plasma. Clin. Biochem. *1*:75–81, 1967.

Dickinson, J. C., Rosenblum, H., and Hamilton, P. B.: Ion exchange chromatography of the free amino acids in the plasma of the newborn infant. Pediatrics *36*:2–13, 1965.

Efron, M. L.: Two-way separation of amino acids and other ninhydrin reading substances by high-voltage electrophoresis followed by paper chromatography. Biochem. J. *72*:691–694, 1959.

Efron, M. L.: High voltage paper electrophoresis. In Smith, I., ed., Chromatographic and Electrophoretic Techniques, Vol. II, 2nd edition. Interscience, New York, pp. 166–193, 1968.

Efron, M. L., Young, D., Moser, H. W., and MacCready, R. A.: A simple chromatographic screening test for the detection of disorders of amino acid metabolism: A technique using white blood or urine collected on filter paper. New Eng. J. Med. *270*:1378–1383, 1964.

Evered, D. F.: Ionophoresis of acidic and basic amino acids on filter paper using low voltages. Biochim. Biophys. Acta *36*:14–19, 1959.

Farriaux, J. P., and Delabre, M.: Le dépistage des hétérozygotes de la phénylcétonurie typique. Arch. Franc. Pediat. *29*:365–372, 1972.

Fogarty International Centre Proceedings No. 6, May 1970. In Harris R., ed., Early Diagnosis of Human Genetic Defects: Scientific and Ethical Considerations. U.S. Department of Health, Education and Welfare, U.S. Government Printing Office, Washington, D.C., pp. 72–75, 1972.

Garrod, A. E.: The Croonian lectures. Lancet (ii), 1, 73, 142, 214, 1908.

Gerritsen, T., Rekberg, M. L., and Waisman, H. A.: On the determination of free amino acids in serum. Anal. Biochim. *11*:460–466, 1965.

Gold, R. J. M., Maag, U., Neal, J., and Scriver, C. R.: Analysis of biochemical data for genetic screening. (Abstract.) Amer. J. Hum. Genet. *24*:24a, 1972.

Grimble, R. F., and Whitehead, R. G.: An automated method for rapid chromatographic analysis of serum, valine, alanine and glycine. Clin. Chim. Acta *31*:355–361, 1971.

Guthrie, R.: Personal communication, 1972.

Guthrie, R., and Susi, A.: A simple phenylalanine method for detecting phenylketonuria in large populations of newborn infants. Pediatrics *32*:338–343, 1963.

Guthrie, R., and Whitney, S.: Phenylketonuria detection in the newborn infant as a routine hospital procedure. Children's Bureau Publication No. 419, U.S. Department of Health, Education and Welfare, Welfare Administration, Washington, D.C., 1964.

Hais, I. M., and Macek, K., eds.: Paper Chromatography: A Comprehensive Treatise, 3rd edition. Academic Press, New York, and Publishing House of the Czechoslovakian Academy of Sciences, Prague, 1963.

Hamilton, P. B.: Ion exchange chromatography of amino acids. a single column high resolving, fully automatic procedure. Anal. Chem. *35*:2055–2064, 1963.

Hansen, S., Perry, T. L., Lesk, D., and Gibson, L.: Urinary bacteria: Potential source of some organic acidiurias. Clin. Chim. Acta *39*:71–74, 1972.

Hill, J. B., Summer, G. K., Pender, M. W., and Roszel, N. O.: An automated procedure for blood phenylalanine. Clin. Chem. *11*:541–546, 1965.

Hochella, N. J.: Automated fluorometric determination of tyrosine in blood. Anal. Biochem. *21*:227–234, 1967.

Horning, E. C., and Horning, M. G.: Human metabolic profiles obtained by GC and GC/MS. J. Chrom. Sci. *9*:129–140, 1971.

Hsia, D. Y. Y.: The detection of heterozygous carriers. Med. Clin. N. Amer. *53*:857–874, 1969.

Jackson, S. H., Sardharwalla, I. B., and Ebers, G. C.: Two systems of amino acid chromatography suitable for mass screening. Clin. Biochem. *2*:163–167, 1968.

Jellum, E., Stokke, O., and Eldjarn, L.: Screening for metabolic disorders using gas-liquid chromatography, mass spectrometry and computer technique. Scand. J. Clin. Lab. Invest. 27:273–285, 1971.

Jellum, E., Stokke, O., and Eldjarn, L.: Combined use of gas chromatography mass spectrometry and computer in diagnosis and studies of metabolic disorders. Clin. Chem. 18:800–809, 1972.

Jørgensen, O. S., Kofod, B., and Rafaelson, O. J.: Amino acid excretion in urine of normal children. Danish Med. Bull. 17:161–165, 1970.

Juvet, R. S., Jr., and Cram, S. P.: Gas chromatography. Anal. Chem. (Annual review) 42:1R–22R, 1970.

Knipfel, J. E., Christensen, D. A., and Owen, B. D.: Effect of deproteinating agents (picric acid and sulfosalicylic acid) on analysis for free amino acids in swine blood and tissue. Ass. Official Anal. Chem. J. 52:981–984, 1969.

Komrower, G. M., Fowler, B., Griffiths, M. J., and Lambert, A. M.: A prospective community survey for aminoacidemias. Proc. Roy. Soc. Med. 61:294–296, 1968.

Komrower, G. M., and Robins, A. J.: Plasma amino acid disturbance in infancy. Arch. Dis. Child. 44:418–421, 1969.

Levy, H. L.: Genetic screening. In Harris, H., and Hirschkorn, K., eds., Advances in Human Genetics, Vol. 3. Plenum Press, New York, 1972.

Levy, H. L., and Barkin, E.: Comparison of amino acid concentrations between plasma and erythrocytes studies in normal human subjects and those with metabolic disorders. J. Lab. Clin. Med. 78:517–523, 1971.

Levy, H. L., Baullinger, P. C., and Madigan, P. M.: A rapid procedure for the determination of phenylalanine and tyrosine from blood filter paper specimens. Clin. Chim. Acta 31:447–452, 1971.

Levy, H. L., Madigan, P. M., and Shih, V. E.: Massachusetts Metabolic Disorders Screening Program 1. Technics and results of urine screening. Pediatrics 49:825–836, 1972.

Levy, H. L., Shih, V. E., and MacCready, R. A.: Massachusetts metabolic screening program. In Harris, R., ed., Early Diagnosis of Human Genetic Defects. Scientific and Ethical Considerations. Fogarty International Centre Proceedings No. 6, May 1970, U.S. Department of Health, Education and Welfare, Publ. No. 72–75, Washington, D.C., pp. 47–54, 1972.

Levy, H. L., Shih, V. E., Madigan, P. M., Karolkewics, V., and MacCready, R. A.: Results of a screening method for free amino acids. I. Whole blood. Clin. Biochem. 1:200–207, 1968a.

Levy, H. L., Shih, V. E., Madigan, P. M., Karolkewicz, V., and MacCready, R. A.: Results of a screening method for free amino acids. II. Urine. Clin. Biochem. 1:208–215, 1968b.

Mabry, C. C., and Karam, E. A.: Measurement of free amino acids in plasma and serum by means of high-voltage paper electrophoresis. Amer. J. Clin. Path. 42:421–430, 1964.

Mamer, O. A., Crawhall, J. C., and Tjoa, S. S.: The identification of urinary acid by coupled gas chromatography-mass spectrometry. Clin. Chim. Acta 32:171–184, 1971.

McCaman, M. W., and Robins, E.: Fluorometric method for the determination of phenylalanine in serum. J. Lab. Clin. Med. 59:885–890, 1962.

Milunsky, A., Littlefield, J. W., Kanfer, J. N., Kolodny, E. H., Shih, V. E., and Atkins, L.: Prenatal genetic diagnosis. New Eng. J. Med. 283: Pt. I, 1370–1381; Pt. II, 1441–1447; Pt. III, 1498–1504, 1970.

Moore, S., Spackman, D. H., and Stein, W. H.: Chromatography of amino acids on sulfonated polystyrene resins. Anal. Chem. 30:1185–1190, 1958.

Moore, S., and Stein, W. H.: Procedures for the chromatographic determination of amino acids on four percent cross-linked sulfonated polystyrene resins. J. Biol. Chem. 211:893–906, 1954.

Murphy, E. A., and Mutalik, G. S.: The application of Bayesian methods in genetic counseling. Hum. Hered. 19:126–151, 1969.

Nadler, H. L., and Hsia, D. Y. Y.: Utilization of white blood cells for study of clinical genetic disorders. Clin. Biochem. 1:192–199, 1968.

O'Brien, D.: Rare inborn errors of metabolism in children with mental retardation. Part B. Technical procedures. Children's Bureau Publication No. 429, U.S. Department of Health, Education and Welfare, U.S. Government Printing Office, Washington, D.C., pp. 70–100, 1965.

Partington, M. W.: Case finding in phenylketonuria. III. One-way paper chromatography of the amino acids in blood. Canad. Med. Ass. J. 99:638–644, 1968.

Perry, T. L., and Hansen, S.: Technical pitfalls leading to errors in the quantitation of plasma amino acids. Clin. Chim. Acta 25:53–58, 1969.

Perry, T. L., Hansen, S., and MacDougall, L.: Urinary screening tests in the prevention of mental deficiency. Canad. Med. Ass. J. 95:89–95, 1966.

Peters, H. J., and Berridge, B. J., Jr.: The determination of amino acids in plasma and urine by ion-exchange chromatography. Chromatogr. Rev. 12:157–165, 1970.

Piez, K. A., and Morris, L.: A modified procedure for the automatic analysis of amino acids. Anal. Biochem. 1:187–201, 1960.

Raine, D. N., Cooke, J. R., Andrews, W. A., and Mahon, D. F.: Screening for inherited metabolic disease by plasma chromatography (Scriver) in a large city. Brit. Med. J. 3:7–14, 1972.

Rook, A.: Hair colour in clinical diagnosis. Irish J. Med. Sci. VII Series 2:415–427, 1969.

Rosenberg, L. E.: Diagnosis and management of inherited aminoacidopathies in the newborn and the unborn. In Genetics and the Perinatal Patient. A Scientific, Clinical and Ethical Consideration. Mead Johnson Symposium on Perinatal and Developmental Medicine #1, p. 45, 1972.

Rosenblatt, D., and Scriver, C. R.: Heterogeneity in genetic control of phenylalanine metabolism in man. Nature (London) 218:677–678, 1968.

Rouser, G., Jelinek, B., Samuels, A. J., and Kinugasa, K.: Free amino acids in the blood of man and animals. I. Method of study and the effects of venipuncture and food intake on blood free amino acids. In Holden, J. T., ed., Amino Acid Pools. Elsevier, New York, pp. 350–372, 1962.

Ruddle, F., Ricciuti, F., McMorris, F. A., Tischfield, J., Creagan, R., Darlington, G., and Chen, T.: Somatic cell genetic assignment of peptidase C and the Rh linkage group to chromosome A-1 in man. Science 176:1429–1431, 1972.

Scriver, C. R.: Hereditary aminoaciduria. In Bearn, A., and Steinberg, A. G., Progress in Medical Genetics, Vol. 2. Grune & Stratton, New York, pp. 83–186, 1962.

Scriver, C. R.: Screening newborns for hereditary metabolic disease. Pediat. Clin. N. Amer. 12: 807–821, 1965.

Scriver, C. R.: Treatment of inherited disease: Realized and potential. Med. Clin. N. Amer. 53: 941–963, 1969.

Scriver, C. R.: Mutants: Consumers with special needs. Nutr. Rev. 29:155–158, 1971.

Scriver, C. R.: Screening and treatment of hereditary metabolic disease. Proceedings of the IV International Congress on Human Genetics, Paris, 1971. Excerpta Medica Foundation, Amsterdam, 1972.

Scriver, C. R., Clow, C. L., and Lamm, P.: Plasma amino acids: Screening quantitation and interpretation. Amer. J. Clin. Nutr. 24:876–890, 1971.

Scriver, C. R., and Davies, E.: Endogenous renal clearance rates of free amino acids in pre-pubertal children. Pediatrics 32:592–598, 1965.

Scriver, C. R., Davies, E., and Cullen, A. M.: Application of a simple method to the screening of plasma for a variety of aminoacidopathies. Lancet (ii), 230–232, 1964.

Scriver, C. R., Davies, E., and Lamm, P.: Accelerated selective short column chromatography of neutral acidic amino acids on a Bechman-Spinco Analyzer, modified for simultaneous analysis of two samples. Clin. Biochem. 1:179–181, 1968.

Shih, V., Efron, M. L., and Mechanic, G. L.: Rapid short column chromatography of amino acids: A method for blood and urine specimens in the diagnosis and treatment of metabolic diseases. Anal. Biochem. 20:299–311, 1967.

Smith, A. J., and Strang, L. B.: An inborn error of metabolism with the urinary excretion of α-hydroxybutyric acid and phenylpyruvic acid. Arch. Dis. Child. 33:109–113, 1958.

Smith, I., ed.: Chromatographic and Electrophoretic Techniques. Vol. I. Chromatography, 3rd edition, 1969. Vol. II. Electrophoresis, 2nd edition, 1968. Heinemann, London.

Snyderman, S. E.: Diagnosis of metabolic disease. Pediat. Clin. N. Amer. 18:199–208, 1971.

Soupart, P.: Free amino acids of blood and urine in the human. In Holden, J. T., ed., Amino Acid Pools. Elsevier, New York, pp. 220–262, 1962.

Spackman, D. H., Stein, W. H., and Moore, S.: Automatic recording apparatus for use in the chromatography of amino acids. Anal. Chem. 30:1190–1206, 1958.

Szeinberg, A., Szeinberg, B., and Cohen, B. E.: Screening method for detection of specific amino-acidemias. Clin. Chim. Acta 23:93–95, 1969.

Tocci, P. M.: The biochemical diagnosis of metabolic disorders by urinalysis and paper chromatography. In Nyhan, W. L., ed., Amino Acid Metabolism and Genetic Variation. McGraw-Hill, New York, pp. 461–490, 1967.

Wilson, J. M. G., and Jungner, G.: Principles and practice of screening for disease. Public Health Papers, No. 34, World Health Organization, Geneva, 1968.

Winter, C. G., and Christensen, H. N.: Migration of amino acids across the membrane of the human erythrocyte. J. Biol. Chem. 239:872–878, 1964.

World Health Organization, Technical Report Series, No. 401: Screening for Inborn Errors of Metabolism. Geneva, 1968.

World Health Organization, Technical Report Series, No. 497: Genetic Disorders: Prevention, Treatment and Rehabilitation. Geneva, 1972.

Yeh, H. L., Frankl, W., Dunn, M. S., Parker, P., Hughes, B., and Gyorgy, P.: The urinary excretion of amino acids by a cystinuric subject. Amer. J. Med. Sci. 214:507–512, 1947.

Zumwalt, R. W., Kuo, K., and Gehrke, C. W.: Applications of a gas-liquid chromatographic method for amino acid analysis. A system for analysis of nanogram amounts. J. Chromatogr. 55:267–280, 1971.

Zweig, G., Moore, R. B., and Sherma, J.: Chromatography. Anal. Chem. (Annual review) 42:349R–362R, 1970.

Appendix to Chapter 5

URINE SCREENING: OFFICE AND LABORATORY PROCEDURES FOR DIAGNOSIS OF DISORDERS OF AMINO ACID METABOLISM

General Considerations

A random urine sample is satisfactory for screening purposes. The early morning specimen is preferred to avoid dietary artifacts which may influence amino acid content of the urine. The urine sample should be preserved with a few crystals of thymol or acidified to below pH 4 with a few drops of 3N HCl, and stored at $-20°C$, if it is not to be analyzed immediately.

Simple chemical tests can be done on the urine to reveal the diagnosis.

The amount of amino acids visible in a partition chromatogram is influenced not only by disease processes but also by the concentration of the urine. Application of a fixed volume will cause considerable variation in the intensity of the amino acid pattern. It is better to apply an amount of urine in relation to some excretion coefficient such as total nitrogen content which can be determined either by the Kjeldahl method for nonprotein nitrogen or by a modification of the urea-nitrogen method adapted for the Technicon auto analyser. An aliquot of urine equivalent to 250 micrograms total nitrogen can be used for two-dimensional chromatography on filter paper sheets (25 × 25 cm squares). Only half of this amount is required on one-dimensional partition chromatograms. Creatinine content can also be used as the coefficient, but creatinine excretion is more variable and less relevant to amino acid content of urine.

Cleanliness of the working area and of the hands is important to avoid artifacts.

Spot separation on chromatograms is improved when the sample is applied to the origin in small aliquots (10 μl max.). However, large volumes, when applied in small aliquots, tend to build up sediment at the origin and to distort the development of the chromatogram. Larger applications (more than 10 μl) produce diffuse spots. When a large volume of sample must be applied, it can be measured out into a watchglass and dried down with a current of air. The residue is then taken up on a small volume of water and applied to the paper.

Chemical Tests

Screening of the urine begins with inspection of the sample. Unusual color or smell may be a clue to diagnosis (Table 5A–1). The presence of crystals should be noted (Fig. 5A–1) and an interpretation pursued. Inappropriate diluteness of urine may indicate tubular damage and failure of the urine-concentrating mechanisms.

Table 5A–1   Interpretation of Positive Chemical Screening Tests on Urine When Applied to the Aminoacidopathies[a]

Positive Benedict's Test
    Glucose, in Fanconi syndrome(s)
    Homogentisic acid, in alcaptonuria
    p-*Hydroxyphenylpyruvate*, in tyrosinemia
Other causes
    Fructose
    Galactose
    Xylulose
    Lactose
    Lactulose
    Phenols

Positive Ferric Chloride Reaction
    Phenylpyruvate (blue-green), in phenylketonuria and variants
    p-*Hydroxyphenylpyruvate* (transient blue-green), in tyrosinemia
    Imidazolpyruvate (gray-green), in histidinemia
    Branched-chain keto acids (blue, yellow, blue-green), in MSUD
    α-*Ketobutyrate* (purple $\rightarrow$ red-brown), in methionine malabsorption
    Homogentisic acid (transient blue-green), in alcaptonuria
    Pyruvic acid (yellow), in *hyper*alaninemia
    Xanthurenic acid (green $\rightarrow$ brown), in xanthurenicaciduria
Other common causes
    Salicylates (purple)
    Phenothiazines (purple-brown)
    Acetoacetic acid (brown)
    Conjugated bilirubin (blue-green)
    Isonicotinic acid hydrazide (grey)

Positive Cyanide-Nitroprusside Test
    Cystine, in cystinurias (classical and variants), *hyper*cystinuria and Fanconi syndrome(s)
    Homocystine, in homocystinuria (cystathionine synthase deficiency), and due to remethylation
        defects
    Cysteine-homocysteine disulfide, in cystinuria and homocystinuria
    β-*mercaptolactate-cysteine disulfide*, in defect of its metabolism
    Penicillamine-cysteine disulfide, in treatment of cystinuria
    Glutathione, in glutathioninemia

Table 5A–1 Interpretation of Positive Chemical Screening Tests on Urine When Applied to the Aminoacidopathies (*Continued*)

Positive Test for Acetone (Acetest [Ames])
    Acetone (purple) ⎱
    Acetoacetate (purple) ⎰ in ketonuria from any cause
    Butanone (red), in α-methylacetoacetate thiolase deficiency and propionicaciduria
    2-Hexanone (yellow) ⎱
    3-Hexanone (faint yellow) ⎰ as for butanone, plus methylmalonicaciduria

Turbidity Test with Sulfosalicylic Acid (20% w/v)
    Protein — clearing with heat, in tubular disease
            — no clearing with heat, in glomerular (with or without tubular) disease

Physical Aspects of Urine

	Condition	Feature
Odor	Maple syrup urine disease	maple syrup, caramel, curry
	Phenylketonuria	musty, mousy
	Hereditary tyrosinemia	cabbage-like, fishy
	Liver failure	cabbage-like, fishy
	Isovaleric acidemia	cheesy
	Oast-house syndrome	hop-like
	Methionine malabsorption	cabbage-like
Color	Alcaptonuria	darkens on standing
	Blue-diaper syndrome	indigo blue stain
Crystals	Cystinuria(s)	cystine crystals
	Liver failure	tyrosine crystals
	Hyperammonemia (OCT defic.)	orotic acid crystals

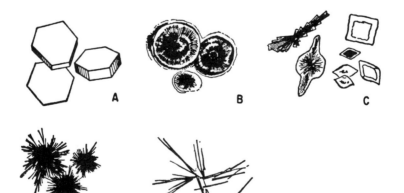

Figure 5A–1 Urinary constituents, visible by light microscopy, which may be found in the spun urine sediment of patients with hereditary or acquired aminoacidopathies and other aberrations of metabolism.
    A. Cystine crystals (birefringent in polarized light).
    B. Leucine crystals.
    C. Uric acid crystals (may occur in some patients with Fanconi syndrome, as well as in the hyperuricemias).
    D. Tyrosine crystals.
    E. Orotic acid crystals (found in X-linked ornithine carbamyl transferase deficiency with hyperammonemia).
(Adapted from Buist: Brit. Med. J. *2*:745–749, 1968.)

Cyanide/Nitroprusside (CN/NP) Test for Disulfides (Including Cystine and Homocystine)

Reagents

Sodium cyanide, 5% (w/v) in water

Sodium nitroprusside, a freshly made solution containing a few crystals in water

An equal quantity of water is mixed with the sodium cyanide reagent and allowed to stand for 10 minutes. Three to four drops of the nitroprusside reagent are added with the aid of a Pasteur pipet. The resulting color is noted.

INTERPRETATION OF TEST. A magenta color is produced by a positive test; the nitroprusside reagent itself produces a weak pink-orange color with urine. In dilute urine, a weak color is produced by a positive test; the color of the latter persists, whereas a false-positive test quickly fades, yielding a brown color.

Compounds with a disulfide group yield a positive test which may be obtained in the cystinurias, the homocystinurias, in generalized aminoacidurias and also with the excretion of unusual disulfides including drugs.

Modified Test for Homocystine (Barber)

The following modification of the cyanide nitroprusside test will differentiate between cystine and homocystine reagents.

Test A.   Add 5 ml urine to a test tube. Saturate with sodium chloride. Add 0.5 ml of 1% $AgNO_3$ (w/v) in 3% NH_3 (v/v). Mix and allow to stand for one minute. Add 0.5 ml freshly prepared sodium nitroprusside solution. Add 0.5 ml sodium cyanide reagent.

Test B.   A control sample is set up similarly, but 3% NH_3 (v/v) is used in place of the silver nitrate reagent.

INTERPRETATION OF TEST. The immediate appearance of a pink-purple color in Test A indicates a positive homocystine test. A slow reaction indicates cystine or some other compound.

Benedict's Test for Reducing Substances

Reagents

Clinitest (Ames) tablets. Follow the instructions supplied with the tablets. Beware of the "pass-through" reaction.

Clinistix (Ames). Follow the instructions. A positive test confirms the presence of glucose.

INTERPRETATION OF TEST. A positive *Clinitest* (appearance of green, yellow or red color) indicates the presence of a reducing substance. A positive *Clinistix* indicates glucose.

A positive *Clinistix* (glucose-oxidase) test does *not* rule out the presence of reducing sugars and substances in urine other than glucose. For example, glucosuria occurs in galactosemia secondary to renal tubular damage; the presence of galactosuria (an important diagnostic clue) will be missed if the *Clinistix* test is used exclusively.

A positive Benedict's test should be followed up by one-dimensional chromatography either on filter paper or on thin-layer to identify the reducing substance in the sample. A differential diagnosis of the positive test is listed in Table 5A–1.

Ferric Chloride Test for Keto Acids (and Other Substances)

Reagents

Ferric chloride ($FeCl_3 \cdot 6H_2O$), 10% (w/v) in 0.25N HCl

1% (w/v) Ferric chloride, 1% (w/v) ferrous ammonium sulfate [$Fe(NH_4)_2(SO_4)_2 \cdot 6H_2O$] dissolved in 0.02N HCl

The second reagent does not detect *p*-hydroxyphenylpyruvic acid.

To perform the test, fresh urine or urine which has been frozen immediately after collection should be used.

With the first reagent, the ferric chloride solution is added dropwise to 1 ml urine, and the color is observed. With the second reagent, the urine is added dropwise to 1 ml of the ferric chloride reagent, and the color is observed.

INTERPRETATION OF TEST. Color develops within the first minute and should be observed between 1 and 3 minutes. The development of any color different from the ferric chloride solution itself is indicative of a positive test. The causes of a positive test are listed in Table 5A–1.

Sulfosalicylic Acid Precipitation Test for Protein

Reagent

Sulfosalicylic acid, 20% (w/v) in water

The reagent is added dropwise to urine; absence of turbidity indicates a negative test. If turbidity appears, the urine is heated; the turbidity may clear to reappear on cooling again.

INTERPRETATION OF TEST. Turbidity unaffected by heat indicates glomerular proteinuria with a molecular weight more than 40,000 daltons. Turbidity which clears with heat indicates tubular proteinuria in which the protein has low molecular weight (30,000–40,000 daltons). The latter is found in the Fanconi syndrome and Lowe's syndrome and with Bence-Jones proteinuria.

2,4-Dinitrophenylhydrazine Reaction for Keto Acids

Reagent

2,4-dinitrophenylhydrazine, 0.5% (w/v) in 2N HCl

Mix equal volumes of urine and reagent.

INTERPRETATION OF TEST. A yellow or red precipitate formed within a minute indicates a large quantity of keto acid. A small precipitate or turbidity after 60 minutes at room temperature is normal. The precipitate produced by acetone disappears if the urine is heated briefly at 100°C before performing the test.

Nitrosonaphthol Test for Tyrosyluria

Reagents

Nitric acid, 2.63N (prepared by mixing 1 vol. conc. nitric acid with 5 vol. H_2O)

Sodium nitrite, 2.5% (w/v) in H_2O (keep in refrigerator)

Nitrosonaphthol, 0.1% (w/v) in 95% ethanol

Pipette 1 ml nitric acid reagent into a small test tube. Add 1 drop sodium nitrite solution and 10 drops nitrosonaphthol. Add 3 drops of urine, and mix. Leave for 2 to 3 minutes. Orange/red color indicates a positive test. Always run a sample containing p-hydroxyphenylacetic acid as control. The reaction mixture must be prepared and used immediately.

INTERPRETATION OF TEST. A positive reaction is obtained with p-hydroxyphenylpyruvic aicd, p-HPLA and p-HPAA; o-HPAA does not give a positive test.

Acetest (Ames) for Acetone

Reagent

Acetest tablets (Ames)

Place one drop of urine on Acetest tablet and read as directed on the bottle.

INTERPRETATION OF TEST. A purple color indicates the presence of acetone in urine. Other substances such as butanone and hexanone also react to give color.

Note: If the test for acetone is positive, the dinitrophenylhydrazine test for keto acids will also be positive. Bringing the urine to 100°C will drive off the volatile acetone and allow further testing.

Supplementary Tests

Additional, relatively simple tests to screen for other metabolic disorders can be done in most clinical laboratories. Papers by Perry et al. (1966), Berry et al. (1968), Buist (1968) and Snyderman (1971) should also be consulted for additional information about these screening tests. The manual by O'Brien (1965) is another source of useful laboratory methods.

The further investigation of urine, blood and plasma is best accomplished with the chromatographic methods described in the Chapter 5. One dimensional partition chromatography (Levy et al., 1972), two-dimensional chromatography (Dent, 1948; Smith, 1968; Berry et al., 1968) and electrochromatography (Efron, 1966) are the preferred methods for further investigation.

Further studies are preferably carried out in collaboration with investigators who are familiar with the type of problem tentatively identified in the preliminary stages of investigation.

REFERENCES

Berry, H. K., Leonard, C., Peters, H., Granger, M., and Chunekanrai, N.: Detection of metabolic disorders. Chromatographic procedures and interpretation of results. Clin. Chem. *14*:1033–1065, 1968.

Buist, N. R. M.: Set of simple side-room urine tests for detection of inborn errors of metabolism. Brit. Med. J. *2*:745–749, 1968.

O'Brien, D.: Rare inborn errors of metabolism in children with mental retardation. Part B. Technical procedures. Children's Bureau Publication No. 429–1965, U.S. Department of Health, Education and Welfare, U.S. Govt. Printing Office, Washington, D.C., pp. 70–100, 1965.

Perry, T. L., Hansen, S., and MacDougall, L.: Urinary screening tests in the prevention of mental deficiency. Canad. Med. J. *95*:89–95, 1966.

Snyderman, S. E.: Diagnosis of metabolic disease. Pediat. Clin. N. Amer. *18*:199–208, 1971.

Membrane Transport of Amino Acids and Its Disorders

Chapter Six

BIOLOGICAL BASIS OF MEMBRANE TRANSPORT: MECHANISMS OF IMPAIRMENT

SCIENTIFIC PERSPECTIVE

Functional Significance of Transport

One of the unique characteristics of living cells is their capacity to maintain an internal composition different from that of their external environment. This is true not only for nucleic acid and protein macromolecules confined to the intracellular compartment, but for small organic and inorganic chemicals as well. Thus, the mammalian cell regularly contains large amounts of potassium, magnesium and organic phosphates but very little sodium and chloride, while the extracellular fluid which surrounds it is very rich in sodium and chloride and very poor in potassium and magnesium. Cells also accumulate sugars, amines, neurohumoral effectors and the substances of particular interest to this discussion — free amino acids. The capacity of mammalian cells to maintain concentrations of amino acids considerably greater than those in their surrounding extracellular media enables cells to control more efficiently those intracellular reactions which amino acids participate in and which are vital to normal cellular homeostasis: activation and incorporation into new protein molecules; conversion to glucose or fatty acids in gluconeogenic or lipogenic pathways; and catabolism to other amino acids, keto acids, urea, ammonia or sulfate.

Another group of transport processes is concerned, not with the maintenance of the intracellular milieu, but with the transfer of solutes from one surface of a sheet of cells to the other. Such processes as the formation of aqueous humor, cerebrospinal fluid and gastrointestinal secretions, the absorption of nutrients from the intestinal tract and the conversion of glomerular filtrate into urine fall into this category of transfer function. With regard to amino acids, this type of transport assumes great importance in the gut and the kidney. The absorption of amino acids by the small intestine plays a key role in nutrition, particularly for those amino acids which the mammalian organism cannot synthesize de novo (the "essential" amino acids). In like fashion, the proximal renal tubule conserves these important substrates by reabsorbing 95 to 100 per cent of the free amino acids filtered. These specialized functions are carried out by cells with equally specialized structure. The mucosal cells of the small intestine and the proximal tubule are lined by countless microvillous processes which provide a huge area of membrane surface capable of interacting with solute molecules. Throughout this discussion we shall emphasize these two tissues, which share so many common anatomical and functional characteristics.

Cellular Mechanisms

The maintenance of differences in concentration of many small molecules requires that some kind of barrier to diffusion exist between the intracellular and extracellular space. If this were not the case, the composition of these two compartments would soon become equalized. This barrier to diffusion is the cell membrane, and the barrier function is relative, not absolute. For many years it was supposed that the composition of cells was established when they were formed and thereafter was maintained by the impermeability of the membranes. The introduction of radioactive isotopes into the study of cellular physiology, however, demonstrated convincingly that this was not the case. Ions were shown to move into and out of cells at a rapid rate. How, then, was the concentration of sodium inside the cell kept at a very low value? Since sodium could be shown to enter cells readily, it became apparent that a mechanism must exist for its extrusion—a mechanism by which this positively charged cation could be moved against both a chemical and an electric gradient (the cell interior is electrically negative). Such a mechanism could not occur spontaneously and was shown to require energy derived from the metabolic activity of the cell. Thus was born the concept of *active transport* as distinguished from *passive diffusion*. The active transport process for sodium (and potassium) is the most widely distributed and, in its energy requirements, the most important mechanism of its kind, but the arguments which were responsible for its identification are equally pertinent to the transmembrane movement of amino acids and other solutes.

The mechanism by which amino acids are transported into mammalian cells and across epithelial cell layers in vitro has been explored extensively during the past 20 years. Tissue preparations and methodology have varied greatly. Some investigators have studied amino acid uptake in suspensions of ascites tumor cells (Christensen, 1966), reticulocytes (Wheeler and Christensen, 1967), human leukocytes (Rosenberg and Downing, 1965), cultured skin fibroblasts (Groth and Rosenberg, 1972) or renal tubules (Hillman et al., 1968b), while others have carried out experiments with organized tissue preparations including diaphragm muscle (Kipnis and Noall, 1958; Elsas et al., 1968), kidney cortex (Rosenberg et al., 1961; Wilson and Scriver, 1967), fetal bone (Finerman and Rosenberg, 1966), brain (Levi et al., 1966), intestinal mucosa (Wilson, 1962; Thier et al., 1965), pancreas (Begin and Scholefield, 1964) or adipose tissue (Goodman, 1966). Labeled and unlabeled amino acids, naturally occurring and synthetic, have contributed to these investigations. Despite great diversity of experimental method and design, many common features of transport processes for amino acids have been defined (Wilson, 1962; Scriver, 1967a; Smyth, 1960; Christensen et al., 1961; Christensen, 1962): L(levo) amino acids, the naturally occurring steroisomers, are transported much more efficiently than their D (dextro) forms; transport occurs against chemical and electrochemical concentration gradients by processes which are dependent on the sodium ion concentration of the incubation medium and on a supply of metabolic energy; intracellular accumulation depends on saturable processes which exhibit substrate specificity, competitive inhibition and noncompetitive inhibition; the transport processes for individual substrates vary with the length and composition of aliphatic side chains, their cationic or anionic properties in solution and the alpha or beta position of the amino groups.

These complex functional characteristics of mammalian transport systems for amino acids demand the existence of equally complex integrated biochemical mechanisms in or near the cell membrane. Although a great deal has been learned about the chemical structure and organization of biological membranes in recent years (Korn, 1966; Stoeckinius and Engelman, 1969; Singer and Nicolson, 1972), it is still not possible to understand the relationship between membrane structure and transport function in more than a highly speculative way. Cell membranes are composed primarily of phospholipids and protein. Robertson (1959) proposed the widely accepted, but still unproved, "unit membrane" concept of membrane structure based on electron microscopic and x-ray diffraction studies of the myelin sheath. This concept states that membranes consist of a bimolecular leaflet of phospholipids whose nonpolar, fatty acid chains are inwardly oriented perpendicular to the plane of the membrane, and whose polar moieties compose the external surface of the phospholipid layer and are covered by a layer of protein. The theory supposes that the phospholipid composition of membranes varies greatly and that significant amounts of cholesterol and other neutral lipids may also be present. The protein layer is presumed to consist of both "structural" components and a variety of different binding proteins and enzymes.

Membranes isolated from erythrocytes (Maddy, 1966; Bakerman and Wasemiller, 1967), ascites tumor cells (Wallach and Kamat, 1964), hepatic cells (Emmelot et al., 1964; Ashworth and Green, 1966) and intestinal epithelium (Eichholz, 1967) have been shown to contain phospholipids, sterols, carbohydrate and a variety of protein species including enzymes, but there is, as yet, no conclusive information about the organization of these components or their site of origin. One of these membrane-bound enzymes, sodium-potassium activated adenosine triphosphatase (Na-K ATPase) has been shown to be intimately involved with sodium and potassium transport and, hence, may be particularly relevant to our discussion. Recent studies with microorganisms have produced more exciting results. Investigators have isolated specific proteins present in or near the cell membrane which selectively bind galactosides (Fox et al., 1967), sulfate (Pardee, 1967) and leucine (Penrose et al., 1968). These binding proteins are genetically controlled and possess many of the kinetic features of the long sought permeases, making them attractive candidates for specific transport mediators. Furthermore, the active transport of many amino acids and sugars has been shown to be enhanced in bacteria by D-lactate, suggesting that D-lactate dehydrogenase may act as an important energy source for transport by coupling the electron transport system of the cell with configurational alteration of membrane carrier molecules (Kaback, 1972).

These still disjointed facets of membrane chemistry fail to provide a satisfactory foundation for the previously mentioned physiological characteristics of amino acid transport. Until such a confirmed structure does exist, we must resort to conceptual models, recognizing that any proposed model must be consistent with the evolving biochemistry and will almost surely be altered by future findings in this evolving field. Such a conceptual model is shown in Figure 6–1, without regard to tissue or specific amino acid substrate. Let us postulate the existence of a molecular species (C) in or near the cell membrane which reversibly binds an amino acid (A). The isolation of binding proteins from bacterial membranes, the existence of specific inborn errors of transport and the great specificity which these binding molecules must have imply that they are macromolecules, probably proteins.

Some investigators have used the terms "permease," "translocase" or, more whimsically, "here-to-there-ase" to describe these postulated proteins, while other workers have preferred functional nomenclature such as "reactive site," "pump" or "carrier." Since amino acid influx has been shown to be sodium-dependent (Curran et al., 1967), we can next postulate that the amino acid-carrier complex (AC) interacts with a sodium ion (Na) to yield a ternary amino acid-carrier-sodium complex (ACNa) which then traverses the cell membrane in some as yet totally undefined way. At the inner surface of the membrane, the ACNa complex dissociates, the amino acid and sodium molecules enter the cell and the carrier undergoes some physical or chemical change (C′) which reduces its affinity for the substrate. Metabolic energy (~P) may be required for the reaction in which the carrier's affinity is reduced or, alternatively, for that in which the carrier is reconverted to its "high affinity" form. Other models have been proposed which also explain reversible substrate binding, interaction with the sodium ion, transport against a concentration gradient and coupling with metabolic energy, but their fundamental features are similar to those presented here.

The proposed model accounts for mediated or active transport of amino acids, but these small molecules are almost surely moved by passive forces as well. Such passive diffusion is postulated to occur through aqueous channels or "pores" in the cell membrane and to obey the usual laws of diffusion through semipermeable membranes. The cardinal feature of this form of transport is that the net flow of amino acid is "downhill," that is, from an area of high concentration to one of lower concentration. Passive diffusion plays a very im-

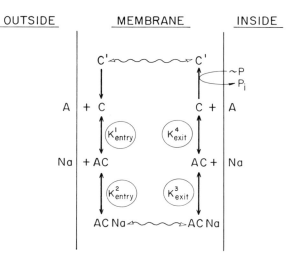

Figure 6–1 Schematic model of carrier-mediated transport of amino acids. A = amino acid; C = carrier molecule; Na = sodium ion; K^{1-4} = association and dissociation constants for entry and exit; C' = "inactivated" carrier molecule; P = high-energy phosphate.

portant role in urine formation and intestinal absorption. Since large "downhill" concentration gradients for amino acids exist between the luminal content of the small bowel and the plasma after a protein meal, it seems likely that passive diffusion plays a more important part in amino acid nutrition and metabolism than is generally supposed. Passive forces may account for a much greater fraction of the net flow of amino acids across the intestinal membrane than active transport processes do, but the relative importance of these two mechanisms will depend on the frequency of food ingestion, the quantity and quality of dietary protein and the functional integrity of the intestinal epithelium.

Genetic Control

The hypothesis that specific reactive sites or carriers in the cell membrane are responsible for the mediated transport of amino acids leads logically to questions pertaining to the functional organization and control of these transport systems. As has so often been the case during the past 20 years, the study of nature's experiments has done much to answer these questions. Thus, investigation of patients with hyperprolinemia (Scriver et al., 1964) and iminoglycinuria (Scriver and Wilson, 1967) was directly responsible for the idea that glycine and the imino acids share a common renal tubular transport system. In like fashion, the study of two other inborn errors of amino acid transport, cystinuria (Dent and Rose, 1951) and Hartnup disease (Baron et al., 1956), revealed that specific transport systems existed for the dibasic amino acids and a large group of neutral amino acids, respectively. The identification and examination of these and many other disorders of amino acid metabolism have done more than point out that transport systems are genetically controlled (Slayman, 1972). They have helped to explain renal clearance and infusion studies in dogs and man which showed selective competition between amino acids of similar structure (Beyer et al., 1947; Webber et al., 1961). They have indicated that marked differences in affinity and capacity for a common transport site exist *within* a group of structurally related amino acids (Scriver and Wilson, 1967; Rosenberg et al., 1962). They have demonstrated that a single amino acid may be transported by two, three or even more specific mechanisms, one of which may be shared with related compounds while others are specific for a single substrate (Scriver and Wilson, 1967; Rosenberg et al., 1967; Hillman et al., 1968a). Finally, they have pointed the way to new experiments by demonstrating how little we understand about the chemical and physiological organization of these transport systems.

The study of inborn errors of amino acid transport coupled with our current concepts of molecular genetics indicates that structural genes code for the synthesis of carrier proteins, permeases or other polypeptide species which catalyze the movement of amino acids across cell membranes. This simple genetic framework may be sufficient to explain most observed transport phenomena in microorganisms. It requires much modification in mammalian systems, as demonstrated by the following observations: Insulin stimulates the uptake of amino acids by skeletal muscle (Kipnis and Noall, 1958; Elsas et al., 1968), but has no such effect in the gut, kidney or brain; dibasic amino acid transport is defective in the kidney and gut in cystinuria but not in circulating leukocytes (Rosenberg and Downing, 1965); some patients with inherited iminoglycinuria have transport defects in the gut and kidney, whereas others have a defect in the kidney only (Rosenberg et al., 1968). These and other observations indicate that the process of tissue differentiation in the mammalian organism exerts profound alterations on transport systems as it does on all other vital functions.

We have no explanations for the phenomena just cited but numerous possibilities are apparent. Perhaps the muscle cell is insulin-responsive because its membrane contains a specific protein which binds the hormone and promotes interaction with amino acid carrier systems which it then modifies. Conversely, gut and kidney cells may contain enzymes which rapidly denature insulin and render it inactive. The remarkable tissue specificity in cystinuria indicates that dibasic amino acids are not transported by the same system in all tissues and implies that certain systems are "turned on" in one tissue and "turned off" in others. Induction, repression and feedback inhibition may influence transport systems as they do intracellular enzymatic reactions and thus add to the organizational complexity and metabolic flexibility of membrane systems.

Environmental Modification

The transport of amino acids is controlled by environmental as well as genetic factors. As pointed out earlier, nutritional influences are significant. Free amino acid excretion in the urine rises modestly as dietary protein goes up, probably as a result of an increased renal filtered load. The episodic eating pattern of man influences intestinal absorption by presenting to the gut mucosa very large concentrations of free amino acids several times daily. Wide fluctuations in plasma amino acids occur after protein ingestion as the large quantity of free amino acids liberated by digestive enzymes is transferred across the gut mucosa by passive and active forces. Nutritional deficiency is also important. Vitamin C and vitamin D deficiency each result in a generalized aminoaciduria (Huisman, 1957) which is rapidly reversible with appropriate vitamin therapy. It seems likely that these aminoacidurias are caused by impaired renal tubular reabsorption, but the exact role of the vitamins in tubular transport systems is unclear. It has not been demonstrated satisfactorily that the transport abnormalities reflect a primary role of the vitamins on membrane transport as opposed to secondary effects either on energy metabolism or on related hormonal systems (Fraser et al., 1967).

Numerous physical or chemical insults may alter amino acid transport. Intestinal absorption can be impaired by neomycin (Huidt and Kjeldsen, 1963), and renal tubular resorption may be profoundly depressed by x-irradiation, heavy metal intoxication, outdated tetracycline and maleic acid (Leaf, 1966). Such environmental insults almost surely affect transport in tissues other than the gut and the kidney, but the external evidence for such effects is much more difficult to perceive and little investigative effort has thus far been invested.

METHODS OF INVESTIGATION

We shall continue to place emphasis on the gut and the kidney in this discussion of disorders of transport of amino acids because they are the only organs which have been implicated clearly in human disease states. This may reflect the propensity of these specialized tissues to undergo mutations or to suffer environmental insults which alter transport. It also reflects the relative ease with which transport can be studied in the gut and the kidney compared to less accessible tissues. Many different experimental techniques, in vitro and in vivo, have contributed to our understanding of disordered amino acid transport in the gut and the kidney. Intestinal absorption of amino acids has been studied by measuring the free amino acid content of feces (Scriver, 1965; Morikawa et al., 1966). Interpretation of such studies may be complicated because intestinal microorganisms modify the intestinal contents. However, in selected instances this very shortcoming has been responsible for important contributions. Thus, Milne and his colleagues (1961) demonstrated an intestinal defect in cystinuria by showing that the products of bacterial decarboxylation of dibasic amino acids were increased in the feces of cystinuric patients. They proposed correctly that malabsorption of the dibasic amino acids had made available to the microorganisms increased amounts of the appropriate substrates for these decarboxylation reactions.

In other instances, an oral load of a single amino acid followed by serial plasma determinations has yielded valuable data on intestinal absorption (London and Foley, 1965; Rosenberg, Durant and Holland, 1965). This approach has two kinds of limitations. First, amino acids absorbed into the mesenteric circulation are carried to the liver, which extracts a significant proportion of these substrates and hence modifies greatly the plasma amino acid profile subsequently sampled in a peripheral vein. Second, the large quantities of an amino acid usually used in such studies may produce such a high intestinal concentration of that amino acid that the observed plasma changes reflect absorption via passive diffusion rather than by the mediated processes being investigated. The technique of small intestinal perfusion would seem to obviate these objections to oral amino acid tolerance tests, but this approach has, thus far, not been extensively used to study intestinal abnormalities in amino acid transport.

Renal amino acid transport has likewise been studied in several ways. The study of the qualitative and quantitative pattern of free amino acids in random or 24-hour urine samples has been extraordinarily profitable since its initial description by Dent (1946). When increased amounts of one or more amino acids are demonstrated in this way, more detailed studies have been done. Renal clearance determinations for individual amino acids have shown that excessive amino acid excretion may reflect either a primary renal tubular abnormality or saturation of normal renal transport systems by an excessive filtered load or a combination thereof. In selected instances, valuable contributions have been made by combining such renal clearance determinations with intravenous administration of amino acid loads (Scriver et al., 1964; Scriver and Wilson, 1967). In this way the maximum tubular transport capacity for selected amino acids in normal subjects and in patients with specific tubular defects has been evaluated (see Chapter 8).

The technique of stop-flow analysis (Malvin et al., 1958) has been used to further localize amino acid transport within the renal tubule. These studies showed that amino acids are reabsorbed in the proximal tubule, in a segment coextensive with that used for glucose reabsorption and p-aminohippurate secretion (Brown et al., 1961; Gayer and Gerok, 1961; Ruskowski et al., 1962; Young and Edwards, 1966). The most direct evidence for localization of amino acid reabsorption to the proximal tubule has been obtained from recent micropuncture and microperfusion experiments. Bergeron (1966) injected isotopically labeled leucine and lysine into the lumen of the proximal tubule and, using radioautographic techniques, demonstrated uptake of the labeled compounds by the cells of the entire proximal tubule. Subsequent studies demonstrated uptake of radioactive amino acids in both the proximal convolution and the pars recta (Bergeron and Morel, 1969). Although these studies have unambiguously identified the proximal tubule as the major site of amino acid reabsorption, they have not excluded the possibility that a small fraction of amino acid reabsorption occurs in the distal nephron.

In a modification of this microinjection technique, Bergeron and Vadeboncoeur (1971) injected ^{14}C-labeled arginine and leucine into the peritubular capillary and demonstrated antiluminal transport of these amino acids in rat kidney. Subsequent studies, using intravenous injection of labeled amino acids followed by radioautographic and quantitative localization within the renal parenchyma, have confirmed the existence of transport mechanisms on the antiluminal border of the tubular cell which appear to be distinct from those on the luminal brush border (Wedeen and Thier, 1971; Ausiello et al., 1972; Greth et al., 1971). Thus, amino acid accumulation within the tubular cell reflects uptake at both the luminal and antiluminal surfaces, thereby complicating the interpretation of in vitro analyses using kidney slices or isolated renal tubules.

Valuable insights have also been obtained using human tissues in vitro. Studies of uptake of labeled amino acids by pieces of jejunal mucosa, slices of kidney cortex or intact leukocytes have yielded data on the transport of amino acids which is unobtainable with any kind of study in intact subjects. The obvious advantages of this investigative technique relate to the controlled environment in which single variables may be altered in the search for specific facets of the transport mechanisms of one amino acid or a group of related compounds. As stated previously, the physiologic significance of such in vitro analysis is limited by the asymmetry of renal and intestinal cells. To date, these in vitro techniques have received wide use only in the study of cystinuria and iminoglycinuria, but they have contributed significantly to current genetic and biochemical concepts. These methods are also applicable to an analysis of hormonal, drug and cofactor modifications of transport processes in man and will surely be so used in the future. For more detailed information on renal tubular transport of amino acids, the interested reader should consult two recent, excellent reviews: Young and Freedman, 1971; Segal and Thier, 1973.

THE PATHOLOGICAL AMINOACIDURIAS

Definition and Scope

As mentioned earlier, the free amino acid content of plasma is filtered at the glomerulus and reabsorbed in the renal tubule. Normally, amino acids account for only 1 to 3 per cent of the total urinary nitrogen. Since normal subjects do excrete finite amounts of amino acids, "aminoaciduria" is a normal finding. The pattern of amino acid excretion varies greatly between individuals, but certain generalizations hold. With the exception of glycine and histidine, 97 to 100 per cent of the filtered load of each amino acid found in protein is reabsorbed. The latter two substances usually account for more than 50 per cent of the urinary amino acids, but their reabsorptive fraction still ranges from 93 to 96 per cent. Pathological aminoaciduria or "hyperaminoaciduria" has been defined in many ways: by an excessive fraction of total urinary nitrogen; by an increase in the total 24-hour excretion value; or by an exaggerated renal clearance. Many specific or generalized pathological aminoacidurias exist in which 10 to 100 times normal amounts of one or more amino acids appear in the urine. At first glance, therefore, it is surprising that these conditions are not characterized by nutritional deficits and growth aberrations. The absence of such clinical manifestations is understandable, however, since most pathological aminoacidurias, even those described as "massive," result in the loss of less than 50 per cent of the filtered load. Such losses must be easily compensated for by enhanced intestinal absorption, accelerated protein turnover, augmented amino acid synthesis and other homeostatic mechanisms which maintain plasma and tissue amino acid concentrations adequate for protein synthesis and growth.

Mechanisms of Pathological Aminoacidurias

The pathological aminoacidurias were formerly assigned to "prerenal" or "renal" categories (Dent and Walshe, 1954). Those conditions in which the exaggerated urinary loss resulted from an excessive filtered load were termed "prerenal" or "overflow" aminoacidurias; the "renal" aminoacidurias were those in which a defect in tubular reabsorption was responsible for the increased urinary loss. This classification is no longer adequate to encompass the many disorders described. Scriver (1967b) has proposed a classification for the pathological aminoacidurias based on the cellular mechanisms which mediate amino acid transport. This classification describes four major types of pathological aminoaciduria (see Table 5–5).

Saturation ("Overflow" Aminoaciduria)

This mechanism underlies the specific aminoaciduria so often associated with enzymatic defects leading to increased plasma concentrations of the amino acid(s) involved. Because of the hyperaminoacidemia, the filtered load of the amino acid exceeds the capacity of its reabsorptive system. An amino acid(s) with a great affinity for its transport system will be cleared in very small amounts until saturation conditions obtain. An amino acid with a lesser affinity for its transport system may show a more exaggerated aminoaciduria under saturation conditions, depending on the capacity of the system.

Competition (Combined Aminoaciduria)

If more than one amino acid shares a common transport system, an increase in the filtered load of one substrate may inhibit the binding and reabsorption of other substrates in the group. The specificity of the aminoaciduria reflects the site involved, while the magnitude of the urinary loss will be dependent on the affinity of the saturating amino acid for the shared system and on the capacity of both the shared system and other systems which mediate tubular reabsorption of the substrates involved. Hence, one amino acid is excreted in excess by an overflow mechanism, the others by the process of competitive inhibition producing an increased renal clearance.

Modification of Tubular Reactive Site (Specific Renal Aminoaciduria)

A mutation of the reactive site or carrier ablates or impairs binding of its substrate(s). The aminoaciduria is specific for one substrate or a group of structurally related substrates.

Inhibition of Substrate Transfer (Generalized Renal Aminoaciduria)

Tubular reabsorption of amino acids against a chemical concentration gradient is impaired by interference with the ion-dependent or energy-requiring steps in the transport processes. A generalized aminoaciduria results which may be accompanied by excessive losses of other substances reabsorbed in the tubule.

Classification of Group-Specific Transport Systems

The study of the pathological aminoacidurias has defined a number of group-specific amino acid transport systems in the kidney. Some of these systems are also present in the gut, but there is little information about their organization in other tissues. The evidence for such group specificity has come from three related lines of investigation: study of the inborn errors of renal tubular transport of amino acids; information gained from renal clearance or combined renal clearance-infusion studies in man and other mammalian species; experiments in vitro with kidney cortex slices or isolated renal tubules. Group-specific systems have been identified for the following five classes of amino acids: the dicarboxylic amino acids; the dibasic amino acids; the imino acids and glycine; the neutral aliphatic and aromatic amino acids; and the β-amino acids. The characteristics of the last four of these systems will be discussed in subsequent chapters devoted to specific disease processes. The evidence for a specific system for the dicarboxylic amino acids (glutamic acid and aspartic acid) rests on renal clearance experiments in dogs (Webber, 1963). No disease has been identified in man which implicates this system.

REFERENCES

Ashworth, L. A. E., and Green, C.: Plasma membranes: Phospholipid and sterol content. Science *151*:210–211, 1966.

Ausiello, D. A., Segal, S., and Thier, S. O.: Cellular accumulation of L-lysine in rat kidney cortex in vivo. Amer. J. Physiol. *222*:1473–1478, 1972.

Bakerman, S., and Wasemiller, G.: Studies on structural units of human erythrocyte membrane. I. Separation, isolation, and partial characterization. Biochemistry 6:1100–1113, 1967.

Baron, D. N., Dent, C. E., Harris, J., Hart, E. W., and Jepson, J. B.: Hereditary pellagra-like skin rash with temporary cerebellar ataxia, constant renal amino-aciduria, and other bizarre biochemical features. Lancet (i), 421–428, 1956.

Begin, N., and Scholefield, P. G.: The uptake of amino acids by mouse pancreas in vitro. I. General characteristics. Biochim. Biophys. Acta 90:82–89, 1964.

Bergeron, M.: Microinjection intratublaire associée à la radioautographic en microscopie électronique: Réabsorption des acides aminés dans le tube contourné proximal du rein. (Abstract.) J. Microscopie 5:32, 1966.

Bergeron, M., and Morel, F.: Amino acid transport in rat renal tubules. Amer. J. Physiol. *216*: 1139–1149, 1969.

Bergeron, M., and Vadeboncoeur, M.: Antiluminal transport of L-arginine and L-leucine following microinjections in peritubular capillaries of the rat. Nephron 8:355–366, 1971.

Beyer, K. H., Wright, L. D., Skeggs, H. R., Russo, H. F., and Shaner, G. A.: Renal clearance of essential amino acids: Their competition for reabsorption by the renal tubules. Amer. J. Physiol. *151*:202–210, 1947.

Brown, J. L., Samiy, A. H., and Pitts, R. F.: Localization of amino nitrogen reabsorption in the nephron of the dog. Amer. J. Physiol. *200*:370–372, 1961.

Christensen, H. N.: Biological Transport. W. A. Benjamin, Inc., New York, 1962.

Christensen, H. N.: Methods for distinguishing amino acid transport systems of a given cell or tissue. Fed. Proc. *25*:850–853, 1966.

Christensen, H. N., Akedo, H., Oxender, D. L., and Winter, C. G.: On the mechanism of amino acid transport into cells. *In* Holden, J. T., ed., Amino Acid Pools. Elsevier, Amsterdam, pp. 527–538, 1961.

Curran, P. F., Schultz, S. G., Chez, R. A., and Fuisz, R. E.: Kinetic relations of the Na-amino acid interaction at the mucosal border of intestine. J. Gen. Physiol. *50*:1261–1286, 1967.

Dent, C. E.: Detection of amino acids in urine and other fluids. Lancet (ii), 637–639, 1946.

Dent, C. E., and Rose, G. A.: Amino acid metabolism in cystinuria. Quart. J. Med. *20*:205–219, 1951.

Dent, C. E., and Walshe, J. M.: Amino-acid metabolism. Brit. Med. Bull. *10*:247–250, 1954.

Eichholz, A.: Structural and functional organization of the brush border of intestinal epithelial cells. III. Enzymatic activities and chemical composition of various fractions of tris-disrupted brush border. Biochim. Biophys. Acta *135*:475–482, 1967.

Elsas, L. J., Albrecht, I., and Rosenberg, L. E.: Insulin stimulation of amino acid uptake in rat diaphragm: Relationship to protein synthesis. J. Biol. Chem. *243*:2846–2853, 1968.

Emmelot, P., Bos, C. J., Benedetti, E. L., and Rümke, P. H.: Studies on plasma membranes. I. Chemical composition and enzyme content of plasma membranes isolated from rat liver. Biochim. Biophys. Acta 90:126–145, 1964.

Finerman, G. A. M., and Rosenberg, L. E.: Amino acid transport in bone: Evidence for separate transport systems for neutral amino and imino acids. J. Biol. Chem. *241*:1487–1493, 1966.

Fox, C. F., Carter, J. R., and Kennedy, E. P.: Genetic control of the membrane protein component of the lactose transport system of Escherichia coli. Proc. Nat. Acad. Sci. U.S.A. *57*:698–705, 1967.

Fraser, D., Kooh, S. W., and Scriver, C. R.: Hyperparathyroidism as the cause of hyperaminoaciduria and phosphaturia in human vitamin D deficiency. Pediat. Res. *1*:425–435, 1967.

Gardner, J. D., and Levy, A. G.: Transport of dibasic amino acids by human erythrocytes. Metabolism *21*:413–431, 1972.

Gayer, J., and Gerok, W.: Die Lokalisierung der L-amino Sauren in der Nieve durch stop-flow Analysen. Klin. Wschr. *39*:1054–1055, 1961.

Goodman, H. M.: Alpha amino isobutyric acid transport in adipose tissue. Amer. J. Physiol. *211*: 815–820, 1966.

Greth, W. E., Thier, S. O., and Segal, S.: Transport of cystine in rat kidney cortex: Independent luminal and contraluminal mechanisms. (Abstract.) Clin. Res. *19*:742, 1971.

Groth, U., and Rosenberg, L. E.: Transport of dibasic amino acids, cystine, and tryptophan by cultured human fibroblasts: Absence of a defect in cystinuria and Hartnup disease. J. Clin. Invest. *51*:2130–2142, 1972.

Herring, L. C.: Observations on the analysis of ten thousand urinary calculi. J. Urol. *88*:545–562, 1962.

Hillman, R. E., Albrecht, I., and Rosenberg, L. E.: Identification and analysis of multiple glycine transport systems in isolated mammalian renal tubules. J. Biol. Chem. *243*:5566–5571, 1968a.

Hillman, R. E., Albrecht, I., and Rosenberg, L. E.: Transport of amino acids by isolated rabbit renal tubules. Biochim. Biophys. Acta *150*:528–530, 1968b.

Huidt, S., and Kjeldsen, C.: Malabsorption induced by small doses of neomycin sulfate. Acta Med. Scand. *173*:699–705, 1963.

Huisman, T. H. J.: L'élimination des acides aminés chez des enfants normaux d'âges différents. Arch. Franc. Pediat. *14*:166–180, 1957.

Kaback, H. R.: Transport across isolated bacterial cytoplasmic membranes. Biochim. Biophys. Acta *265*:367–416, 1972.

Kipnis, D. M., and Noall, M. W.: Stimulation of amino acid transport by insulin in the isolated rat diaphragm. Biochim. Biophys. Acta *28*:226–227, 1958.

Korn, E. D:: Structure of biological membranes. Science *153*:1491–1498, 1966.

Leaf, A.: The syndrome of osteomalacia, renal glycosuria, aminoaciduria, and increased phosphorus clearance (the Fanconi syndrome). *In* Stanbury, J. B., Wyngaarden, J. B., and Fredrickson, D. S., eds., The Metabolic Basis of Inherited Disease, 2nd edition. McGraw-Hill, New York, pp. 1205–1220, 1966.

Levi, G., Blasberg, R., and Lajtha, A.: Substrate specificity of cerebral amino acid exit in vitro. Arch. Biochem. Biophys. *114*:339–351, 1966.

London, D. R., and Folcy, J. H.: Cystine metabolism in cystinuria. Clin. Sci. *29*:129–141, 1965.

Maddy, A. H.: The properties of the protein of the plasma membrane of ox erythrocytes. Biochim. Biophys. Acta *117*:193–200, 1966.

Malvin, R. L., Wilde, W. S., and Sullivan, L. P.: Localization of nephron transport by stop-flow analysis. Amer. J. Physiol. *194*:135–142, 1958.

Milne, M. D., Asatoor, A. M., Edwards, K. D. G., and Loughridge, L. W.: The intestinal absorption defect in cystinuria. Gut *2*:323–337, 1961.

Morikawa, T., Tada, K., Ando, T., Yoshida, T., Yokoyama, Y., and Arakawa, T.: Prolinuria: Defect in intestinal absorption of imino acids and glycine. Tohoku J. Exp. Med. *90*:105–116, 1966.

Pardee, A. B.: Crystallization of a sulfate-binding protein (permease) from Salmonella typhimurium. Science *156*:1627–1628, 1967.

Penrose, W. R., Nichoalds, G. E., Piperno, J. R., and Oxender, D. L.: Purification and properties of a leucine-binding protein from E. coli. J. Biol. Chem. *243*:5921–5928, 1968.

Robertson, J. D.: The ultrastructure of cell membranes and their derivatives. Symp. Biochem. Soc. *16*:3–44, 1959.

Rosenberg, L. E., Albrecht, I., and Segal, S.: Lysine transport in human kidney: Evidence for two systems. Science *155*:1426–1428, 1967.

Rosenberg, L. E., Blair, A., and Segal, S.: Transport of amino acids by slices of rat-kidney cortex. Biochim. Biophys. Acta *54*:479–488, 1961.

Rosenberg, L. E., and Downing, S. J.: Transport of neutral and dibasic amino acids by human leukocytes: Absence of defect in cystinuria. J. Clin. Invest. *44*:1382–1393, 1965.

Rosenberg, L. E., Downing, S. J., and Segal, S.: Competitive inhibition of dibasic amino acid transport in rat kidney. J. Biol. Chem. *237*:2265–2270, 1962.

Rosenberg, L. E., Durant, J. L., and Elsas, L. J.: II: Familial imino-glycinuria: An inborn error of renal tubular transport. New Eng. J. Med. *278*:1407–1412, 1968.

Rosenberg, L. E., Durant, J. L., and Holland, J. M.: Intestinal absorption and renal extraction of cystine and cysteine in cystinuria. New Eng. J. Med. *273*:1239–1245, 1965.

Ruszkowski, M., Arasimowicx, C., Knapowski, J., Steffen, J., and Weiss, K.: Renal reabsorption of amino acids. Amer. J. Physiol. *203*:891–896, 1962.

Scriver, C. R.: Amino acid transport in mammalian kidney. *In* Nyhan, W. L., ed., Amino Acid Metabolism and Genetic Variation. McGraw-Hill, New York, pp. 327–340, 1967a.

Scriver, C. R.: Hartnup disease: A genetic modification of intestinal and renal transport of certain neutral alpha-amino acids. New Eng. J. Med. *273*:530–532, 1965.

Scriver, C. R.: Hyperaminoaciduria. *In* Beeson, P. B., and McDermott, W., eds., Textbook of Medicine, 12th edition. W. B. Saunders Company, Philadelphia, pp. 1219–1225, 1967b.

Scriver, C. R., Efron, M. L., and Schafer, I. A.: Renal tubular transport of proline, hydroxyproline, and glycine in health and in familial hyperprolinemia. J. Clin. Invest. *43*:374–385, 1964.

Scriver, C. R., and Wilson, O. H.: Amino acid transport: Evidence for genetic control of two types in human kidney. Science *155*:1428–1430, 1967.

Segal, S., and Thier, S. O.: The renal handling of amino acids. *In* Orloff, J., ed., Handbook of Physiology. (In press.)

Singer, S. J., and Nicolson, G. L.: The fluid mosaic model of the structure of membranes. Science *175*:720–731, 1972.

Slayman, C. W.: Genetic control of membrane transport. *In* Bronner, F., and Kleinzeller, A., eds., Current Topics in Membranes and Transport. Academic Press, New York, 1972.

Smyth, D. H.: Studies on the transport of amino acids and glucose by the intestine. *In* Kleinzeller, A., and Kotyk, A., eds., Membrane Transport and Metabolism. Academic Press, New York, pp. 488–499, 1960.

Stoeckinius, W., and Engelman, D. M.: Current models for the structure of biological membranes. J. Cell Biol. *42*:613–646, 1969.

Thier, S. O., Segal, S., Fox, M., Blair, A., and Rosenberg, L. E.: Cystinuria: Defective intestinal transport of dibasic amino acids and cystine. J. Clin. Invest. *44*:442–448, 1965.

Wallach, D. F. H., and Kamat, V. B.: Plasma and cytoplasmic membrane fragments from Ehrlich ascites carcinoma. Proc. Nat. Acad. Sci. U.S.A. *52*:721–728, 1964.

Webber, W. A.: Characteristics of acidic amino acid transport in mammalian kidney. Canad. J. Biochem. *41*:131–137, 1963.

Webber, W. A., Brown, J. L., and Pitts, R. F.: Interactions of amino acids in renal tubular transport. Amer. J. Physiol. *200*:380–386, 1961.

Wedeen, R. P., and Thier, S. O.: Intrarenal distribution of nonmetabolized amino acids in vivo. Amer. J. Physiol. *220*:507–512, 1971.

Wheeler, K. P., and Christensen, H. N.: Role of Na^+ in the transport of amino acids in rabbit red cells. J. Biol. Chem. *242*:1450–1457, 1967.

Wilson, O. H., and Scriver, C. R.: Specificity of transport of neutral and basic amino acids in rat kidney. Amer. J. Physiol. *213*:185–190, 1967.

Wilson, T. H.: Intestinal Absorption. W. B. Saunders Company, Philadelphia, 1962.

Young, J. A., and Edwards, K. D. G.: Clearance and stop-flow studies on histidine and methyldopa transport by rat kidney. Amer. J. Physiol. *210*:667–675, 1966.

Young, J. A., and Freedman, B. S.: Renal tubular transport of amino acids. Clin. Chem. *17*:245–266, 1971.

Chapter Seven

NATURE AND DISORDERS OF CYSTINE AND DIBASIC AMINO ACID TRANSPORT

At first glance it may seem strange to discuss disorders of cystine and "dibasic" amino acid transport together. Cystine has two carboxyl groups and two amino groups, whereas the dibasic amino acids lysine, arginine and ornithine have two amino groups but only one carboxyl. In accord with these chemical differences, the pK values of the dibasic amino acids and their aqueous solubilities differ markedly from that for cystine. The logic of discussing these chemically distinct substances together stems from their association in the inherited disorder cystinuria. In this disease the renal and intestinal transport of cystine *and* the dibasic amino acids are impaired, implying that, despite apparent chemical differences, cystine shares a transport process in gut and kidney with lysine, arginine and ornithine. Two other inherited transport defects demonstrate equally clearly that this common transport system is not the only

155

one used by the four amino acids in question. In dibasicaminoaciduria, only the transport of lysine, arginine and ornithine is defective. Conversely, in isolated hypercystinuria, only the transport of cystine is impaired. These disorders provide the keystone for the theses that some — perhaps all — amino acids are transported by substrate-specific as well as group-specific mechanisms and that these mechanisms are expressed differently in different tissues.

CYSTINURIA

Cystinuria is one of the oldest recognized and most common inborn errors of metabolism. The disease is inherited as an autosomal recessive trait and is characterized chemically by a specific dibasic aminoaciduria. Cystine, lysine, arginine and ornithine are excreted in great excess by patients homozygous for the defect, but it is the exaggerated cystine excretion which is responsible for the clinical manifestations of this disorder. Since cystine is the least soluble of the naturally occurring amino acids, the appearance of large amounts of this amino acid in the urine predisposes to the formation of renal, ureteral and bladder calculi. Cystine stones account for one to two per cent of all urinary tract calculi (Herring, 1962), ranking behind calcium oxalate, calcium phosphate, magnesium ammonium phosphate and urate in frequency. The significance of this disorder, however, exceeds its clinical impact. It has been of interest to pathologists, biochemists, geneticists and renal physiologists as well as clinicians for 160 years, as attested to by the historical survey shown in Table 7–1.

Biochemical Abnormality and Pathophysiology

Early Description, Historical Development and Definition

In 1810 Wollaston described "a new species of urinary calculus" composed of "flat hexagonal plates" which were soluble in strong acid or alkali. He thought the substance was an oxide and, because of its occurrence in the bladder (Greek, *kystis*), gave it the name *cystic oxide*. Twenty years later Berzelius (1830) demonstrated that this substance was not an oxide and suggested it be called *cystin*. Marcet recognized in 1817 that cystine stones occurred in the kidney as well as the bladder and noted the familial nature of the disorder. Prout (1823) and Stromeyer (1824) observed typical cystine crystals in the urine of patients who formed cystine stones and suggested that excessive excretion of cystine was responsible for the crystalluria and the lithiasis. This suggestion was confirmed by Toel in 1855, who reported that patients with cystinuria excreted up to 1.5 gm. of cystine per day. In 1876 Neimann published the first extensive review of cystinuria and documented 52 cases. He confirmed that the disease was familial and assumed that it was hereditary because one of his patients was less than two years old. He defined cystinuria as a specific disease entity in which a lifelong, familial predisposition to excessive cystine excretion predisposed to crystalluria and cystine stone formation, but it took nearly an additional century for this definition to culminate in our current concept of cystinuria as an inborn error in the intestinal and renal transport of cystine and the dibasic amino acids.

In 1889 von Udransky and Baumann noted that cystinuric patients also excreted large quantities of cadaverine and putrescine in the urine. The presence of these diamines, now known to be produced by bacterial decarboxylation of lysine and ornithine, respectively, was the first hint that dibasic amino acids

Table 7-1 Historical Landmarks in the Study of Cystinuria

Date	Investigator	Renal Defect	Intestinal Defect	Genetics
1810	Wollaston	Described cystine bladder calculi		
1818	Marcet	Identified cystine renal calculi		Noted familial occurrence
1855	Toel	Documented excessive urine cystine		
1891	von Udransky and Baumann		Noted urinary diamines	
1908	Garrod			Postulated inborn error
1935	Brand and Cahill	Failed to define catabolic block		
1947	Yeh et al.	Noted excessive urinary lysine and arginine		
1951	Dent and Rose	Postulated inborn error of renal transport		
1955	Harris et al.			Documented recessive inheritance
1961	Milne et al.		Demonstrated intestinal malabsorption of diabasic amino acids	
1964	Fox et al.	Reported defect in uptake of dibasic amino acids by kidney slices		
1964	Thier et al.		Reported defect in uptake of cystine and dibasic amino acids by gut mucosa	
1967	Rosenberg and Segal	Identified two lysine transport systems		Confirmed genetic heterogeneity

other than cystine were implicated in the pathogenesis of cystinuria. However, the significance of these and related observations was not appreciated for many years. Between 1905 and 1910 Alsberg and Folin (1905) and Wolff and Shaffer (1908) reported an abnormal urinary excretion of "undetermined nitrogen" in cystinuric patients and suggested that this was due, at least in part, to other amino acids. Ackermann and Kutscher actually isolated crystalline derivatives of lysine from cystinuric urine in 1911, but these observations went unnoticed. Garrod commented on some of these findings in 1908 in his famous Croonian lectures, which formally introduced the concept of "inborn errors of metabolism." He concluded that the excessive urinary excretion of cystine in cystinuric patients was due to a block in the catabolism of cystine and assumed that elucidation of the pathway of sulfur amino acid catabolism would account for the confusing observations referable to other amino acids.

Two seemingly unrelated studies began to draw together these divergent investigative pathways. In 1935 Brand and Cahill performed a series of feeding experiments on two cystinuric patients which were responsible for our current concept of the metabolic pathway of the sulfur-containing amino acids but which argued against a catabolic block in cystinuria. Methionine, a recently discovered sulfur-containing amino acid, was identified as a precursor of cystine (Brand et al., 1935). Administration of methionine led to increased cystine output by the cystinuric patients, but administration of cystine did *not*. Furthermore, the ingestion of cystine augmented inorganic sulfate excretion significantly, an observation inconsistent with a block in cystine catabolism (Brand and Cahill, 1934). These detailed observations failed to support the Garrodian concept of cystinuria but offered no satisfactory alternative. In 1947 Yeh and his coworkers, using microbiological techniques, documented excessive lysine and arginine in the urine of cystinuric subjects, and shortly thereafter, Stein (1951) reported that ornithine was also excreted in excess.

The Renal Tubular Theory and Its Aftermath.   It remained for Dent and his colleagues to seize these myriad observations and synthesize a correct interpretation. In 1951 Dent and Rose pointed out in their classic paper that cystine, lysine, ornithine and arginine each had two amino (or guanidine) groups separated by four to six carbon or sulfur atoms (Fig. 7–1). They suggested that these structurally related amino acids were reabsorbed by a common renal tubular mechanism which was defective in cystinuria. This simple and elegant hypothesis was important not only because it explained correctly the pattern of the aminoaciduria in cystinuric patients; its broader significance lay in the understanding that renal tubular reabsorption was accomplished by specific mechanisms under genetic control. Thus was born the concept of "inborn errors of transport" which we now recognize as one class of inborn metabolic diseases. Renal clearance studies performed by Dent et al. (1954), Arrow and Westall (1958), Robson and Rose (1957) and Doolan et al. (1957) amply confirmed the presence of a specific tubular reabsorptive defect in cystinuria.

The elucidation of a renal tubular defect in cystinuria ushered in many subsequent studies of the biochemical and genetic abnormalities in this disease. In 1955 Harris and coworkers (1955a, 1955b) analyzed 27 pedigrees containing one or more cystinuric subjects, using quantitative amino acid determinations in the urine, and concluded that cystinuria is inherited as an autosomal recessive trait. Their data also provided the first suggestion of genetic heterogeneity in cystinuria. Milne and his associates demonstrated in 1961 that, like Hartnup disease, cystinuria is characterized by an intestinal as well as a renal transport defect for the dibasic amino acids. These workers applied the knowledge that lysine and ornithine are decarboxylated by colonic bacteria to yield cadaverine and putrescine, respectively (Fig. 7–2). These diamines then undergo cyclization and deamination to piperidine and pyrrolidine. These investigators fed large amounts of lysine and ornithine to cystinuric patients and noted significant diaminuria and the excretion of specific heterocyclic amines. Analogous results were noted following arginine ingestion (Asatoor et al., 1962). Furthermore, the fecal organisms isolated from cystinuric patients produced about four times more diamines from lysine and ornithine than did organisms from controls. Milne and coworkers concluded that the dibasic amino acids are malabsorbed from the small intestine in cystinuria and are, therefore, present in high concentration in the colon where they are decarboxylated to the diamines, absorbed

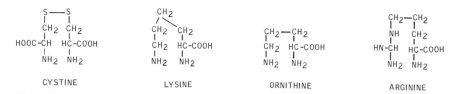

Figure 7–1 Amino acids involved in cystinuria. Structures drawn to emphasize molecular similarities.

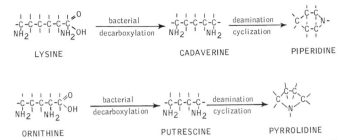

Figure 7–2   Biochemical basis for diaminuria in cystinuria. Arginine may be catabolized by intestinal bacteria by reactions similar to those shown for lysine and ornithine.

into the circulation, cyclized and excreted. In 1964 Fox, Thier, Segal and Rosenberg demonstrated in vitro a defect in renal and intestinal transport of cystine and the dibasic amino acids (Fox et al., 1964; Thier et al., 1964). Finally, in 1966 and 1967 Rosenberg and Segal used in vivo and in vitro techniques to demonstrate that lysine transport in the human kidney is mediated by more than a single transport system (Rosenberg et al., 1967a) and to confirm the existence of genetic heterogeneity in this disorder (Rosenberg et al., 1966a).

Organization and Regulation of Dibasic Amino Acid Transport

The tortuous research trail just summarized begins to present a picture of the mammalian transport systems for the dibasic amino acids and cystine. Since data are now available on these systems in the gut, kidney, leukocytes and cultured fibroblasts, and since important differences exist between these tissues, the organ specific systems will be discussed individually.

Intestine.   In the gut the transport system for the dibasic amino acids and cystine appears to be relatively simple. Cystine, lysine, arginine and ornithine are transported by a common process. This conclusion is based on studies of intestinal absorption in cystinuria (Milne et al., 1961; Asatoor et al., 1962) and on uptake experiments in vitro (Thier et al., 1964; 1965). This common transport system is sodium- and energy-dependent (Thier et al., 1965) and exhibits striking substrate specificity as demonstrated by the failure of glycine or cysteine to compete with the dibasic amino acids for uptake (Thier et al., 1964; Rosenberg et al., 1967b). Furthermore, the absence of mediated uptake of cystine and the dibasic amino acids by gut mucosa from most cystinuric patients (Rosenberg et al., 1966a) implies that the common transport system defective in cystinuria is the *only* mediated process in the gut with appreciable affinity for these free amino acids. More recently, however, it has been demonstrated that lysine-containing dipeptides are absorbed normally by cystinuric patients, implying that such dipeptides are transported by a system not identical with that utilized by their free amino acid constituents (Hellier et al., 1970).

Kidney.   A much more complex picture emerges from detailed examination of the renal transport systems for these amino acids. That the group-specific system identified in the gut also exists in the kidney is assured by the mere existence of the disease cystinuria, with its demonstrable abnormalities in tubular reabsorption and cellular transport. It now seems equally certain that this common mechanism is *not* the only process which facilitates the transtubular flux of the dibasic amino acids. This conclusion rests on the following observations: First, the renal clearance of cystine in most cystinuric patients approximates the glomerular filtration rate (GFR) or even exceeds it (Dent et al., 1954;

Arrow and Westhall, 1958; Frimpter et al., 1962; Crawhall et al., 1967), while the clearance of the dibasic amino acids is variable but almost always less than the GFR (Arrow and Westhall, 1958; Frimpter et al., 1962; Crawhall et al., 1967). Second, lysine infusion augments the clearance of cystine, arginine and ornithine in normal subjects but fails to affect these clearances measurably in cystinuric patients (Robson and Rose, 1957). Third, experiments in vitro with kidney slices from cystinuric subjects have demonstrated only a *partial* defect in the transport of the dibasic amino acids and *no* abnormality in the uptake of cystine (Fox et al., 1964). Fourth, cystine does not compete for uptake with the other dibasic amino acids in human or rat kidney (Rosenberg et al., 1962; Fox et al., 1964). Fifth, two kinetically distinct transport mechanisms for lysine have been demonstrated in vitro (Rosenberg et al., 1967a). Sixth, the efflux of cysteine is inhibited by lysine, arginine and ornithine in vitro whereas the efflux of cystine is unaffected by the dibasic amino acids (Schwartzman et al., 1966). Finally, single families have been reported with a tubular defect for cystine *only* (Brodehl et al., 1966) or with a reabsorptive defect for lysine, arginine and ornithine but *not* cystine (Perheentupa and Visakorpi, 1965).

These results effectively exclude the hypothesis that dibasic amino acids and cystine are reabsorbed by only a single, common renal tubular system. They suggest (see Fig. 7–3) that cystine does, indeed, share a transport system with the dibasic amino acids, but that at least two other transport mechanisms for these substances also exist in the kidney: one is responsible for reabsorption and secretion of cystine (or cysteine); the second is responsible for reabsorption of dibasic amino acids but not cystine. Such a schema has ample biological precedent (Ames, 1964) and can account for the in vivo and in vitro observations made thus far. A genetic defect in the transport process shared by cystine and the dibasic amino acids, with sparing of the other systems, can explain the clearance data in cystinuria and the partial defect demonstrable in vitro. The presence of two dibasic amino acid transport systems provides an explanation for the failure to demonstrate in vitro competition between cystine and the dibasic amino acids. The presence of a specific cystine (or cysteine) transport process accounts for both the apparent absence of an in vitro defect for cystine uptake in cystinuric kidney (since its directional component would not be dis-

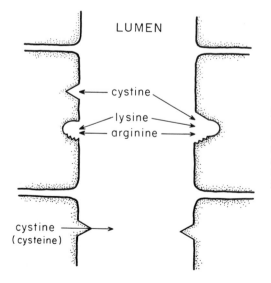

Figure 7–3 Postulated transport systems for dibasic amino acids and cystine in the renal tubule. Ornithine is excluded for artistic convenience, but it appears to be transported by the same mechanisms utilized by lysine and arginine. The arrows directed from the lumen to the cell indicate reabsorption, while those from the cell to the lumen depict secretion.

tinguishable in such a system) and the presence of net tubular secretion of cystine in some cystinuric subjects. Finally, the families with abnormalities in tubular reabsorption of cystine only or of dibasic amino acids only may represent mutations of the postulated specific transport mechanisms for cystine and the dibasic amino acids, respectively. It is, of course, possible that other transport systems exist which are specific for lysine or arginine or ornithine, but there is no clinical or experimental data which demands such a thesis at this time.

Leukocytes, Erythrocytes and Fibroblasts. A still different picture emerges from the study of dibasic amino acid transport in leukocytes (Rosenberg and Downing, 1965) and erythrocytes (Gardner and Levy, 1972) isolated from the peripheral blood and in skin fibroblasts propagated in tissue culture (Groth and Rosenberg, 1972). These cells accumulate lysine, arginine and ornithine by a common, mediated process not shared with cystine. Furthermore, *no* defect in the transport of dibasic amino acids or cystine has been demonstrable in any of these tissues obtained from cystinuric patients (Rosenberg and Downing, 1965; Gardner and Levy, 1972; Groth and Rosenberg, 1972; Becker and Green, 1958). These results attest to the variation of transport systems for a single group of substances which exist in tissues with different morphological and functional characteristics. They also emphasize that the expression of the common genetic information inherent in all human cell types differs with regard to the control of transport processes just as it does for so many other biochemical mechanisms.

Genetics

The earliest descriptions of cystinuria indicated that it was an inherited disorder. Marcet (1817) and Niemann (1876) documented the occurrence of cystine stones in two or more siblings. Niemann also reported a patient who presented with cystine stones at two years of age, and he suggested that the disease was probably present from birth on. In his study of the inborn errors of metabolism, Garrod (1908) pointed out that the disease rarely occurred in successive generations and that consanguinity was frequently observed among the parents of affected offspring. He proposed that stone-forming patients were homozygous for a rare autosomal mutation and that the disease was inherited as an autosomal recessive trait. This genetic hypothesis was based on the assumption that the formation of cystine stones was the hallmark of the abnormal phenotype in cystinuria, a definition subsequently shown to be inadequate. Thus, the studies of Yeh et al. (1947), Stein (1951) and Dent and Rose (1951) indicated that phenotypic cystinuria was characterized by the excretion of large amounts of the dibasic amino acids as well as cystine and that all patients with this biochemical disturbance did *not* form demonstrable calculi.

Autosomal Recessive Inheritance

These observations led Harris and his colleagues (1955a, 1955b) to their definitive study of the genetics of cystinuria. They tested the hypothesis of autosomal recessive inheritance in 27 pedigrees by assuming that patients homozygous for the mutant gene excreted more than 400 mg of cystine per gram of urinary creatinine and equally large excesses of lysine, arginine and ornithine. Cystine was assayed polarigraphically, and microbiological assays were used to quantitate the urinary excretion of dibasic amino acids. Two kinds of families were observed. In 18 of their pedigrees all parents and children of affected subjects excreted normal amounts of cystine and the dibasic amino acids.

Statistical analysis in this group was compatible with autosomal recessive inheritance. In the remaining families, however, moderate excesses of cystine and lysine were found in each parent and child of cystinuric patients, suggesting that the disorder was "incompletely recessive" in these families. Since these detectable heterozygotes failed to excrete abnormal amounts of arginine or ornithine with the methods used, Harris postulated that these amino acids had a greater affinity for the common mechanism which they shared with lysine and cystine. This thesis was confirmed several years later in rat kidney slices (Rosenberg et al., 1962). These interfamilial differences were taken as evidence that the abnormal phenotype in cystinuria could be produced by two different mutations.

Genetic Heterogeneity and Allelism

Additional evidence for genetic heterogeneity in cystinuria followed the demonstration in vitro of a gut transport defect (Thier et al., 1965). In ten of 12 stone-forming cystinuric patients, mediated uptake of cystine, lysine and arginine by jejunal mucosa was absent, but in two other affected subjects gut transport of the three substrates was impaired but present. These differences in gut transport were not associated with differences in urinary amino acid excretion among the affected patients, but they seemed to correlate well with urinary findings in heterozygotes. Three genetically distinct types of cystinuria were defined by Rosenberg, Segal and their colleagues (Rosenberg et al., 1966a), who studied gut transport and urinary excretion in affected families (Table 7–2). "Type I" cystinuria was characterized by the absence of active transport of cystine, lysine or arginine in gut mucosa from affected subjects, by failure of affected subjects to elevate plasma cystine after an oral cystine load and by normal urinary excretion of dibasic amino acids in heterozygotes. "Type II" cystinuria differed in that active transport of cystine but not of lysine was retained by gut mucosa from affected patients and in that heterozygotes excreted distinctly increased quantities of all four dibasic amino acids. In "Type III" cystinuria, intestinal transport of cystine, lysine and arginine was reduced, but not absent, in gut mucosa of affected subjects; plasma cystine rose almost normally after oral cystine loads; and heterozygotes excreted modest excesses of cystine, lysine, arginine and ornithine. Of 13 families studied in this way, seven were Type I, two were Type II and four were Type III. Figure 7–4 demonstrates typical urinary findings in heterozygotes of families designated Type I, II and III, respectively. The probands in these and the other families studied could not be differentiated on clinical grounds or by quantitative 24-hour urinary amino acid determinations.

These data, coupled with those of Harris (1955a, 1955b), suggested that there are at least three different mutations which lead to a common clinical

Table 7–2   Evidence for Three Genetically Distinct Types of Cystinuria*

Cystinuria Designation	Active Intestinal Transport in Affected Patients			Excretion of Dibasic Amino Acids and Cystine by Heterozygotes
	Cystine	Lysine	Arginine	
Type I	Absent	Absent	Absent	Normal
Type II	Present	Absent	Not studied	++Increased
Type III	Present	Present	Present	+Increased

*From Rosenberg et al., 1966a.

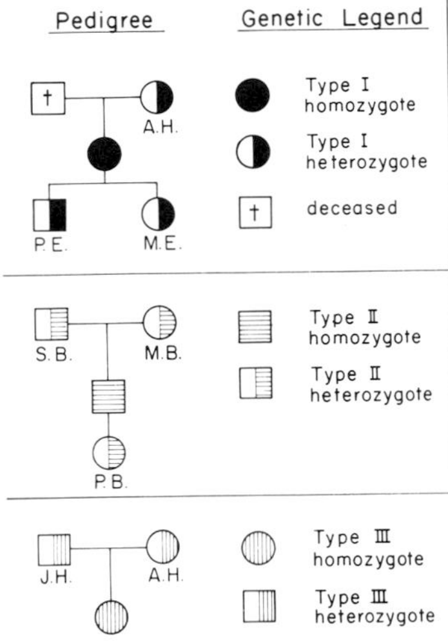

Pedigree	Genetic Legend	Hetero-zygote	Urinary Dibasic Amino Acids (mg/gm creatinine)			
			cystine	lysine	arginine	ornithine
	Type I homozygote	A.H.	36	54	2.2	4.9
	Type I heterozygote	P.E.	28	29	0.5	3.1
	deceased	M.E.	29	36	2.0	3.3
	Type II homozygote	S.B.	177	276	33	175
	Type II heterozygote	M.B.	213	432	13	36
		P.B.	285	792	70	99
	Type III homozygote	J.H.	88	92	5.4	8.3
	Type III heterozygote	A.H.	114	220	7.6	16.4

Figure 7-4   Urinary excretion of dibasic amino acids and cystine by heterozygotes for cystinuria. Note interfamilial differences. (From Rosenberg, L. E.: *In* Nyhan, W. L., ed., Amino Acid Metabolism and Genetic Variation. McGraw-Hill, New York, 1967.)

phenotype in cystinuria, but they did not determine if the observed genetic heterogeneity is due to homoallelic, heteroallelic or nonallelic mutations. Harris (1955a, 1955b) and Crawhall (Crawhall et al., 1966a; Crawhall et al., 1969) noted that all heterozygotes *within* a single cystinuric pedigree showed very similar values for urinary dibasic amino acid excretion: that is, only a single genetic type of heterozygote was found in any single pedigree. Subsequently, Hershko and coworkers (1965), Rosenberg (1967) and Morin and his colleagues (1971) described six important families, each containing at least one stone-forming, cystinuric subject who could not be distinguished from other affected patients by differences in clinical course or urinary findings. Their pedigrees, however, were unique (Fig. 7–5). In one family (G. F., proband) the father of the affected subject (F. F.) showed a urinary amino acid pattern typical of a Type III heterozygote, while his mother (M. F.) and another son had normal urine patterns characteristic of Type I heterozygotes. These data were strengthened by finding other Type I and Type III heterozygotes in the pedigree. Similar results were noted in the other families. J. P.'s father (H. P.) was a type II heterozygote, but his mother was a Type I heterozygote. Analyses of urine from each of B. B.'s five children indicated that three were Type II heterozygotes and two were Type III heterozygotes. These findings suggested that J. B., B. B., and G. F. were not homozygous for a single mutant gene leading to phenotypic cystinuria but, rather, were each genetic compounds, heterozygous for two different mutations. Since double heterozygotes for nonallelic mutations should be no more seriously affected than heterozygotes for a single mutant gene (Rosenberg et al., 1966b), these data were interpreted as evidence for multiple allelic mutations. In their study of 10 cystinuric pedigrees, Morin et al. (1971) identified two families, each containing one or more genetic compounds of genotype I/II. Clinical and biochemical findings in these patients were less severe than those found in either Type I or Type II homozygotes.

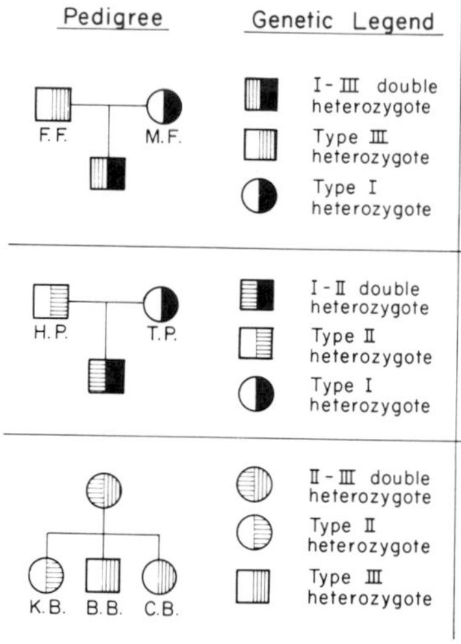

Pedigree	Genetic Legend	Hetero-zygote	Urinary Dibasic Amino Acids (mg/gm creatinine)			
			cystine	lysine	arginine	ornithine
	I-III double heterozygote	F.F.	113	141	6.5	11.7
	Type III heterozygote	M.F.	24	35	3.0	3.9
	Type I heterozygote					
	I-II double heterozygote	H.P.	285	280	36.7	103.8
	Type II heterozygote	T.P.	49	35	2.5	6.0
	Type I heterozygote					
	II-III double heterozygote	K.B.	254	800	64.6	207
	Type II heterozygote	B.B.	44	80	3.6	3.1
	Type III heterozygote	C.B.	69	103	6.5	21

Figure 7–5 Partial pedigrees demonstrating intrafamilial differences in urinary excretion of dibasic amino acids and cystine by heterozygotes for cystinuria. The evidence for allelic mutations is discussed in the text. (From Rosenberg, L. E.: *In* Nyhan, W. L., ed., Amino Acid Metabolism and Genetic Variations. McGraw-Hill, New York, 1967.)

Genotypes and Phenotypes in Cystinuria

These findings suggest that the group-specific transport of cystine, lysine, arginine and ornithine in gut and kidney is catalyzed by a specific carrier protein whose synthesis is controlled by a single pair of allelic genes. If the normal allele is denoted by "n" and the three proposed mutant alleles by "I," "II" and "III," 10 possible genotypes may be defined (Table 7–3). Six genotypes (I-I, II-II, III-III, I-II, II-III and I-III) lead to phenotypic cystinuria. Only subjects with genotype n-I (Type I heterozygotes) are indistinguishable from normals (n-n) using urinary excretion data, and these heterozygotes may be detected by appropriate studies of intestinal transport or absorption (Rosenberg, 1967). Other

Table 7–3   Genotypes and Phenotypes in Cystinuria

Proposed Genotype	Genetic Designation	Phenotype*
n-n	Normal homozygote	normal
n-I	Type I heterozygote	normal
n-II	Type II heterozygote	++increased
n-III	Type III heterozygote	+increased
I-I	Type I homozygote	++++increased
II-II	Type II homozygote	++++increased
III-III	Type III homozygote	++++increased
I-II	Genetic compound	++++increased
II-III	Genetic compound	++++increased
I-III	Genetic compound	++++increased

*Refers to urinary excretion of dibasic amino acids and cystine. From Rosenberg, 1967.

genetic variants will almost surely be found as more families are investigated. Identification and characterization of the postulated dibasic amino acid carrier will provide the link between this genetic hypothesis and the molecular events responsible for the altered phenotypes in cystinuria.

Hereditary Pancreatitis and Cystine-Lysinuria

Gross and coworkers (1957, 1964) described cystine-lysinuria in 17 members of four pedigrees with hereditary pancreatitis. The amino acid pattern in the urine was similar to that found in heterozygotes for "incompletely recessive" (or Types II and III) cystinuria in that lysine and cystine were excreted in considerable excess, whereas arginine and ornithine were present in normal or near normal amounts. Renal clearance studies confirmed that the lysinuria was due to defective tubular reabsorption (Gross et al., 1964). This specific aminoaciduria was found in about half of the 20 patients with pancreatitis but was present with equal frequency in 14 clinically unaffected relatives. Hence, no etiological or pathogenetic relationship between the aminoaciduria and the pancreatitis was found. Nonetheless, the finding of the same renal aminoaciduria in four kindreds with hereditary pancreatitis suggests more than chance association.

Incidence

The foregoing discussion of the genetics of cystinuria indicates that patients with several different genotypes may excrete excessive amounts of cystine and the dibasic amino acids. This genetic complexity complicates the interpretation of studies aimed at defining the incidence of cystinuria, all of which have relied on urinary amino acid determinations. If all patients homozygous for one of the mutant genes or heterozygous for two of them formed cystine calculi, it might be possible to estimate the frequency of the disorder using this discriminant. This is, unfortunately, not the case, and even if it were it would not solve the problem, since some Type II heterozygotes may excrete sufficient cystine to form calculi on rare occasions. Lewis (1932b) found that the urine of 1:600 asymptomatic college students gave a positive nitroprusside test for cystine, but this test will give positive results if the concentration of cystine in the urine exceeds 75 mg per liter and, hence, cannot distinguish between homozygotes and many heterozygotes.

Boström and Tottie (1959) used the nitroprusside test as a preliminary screening procedure in their study of 7793 Swedish schoolchildren and examined all specimens which gave a positive result by chromatographic or electrophoretic methods. They found three children who excreted excessive amounts of cystine, lysine, arginine and ornithine (1:2600) and who were, therefore, considered to have homozygous cystinuria. On the basis of these figures, thousands of Swedish citizens should have cystinuria, but only 98 cases of the disease have been reported in that country between 1870 and 1962 (Boström and Hambraeus, 1964) despite a virtually continuous survey of the disease by Mörner and his successors. A ready explanation for this discrepancy is not at hand, but two likely possibilities exist: the reported incidence of 1:2600 is artifactually elevated by the failure to distinguish between homozygotes and those heterozygotes with distinctly increased urinary arginine and ornithine (see Fig. 7–4), or else the case finding in Sweden, despite its excellent health records, is incomplete.

Crawhall and coworkers (1967) found that 1:200 patients who presented themselves to a medical clinic of a large general hospital in London excreted excessive cystine and lysine. They assumed that these subjects were heterozygotes for the "incompletely recessive" form of cystinuria (Types II and III) and that an equal number of heterozygotes exist who cannot be detected by urinary abnormalities (Harris et al., 1955a, 1955b; Rosenberg, 1967). These figures lead to an estimate of heterozygote frequency of 1:100, suggesting that homozygous cystinuria occurs in about 1:40,000. This is almost surely an underestimate, since families in which the heterozygotes are not detectable are probably twice as common as those in which heterozygotes excrete excessive cystine and dibasic amino acids (Harris et al., 1955a, 1955b). Hence, these data suggest that homozygous cystinuria may be as common as 1:20,000 in the British population. In the most comprehensive population survey reported to date, Levy and co-workers (1972) carried out chromatographic analyses on urine specimens from 141,903 newborns. They found homozygous cystinurics with a frequency of 1: 17,738. Phenylketonuria, histidinemia, Hartnup disease and iminoglycinuria were the only other aminoacidopathies with a frequency as high as that found for cystinuria. Scriver et al. (1970) predicted a similar prevalence.

Signs and Symptoms

Detailed reviews of the clinical consequences of cystinuria have been presented by Niemann (1876), Mörner (1925), Renander (1941) and more recently by Boström and Hambraeus (1964). As in most conditions involving increased amino acid excretion, the urinary loss of amino acids in cystinuria is probably of negligible nutritional significance. Lysine is the only essential amino acid excreted in excess. Although losses of this amino acid may exceed the minimal daily requirement in an adult (1.6 g per day), an adequate protein diet usually provides 5 to 7 g of lysine daily — more than enough to prevent lysine deficiency. Collis et al. (1963), however, have reported that the mean height of 44 British cystinurics was statistically less than the corresponding height in the general population. These authors attributed this difference to the combined effects of excessive urinary loss of lysine and impaired intestinal absorption of this essential amino acid, but urinary tract infections, surgical intervention and renal insufficiency could also be partially or totally responsible for the height difference. Scriver et al. (1970) have recently called attention to another possible clinical consequence of homozygous cystinuria: impaired cerebral function. Previous workers (Berry, 1962) had noted an incidence of cystinuria of about 1:1000 in patients with disturbed cerebral function, but the meaning of this observation was not clear because the incidence of cystinuria in the general population was not known. In their recent study, Scriver et al. confirmed an incidence of cystinuria of 1:1000 in a population with mental illness, a frequency 10 times greater than that in the population at large. This potentially important observation must now be subjected to additional study.

The physical properties of cystine are responsible for the major clinical impact of this disorder. Cystine is quite soluble below pH 3, but its maximum solubility between pH 4.5 and 7 is about 300 mg per liter (Fig. 7–6). Since this is the pH range usually found in the urine, and since cystinuric "homozygotes" commonly excrete 600 to 1300 mg of cystine in a 24-hour period, crystalluria and calculus formation are a constant threat (Fig. 7–7). This is particularly true during the night, when the urine tends to become more concentrated and water intake is minimal (Dent and Senior, 1955). Cystine calculi have been reported during the first year of life and as late as age 80, but the initial symptoms of lithiasis are most common during the third and fourth decades (Boström and Hambraeus, 1964). Males and females appear to be affected with about

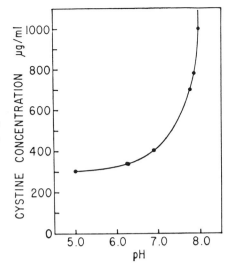

Figure 7–6 Effect of urinary pH on solubility of cystine. (From Dent, C. E., and Senior, B.: Brit. J. Urol. *27*:317–332, 1955.)

equal frequency, but, as is true of all types of renal lithiasis, morbidity is accentuated in males. Pure cystine stones are not difficult to recognize. They are sand-colored and granular and may be recovered from the renal pelvis, ureter or bladder. They are radiopaque owing to their sulfur content, but their roentgenologic density is less than that of calcium or magnesium stones. Cystine stones have a tendency to grow to a large size and may form a cast of the entire pelvic system or grow to the size of a large egg in the bladder. Cystinuric patients may, however, form mixed calculi, and this has great clinical significance. In their extensive review of 56 stone-forming cystinurics, Boström and Hambraeus (1964) noted that only about 50 per cent of the stones passed by their patients were pure cystine, an additional 40 per cent being composed of cystine and calcium oxalate, calcium phosphate or magnesium ammonium phosphate. Nearly 10 per cent of the stones passed by these documented cystinurics contained *no* detectable cystine, and of even greater significance, the initial stone analyzed in about 10 per cent of the cases was reportedly cystine free. Thus, stone analysis, per se, is an unsatisfactory means of excluding cystinuria in patients with renal lithiasis, *all* of whom should have a urinary nitroprusside test to exclude this condition.

As with all forms of renal lithiasis, the formation of cystine calculi predisposes to urinary tract obstruction and secondary infection. The latter complication plus repeated surgical intervention may lead to nephrectomy or renal insufficiency. Boström and Hambracus (1964) reported that about 50 per cent of the deceased cystinuric patients whom they surveyed had died of renal failure. The average life span of those cystinurics dying from renal insufficiency was 20 to 30 years shorter than that of cystinurics who died from other causes. This applied to both sexes, but the average life span of affected male patients was about 10 years shorter than that of females.

Diagnosis and Differential Diagnosis

The diagnosis of cystinuria is not difficult to establish. The appearance of hexagonal, flat crystals in the urine (Fig. 7–7) in a patient who has not been taking sulfa drugs is pathognomonic. These crystals should be looked for in con-

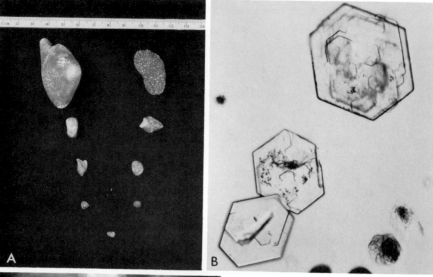

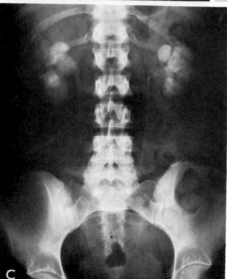

Figure 7–7 Cystine crystalluria and lithiasis. *A*, renal and ureteral calculi composed of cystine; *B*, hexagonal crystals of cystine in urine; and *C*, bilateral nephrolithiasis due to radiopaque cystine calculi.

centrated urine specimens, but since they will be present only if the cystine concentration exceeds its maximum solubility, other approaches are needed. The cyanide-nitroprusside test, originally described by Lewis (1932a), is simple and very valuable. The addition of sodium cyanide to a urine sample made alkaline with ammonium hydroxide leads to reduction of cystine to cysteine. The cysteine forms a magenta-red color complex when sodium nitroprusside is added. The intensity of the color is proportional to the free sulfhydryl content and, hence, will be weakly positive in those heterozygotes who excrete modest or moderate excesses of cystine. Positive tests will also be obtained in patients with homocystinuria and a new metabolic disorder characterized by the excretion of cystine-β-mercaptolactate mixed disulfide (Ampola et al., 1968), but these disorders can easily be differentiated on clinical grounds. Acetone and other drugs may give false positive results. Diagnostic confirmation depends on the demonstration of the characteristic amino acid pattern in the urine. Selective excessive excretion of cystine, lysine, arginine and ornithine is not observed in other pathological aminoacidurias and can be detected easily by paper chromatographic or electrophoretic techniques. In those instances in which it is important to differentiate between homozygotes and heterozygotes for cystinuria, quantitative amino acid determinations obtained by column chromatography may be necessary.

Cystinuria has long been confused with another disorder of cystine metabolism—cystinosis. With the exception of their names, however, these disorders are very different (Table 7–4). Cystinosis is characterized by the accumulation of intracellular cystine in the cornea, leukocytes, bone marrow, liver and kidney, *not* by the formation of cystine renal calculi. Renal insufficiency and uremia are early manifestations in most patients with cystinosis, probably secondary to the intracellular deposits of cystine in renal tubular cells. In cystinosis, a generalized renal aminoaciduria occurs along with glycosuria, phosphaturia and proteinuria. Cystine excretion is not more prominent than that of other amino acids, and no selective dibasic aminoaciduria is observed.

There should be even less trouble distinguishing cystinuria from homocystinuria. These conditions both give a positive urinary nitroprusside test and result in the excretion of the mixed disulfide of cysteine and homocysteine, originally described by Frimpter (1961). They are similar in no other way. Homocystinuria is featured clinically by dislocated lenses, mental retardation and cutaneous flushing. Renal calculi do not occur, because homocystine is excreted in relatively small amounts compared to the excretion of cystine in cystinuria. Finally, the urinary amino acid pattern in the two disorders is very different.

Treatment

The object of treatment in cystinuria is simple: to keep the concentration of cystine in the urine below saturation and thus prevent precipitation and stone formation. This goal may be sought by reducing the amount of cystine excreted in the urine, by increasing the volume of urine in which the cystine is dissolved, by increasing the solubility of cystine in urine or by changing cystine to a chemically more soluble form. Each of these approaches has been used in cystinuria

Table 7–4 Differential Diagnosis of Cystinuria, Cystinosis and Homocystinuria

Parameter	Cystinuria	Cystinosis	Homocystinuria*
Clinical			
Renal calculi	Yes	No	No
Tissue deposits of cystine	No	Yes	No
Renal insufficiency	Late	Early	No
Dislocated lenses	No	No	Yes
Fanconi syndrome	No	Yes	No
Laboratory			
Nitroprusside test	++++	(±)	++++
Crystalluria	Yes	No	No
Pathologic aminoaciduria	Specific (cystine, dibasics, cysteine-homocysteine disulfide)	Generalized (cystine not prominent)	Specific (homocystine)

*Due to cystathionine synthase deficiency.

with variable success. Many investigators have attempted to reduce cystine excretion by limiting dietary protein and methionine. Dent and Senior (1955) reported that urinary cystine was lowered by 30 per cent when dietary protein was limited to 20 g per day, an intake too low to maintain nitrogen balance. More enthusiastic results were obtained by Smith et al. (1959) in two patients fed a low methionine diet containing largely vegetable protein. Lotz (1966), Kolb (1967) and their colleagues have also reported beneficial effects of a low protein diet, but other workers (Zinneman and Jones, 1966) have reported disappointing results. These conflicting results indicate that while dietary restriction may be useful in some patients, it cannot be considered a principal or definitive form of therapy in cystinuria.

The most important single aspect of treatment is the maintenance of a high urine volume by a large fluid intake. Weinberg and Tabenkin (1952) and Dent and his colleagues (1965) have reported cystine stone dissolution as well as prevention with this regimen alone. Effective use of this form of therapy, however, demands continuous cooperation by the patient and support from the physician. Fluid administration must be continued throughout the 24-hour period. To prevent urinary concentration during the nighttime hours, Dent and colleagues (1965) recommend the ingestion of 500 ml of water at bedtime and another 500 ml at 2:00 A.M. Fluid ingestion should exceed four liters in a 24-hour period, and the intake of five to seven liters is optimal. Over a 10-year period, Dent (1965) reported that six of 18 patients treated in this way formed new calculi, but attributed the poor results in these patients to their failure to follow the regimen appropriately.

The solubility of cystine in urine rises sharply above pH 7.5 (see Figure 7–6), and therefore, alkalinization therapy has also been tried. To be effective, however, the day and night urine must be kept above pH 7.5. This can sometimes be accomplished by combining day-long sodium bicarbonate therapy (10 g per day) with acetazolamide (250 to 500 mg) at bedtime. The potential advantage of this form of therapy is minimized by the tendency of calcium phosphate to precipitate in an alkaline medium, thus predisposing to nephrocalcinosis or to deposition of calcium salts on existing cystine stones.

In 1963 Crawhall and coworkers proposed a new form of therapy in cystinuria based on thioldisulfide exchange. It is known that thiols dissociate like acids to yield active anions which may undergo exchange reactions with disulfides (Ryle and Sanger, 1955; Pihl et al., 1958).

$$R' \ S \ H \leftrightharpoons R' \ S^- + H^+$$
$$R\text{-}S\text{-}S\text{-}R + R' \ S^- \leftrightharpoons R\text{-}S\text{-}S\text{-}R' + R \ S^-$$

When D-penicillamine (β, β-dimethyl cysteine) was fed to cystinuric patients, cystine excretion fell markedly (Fig. 7–8), and the mixed disulfide of cystine and penicillamine was noted in the urine, as was the symmetrical disulfide of penicillamine. These authors subsequently observed that long-term treatment with penicillamine controlled cystine excretion (Crawhall et al., 1964) — findings confirmed by several other investigators (Bartter et al., 1965; McDonald and Henneman, 1965; McDonald and Fellows, 1966).

Several reports have appeared subsequently indicating that dissolution of cystine stones as well as prevention of new calculi has been achieved with administration of 1 to 3 g of D-penicillamine daily in divided doses. The efficacy of therapy can be monitored effectively, using either colorimetric (Coxon and Kolb, 1954) or chromatographic procedures (Crawhall et al., 1966b), the aim of treatment being to keep urine cystine between 200 and 300 mg per 24 hours.

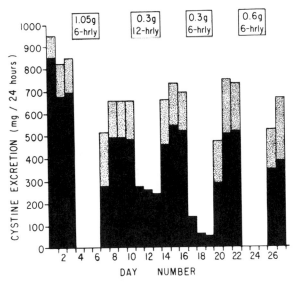

Figure 7–8 Effect of oral administration of D-penicillamine on urinary excretions of cystine in cystinuria. Cystine content was estimated by gravimetric (black bars) and isotope dilution (stippled bars) techniques. D-Penicillamine was administered according to dosage schedule shown at the top of the graph. (From Crawhall, J. C., et al.: Brit. Med. J. *1*:588–590, 1963.)

Unfortunately, this very promising form of therapy has important drawbacks. Penicillamine is a potent vitamin B_6 antagonist (Jaffe et al., 1964), and patients on long-term therapy should receive supplements of pyridoxine. Penicillamine also increases the ratio of soluble to insoluble collagen (Harris and Sjoerdsma, 1966) and impairs wound healing in animals and man. Serum sickness-like reactions have been observed in nearly half of the cystinuric patients treated with penicillamine thus far (McDonald and Fellows, 1966; Rosenberg and Hayslett, 1967). These reactions usually appear between the seventh and tenth day of treatment and are characterized by fever, erythematous skin rash, arthralgia and adenopathy. Transient leukopenia has been observed rarely, as has fatal agranulocytosis (Corcos et al., 1964). A less frequent complication is delayed renal injury.

Rosenberg and Hayslett (1967) reported that four of 20 cystinuric patients treated with penicillamine for periods ranging from three months to three years developed significant proteinuria which progressed to the nephrotic syndrome in one patient and which disappeared when the drug was stopped. Renal biopsies in three patients with proteinuria demonstrated a focal glomerulitis and electron-dense deposits in the glomerular basement membrane (Hayslett et al., 1968). These morphological findings suggested that the nephropathy was due to a hypersensitivity reaction affecting the kidney—a conclusion strengthened by immunofluorescent techniques which demonstrated gamma globulin in the glomeruli of affected patients. These findings have been confirmed by others (Felts et al., 1968) and indicate that all patients being treated with penicillamine must be watched constantly for both early and late toxic reactions. Patients should probably be hospitalized when therapy is instituted to detect the earliest signs of toxicity, which respond to adrenal steroids but not to salicylates or antihistamines. Stokes et al. (1968) reported that N-acetyl-D-penicillamine also reduces cystine excretion, but this penicillamine analogue appears to share the latter agent's propensity for initiating hypersensitivity reactions and is slightly less effective in lowering urinary cystine (Stephens and Watts, 1971).

Animal Models of Cystinuria

Cystine calculi have been recovered from the kidney, ureter and bladder of dogs (White, 1944) and minks (Oldfield et al., 1956). Brand (1940), Hess (1942) and their colleagues demonstrated that canine cystinuria is an inherited disorder. In contrast to the human disease, only males were affected, suggesting that canine cystinuria was X-linked. Treacher (1962, 1964) reported that urine samples from dogs with cystinuria also contained large amounts of lysine, arginine and ornithine, but Holtzapple et al. (1971) noted only excess of urinary lysine and cystine. The latter group failed to demonstrate in vitro transport defects in the gut or kidney of these animals, indicating that canine cystinuria is distinctly different from the human disease. The blotched Kenya genet was also reported to excrete very large quantities of cystine (Datta and Harris, 1953), but Crawhall and Segal (1965) have demonstrated that the sulfur-containing amino acid excreted by this species is S-sulfo-L-cysteine, not cystine.

HYPERDIBASICAMINOACIDURIA

Since 1965, several pedigrees from three countries have been described with an isolated defect in renal and intestinal transport of the three dibasic amino acids (lysine, arginine and ornithine). Since none of these patients excrete excess cystine, this disorder can be distinguished clinically and chemically from classic cystinuria and almost surely reflects a mutation in the renal and intestinal transport system used by the dibasic amino acids but *not* by cystine.

Biochemical Features

Considerable interfamilial variability has been noted despite the paucity of involved cases. In the Finnish patients reported by Kekkomaki et al. (1967b) and Perheentupa and Visakorpi (1965), renal clearance of lysine was distinctly increased, arginine clearance was modestly exaggerated and ornithine clearance was not measured. Fasting plasma arginine and lysine concentrations were reduced, but concentrations of other free amino acids were normal. No studies of intestinal absorption of amino acids were conducted. The concentration of urea and ammonia in fasting blood samples was unremarkable, but distinct abnormalities were observed after intravenous infusion of L-alanine. In normal subjects alanine infusion was followed by a prompt increase in blood urea and by no change in blood ammonia. In these affected patients, however, the infusion produced a marked increase in blood ammonia and little or no rise in blood urea, indicating a defect in urea synthesis. When arginine was infused with alanine, the patients responded normally with a rise in blood urea and no increase in ammonia. These findings suggested that arginine deficiency, rather than a primary defect in the enzymes of the urea cycle, was responsible for the observed defect in urea synthesis. This hypothesis was confirmed by in vitro studies of the urea cycle enzymes in liver biopsies from two affected patients (Kekkomaki et al., 1967a). The activity of each of the urea cycle enzymes was normal (carbamyl phosphate synthetase, argininosuccinic acid synthetase, arginase) or increased (ornithine transcarbamylase and argininosuccinase). Furthermore the K_m for arginase in affected patients was not increased, nor was its response to lysine addition atypical. These enzymatic findings are consistent with normal adaptive changes to arginine deficiency.

In the French Canadian pedigree (Whelan and Scriver, 1968), 13 individuals had hyperdibasicaminoaciduria and increased renal clearances of lysine, arginine and ornithine. Each of three affected members also demonstrated impaired intestinal absorption of lysine. The two affected female siblings in the Japanese pedigree (Oyanagi et al., 1970) also demonstrated impaired renal and intestinal transport of dibasic amino acids, but neither of these girls nor the affected members of the French Canadian family had disturbances in ammonia or urea metabolism.

Signs and Symptoms

All 10 Finnish patients tolerated breast milk well. Shortly after they were weaned, however, vomiting and diarrhea commenced and the patients failed to thrive. Diarrhea and vomiting were produced even by diluted cow's milk. When old enough to select their own food, all patients rejected cow's milk, meat, fish, liver and eggs and chose a diet consisting mainly of grains, vegetables and juices. Diarrhea subsided on this self-restricted diet. All patients demonstrated distinct growth failure, but mental development was apparently normal in eight of them. Hepatomegaly was a regular finding, and splenomegaly was observed in four patients. Liver biopsies in three patients revealed round cell infiltration in the portal triads and early fibrous change.

The French Canadian female proband and the affected Japanese sibs also demonstrated mild intestinal malabsorption and growth retardation, but only the Japanese girls evidenced distinct mental retardation as well. Significantly, none of the other affected French Canadians had any clinical abnormalities.

Genetics

No consistent family pattern has emerged: consanguinity was reported in the Japanese and one of the Finnish pedigrees but not in the French Canadian family; none of the parents of affected children from Finland or Japan had hyperdibasicaminoaciduria, but several instances of direct parent-child transmission of the trait were noted in the Canadian kindred. It seems likely that isolated hyperdibasicaminoaciduria represents the heterozygous manifestation of a trait which causes more profound biochemical and clinical disturbances (hyperammonemia, mental retardation) in affected homozygotes. Since only some heterozygotes appear to express the trait, however, the strong possibility of genetic heterogeneity, similar to that noted in cystinuria or iminoglycinuria, must be entertained.

Diagnosis

This disease should be considered in any patient with protein intolerance or increased urinary excretion of dibasic amino acids. Amino acid excretion in the early months is so variable that the diagnosis of hyperdibasicaminoaciduria will not be made unless the disease is specifically considered. Since postprandial hyperammonemia may be a problem in these patients, the disorder must be included in the differential diagnosis of hyperammonemia during the first year of life. (See Chapter 12.)

Treatment

A low-protein diet seems necessary to prevent the impressive gastrointestinal symptoms noted in some patients with this disorder, but such a diet may also lead to growth failure and central nervous system abnormalities. A low-protein diet supplemented with lysine or arginine may be helpful if arginine deficiency, per se, is responsible for the hyperammonemia or if lysine deficiency is etiologically related to the mental retardation.

ISOLATED HYPERCYSTINURIA

In 1966 Brodehl and his colleagues reported that a four-year-old girl and her two-year-old brother excreted markedly increased amounts of cystine in their urine but *no* excessive quantities of lysine, arginine or ornithine. Cystine clearance in these children was about 30 ml per minute, with dibasic amino acid clearances all less than 1 ml per minute. Renal lithiasis was not reported in either patient. Both parents and one sibling excreted normal amounts of cystine. These intriguing results are not like those reported in patients homozygous or heterozygous for classic cystinuria. They suggest that cystine is transported by a renal tubular mechanism unshared with lysine, arginine or ornithine and that this cystine-specific system is defective in the two children studied. To distinguish this disorder from classic cystinuria, Brodehl suggested the name "isolated hypercystinuria."

REFERENCES

Ackermann, D., and Kutscher, F.: Ueber das Vorkommen von Lysin im harn bei Cystinurie. Z. Biol. *57*:355, 1911.

Alsberg, A., and Folin, O.: Protein metabolism in cystinuria. Amer. J. Physiol. *14*:54–72, 1905.

Ames, G. F.: Uptake of amino acids by Salmonella typhimurium. Arch. Biochem. Biophys. *104*: 1–18, 1964.

Ampola, M., Bixby, E. M., Crawhall, J. C., Efron, M. L., Parker, R., Sneddon, W., and Young, E. P.: Isolation of a new sulphur-containing amino acid. Biochem. J. *107*:16P, 1968.

Arrow, U. K., and Westall, R. G.: Amino acid clearances in cystinuria. J. Physiol. *142*:141–146, 1958.

Asatoor, A. M., Lacey, B. W., London, D. R., and Milne, M. D.: Amino acid metabolism in cystinuria. Clin. Sci. *23*:285–304, 1962.

Bartter, F. C., Lotz, M., Thier, S., Rosenberg, L. E., and Potts, J. T.: Cystinuria. Combined clinical staff conference at the National Institutes of Health. Ann. Intern. Med. *62*:796–822, 1965.

Becker, F. F., and Green, H.: Incorporation of cystine and lysine by normal and "cystinuric" leukocytes. Proc. Soc. Exp. Biol. Med. *99*:694–696, 1958.

Berry, H. K.: Detection of metabolic disorders among mentally retarded children by means of paper spot tests. Amer. J. Ment. Defic. *66*:555–560, 1962.

Berzelius, J. J.: Lärobok i kemien *6*:479, 1830.

Boström, H., and Hambraeus, L.: Cystinuria in Sweden. VII. Clinical, histopathological and medico-social aspects of the disease. Acta Med. Scand. Supplement. 411, 1964.

Boström, H., and Tottie, K.: Cystinuria in Sweden. II. The incidence of homozygous cystinuria in Swedish school children. Acta Paediat. Scand. *48*:345–352, 1959.

Brand, E., and Cahill, G. F.: Further studies on metabolism of sulfur compounds in cystinuria. Proc. Soc. Exp. Biol. Med. *31*:1247, 1934.

Brand, E., Cahill, G. F., and Harris, M. M.: Cystinuria. II. The metabolism of cysteine, methionine and glutathione. J. Biol. Chem. *109*:69–83, 1935.

Brand, E., Cahill, G. F., and Kassell, B.: Canine cystinuria. V. Family history of two cystinuric Irish terriers and cystine determinations in dog urine. J. Biol. Chem. *133*:431–436, 1940.

Brodehl, J., Gellissen, K., and Kowalewsko, S.: Isolated cystinuria (without lysine-ornithine-argininuria) in a family with hypocalcemic tetany. Proceedings of the Third International Congress on Nephrology, Washington, 1966.

Collis, J. E., Levi, A. J., and Milne, M. D.: Stature and nutrition in cystinuria and Hartnup disease. Brit. Med. J. *1*:590–592, 1963.

Corcos, J. M., Soler-Bechera, J., Mayer, K., Freyberg, R. H., Goldstein, R., and Jaffe, I.: Neutrophilic agranulocytosis during administration of penicillamine. J.A.M.A. *189*:265–268, 1964.

Coxon, U., and Kolb, F. O.: The use of oral choline in cystinuria. Metabolism *3*:255–261, 1954.

Crawhall, J. C., Purkiss, P., Watts, R. W. E., and Young, E. P.: The excretion of amino acids by cystinuric patients and their relatives. Ann. Hum. Genet. *33*:149–169, 1969.

Crawhall, J. C., Saunders, E. P., and Thompson, C. J.: Heterozygotes for cystinuria. Ann. Hum. Genet. *29*:257–269, 1966a.

Crawhall, J. C., Scowen, E. F., Thompson, C. J., and Watts, R. W. E.: The renal clearance of amino acids in cystinuria. J. Clin. Invest. *46*:1162–1171, 1967.

Crawhall, J. C., Scowen, E. F., and Watts, R. W. E.: Effect of penicillamine on cystinuria. Brit. Med. J. *1*:588–590, 1963.

Crawhall, J. C., Scowen, E. F., and Watts, R. W. E.: Further observations on use of D-penicillamine in cystinuria. Brit. Med. J. *1*:1411–1413, 1964.

Crawhall, J. C., and Segal, S.: Sulphocysteine in the urine of the blotched Kenya genet. Nature *208*:1320–1322, 1965.

Crawhall, J. C., Thompson, C. J., and Bradley, K. H.: Separation of cystine, penicillamine disulfide and cysteine-penicillamine mixed disulfide by automatic amino acid analysis. Anal. Biochem. *14*:405–413, 1966b.

Datta, S. P., and Harris, H.: Urinary amino acid patterns of some mammals. Ann. Eugen. (London) *18*:106–115, 1953.

Dent, C. E., Friedmann, M., Green, H., and Watson, L. C. A.: Treatment of cystinuria. Brit. Med. J. *1*:403–408, 1965.

Dent, C. E., and Rose, G. A.: Amino acid metabolism in cystinuria. Quart. J. Med. *20*:205–219, 1951.

Dent, C. E., and Senior, B.: Studies on the treatment of cystinuria. Brit. J. Urol. *27*:317–332, 1955.

Dent, C. E., Senior, B., and Walshe, J. M.: The pathogenesis of cystinuria. II. Polarographic studies of the metabolism of sulphur-containing amino acids. J. Clin. Invest. *33*:1216–1226, 1954.

Doolan, P. D., Harper, H. A., Hutchin, M. E., and Alpen, E. L.: Renal clearance of lysine in cystinuria. Amer. J. Med. *23*:416–425, 1957.

Felts, J. H., King, J. S., and Boyce, W. H.: Nephrotic syndrome after treatment with D-penicillamine. Lancet (i), 53–54, 1968.

Fox, M., Thier, S., Rosenberg, L. E., Kiser, W., and Segal, S.: Evidence against a single renal transport defect in cystinuria. New Eng. J. Med. *270*:556–561, 1964.

Frimpter, G. W.: The disulfide of L-cysteine and L-homocysteine in urine of patients with cystinuria. J. Biol. Chem. *236*:PC51–53, 1961.

Frimpter, G. W., Horwith, M., Furth, E., Fellows, R. E., and Thompson, D. D.: Inulin and endogenous amino acid renal clearances in cystinuria: Evidence for tubular secretion. J. Clin. Invest. *41*:281–288, 1962.

Gardner, J. D., and Levy, A. G.: Transport of dibasic amino acids by human erythrocytes. Metabolism *21*:413–431, 1972.

Garrod, A. E.: The Croonian lectures. Lancet (ii), 1, 73, 142, 214, 1908.

Gross, J. B., Comfort, M. W., and Ulrich, J. A.: Abnormalities in serum and urinary amino acids in hereditary and non-hereditary pancreatitis. Trans. Ass. Amer. Physicians *70*:127–139, 1957.

Gross, J. B., Ulrich, J. A., Jones, J. D., and Maher, F. T.: Endogenous renal clearances of 12 individual amino acids in four apparently healthy subjects and in four aminoaciduric persons of a kindred with hereditary pancreatitis. J. Lab. Clin. Med. *63*:933–944, 1964.

Groth, U., and Rosenberg, L. E.: Transport of dibasic amino acids, cystine, and tryptophan by cultured human fibroblasts: Absence of a defect in cystinuria and Hartnup disease. J. Clin. Invest. *51*:2130–2142, 1972.

Harris, E. D., and Sjoerdsma, A.: Effect of penicillamine on human collagen and its possible application to treatment of scleroderma. Lancet (ii), 996–999, 1966.

Harris, H., Mittwoch, U., Robson, E. B., and Warren, F. L.: Pattern of amino acid excretion in cystinuria. Ann. Human. Genet. *19*:195–208, 1955.

Harris, H., Mittwoch, U., Robson, E. B., and Warren, F. L.: Phenotypes and genotypes in cystinuria. Ann. Hum. Genet. *20*:57–91, 1955.

Hayslett, J. P., Bensch, K. G., Kashgarian, M., and Rosenberg, L. E.: Focal glomerulitis due to penicillamine. Lab. Invest. *19*:376–381, 1968.

Hellier, M. D., Perrett, D., and Holdsworth, C. D.: Dipeptide absorption in cystinuria. Brit. Med. J. *4*:782–783, 1970.

Herring, L. C.: Observations on the analysis of ten thousand urinary calculi. J. Urol. *88*:545–562, 1962.

Hershko, L., Ben-Ami, E., Paciorkovski, J., and Levin, N.: Allelomorphism in cystinuria. Proc. Tel-Hashomer Hosp. *4*:21–23, 1965.

Hess, W. C., and Sullivan, M. X.: Canine cystinuria: The effect of feeding cystine, cysteine and methionine at different protein levels. J. Biol. Chem. *143*:545–550, 1942.

Hillman, R. E., Albrecht, I., and Rosenberg, L. E.: Identification and analysis of multiple glycine transport systems in isolated mammalian renal tubules. J. Biol. Chem. *243*:5566–5571, 1968.

Holtzapple, P. G., Rea, C., Bovee, K., and Segal, S.: Characteristics of cystine and lysine transport in renal and jejunal tissue from cystinuric dogs. Metabolism *20*:1016–1022, 1971.

Jaffe, I. A., Altman, K., and Merryman, P.: The antipyridoxine effect of penicillamine in man. J. Clin. Invest. *43*:1869–1873, 1964.

Kekkomaki, M., Raiha, C. R., and Perheentupa, J.: Enzymes of urea synthesis in familial protein intolerance with deficient transport of basic amino acids. Acta Paediat. Scand. *56*:631–636, 1967a.

Kekkomaki, M., Visakorpi, J. K., Perheentupa, J., and Saxen, L.: Familial protein intolerance with deficient transport of basic amino acids. An analysis of ten patients. Acta Paediat. Scand. *56*:617–630, 1967b.

Kolb, F. O., Earll, J. M., and Harper, H. A.: "Disappearance" of cystinuria in a patient treated with prolonged low methionine diet. Metabolism *16*:378–381, 1967.

Levy, H. J., Shih, V. E., and MacCready, R. A.: Massachusetts metabolic disorders screening program. *In* Harris, M., ed., Early Diagnosis of Human Genetic Defects. U.S. Government Printing Office, Washington, D.C., pp. 47–66, 1972.

Lewis, H. B.: Cystinuria. A review of some recent investigations. Yale J. Biol. *4*:437–499, 1932a.

Lewis, H. B.: The occurrence of cystinuria in healthy young men and women. Ann. Intern. Med. *6*:183–192, 1932b.

Lotz, M., Potts, J. T., Holland, J. M., Kiser, W. S., and Bartter, F. C.: D-penicillamine therapy in cystinuria. J. Urol. *95*:257–263, 1966.

Marcet, A.: An essay on the chemical history and medical treatment of calculus disorders. London, 1817.

McDonald, J. E., and Fellows, L. E.: Penicillamine in the treatment of patients with cystinuria. J.A.M.A. *187*:396–402, 1966.

McDonald, J. E., and Henneman, P. H.: Stone dissolution in vivo and control of cystinuria with D-penicillamine. New Eng. J. Med. *273*:578–583, 1965.

Milne, M. D., Asatoor, A. M., Edwards, K. D. G., and Loughridge, L. W.: The intestinal absorption defect in cystinuria. Gut *2*:323–337, 1961.

Morin, C. L., Thompson, M. W., Jackson, S. H., and Sass-Kortsak, A.: Biochemical and genetic studies in cystinuria: Observations on double heterozygotes of Genotype I/II. J. Clin. Invest. *50*:1961–1975, 1971.

Mörner, C. T.: On present knowledge of cystinuria. Uppsala Läk.-foren. Förh. *31*:171, 1925.

Niemann, A.: Beitrag zur Lehre von Cystinurie beim Menschen. Deutsch. Arch. Klin. Med. *18*:232, 1876.

Oldfield, J. E., Allen, P. H., and Adair, J.: Identification of cystine calculi in mink. Proc. Soc. Exp. Biol. Med. *91*:560–562, 1956.

Oyanagi, K., Miura, R., and Yamanouchi, T.: Congenital lysinuria: A new inherited transport disorder of dibasic amino acids. J. Pediat. *77*:259–266, 1970.

Perheentupa, J., and Visakorpi, J. K.: Protein intolerance with deficient transport of basic amino acids: Another inborn error of metabolism. Lancet (ii), 813–816, 1965.

Pihl, A., Eldjarn, L., and Nakken, K. F.: The nucleophilic reactivity of biological thiols with respect to thiol-disulphide exchange reactions. Acta Chem. Scand. *12*:1357–1358, 1958.

Prout, W.: Traite de la gravelle. Paris, p. 278, 1823.

Renander, A.: The roentgen density of the cystine calculus: A roentgenographic and experimental study including a comparison with more common uroliths. Acta Radiol. (Stockholm) Supplement. *41*:1–148, 1941.

Robson, E. B., and Rose, G. A.: The effect of intravenous lysine on the renal clearances of cystine, arginine and ornithine in normal subjects, in patients with cystinuria and Fanconi syndrome and in their relatives. Clin. Sci. *16*:75–91, 1957.

Rosenberg, L. E.: Genetic heterogeneity in cystinuria. *In* Nyhan, W. L., ed., Amino Acid Metabolism and Genetic Variation. McGraw-Hill, New York, pp. 341–349, 1967.

Rosenberg, L. E., Albrecht, I., and Segal, S.: Lysine transport in human kidney: Evidence for two systems. Science *155*:1426–1428, 1967a.

Rosenberg, L. E., Crawhall, J. L., and Segal, S.: Intestinal transport of cystine and cysteine in man: Evidence for separate mechanisms. J. Clin. Invest. *46*:30–34, 1967b.

Rosenberg, L. E., and Downing, S. J.: Transport of neutral and dibasic amino acids by human leukocytes: Absence of defect in cystinuria. J. Clin. Invest. *44*:1382–1393, 1965.

Rosenberg, L. E., Downing, S. J., Durant, J. L., and Segal, S.: Cystinuria: Biochemical evidence for three genetically distinct diseases. J. Clin. Invest. *45*:365–371, 1966a.

Rosenberg, L. E., Downing, S. J., and Segal, S.: Competitive inhibition of dibasic amino acid transport in rat kidney. J. Biol. Chem. *237*:2265–2270, 1962.

Rosenberg, L. E., Durant, J. L., and Albrecht, I.: Genetic heterogeneity in cystinuria: Evidence for allelism. Trans. Ass. Amer. Physicians *79*:284–296, 1966b.

Rosenberg, L. E., and Hayslett, J. P.: Nephrotoxic effects of penicillamine in cystinuria. J.A.M.A. *201*:698–699, 1967.

Ryle, A. P., and Sanger, F.: Disulphide interchange reactions. Biochem. J. *60*:535–540, 1955.

Schwartzman, L., Blair, A., and Segal, S.: A common renal transport system for lysine, ornithine, arginine and cysteine. Biochem. Biophys. Res. Commun. *23*:220–226, 1966.

Scriver, C. R., Whelan, D. T., Clow, C. L., and Dallaire, L.: Cystinuria: Increased prevalence in patients with mental disease. New Eng. J. Med. *283*:783–786, 1970.

Smith, D. R., Kolb, F. O., and Harper, H. A.: Management of cystinuria and cystine-stone disease. J. Urol. *81*:61–69, 1959.

Stein, W. H.: Excretion of amino acids in cystinuria. Proc. Soc. Exp. Biol. Med. *78*:705–708, 1951.

Stephens, A. D., and Watts, R. W. E.: The treatment of cystinuria with N-acetyl-D-penicillamine; a comparison with the results of D-penicillamine treatment. Quart. J. Med. *40*:355–370, 1971.

Stokes, G. S., Potts, J. T., Lotz, M., and Bartter, F. C.: New agent in the treatment of cystinuria: N-acetyl-D-penicillamine. Brit. Med. J. *1*:284–288, 1968.

Stromeyer, L.: Ann. Chim. et Phys. *27*:221, 1824.

Thier, S. O., Fox, M., Segal, S., and Rosenberg, I. E.: Cystinuria: In vitro demonstration of an intestinal transport defect. Science *143*:482–484, 1964.

Thier, S. O., Segal, S., Fox, M., Blair, A., and Rosenberg, L. E.: Cystinuria: Defective intestinal transport of dibasic amino acids and cystine. J. Clin. Invest. *44*:442–448, 1965.

Toel, F.: Beobachtungen ueber cystinbildung. Ann. Chem. Pharmakol. *96*:247, 1855.

Treacher, R. J.: Amino acid excretion in canine cystine stone disease. Vet. Res. *74*:503–504, 1962.

Treacher, R. J.: Quantitative studies on the excretion of the basic amino acids in canine cystinuria. Brit. Vet. J. *120*:178–185, 1964.

von Udransky, L., and Baumann, E.: Ueber das Vorkommen von Diaminen, sogenannten Ptomainen, bei Cystinurie. Z. Physiol. Chem. *13*:562–594, 1899.

Weinberg, S. R., and Tabenkin, P. A.: Observations on therapy of cystine calculus disease. Arch. Intern. Med. *90*:850–857, 1952.

Whelan, D. T., and Scriver, C. R.: Hyperdibasicaminoaciduria: An inherited disorder of amino acid transport. Pediat. Res. *2*:525–534, 1968.

White, E. G.: Urinary calculi in the dog, with special reference to cystine stones. J. Comp. Path. *54*:16–25, 1944.

Wolff, C. G. L., and Shaffer, P. A.: Protein metabolism in cystinuria. J. Biol. Chem *4*:439–472, 1908.

Wollaston, W. H.: On cystic oxide, a new species of urinary calculus. Phil. Trans. B. *100*:223–230, 1810.

Yeh, H. L., Frankl, W., Dunn, M. S., Parker, P., Hughes, B., and György, P.: The urinary excretion of amino acids by a cystinuric subject. Amer. J. Med. Sci. *214*:507–512, 1947.

Zinneman, H. H., and Jones, J. E.: Dietary methionine and its influence on cystine excretion in cystinuric patients. Metabolism *15*:915–921, 1966.

Chapter Eight

NATURE AND DISORDERS OF IMINO ACID AND GLYCINE TRANSPORT

FAMILIAL IMINOGLYCINURIA

In 1961 Scriver, Schafer and Efron observed that patients with elevated plasma proline concentrations due to an inherited disorder of proline catabolism excreted increased quantities of glycine and hydroxyproline in the urine. They reasoned that the hyperglycinuria and hydroxyprolinuria resulted from competitive inhibition of tubular reabsorption of glycine and hydroxyproline by proline and proposed that glycine and the imino acids (proline and hydroxyproline) shared a common transport mechanism in the kidney. This thesis was strengthened by renal clearance and infusion studies in normal humans (Scriver et al., 1964) and by experiments with kidney slices in vitro (Wilson and Scriver, 1967; Scriver and Wilson, 1964). Since 1958, more than 20 patients have been described who demonstrate that this shared tubular mechanism is under specific genetic control. Several groups have reported patients with iminoglycinuria due to a specific inherited defect in tubular reabsorption of these substances (Scriver and Wilson, 1967; Rosenberg et al., 1968; Morikawa et al., 1966; Scriver, 1968; Tada et al., 1965; Goodman et al., 1967; Whelan and Scriver, 1968; Fraser et al., 1968; Mardens et al., 1968; Joseph et al., 1958). An intestinal transport defect for the imino acids and glycine has been described in some (Tada et al., 1965; Goodman et al., 1967), but not all, of these patients (Rosenberg et al., 1968; Scriver, 1968; Tancredi et al., 1970). Scriver and Wilson (1967) postulated that patients with inherited iminoglycinuria are homozygous for an autosomal mutation and that most heterozygotes for this defect

178

excrete increased quantities of glycine only. This mutation does not appear to produce any clinical abnormalities, but it has done much to clarify the mechanisms by which glycine and the imino acids cross cell membranes.

Transport of Imino Acids and Glycine

Normal Mechanisms

Glycine, the simplest of all the naturally occurring amino acids, and the imino acids proline and hydroxyproline have been the subject of intense biochemical investigation. These three substances are the most abundant amino acids in collagen. In addition, glycine and imino acids have other important and complex intracellular fates which will be discussed in subsequent chapters. Their transport mechanisms are equally complex and equally significant. In ascites tumor cells (Oxender and Christensen, 1963) and mature erythrocytes (Winter and Christensen, 1965), glycine is accumulated by a mediated system(s) with preference for many other neutral, aliphatic amino acids (the so-called "alanine-preferring" or A system). In kidney slices (Wilson and Scriver, 1967; Scriver and Wilson, 1964; Fox et al., 1964), fetal bone (Finerman and Rosenberg, 1966) and intestinal segments (Lin et al., 1962; Munck, 1966), the transport of the imino acids and glycine is mediated by sodium-dependent, energy-requiring, ouabain-sensitive systems which have a greater affinity for the imino acids than for glycine (Wilson and Scriver, 1967; Scriver and Wilson, 1964). These in vitro observations are reflected in the transport of these compounds in vivo. Glycine and the imino acids are excreted abundantly by the premature and the newborn human infant. However, by six to 12 months of age, no free proline and hydroxyproline are excreted in the urine of normal subjects, and their presence thereafter is pathological. In contrast, glycine is excreted throughout life. The normal human adult excretes 50 to 300 mg of free glycine per day, this substance accounting for 30 or more per cent of the total daily amino acid nitrogen (Soupart, 1962). Although 93 to 98 per cent of the filtered glycine is reabsorbed by the renal tubule, it is one of the few amino acids with renal clearances above 2 ml per minute (normal values for glycine range from 1.5 to 8.0 ml per minute). Glycine, proline and hydroxyproline are also excreted in the form of conjugates or small peptides. The excretion of these substances in bound form provides an important index of collagen and bone turnover but is *not* relevant to this discussion of free amino acid transport.

The Common Imino Acid-Glycine System

We have already alluded to the initial evidence for a common renal transport system for glycine and the imino acids. The urinary pattern of patients with hyperprolinemia led Scriver and his colleagues to other experiments. They showed that the excretion and clearance of glycine and hydroxyproline could be selectively increased by proline infusion and that the clearance of glycine, but not of proline, was augmented by hydroxyproline administration (Scriver et al., 1964). Wilson and Scriver (1967) demonstrated mutual inhibition between this substance in kidney slices, an observation confirmed by Lin et al. (1962) and Finerman and Rosenberg (1966) in intestinal segments and fetal rat bone, respectively. These experiments supported the hypothesis that glycine, proline and hydroxyproline shared a common transport system in many mammalian tissues but also raised important questions. Thus, it was not clear why glycine transport was *competitively* inhibited by proline and hydroxyproline in the kidney slice, whereas the transport of proline was inhibited *noncompetitively* by glycine (Wilson and Scriver, 1967). Similar complexities were apparent in the fetal bone: glycine transport was partially dependent on the sodium ion, but imino acid transport was completely dependent on this cation; neither glycine nor proline inhibited each other's transport competitivity; and no exchange diffusion would be demonstrated between these compounds (Finerman and Rosenberg, 1966). As has so often been the case in human biochemistry, the resolution of these disparate findings came from the identification of a mutant phenotype.

The Defect in Iminoglycinuria

Joseph et al. (1958) described familial iminoglycinuria for the first time and attributed it to a defect in renal tubular transport. In 1965 Tada and his colleagues described two unrelated children with distinctly increased urinary concentrations of glycine and the imino acids. Since plasma concentrations of these substances were normal, they also suggested that the iminoglycinuria was due to a renal tubular reabsorptive defect. Scriver and Wilson (1967) detected similar abnormalities in a Canadian adult and subsequently studied this abnormality in nine affected patients in three kindreds (Scriver, 1968). They found that patients with iminoglycinuria reabsorbed about 60 per cent of the filtered glycine and that infusion of proline or hydroxyproline did not reduce glycine reabsorption further. In addition, the tubular maxima (T_m) for the imino acids was reduced to about 10 per cent of normal in these patients (Fig. 8–1), some of whom had distinctly elevated imino acid clearances as well. The parents and children of the patients reported by Scriver (1968) exhibited distinct hyperglycinuria but no iminoaciduria. Clearance studies in these individuals revealed a glycine clearance intermediate between that observed in normals and the patients with iminoglycinuria. Furthermore, these hyperglycinuric relatives had a distinctly reduced T_m for proline and hydroxyproline without an exaggerated splay in the titration curve (Fig. 8–1). Many of these observations have been confirmed by Rosenberg and coworkers (1968) in their study of a family with iminoglycinuria. A summary of these renal findings is presented in Table 8–1.

A particularly interesting form of hyperglycinuria without endogenous iminoaciduria has been discovered recently (Green et al., 1972). The renal clearance of glycine in the healthy, teenage proband and his brother were in the range noted for individuals presumably homozygous for iminoglycinuria. The proband had a normal T_m for proline but a markedly exaggerated "splay" (Fig. 8–1). As with the patients previously described, glycine reabsorption was not further depressed by proline infusion. The father of these boys was modestly hyperglycinuric, but their mother was not. These findings are compatible with the thesis that the affected brothers are either homozygous or doubly heterozygous for a mutation(s) which alters the affinity rather than the capacity of the shared system which transports imino acids and glycine.

Morikawa (1966), Goodman (1967) and their colleagues reported that patients with renal iminoglycinuria may also have an intestinal defect. They showed increased fecal concentrations of glycine and the imino acids in two affected patients and reported that plasma proline increased less after oral proline loads in these patients than in controls. It is clear, however, that a gut defect does not exist in all patients with this renal tubular abnormality, since many groups have been unable to find in vivo or in vitro evidence for an intestinal defect in other patients with iminoglycinuria.

Table 8-1 Renal Clearance, Fractional Tubular Reabsorption and T_m of Imino Acids and Glycine in Familial Iminoglycinuria*

Phenotype	Proline			Hydroxyproline			Glycine	
	Endog. Clearance (ml/min/1.73m²)	% Reabsorbed	T_m (μmoles/min/1.73m²)	Endog. Clearance (ml/min/1.73m²)	% Reabsorbed	T_m (μmoles/min/1.73m²)	Endog. Clearance (ml/min/1.73m²)	% Reabsorbed
Normal	0–0.03	>99.8	180–300	0	100	60–135	1.2–8.6	93–99
Homozygous	0.5–19.6	77–99.5	10–18	1–33.6	65–99	6	17.0–41.6	61–77
Heterozygous								
"Hyperglycinuric"	0	100	35–117	0	100	50	8.6–26.2	82–95
"Normoglycinuric"	0	100	– – –	0	100	– – –	3.1–6.7	>93

*Adapted from Scriver, 1972. Values shown represent range of reported observations.

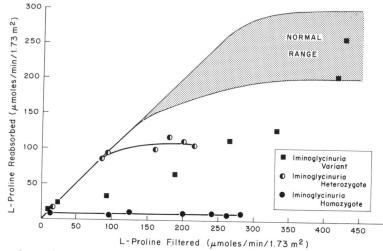

Figure 8–1 Plot of filtered vs. reabsorbed L-proline in normal subjects (hatched area) and subjects with iminoglycinuric phenotypes. Note the reduced T_m and absence of exaggerated splay in the iminoglycinuric homozygote and heterozygote as compared with the exaggerated splay and normal T_m in the iminoglycinuric variant. (Redrawn from Scriver, 1968, and Greene et al., 1973.)

Shared but Not Exclusive Systems

The findings described previously indicate that glycine and the imino acids are transported in the renal tubules and the intestine by a genetically controlled system with selective affinity for these substances. The proposed common system has a higher affinity for the imino acids than for glycine as evidenced by the in vitro findings and by the results in obligate heterozygotes for iminoglycinuria. This shared mechanism is responsible for the reabsorption of about 40 per cent of the filtered glycine at normal plasma concentrations but probably accounts for the reabsorption of more than 90 per cent of the filtered imino acids under these conditions. The following observations make it equally certain that this common system is not the only transport process for glycine or the imino acids in the kidney and the gut: the inability to demonstrate mutual competitive inhibition in vitro; the identification of at least three separate glycine transport systems and two separate proline systems in isolated renal tubules (Hillman et al., 1968; Hillman and Rosenberg, 1969) and kidney slices (Mohyuddin and Scriver, 1970); and the failure of proline infusion to reduce fractional glycine reabsorption below 60 per cent of that filtered in subjects with iminoglycinuria, their relatives or normals. Such in vivo and in vitro analyses have led to the following descriptions of transport systems for the imino acids and glycine: a high-capacity, low-affinity system shared by all three compounds; a low-capacity system for glycine which is not shared by proline or hydroxyproline; and a low-capacity system utilized by the imino acids but not glycine. Glycine undoubtedly also shares a transport process with other neutral amino acids in the kidney (Scriver et al., 1964), and its clearance is increased by infusions of dibasic amino acids as well (Webber et al., 1961), suggesting that this simple molecule may be transported in part by all the tubular transport systems for amino acids.

Transport Studies in Other Tissues

Tada et al. (1966) examined the uptake of proline and its incorporation into collagen in both peripheral blood leukocytes and cultured skin fibroblasts from a patient with iminoglycinuria. No differences from normal were observed, once again demonstrating that transport defects found in kidney and intestine are generally not expressed in other tissues.

Genetics

Recessive Inheritance

As shown in Figure 8-2, familial iminoglycinuria has been observed in more than 10 pedigrees, several of which contain more than a single affected member. Approximately equal numbers of affected males and females have been reported. No instance of parent to child transmission of the complete mutant phenotype (iminoaciduria and hyperglycinuria) has been reported. Close consanguinity in the parents of iminoglycinuric children has been observed in two families, but not in the others. These features, plus the distinct hyperglycinuria without iminoaciduria in many parents and offspring of affected probands, indicate that familial iminoglycinuria is inherited as an autosomal recessive trait. The study of Levy et al. (1972), in which iminoglycinuria was found with a population frequency of 1:20,000, indicates that this transport defect is about as common as cystinuria or Hartnup disease.

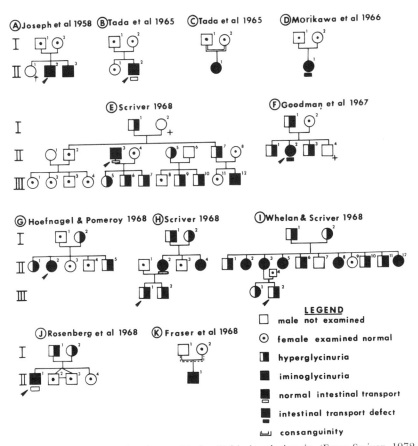

Figure 8-2 Pedigrees of patients with familial iminoglycinuria. (From Scriver, 1972.)

Genetic Heterogeneity

Three kinds of evidence indicate that more than one genotype can produce the mutant phenotype characteristic of this disorder (Table 8–2). First, an intestinal defect has been described in some affected patients but not in others, their renal tubular defects being indistinguishable. Second, all obligate heterozygotes have exhibited hyperglycinuria in some pedigrees, but no heterozygotes have been thus detected in others. In still other families, one parent of an affected patient excreted increased glycine, whereas the other parent did not. Third, some affected patients have a very low T_m for proline, while others have a normal T_m with an increased splay. These observations, reminiscent of those reported earlier in cystinuria, suggest that the two or more mutations responsible for the mutant phenotype in this disorder may be allelic.

Familial Hyperglycinuria

In 1957 de Vries and his colleagues described four females in three generations of an Ashkenazic Jewish family who had hyperglycinuria but not iminoaciduria. Three of the four affected subjects had formed calcium oxalate kidney stones, but the pathophysiological relationship between the lithiasis and the hyperglycinuria was not defined. It seems very likely that such affected individuals are heterozygous for the mutant gene responsible for iminoglycinuria. Such a hypothesis can explain both the urinary findings and the apparently "dominant" mode of inheritance. It is, of course, possible that these hyperglycinuric individuals have a mutation for a glycine-specific transport system—a thesis which can be excluded only by appropriate clearance and infusion studies.

A very different kind of familial hyperglycinuria has also been reported by Kaser et al. (1962). They described a nine-year-old boy with renal glycosuria and an elevated glycine clearance. The patient's father, one of six siblings and 11 of 37 relatives also exhibited glucosuria and hyperglycinuria. Neither of the two conditions occurred alone. The glucoglycinuria was inherited in a dominant fashion, but the nature of the mutation and its relationship to iminoglycinuria remains obscure.

Signs and Symptoms

No reproducible clinical picture has emerged from the study of the reported patients with iminoglycinuria. Affected patients have ranged from one to 42 years. Several patients have been mentally retarded, but they were detected by urinary screening programs in retarded children, suggesting that the association between the retardation and the iminoglycinuria is fortuitous, not eti-

Table 8–2   Evidence for Genetic Heterogeneity in Familial Iminoglycinuria*

Iminoglycinuria Type	Urinary Glycine and Imino Acids in Homozygotes	Intestinal Absorption of Proline in Homozygotes	Urinary Glycine in Heterozygotes
I	increased	impaired	normal
II	increased	normal	normal
III	increased	normal	increased

*Findings obtained from reports by Tada (1965), Morikawa (1966), Scriver (1968), Rosenberg (1968) and their colleagues.

ological. Two boys had congenital nerve deafness, but they also were detected because of this disability, which has not been reported in any of the other patients. Most of the patients with this disorder are living and well. Two of the families studied by Scriver (1972) were investigated for other amino acid disorders: in one family the proband had hyperglycinuria and cystathioninuria; in the other, the proband had hyperglycinuria and cystinosis. Investigation of their families led to the detection of patients with typical iminoglycinuria.

Diagnosis

Since this transport error does not appear to cause reproducible clinical pathology, its detection will necessarily depend on screening programs or amino acid studies for other reasons. Homozygotes will be detected without difficulty by paper chromatographic or electrophoretic studies of urinary amino acids because the appearance of *any* free proline or hydroxyproline is abnormal after the first months of life. Determination of plasma proline and hydroxyproline concentrations is necessary to exclude hyperprolinemia and hydroxyprolinemia, which can produce the same aminoaciduria for very different reasons. Heterozygote detection is more difficult because qualitative methods may not be sensitive enough to define hyperglycinuria.

Treatment

Patients should be told that they suffer from one of "nature's experiments" which will not affect their health or longevity. No other therapy is indicated for this disorder as we now understand it.

REFERENCES

de Vries, A., Kochwa, S., Lazebink, J., Frank, M., and Djaldetti, M.: Glycinuria, a hereditary disorder associated with nephrolithiasis. Amer. J. Med. 23:408–415, 1957.

Finerman, G. A. M., and Rosenberg, L. E.: Amino acid transport in bone: Evidence for separate transport systems for neutral amino and imino acids. J. Biol. Chem. 241:1487–1493, 1966.

Fox, M., Thier, S., Rosenberg, L. E., and Segal, S.: Ionic requirements for amino acid transport in the rat kidney cortex slice. I. Influence of extracellular ions. Biochim. Biophys. Acta 79: 167–176, 1964.

Fraser, G. R., Friedmann, A. I., Patton, V. M., Wade, D. N., and Woolf, L. I.: Iminoglycinuria — a "harmless" inborn error of metabolism? Humangenetik 6:362–367, 1968.

Goodman, S. I., McIntyre, C. A., and O'Brien, D.: Impaired intestinal transport of proline in a patient with familial iminoaciduria. J. Pediat. 71:246–249, 1967.

Greene, M. L., Lietman, P. S., Rosenberg, L. E., and Seegmiller, J. E.: Familial hyperglycinuria: New defect in renal tubular transport of glycine and the imino acids. Amer. J. Med. 54:265–271, 1973.

Hillman, R. E., and Rosenberg, L. E.: Amino acid transport by isolated mammalian renal tubules. II. Transport systems for L-proline. J. Biol. Chem. 244:4494–4498, 1969.

Joseph, R., Ribierre, M., Job, J.-C., and Girault, M.: Maladie familiale associante des convulsions à début très précoce, une hyperalbuminorachie et une hyperaminoacidurie. Arch. Franc. Pediat. 15:374–387, 1958.

Kaser, H., Cottier, P., and Antener, I.: Glucoglycinuria, a new familial syndrome. J. Pediat. 61: 386–394, 1962.

Levy, H. J., Shih, V. E., and MacCready, R. A.: Massachusetts metabolic disorders screening program. In Harris, M., ed., Early Diagnosis of Human Genetic Defects. U.S. Government Printing Office, Washington, D.C., pp. 47–66, 1972.

Lin, E. C. C., Hagihira, H., and Wilson, T. H.: Specificity of the transport system for neutral amino acids in the hamster intestine. Amer. J. Physiol. 202:919–925, 1962.

Mardens, Y., Adriaenssens, K., and Van Sande, M.: Glycinurie et iminoacidurie rénales associées à une oligophrénie. Étude clinique et biochimique. J. Neurol. Sci. 6:333–346, 1968.

Mohyuddin, F., and Scriver, C. R.: Amino acid transport in mammalian kidney. Identification and analysis of multiple systems for imino acids and glycine in rat kidney. Amer. J. Physiol. *219*: 1–8, 1970.

Morikawa, T., Tada, K., Ando, T., Yoshida, T., Yokoyama, Y., and Arakawa, T.: Prolinuria: Defect in intestinal absorption of imino acids and glycine. Tohoku J. Exp. Med. *90*:105–116, 1966.

Munck, B. G.: Amino acid transport by the small intestine of the rat. The existence and specificity of the transport mechanism of imino acids and its relation to the transport of glycine. Biochim. Biophys. Acta *120*:97–103, 1966.

Oxender, D. L., and Christensen, H. N.: Distinct mediating systems for the transport of neutral amino acids by the Ehrlich cell. J. Biol. Chem. *238*:3686–3699, 1963.

Rosenberg, L. E., Durant, J. L., and Elsas, L. J., II: Familial iminoglycinuria: An inborn error of renal tubular transport. New Eng. J. Med. *278*:1407–1412, 1968.

Scriver, C. R.: Familial iminoglycinuria. *In* Stanbury, J. B., Wyngaarden, J. B., and Fredrickson, D. S., eds., The Metabolic Basis of Inherited Disease. McGraw-Hill, New York, pp. 1520–1535, 1972.

Scriver, C. R.: Renal tubular transport of proline, hydroxyproline and glycine. III. Genetic basis for more than one mode of transport in human kidney. J. Clin. Invest. *47*:823–835, 1968.

Scriver, C. R., Efron, M. L., and Schafer, I. A.: Renal tubular transport of proline, hydroxyproline, and glycine in health and in familial hyperprolinemia. J. Clin. Invest. *43*:374–385, 1964.

Scriver, C. R., Schafer, I. A., and Efron, M. L.: New renal tubular amino-acid transport system and a new hereditary disorder of amino-acid metabolism. Nature (London) *192*:672–673, 1961.

Scriver, C. R., and Wilson, O. H.: Amino acid transport: Evidence for genetic control of two types in human kidney. Science *155*:1428–1430, 1967.

Scriver, C. R., and Wilson, O. H.: Possible locations for a common gene product in membrane transport of imino acids and glycine. Nature (London) *202*:92–94, 1964.

Soupart, P.: Free amino acids of blood and urine in the human. *In* Holden, J. T., ed., Amino Acid Pools. Elsevier, Amsterdam, pp. 220–263, 1962.

Tada, K., Morikawa, T., Ando, T., Yoshida, T., and Minagawa, A.: Prolinuria: A new renal tubular defect in transport of proline and glycine. Tohoku J. Exp. Med. *87*:133–143, 1965.

Tada, K., Morikawa, T., and Arakawa, T.: Prolinuria: Transport of proline by leukocytes. Tohoku J. Exp. Med. *90*:189–193, 1966.

Tancredi, R., Guazzi, G., and Auricchio, S.: Renal iminoglycinuria without intestinal malabsorption of glycine and imino acids. J. Pediat. *76*:386–392, 1970.

Webber, W. A., Brown, J. L., and Pitts, R. F.: Interactions of amino acids in renal tubular transport. Amer. J. Physiol. *200*:380–386, 1961.

Whelan, D. T., and Scriver, C. R.: Cystathioninuria and renal iminoglycinuria in a pedigree: A perspective on counselling. New Eng. J. Med. *278*:924–927, 1968.

Wilson, O. H., and Scriver, C. R.: Specificity of transport of neutral and basic amino acids in rat kidney. Amer. J. Physiol. *213*:185–190, 1967.

Winter, C. G., and Christensen, H. N.: Contrasts in neutral amino acid transport by rabbit erythrocytes and reticulocytes. J. Biol. Chem. *240*:3594–3600, 1965.

Chapter Nine

NATURE AND DISORDERS OF NEUTRAL AMINO ACID TRANSPORT

Most natural, protein α-amino acids contain a single amino group and a single carboxyl group and, therefore, carry no net positive or negative charge at physiologic pH. Although these so-called "neutral" amino acids differ strikingly in the length and character of their side chains (see Figure 1–2A), in their solubility properties (see Table 1–1) and in their intracellular fates, most of them appear to be transported across mammalian cell membranes by a group-specific "neutral" amino acid carrier system. In addition, some — perhaps all — of these neutral amino acids are transported by substrate-specific systems (Ames, 1964; Grenson, 1966). The evidence for such group and substrate specificity in man rests largely on information obtained from the study of three inherited human transport disorders: Hartnup disease, in which the group-specific system is defective; and the tryptophan and methionine malabsorption syndromes, in which the substrate-specific systems for tryptophan and methionine, respectively, are impaired.

HARTNUP DISEASE

In 1956 Baron and coworkers described four children in a single sibship with a bizarre illness characterized by a pellagra-like skin rash, temporary cerebellar ataxia and a constant renal aminoaciduria. A total of 43 cases of this disorder, named for the first family in which it was identified, have been described subsequently in England, Belgium, Germany, Holland, Norway, Finland, India, Australia, United States and Japan (Jepson, 1972). The high incidence of parental consanguinity, the frequent occurrence of the disease in siblings of affected patients and the absence of parent to child transmission have confirmed the initial impression that Hartnup disease is an inherited disorder due to a rare autosomal mutation. The renal aminoaciduria is selective for mono-amino-monocarboxylic amino acids with neutral or aromatic side chains. An intestinal transport defect for these same amino acids has been described which, in contrast to cystinuria, is much more important in the pathophysiology of the disease than is the renal tubular abnormality. Although the basic biochemical defect involves the intestinal and renal transport of many amino acids, the clinical abnormalities appear to be secondary to the malabsorption of one of these amino acids: tryptophan.

Biochemical Abnormalities

Tryptophan Transport and Metabolism

Tryptophan is an essential amino acid which is absorbed from the small intestine by active and passive transport processes specific for the natural L-isomer (Orten, 1963). The complex catabolic pathways for tryptophan are shown in Figure 9–1. The major pathway leads to the synthesis of nicotinamide and nicotinamide adenine dinucleotide (NAD)—a reaction sequence which proceeds through several chemical intermediates, including formylkynurenine, kynurenine, 3-OH-kynurenine and 3-OH-anthranilic acid (Jepson, 1972). Quantitatively little nicotinamide is formed from this pathway, since it is estimated that the replacement of 1 mg of dietary nicotinamide in the form of niacin requires 60 mg of tryptophan. Nonetheless, it is this apparently inefficient conversion mechanism which is responsible for the physiological aberrations in Hartnup disease. Two other minor pathways of tryptophan catabolism are known. Normally, little tryptophan is converted to serotonin or to 5-OH-indoleacetic acid, but in the malignant carcinoid syndrome, large amounts of these compounds are formed and excreted in the urine (Varley and Gowenlock, 1963). Armstrong et al. (1958) demonstrated that other indoles, including indoleacetic acid, indolelactic acid and indoleacetylglutamine, are also present in small amounts in normal urine. These indolic products are produced in the tissues, but a more important source appears to be the intestinal bacteria (Weissbach et al., 1959). These microorganisms contain tryptophanase, an enzyme which cleaves tryptophan to indole and pyruvic acid (Happold, 1950). Indole and its methylated derivative skatole (3-methyl indole) are absorbed from the intestine and conjugated with sulfate prior to excretion.

Pellagra is the clinical syndrome produced by dietary niacin deficiency. It is characterized by an erythematous, eczematoid skin rash, dementia and gastrointestinal disturbances. In recent years, however, pellagra-like syndromes have been described in the absence of dietary deficiency of niacin. In each case, the pellagra has resulted from the reduced conversion of tryptophan to nicotinamide. Pellagra has occurred rarely in patients with the carcinoid syndrome because dietary tryptophan is hydroxylated to 5-OH-tryptophan and hence to serotonin (Sjoerdsma et al., 1956). Prolonged treatment with isoniazid may lead to niacin deficiency by competing with pyridoxal phosphate, a coenzyme required in the kynurenine-nicotinamide pathway (Harrison and Feiwel, 1956). Tada et al. (1963) described a child with dwarfism and a pellagra-like rash who

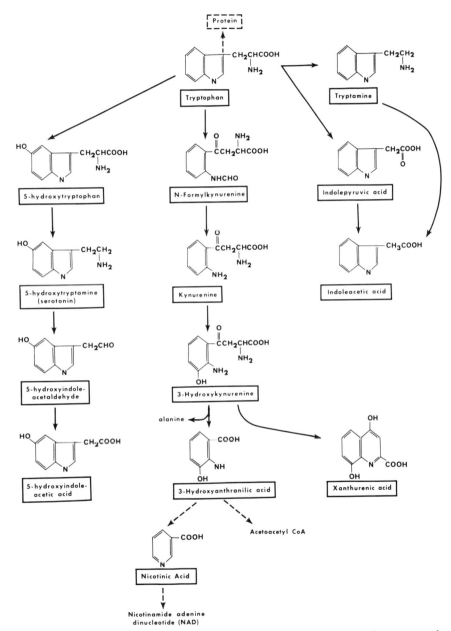

Figure 9–1   Catabolic pathways for tryptophan in man. The pathway from tryptophan to nicotinic acid and NAD represents the major degradative route.

was unable to convert tryptophan to kynurenine. Finally, patients with Hartnup disease develop a syndrome indistinguishable from pellagra because tryptophan is not absorbed from the small intestine and hence cannot be converted in the liver and other tissues to nicotinamide.

The Gut Transport Defect

Although interest in tryptophan absorption has captured the investigative effort in Hartnup disease, there is ample evidence for a gut defect for many other neutral amino acids. Scriver and Shaw (Scriver, 1965; Scriver and Shaw, 1962) reported that the free amino acid content of feces from patients with Hartnup disease is many times normal and that the amino acid pattern closely resembles that of the urine (Fig. 9–2). Shih and coworkers (1971) reported

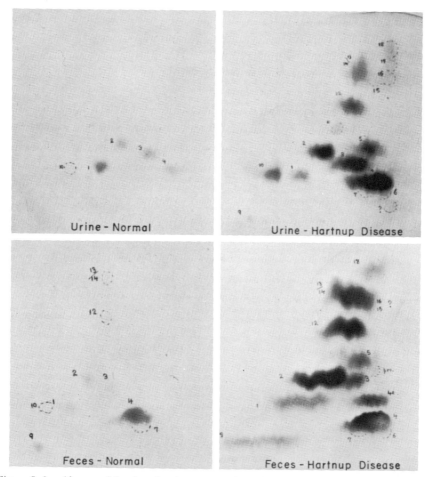

Figure 9–2. Abnormal fecal and urinary excretion of free amino acids in Hartnup disease. Two-dimensional patterns obtained by combined paper electrophoresis and chromatography. Amino acid key: *1*, glycine; *2*, alanine; *3*, serine; *4*, glutamine; *4'*, glutamic acid; *5*, threonine; *6*, aspartic acid; *7*, asparagine; *9*, dibasic amino acids; *10*, histidine; *11*, α-amino-n-butyric acid; *12*, valine; *13/14*, leucine and isoleucine; *15*, methionine; *16*, phenylalanine; *17*, tyrosine; *18*, tryptophan. (From Scriver, C. R.: New Eng. J. Med. *273*:530–532, 1965.)

reduced uptake of tryptophan and methionine by gut mucosa from two brothers with Hartnup disease, thereby providing the first in vitro demonstration of a primary transport defect in this disorder. Since patients with Hartnup disease have been shown to absorb normally oligopeptides containing tryptophan, histidine and phenylalanine (Navab and Asatoor, 1970; Asatoor et al., 1970), it follows that the gut defect is specific for free amino acids and that oligopeptides are absorbed by mechanisms distinct from those used by free amino acids.

The description of indoluria and indicanuria in affected members of the Hartnup family (Baron et al., 1956) suggested an abnormality of tryptophan absorption. This thesis was confirmed by the studies of Milne and his colleagues (1960). They demonstrated defective absorption of tryptophan in four ways. After ingestion of large amounts of L-tryptophan, unchanged tryptophan was detected in the feces of patients with Hartnup disease but not in normal controls. Plasma tryptophan rose less in affected patients after tryptophan loading than in controls. Oral administration of D-tryptophan to normals resulted in limited absorption of the isomer and enzymatic conversion to indolyl-3-pyruvic acid, while patients with Hartnup disease excreted the D-tryptophan in the stools. Finally, patients with Hartnup disease excreted abnormally large amounts of bacterial breakdown products of tryptophan in the urine because significant amounts of this amino acid escaped absorption in the jejunum and reached colonic bacteria. These bacterial degradative products included indican, indolic acids, indoxyl sulfate and indolacetylglutamine. The important role of intestinal bacteria in the observed biochemical abnormalities was confirmed by demonstrating that pretreatment with neomycin, an effective oral antibiotic, almost completely inhibited the excretion of all the indolic compounds in affected patients.

Milne (1972) pointed out that, since half the usual daily requirement for nicotinamide (20 mg) is derived from dietary tryptophan, nicotinamide deficiency (and pellagra) could result from failure of the tryptophan-kynurenine-nicotinamide pathway due to impaired absorption of tryptophan, per se. Jepson (1972) has presented alternatives to this logical schema. He argued that studies in rats (DeLaey et al., 1964) indicated that indoles inhibit tryptophan pyrrolase and other enzymes in the tryptophan to nicotinamide pathway; that nicotinamide prevents the formation of indoles from tryptophan by intestinal bacteria; and that nicotinic acid enhances the uptake of tryptophan into intestinal cells. Accordingly, a "vicious cycle" could occur in Hartnup disease: diminished absorption of tryptophan leading to excessive indole formation; inhibition of nicotinamide synthesis by indole; and subsequent depression of tryptophan uptake due to nicotinamide deficiency. Both these formulations stress the importance of nicotinamide deficiency in the pathophysiology of Hartnup disease and differ only in the proposed route by which such deficiency is produced.

The Renal Defect

A constant pathological aminoaciduria has been the only consistent feature of Hartnup disease. Alanine, serine, threonine, valine, leucine, isoleucine, phenylalanine, tyrosine, tryptophan and histidine are excreted in five to ten times normal amounts, as are glutamine and asparagine (Jepson, 1972). The renal clearances of these amino acids are correspondingly elevated. Histidine clearance approaches the glomerular filtration rate, while those of serine, threonine, alanine and tyrosine indicate that 30 to 60 per cent of the filtered load is reabsorbed (Cusworth and Dent, 1960) compared to normal values of greater than 95 per cent for each of these substances. Plasma amino acid concentrations are normal except for slight and variable reductions in threonine, serine, asparagine and glutamine (Cusworth and Dent, 1960). Urinary excretion of the dibasic, dicarboxylic and β-amino acids is normal, as is the excretion of the imino acids and glycine. The prominent aminoaciduria is of great diagnostic significance and provides the strongest evidence now available for a genetically controlled transport system specific for this group of α-amino acids. The existence of this common system does not mean that these amino acids are not also transported in the kidney and gut by other substrate-specific or group-specific mechanisms. The lessons learned from the study of cystinuria and iminoglycinuria suggest that multiple transport systems for this group of structurally dissimilar α-amino acids also exist.

The aminoaciduria in Hartnup disease is of little or no clinical importance. Tryptophanuria may contribute to the nicotinamide deficiency which results largely from the intestinal malabsorption of tryptophan, but the aminoaciduria has not been shown to result in any other nutritional disturbance. As discussed above, the urine also contains increased quantities of indoles, but this abnormality is secondary to the gut defect and does not appear to reflect an intrinsic tubular abnormality for these substances. All other tests of tubular function and renal clearance have been normal. Specifically, no glucosuria or excess phosphate excretion has been noted (Jepson, 1972).

Transport in Other Tissues

Sweat and saliva from Hartnup patients have a normal amino acid composition. Peripheral blood leukocytes (Tada et al., 1966) and cultured skin fibroblasts (Groth and Rosenberg, 1972) from patients with the disease likewise transport tryptophan normally in vitro. Thus, as with cystinuria, there is evidence that transport systems in different tissues are not expressed identically.

Genetics

Recessive Inheritance and Consanguinity

The 43 reported cases of Hartnup disease have occurred in 28 sibships, 10 of which have contained more than one patient with the disease. The disorder affects both sexes, but females have predominated thus far (25:18). Consanguinity among the parents of affected patients has been documented in seven of the 28 families. In one family, two affected sibs married healthy partners and reproduced unaffected children. The cutaneous, neurological and psychiatric manifestations of the disorder have varied greatly between sibships and within a single family, but the urinary amino acid pattern has been constant in all reported patients. These findings are all consistent with the hypothesis that Hartnup disease is inherited as an autosomal recessive trait and that affected patients are homozygous for a rare mutant gene.

Heterozygote Detection

No reproducible method for detection of heterozygotes has been reported. Parents, children and many relatives of known Hartnup patients have been examined for the characteristic aminoaciduria, but in only one Japanese pedigree have abnormalities been recorded (Oyanagi et al., 1967). Oral loading with casein (Dent, 1954) or tryptophan (Halvorsen and Halvorsen, 1963) has like-wise failed to produce amino acid abnormalities in the urine of all obligate heterozygotes but has been abnormal in some (Wong and Pillai, 1966). Photo-sensitivity has been reported among some relatives of affected patients (Hal-vorsen and Halvorsen, 1963), as have abnormalities in urinary indoles (Varley and Gowenlock, 1963; Halvorsen and Halvorsen, 1963), but these findings have been inconsistent and have not appeared in parents of affected children. In vitro studies of intestinal transport in presumed heterozygotes would be of great interest.

Signs and Symptoms

The clinical manifestations of Hartnup disease are intermittent and vari-able. Recognizable "attacks" occur rarely and appear to grow milder with in-creasing age. The skin changes resemble dietary pellagra; the pigmented rash affects the face and extremities, where it shows a "glove and stocking" distribu-tion. The rash may be eczematoid or dry and is usually made worse by exposure to sunlight. The neurological abnormalities are remarkable for their varia-bility, their transiency and their complete reversibility.

Unsteadiness of gait, clumsiness, nystagmus, tremor and diplopia are characteristic of cerebellar ataxia. No sensory deficit has been noted, but remark-able "falling attacks" have been described in which the patient collapses without loss of consciousness and recovers motor function over a period of days or weeks. The neurological aberrations usually coincide with exacerbation of the skin rash but may follow infectious diseases or nutritional stresses *without* cutaneous worsening. Psychiatric disturbances have ranged from minimal emotional instability to frank delirium, a continuum not unlike that observed in dietary pellagra. Seven of the 43 affected patients are mentally retarded, but this may reflect the bias of screening programs rather than the basic disease process. In the original Hartnup family, the least intelligent sibling was un-affected (Baron et al., 1956).

Although attacks have been precipitated by fever, sunlight, psychiatric stress and sulfonamide therapy (Jepson, 1972), they have invariably been asso-ciated with poor nutrition. This temporal association suggests that patients with Hartnup disease are particularly liable to pellagra when dietary nicotinamide deficiency accentuates their inherent inability to form nicotinamide from its only precursor amino acid: tryptophan. The cause of the cerebellar dysfunction is less certain. It may be due to nicotinamide deficiency, but intoxication with some other bacterial product is a distinct possibility. Bacterial decarboxylation of other unabsorbed amino acids could lead to the formation of tryptamine, phenylethylamine, tyramine and histamine. These amines or the indoles com-mented on previously are potentially toxic substances which must be investigated.

Diagnosis

Hartnup disease should be suspected in patients with pellagra without die-tary deficiency, particularly if the cutaneous and psychiatric abnormalities are accompanied by cerebellar signs. The diagnosis can be established with certainty, however, only by the typical urinary amino acid pattern. Neither dietary pellagra (Baron et al., 1956; Jepson, 1972) nor those disorders capable of producing secondary nicotinamide deficiency (carcinoid syndrome, tryptophanuria) are associated with the excretion of large amounts of monoamino-monocarboxylic amino acids so characteristic of Hartnup disease. The Fanconi syndrome (see later) can be excluded by examination of the urine for glucose and phosphate excess and by the amino acid pattern.

Treatment

The paucity of cases and the intermittent nature of the clinical signs have made it difficult to evaluate therapeutic programs. Nicotinamide (40 to 250 mg per day) has resulted in marked improvement in the cutaneous abnormalities and neurological deficit (Halvorsen and Halvorsen, 1963) and should probably be administered to all patients with Hartnup disease. Undue exposure to sunlight should be avoided since it exacerbates the rash. Milne (1972) has suggested that temporary sterilization of the colon by neomycin may reduce bacterial decarboxylation of unabsorbed dietary amino acids and thus lessen absorption of indoles and other amines. These and other regimens will be modified as more patients are described and as the natural history of this unusual disorder unfolds.

TRYPTOPHAN MALABSORPTION ("THE BLUE-DIAPER SYNDROME")

In 1964 Drummond and his colleagues described a nine-month-old boy whose urine-stained diapers turned a bright indigo blue. This child was hospitalized because of recurrent febrile episodes, growth retardation, irritability and constipation. His unrelated parents and one male sibling were in good health, but his sister's urine also stained her diapers blue. A second brother with "the blue-diaper syndrome" and a clinical picture very similar to that of the proband had died at the age of seven months following a subdural hematoma. Hypercalcemia was noted in both affected males, presumably due to unusual sensitivity to vitamin D. The dye responsible for the blue diapers was shown to be indigotonin (indigo blue), an oxidation product of indican. Other indoles were also present in the urine in large amounts, prompting a detailed study of tryptophan absorption and metabolism. No tryptophan was found in the urine, and amino acid excretion was normal on several occasions. Three kinds of evidence suggested a selective intestinal absorptive defect for tryptophan: large amounts of tryptophan were found in aqueous fecal extracts, and this abnormal finding was accentuated by oral tryptophan loading; the marked indoluria and indicanuria were accentuated by tryptophan ingestion and improved by neomycin; and several metabolites in the tryptophan-kynurenine pathway were also found in increased amounts in the urine.

Tryptophan loading studies in the parents and sister of the proband revealed no reproducible abnormalities. The authors concluded that these affected children, like those with Hartnup disease, excrete indoles and kynurenines in the urine because colonic bacteria catabolize the unabsorbed tryptophan to products which are absorbed from the colon and excreted in the urine. Despite the prominent indoluria, however, no pellagra-like skin rash or neurological deficit was observed, indicating some important difference between the pathophysiology of this disorder and that of Hartnup disease. Conversely, patients with Hartnup disease have not been reported to stain their diapers, presumably because the quantity of indoles in the urine is less than that observed in patients with selective tryptophan malabsorption. The absence of tryptophanuria in patients with "the blue-diaper syndrome" is interesting and suggests that the mechanisms responsible for tryptophan transport in the kidney are not identical to those in the intestine. Finally, the association between the tryptophan malabsorption and the hypercalcemia deserves comment. On two separate occasions tryptophan loading in the proband was followed by episodic hypercalcemia. Similar findings were obtained in normal subjects, but the mechanism involved is totally obscure.

METHIONINE MALABSORPTION SYNDROME ("OASTHOUSE URINE DISEASE")

Smith and Strang described an infant in 1958 with white hair, edema, attacks of hyperpnea, convulsions and mental retardation who died at the age of 10 months. The odor of his urine was unpleasant and unusual, like that of an oasthouse or of dried celery. The urinary ferric chloride test gave a green color, and urine chromatography revealed persistently large amounts of methionine, the branched chain amino acids, phenylalanine and tyrosine. Efron (1965) reported that methionine was the most prominent amino acid in the urine of this patient. Plasma amino acids were not measured. In addition to the prominent aminoaciduria, the urine contained large amounts of α-hydroxybutyric acid. The authors suggested that this hydroxy acid was formed from α-n-butyric acid by transamination and reduction.

Hooft and his colleagues (1965) subsequently reported a two-year-old girl with a similar disorder. This patient also had white hair, convulsions, mental retardation, attacks of hyperpnea and an unusual smell. When the child was on a normal diet, the urine contained α-hydroxybutyric acid but not methionine, while the feces contained large amounts of both α-hydroxybutyric acid and methionine. An oral methionine loading test provoked diarrhea and an increase in urinary and fecal α-hydroxybutyric acid. Oral loads of six other amino acids failed to produce these biochemical findings. In addition to the α-hydroxybutyric aciduria, the patient also excreted branched-chain keto acids in excess. These workers concluded that their patient and the one reported by Smith and Strang were unable to absorb methionine from the intestine. They proposed that α-hydroxybutyric acid is formed from the desulfuration, transamination and reduction of methionine by colonic bacteria and then excreted in the feces and urine. They explained the branched-chain ketoaciduria by suggesting that the unabsorbed methionine competitively inhibited the absorption of branched-chain amino acids, which were subsequently transaminated by colonic organisms and absorbed. This very interesting thesis could not be tested in this family because the parents refused additional investigation of the patient or 11 older siblings.

REFERENCES

Ames, G. F.: Uptake of amino acids by Salmonella typhimurium. Arch. Biochem. Biophys. *104*: 1–18, 1964.

Amstrong, M. D., Shaw, K. N. F., Gortatowski, M. J., and Singer, H.: The indole acids of human urine. Paper chromatography of indole acids. J. Biol. Chem. *232*:17–30, 1958.

Asatoor, A. M., Cheng, B., Edwards, K. D. G., Laut, A. F., Matthews, D. M., Milne, M. D., Navab, F., and Richards, A. J.: Intestinal absorption of two dipeptides in Hartnup disease. Gut *11*:380–387, 1970.

Baron, D. N., Dent, C. E., Harris, H., Hart, E. W., and Jepson, J. B.: Hereditary pellagra-like skin rash with temporary cerebellar ataxia, constant renal amino-aciduria, and other bizarre biochemical features. Lancet (i), 421–428, 1956.

Cusworth, D. C., and Dent, C. E.: Renal clearances of amino acids in normal adults and in patients with aminoaciduria. Biochem. J. *74*:550–561, 1960.

DeLaey, P., Hooft, C., Timmermans, J., and Snoeck, J.: Biochemical aspects of the Hartnup disease. I. Results of intravenous and oral tryptophan loading tests in a case of Hartnup disease. Ann. Paediat. (Basel) 202:145–160, 1964.

Dent, C. E.: The renal amino-acidurias. Exp. Med. Surg. 12:229–232, 1954.

Drummond, K., Michael, A., Ulstrom, A., and Good, R.: Blue diaper syndrome: Familial hypercalcemia with nephrocalcinosis and indicanuria. Amer. J. Med. 37:928–948, 1964.

Efron, M. L.: Aminoaciduria. New Eng. J. Med. 272:1058–1067, 1107–1113, 1965.

Grenson, M.: Multiplicity of the amino acid permeases in Saccharomyces cerevisae. II. Evidence for a specific lysine-transporting system. Biochim. Biophys. Acta 127:339–346, 1966.

Groth, U., and Rosenberg, L. E.: Transport of dibasic amino acids, cystine, and tryptophan by cultured human fibroblasts: Absence of a defect in cystinuria and Hartnup disease. J. Clin. Invest. 51:2130–2142, 1972.

Halvorsen, K., and Halvorsen, S.: Hartnup disease. Pediatrics 31:29–38, 1963.

Happold, F. C.: Tryptophanase-tryptophan reaction. Advances Enzym. 10:51–82, 1950.

Harrison, R. J., and Feiwel, M.: Pellagra caused by isoniazid. Brit. Med. J. 2:852–854, 1956.

Hooft, C., Timmermans, J., Snoeck, J., Antener, I., Oyaert, W., and van den Hende, C.: Methionine malabsorption syndrome. Ann. Paediat. (Basel) 205:73–84, 1965.

Jepson, J. B.: Hartnup disease. In Stanbury, J. B., Wyngaarden, J. B., and Fredrickson, D. S., eds., The Metabolic Basis of Inherited Disease, 3rd edition. McGraw-Hill, New York, pp. 1486–1503, 1972.

Milne, M. D.: Renal tubular dysfunction. In Strauss, M. B., and Welt, L. G., eds., Diseases of the Kidney, 2nd edition. Little, Brown and Company, Boston, pp. 1071–1138, 1972.

Milne, M. D., Crawford, M. A., Girao, C. B., and Loughridge, L.: The metabolic disorder in Hartnup disease. Quart. J. Med. 29:407–421, 1960.

Navab, F., and Asatoor, A. M.: Studies on intestinal absorption of amino acids and a dipeptide in a case of Hartnup disease. Gut 11:373–379, 1970.

Orten, A. U.: Intestinal phase of amino acid nutrition. Fed. Proc. 22:1391–1399, 1963.

Oyanagi, K., Takagi, K., Kitabatake, M., and Nakao, T.: Hartnup disease. Tohoku J. Exp. Med. 91:383–395, 1967.

Scriver, C. R.: Hartnup disease. A genetic modification of intestinal and renal transport of certain neutral alpha-amino acids. New Eng. J. Med. 273:530–532, 1965.

Scriver, C. R., and Shaw, K. N. F.: Hartnup disease: An example of genetically determined defective cellular amino acid transport. Canad. Med. Ass. J. 86:232, 1962.

Shih, V. E., Bixby, E. M., Alpers, D. H., Bartosocas, C. S., and Thier, S. O.: Studies of intestinal transport defect in Hartnup disease. Gastroenterology 61:445–453, 1971.

Sjoerdsma, A., Weissbach, M. S., and Udenfriend, S.: A clinical, physiologic and biochemical study of patients with malignant carcinoid (argentaffinoma). Amer. J. Med. 20:530–532, 1956.

Smith, A. J., and Strang, L. B.: An inborn error of metabolism with the urinary excretion of α-hydroxybutyric acid and phenyl-pyruvic acid. Arch. Dis. Child. 33:109–113, 1958.

Tada, K., Ito, H., Wada, Y., and Arakawa, T.: Congenital tryptophanuria with dwarfism ("H" disease-like clinical features without indicanuria and generalized amino-aciduria: A probably new inborn error of tryptophan metabolism. Tohoku J. Exp. Med. 80:118–134, 1963.

Tada, K., Morikawa, T., and Arakawa, T.: Tryptophan load and uptake of tryptophan by leukocytes in Hartnup disease. Tohoku J. Exp. Med. 90:337–346, 1966.

Varley, H., and Gowenlock, A. H.: The Clinical Chemistry of Monoamines. Elsevier, Amsterdam, pp. 107–172, 1963.

Weissbach, H., King, W., Sjoerdsma, A., and Udenfriend, S.: Formation of indole-3-acetic acid and tryptamine in animals. A method for estimation of indole-3-acetic acid in tissues. J. Biol. Chem. 234:81–86, 1959.

Wong, P. W. K., and Pillai, P. M.: Clinical and biochemical observations in two patients with Hartnup disease. Arch. Dis. Child. 41:383–388, 1966.

Chapter Ten

GENERALIZED DISORDERS OF AMINO ACID TRANSPORT: THE FANCONI SYNDROME

All the disorders in which a pathological aminoaciduria is produced by saturation, competition or modification of a transport site (Chapters 7, 8, 9) have two very important features in common: they are specific for one amino acid or for a group of structurally related substances; and they are inherited. There is another large group of acquired and inherited diseases which lead to pathological aminoacidurias characterized by the excretion of excessive amounts of most, if not all, of the naturally occurring amino acids and amides. In severe hepatic failure, a generalized aminoaciduria may supervene terminally because the liver is no longer capable of extracting free amino acids from the portal and systemic circulation (Walshe, 1953). In this event, the plasma concentrations of virtually all amino acids rise to pathological levels and exceed the capacity of tubular reabsorptive mechanisms. With this single exception, the generalized aminoacidurias result from defective renal tubular reabsorption of amino acids. In some patients the tubular defect apparently involves amino acids only. In others all the functions carried out by the proximal tubule are affected, a constellation referred to as the Fanconi syndrome. Although very little is known about the cellular mechanisms responsible for generalized renal aminoacidurias, it seems likely that the amino acid transport defect is a secondary manifestation of some underlying tubular disorder. Thus, generalized aminoaciduria, like proteinuria or hematuria, should be thought of as a sign of renal injury, not as a diagnosis in and of itself.

CLASSIFICATION OF GENERALIZED RENAL AMINOACIDURIAS

All generalized renal aminoacidurias are probably acquired in the sense that they are secondary to some underlying disease. To aid in their classification, they will be grouped according to the acquired or inherited nature of the underlying pathology (Table 10–1). This classification may be helpful in thinking about the pathophysiology and the differential diagnosis.

Acquired Causes

Chemical or physical intoxication may produce a generalized aminoaciduria. Heavy metal poisoning due to cadmium, uranium, lead or mercury ingestion or inhalation has produced aminoaciduria as part of the diffuse nephrotoxicity of these compounds (Clarkson and Kench, 1956). Chemical toxins, including nitrobenzene (Parker, 1953), Lysol (Spencer and Franglen, 1952), outdated tetracycline (Gross, 1963) and salicylate (Andrews et al., 1961), have likewise been responsible for significant and, in many cases, reversible generalized aminoaciduria. Berliner and coworkers (1950) showed that administration of maleic acid, a potent inhibitor of several enzymatic systems, was followed in dogs by a transient Fanconi-like syndrome. These findings were confirmed by several

Table 10–1   Classification of Generalized Renal Aminoacidurias

	References
Acquired	
Chemical or Physical Intoxication	
Heavy metal poisoning (cadmium, uranium, mercury, lead)	Clarkson and Kench, 1956
Chemical ingestion (nitrobenzene, Lysol, salicylate, maleic acid, outdated tetracycline)	Parker, 1953; Spencer and Franglen, 1952; Gross, 1963; Andrews et al., 1961; Berliner et al., 1950; Harrison and Harrison, 1954; Angielski et al., 1958; Rosenberg and Segal, 1964
Thermal burns	Eades et al., 1955
Nutritional Disturbance	
Vitamin deficiency (vitamins B_{12}, C, D)	Huisman, 1957; Todd, 1959
Kwashiorkor	Schendel and Hansen, 1962
Potassium depletion	Davidson et al., 1960
Manifestation of Renal or Metabolic Disorder	
Hyperparathyroidism	Khachadurian, 1962
Acute tubular necrosis	Smith et al., 1956
Nephrotic syndrome	Woolf and Giles, 1956
Multiple myeloma	Engle and Wallis, 1957
Inherited	
Primary Disease Known	
Galactosemia	Leaf, 1966
Hereditary fructose intolerance	Froesch, 1972
Wilson's disease	Leaf, 1966
Glycogenoses	Leaf, 1966
Cystinosis	Leaf, 1966
Congenital renal tubular acidosis	Harrison and Harrison, 1957
Osteogenesis imperfecta	Chowers et al., 1962
Congenital anemias (sickle cell, spherocytosis, thalassemia)	Choremis et al., 1959; Souchan and Grunau, 1952
Primary Disease Unknown	
Adult Fanconi syndrome	Leaf, 1966
Lowe's syndrome	Scriver, 1962; Lowe et al., 1952
Busby syndrome	Rowley et al., 1961
Luder-Sheldon syndrome	Luder and Sheldon, 1955
Microcephaly and spastic diplegia	Paine, 1960

groups of investigators working with rats (Harrison and Harrison, 1954; Angielski et al., 1958; Rosenberg and Segal, 1964).

Nutritional deficiencies of several kinds cause a generalized aminoaciduria. The mechanisms responsible for this abnormality in scurvy and rickets (Huisman, 1957) and pernicious anemia (Todd, 1959) are unknown, and the aminoaciduria is rapidly reversed with appropriate therapy. Fraser and colleagues (1967) and Grose and Scriver (1968) have suggested that the aminoaciduria found in patients with vitamin D deficiency is due, not to a direct effect of vitamin D on renal tubular reabsorption, but to the secondary hyperparathyroidism which follows vitamin D deficiency. This suggestion is given added weight by the observation that primary hyperparathyroidism may also produce a generalized renal aminoaciduria (Cusworth et al., 1972). Potassium depletion interferes with the ability to concentrate the urine and leads to tubular vacuolization, but the relationship between these defects and the generalized aminoaciduria which may be seen in potassium-depleted patients remains obscure (Davidson et al., 1960). Aminoaciduria has also been described with other diseases which affect the kidney: acute tubular necrosis (Smith et al., 1956), the nephrotic syndrome (Woolf and Giles, 1956) and multiple myeloma (Engle and Wallis, 1957).

Inherited Causes

Several inborn errors of metabolism which lead to accumulation of some specific substance in tissues may produce a generalized aminoaciduria. It seems likely that the aminoaciduria observed in patients with galactosemia, hereditary fructose intolerance, Wilson's disease, glycogenosis Type I and cystinosis (Leaf, 1966) results from deposition in the renal tubule of galactose-1-phosphate, fructose-1-phosphate, copper, glycogen and cystine, respectively. This thesis is supported by the observation that galactosemic patients develop their aminoaciduria only after the first six months of life, implying that some toxic product, presumably galactose-1-phosphate, accumulates during this interval and impairs proximal tubular function. Similarly, in hereditary fructose intolerance aminoaciduria is manifest only after oral or parenteral administration of fructose. Each of these disorders may produce glycosuria, phosphaturia and hyperuricuria as well as aminoaciduria (the Fanconi syndrome).

Another heterogeneous group of disorders exists which lead to a generalized renal aminoaciduria. These disorders have been shown to be familial and are assumed to be inherited, but no clue exists as to the basic etiology or the toxic product. Most adults with the Fanconi syndrome do not have any of the primary disorders enumerated above, yet the occurrence of this syndrome in several generations of the same family certainly suggests a genetic etiology (Leaf, 1966; Ben Ishay et al., 1961). Lowe (1952) and others (Scriver, 1962) have described males with an apparently X-linked oculocerebro-renal syndrome in which buphthalmos, congenital cataracts, growth failure and mental retardation accompany the Fanconi syndrome. In contrast, three siblings with the Busby syndrome (named for the family in which it was described) exhibited a generalized aminoaciduria but no other abnormalities in proximal tubular function (Rowley et al., 1961).

DISORDERED STRUCTURE AND FUNCTION

Morphological Changes

Since generalized renal aminoaciduria may accompany more than 40 different disease processes, it is not surprising that pathological findings have been variable. No proximal tubular lesion has been described which is in any way specific. In 1953 Clay and his colleagues isolated individual nephrons from the kidneys of two patients with the Fanconi syndrome due to cystinosis. They described a characteristic shortening and narrowing of the juxtaglomerular portion of the proximal tubule, which has been called the "swan neck" deformity. This lesion was found in 100 of 101 nephrons examined. Darmady and Straneck (1957) confirmed the swan neck deformity in eight other patients with cystinosis and the Fanconi syndrome and also commented on two patients with the syndrome but no cystinosis, both of whom had the same pathological findings on microdissection. It is difficult to believe that this deformity is the primary abnormality in the Fanconi syndrome. It cannot explain the widespread tissue deposits of cystine in cystinosis and certainly does not account for the metabolic abnormalities in Wilson's disease, galactosemia or many other conditions characterized by aminoaciduria with or without other proximal tubular abnormalities. It seems much more likely that the swan neck deformity is secondary to the primary events responsible for the tubular damage, but this hypothesis lacks experimental confirmation.

Pathophysiology

The wide spectrum of renal functional derangements in patients with generalized aminoaciduria has already been alluded to. The proximal tubular defect may involve amino acids (Rowley et al., 1961), amino acids and sugars (Luder and Sheldon, 1955), amino acids and phosphate (Jonxis, 1961) or a combination of all these plus abnormalities in uric acid reabsorption and acidification (Leaf, 1966). It is important to emphasize that this "spectrum" is based on analysis of random urine samples, 24-hour urine samples and, in some cases, renal clearance studies. However, systematic quantitation of several tubular functions has not been carried out in patients with generalized aminoaciduria. For example, we may say that a patient has isolated, generalized aminoaciduria because his urine contains no glucose and because endogenous phosphate reabsorption is unimpaired. However, to validate such conclusions, glucose and phosphate infusion studies must be performed and estimates of the tubular maxima (T_m) for these substances defined. Only in this way can the true spectrum of the proximal tubular abnormalities observed with generalized aminoaciduria be clarified.

The aminoaciduria usually reflects an exaggeration of the normal pattern rather than an altered one. The renal clearance of most amino acids is distinctly increased, but a very considerable fraction of the filtered load of each amino acid is reabsorbed. In those patients who have glycosuria and hyperphosphaturia as well as aminoaciduria, reduced tubular maxima for glucose have been documented (Sirota and Hamerman, 1954), but virtually no estimates of the T_m for phosphate or individual amino acids are available (Mudge, 1958). Prominent abnormalities in bone mineral metabolism and acid-base balance have also been described in some patients with the Fanconi syndrome. Osteomalacia and pathological fractures appear to be secondary to the renal defect in tubular reabsorption of phosphate and to the acidosis. Metabolic acidosis is caused by several factors: defective tubular reabsorption of bicarbonate; impaired ammonium secretion; reduced titratable acidity; and excessive organic acid excretion. These aspects of the Fanconi syndrome have been reviewed extensively by Leaf (1966).

Possible Mechanisms

In Chapter 6 we presented a conceptual model of amino acid transport (see Figure 6–1) which has four basic features: a lipoprotein cell membrane;

specific reactive sites or carriers; interaction with the sodium ion; and expenditure of metabolic energy. We have presented evidence which supports the thesis that the specific aminoacidurias (cystinuria, Hartnup disease, iminoglycinuria) are caused by genetic disturbances in the group-specific sites or carriers which lead to defective binding of substrate to carrier. The generalized aminoacidurias do not lend themselves to such a simple formulation. The diverse etiologies and the variable spectrum of physiological defects suggest that the tubular abnormalities in each case are *secondary* to some known or unknown toxic substance. A toxic substance could interfere with transport at several different sites. Thus, the transport abnormalities could reflect structural damage to the membrane of the tubule (i.e., the swan neck deformity); damage to each of the carrier systems for amino acids, sugars, phosphate and so forth; or impairment of intracellular reactions which provide energy to active transport processes. The latter explanation is the most attractive one. It requires only a single site of action, a parsimony expected of most biological mechanisms. It is also consistent with some experimental observations.

Since Curran and his colleagues (1967) have shown that the unidirectional flux of amino acids into the intestinal cell is not energy-dependent, it follows that a toxic substance which impairs transport by interfering with energy-yielding reactions need not be expected to alter the affinity between the substrate and its carrier mechanism. This has, indeed, been the case in the few instances in which it has been examined. Rosenberg and Segal (1964) showed that maleic acid inhibited amino acid transport in kidney slices noncompetitively, meaning that the affinity of amino acids for their carrier systems was not altered by the inhibitor. Segal and Blair (1963) demonstrated similar findings in their study of the inhibitory effect of salicylate on amino acid transport. Such findings would not be expected if the toxic substances altered the primary or secondary structure of the postulated carrier proteins in the cell membrane. Although these observations suggest that a variety of toxic substances may limit transport by interfering with energy production, they offer no information about the specific mechanism of such interference and point out the need for additional study.

As suggested earlier, humoral factors may also modulate proximal tubular reabsorption of amino acids. To date, only parathyroid hormone (PTH) has received much attention in this regard. Three kinds of evidence suggest that PTH impairs proximal tubular reabsorption of amino acids. First, some patients with primary hyperparathyroidism demonstrate a generalized renal aminoaciduria which disappears when the parathyroid adenoma is removed (Khachadurian, 1962; Cusworth et al., 1972). Second, patients with secondary hyperparathyroidism due to vitamin D deficiency often develop a reversible, generalized renal aminoaciduria (Fraser et al., 1967; Grose and Scriver, 1968; Arnaud et al., 1972). Third, normal volunteers respond to acute, parenteral administration of PTH with a prompt, short-lived generalized aminoaciduria (Short and Rosenberg, unpublished observations).

The findings of Morris et al. (1971) suggest that this modulatory role of PTH may have unusual significance. They studied a woman with both hereditary fructose intolerance (HFI) and postsurgical hypoparathyroidism. Euparathyroid patients with HFI respond to fructose administration with a prompt appearance of a generalized aminoaciduria, bicarbonaturia and phosphaturia (the Fanconi syndrome). However, none of the features of the Fanconi syndrome were observed in the patient with HFI and hypoparathyroidism until PTH was administered along with fructose. The nature of this "permissive" or "amplificatory" action of PTH is unclear but may have both pathophysiologic and biochemical importance.

SIGNS AND SYMPTOMS

As discussed previously, the aminoaciduria, per se, leads to no clinical disturbance, but this is not true of the other tubular defects present in patients with the Fanconi syndrome. In the infantile syndrome, the disease characteristically has its onset at about four to six months of age. Growth retardation, vomiting, fever, vitamin D-resistant rickets, polyuria and dehydration are the most prominent clinical features. In patients with cystinosis, glomerular insufficiency supervenes, and these children usually die within a few years of uremia or intercurrent infections. In the adult, osteomalacia and pathological fractures dominate the clinical course, but acidosis, hypokalemia and polyuria may also be apparent. Renal insufficiency is the leading cause of death in adults as well as children, but this is by no means a universal consequence of the Fanconi syndrome.

DIAGNOSIS

Since the premature infant and the full-term neonate normally excrete large quantities of free amino acids, it is not easy to define a generalized aminoaciduria before the age of four to six months. After this time, chromatographic techniques should detect generalized aminoacidurias with ease. Hepatic failure must be excluded before the generalized aminoaciduria is ascribed to a tubular defect. Once it is clear that a generalized renal aminoaciduria exists, the specific disorders noted in Table 10–1 must be investigated. A careful history and physical examination will exclude many of the diagnostic possibilities. Urinary assays for heavy metals should be performed if there is any suggestion of intoxication or if no other etiology is found. Most patients with a generalized aminoaciduria (with or without the Fanconi syndrome) will require bone x-rays and determinations of serum calcium, phosphorus and electrolytes to define the presence and importance of bone disease and acidosis.

TREATMENT

No therapy is needed if the generalized aminoaciduria is not accompanied by losses of phosphate or by acidosis. Therapy is aimed at replacing abnormal renal losses. The infantile Fanconi syndrome should be treated with 50,000 to 400,000 units of vitamin D daily and by supplementing the diet with neutral phosphates. The metabolic acidosis usually responds to treatment with Shohl's solution (140 g citric acid and 98 g sodium citrate per liter). Potassium bicarbonate or citrate may be necessary if potassium depletion is a problem. Such a replacement regimen can often control the consequences of the tubular abnormalities but will not affect the underlying pathology or the progression of renal impairment. Since the syndrome may disappear spontaneously if the toxic agent is withdrawn, "cures" produced by specific treatment must be evaluated with caution.

Briggs et al. (1972) reported a 14-year-old boy with the idiopathic Fanconi syndrome and renal insufficiency in whom a renal transplant was performed. All urinary findings of the Fanconi syndrome disappeared immediately after transplantation but reappeared within five weeks, suggesting that a systemic, extrarenal abnormality existed which affected the renal tubule secondarily.

REFERENCES

Andrews, B. F., Bruton, O. C., and Knoblock, E. C.: Aminoaciduria in salicylate intoxication. Amer. J. Med. Sci. *242*:411–414, 1961.

Angielski, S., Niemiro, R., Makarewicz, W., and Rogulski, J.: Aminoacyduria wywolana kwasem maleinowym. Acta Biochem. Polonica *5*:431–436, 1958.

Arnaud, C., Glorieux, F., and Scriver, C. R.: Serum parathyroid hormone levels in acquired vitamin D deficiency of infancy. Pediatrics *49*:837–840, 1972.

Ben-Ishay, D., Dreyfuss, F., and Ullmann, T. D.: Fanconi syndrome with hypouricemia in an adult. Amer. J. Med. *31*:793–800, 1961.

Berliner, R. W., Kennedy, T. J., and Hilton, J. G.: Effect of maleic acid on renal function. Proc. Soc. Exp. Biol. Med. *75*:791–794, 1950.

Briggs, W. A., Kominami, N., Wilson, R. E., and Merrill, J. P.: Kidney transplantation in Fanconi syndrome. New Eng. J. Med. *286*:25–26, 1972.

Choremis, C., Kiossoglou, K., Maounis, F., and Basti, B.: Amino-acid tolerance curves and aminoaciduria in Cooley's and sickle cell anemias. J. Clin. Path. *12*:245–253, 1959.

Chowers, I., Czaczkes, J. W., Ehrenfeld, E. N., and Landau, S.: Familial aminoaciduria in osteogenesis imperfecta. J.A.M.A. *181*:771–775, 1962.

Clarkson, T. W., and Kench, J. E.: Urinary excretion of amino acids by men absorbing heavy metals. Biochem. J. *62*:361–372, 1956.

Clay, R. D., Darmady, E. M., and Hawkins, M.: The nature of the renal lesion in the Fanconi syndrome. J. Path. Bact. *65*:551–558, 1953.

Curran, P. F., Schultz, S. G., Chez, R. A., and Fuisz, R. E.: Kinetic relations of the Na-amino acid interaction at the mucosal border of intestine. J. Gen. Physiol. *50*:1261–1286, 1967.

Cusworth, D., Dent, C. E., and Scriver, C. R.: Primary hyperparathyroidism and hyperaminoaciduria. Clin. Chim. Acta *41*:355–362, 1972.

Darmady, E. M., and Straneck, R.: Microdissection of the nephron in disease. Brit. Med. Bull. *13*: 21–25, 1957.

Davidson, L. A. G., Flear, C. T. G., and Donald, K. W.: Transient amino-aciduria in severe potassium depletion. Brit. Med. J. *1*:911–913, 1960.

Eades, C. H., Pollack, R. L., and Hardy, J. D.: Thermal burns in man. IX. Urinary amino acid patterns. J. Clin. Invest. *34*:1756–1759, 1955.

Engle, R. L., and Wallis, L. A.: Multiple myeloma and the adult Fanconi syndrome. I. Report of a case with crystal-like deposits in the tumor cells and in the epithelial cells of the kidney. Amer. J. Med. *22*:5–12, 1957.

Fraser, D., Kooh, S. W., and Scriver, C. R.: Hyperparathyroidism as the cause of hyperaminoaciduria phosphaturia in human vitamin D deficiency. Pediat. Res. *1*:425–435, 1967.

Froesch, E. R.: Essential fructosuria and hereditary fructose intolerance. *In* Stanbury, J. B., Wyngaarden, J. B., and Fredrickson, D. S., eds., The Metabolic Basis of Inherited Disease, 3rd edition. McGraw-Hill, New York, pp. 131–148, 1972.

Grose, J. H., and Scriver, C. R.: Parathyroid-dependent phosphaturia and aminoaciduria in the vitamin D-deficient rat. Amer. J. Physiol. *214*:370–377, 1968.

Gross, J. J. M.: Fanconi syndrome (adult type) developing secondary to the ingestion of outdated tetracycline. Ann. Intern. Med. *58*:523–528, 1963.

Harrison, H. E., and Harrison H. C.: Aminoaciduria in relation to deficiency diseases and kidney function. J.A.M.A. *164*:1571–1577, 1957.

Harrison, H. E., and Harrison, H. C.: Experimental production of renal glycosuria, phosphaturia and amino acid uria by injection of maleic acid. Science *120*:606–608, 1954.

Huisman, T. H. J.: L'élimination des acides aminés chez des enfants normaux d'âges différents. Arch. Franc. Pediat. *14*:166–180, 1957.

Jonxis, J. H. P.: Some investigations on rickets. J. Pediat. *59*:607–615, 1961.

Khachadurian, A. K.: Amino-aciduria secondary to a functioning parathyroid carcinoma. Ann. Intern. Med. *56*:931–934, 1962.

Leaf, A.: The syndrome of osteomalacia, renal glycosuria, aminoaciduria, and increased phosphorus clearance (the Fanconi syndrome). *In* Stanbury, J. B., Wyngaarden, J. B., and Fredrickson, D. S., eds., The Metabolic Basis of Inherited Disease, 2nd edition. McGraw-Hill, New York, pp. 1205–1220, 1966.

Lowe, C., Terrey, M., and MacLachlan, E. A.: Organic-aciduria, decreased renal ammonia production, hydrophthalmos and mental retardation. A clinical entity. Amer. J. Dis. Child. *83*:164–184, 1952.

Luder, J., and Sheldon, W.: A familial tubular absorption defect of glucose and amino-acids. Arch. Dis. Child. *30*:160–164, 1955.

Morris, R. C., Jr., McSherry, E., and Sebastian, A.: Modulation of experimental renal dysfunction of hereditary fructose intolerance by circulating parathyroid hormone. Proc. Nat. Acad. Sci. U.S.A. *68*:132–135, 1971.

Mudge, G. H.: Clinical patterns of tubular dysfunction. Amer. J. Med. *24*:785–804, 1958.

Paine, R. S.: Evaluation of familial biochemically determined mental retardation in children with special reference to aminoaciduria. New Eng. J. Med. *262*:658–665, 1960.

Parker, W. E.: Acute nitrobenzene poisoning with transient amino-aciduria. Brit. Med. J. *1*:653–655, 1953.

Rosenberg, L. E., and Segal, S.: Maleic acid-induced inhibition of amino acid transport in rat kidney. Biochem. J. *92*:345–352, 1964.

Rowley, P. T., Mueller, P. S., Watkin, D. M., and Rosenberg, L. E.: Familial growth retardation, renal aminoaciduria and cor pulmonale. I. Description of a new syndrome, with case reports. Amer. J. Med. *31*:187–204, 1961.

Schendel, H. E., and Hansen, J. D. L.: Study of factors responsible for the increased aminoaciduria of kwashiorkor. J. Pediat. *60*:290–293, 1962.

Scriver, C. R.: Hereditary aminoaciduria. *In* Steinberg, A. G., and Bearn, A. G., eds., Progress in Medical Genetics. Grune & Stratton, New York, pp. 83–186, 1962.

Segal, S., and Blair, A.: In vitro effect of salicylate on amino-acid accumulation by kidney cortex slices. Nature (London) *200*:139–141, 1963.

Sirota, J. H., and Hamerman, D.: Renal function studies in an adult subject with the Fanconi syndrome. Amer. J. Med. *16*:138–152, 1954.

Smith, E., Johnstone, J. H., Thomson, M., and Lowe, K. G.: Amino-aciduria in acute tubular necrosis. Clin. Sci. *15*:171–176, 1956.

Souchan, R., and Grunau, G.: Zur aminosäurenausscheidung bei liberkranken Kindern. Klin. Wschr. *30*:663, 1952.

Spencer, A. G., and Franglen, G. T.: Gross amino-aciduria following a Lysol burn. Lancet ii, 190–192, 1952.

Todd, D.: Observations on the amino-aciduria in megaloblastic anemia. J. Clin. Path. *12*:238–244, 1959.

Walshe, J. M.: Disturbances of amino acid metabolism following liver injury. Quart. J. Med. *22*:483–505, 1953.

Woolf, L. I., and Giles, H. McC.: Urinary excretion of amino-acids and sugar in the nephrotic syndrome. A chromatographic study. Acta Paediat. Scand. *45*:489–500, 1956.

Metabolism of Specific Amino Acids and Their Disorders

Chapter Eleven

SULFUR AMINO ACIDS

All living organisms require sulfur in some form, and in mammals this need is met by the sulfur-containing amino acids L-cysteine, L-cystine and L-methionine and by the vitamins biotin and thiamine. The sulfur-containing amino acids participate in many vital biochemical systems in addition to their primary role as constituents of proteins. Methionine is one of the chief methyl donors in the body and is, thereby, concerned with the synthesis of choline, acetylcholine, creatine and epinephrine (du Vigneaud, 1942–43). Cysteine is a component of the tripeptide glutathione and is a precursor of coenzyme A and taurine. Inorganic sulfate, one of the end products of sulfur amino acid catabolism, is required for the synthesis of sulfomucopolysaccharides and other conjugated sulfuric acid esters.

The sulfur amino acids and their end products are involved in many human diseases. The fetor of hepatic coma is probably due to the presence in the expired air of methyl mercaptan, a degradative product of methionine which is formed when normal methionine metabolism fails (Challenger and Walshe, 1955). Inorganic sulfate retention contributes to the metabolic acidosis of renal insufficiency. In addition to these acquired disorders of sulfur metabolism, more than 12 different human mutations lead to disorders of the sulfur amino acids. We have already discussed cystinuria and the methionine malabsorption syndrome, diseases characterized by defects in renal and intestinal transport of cystine and methionine, respectively. The other inherited disorders of sulfur amino acid metabolism impair the enzymatic biosynthesis or catabolism containing compounds: methionine; homocysteine; mercaptolactate-cysteine; and sulfite. Much of our present understanding of normal sulfur metabolism has been gained from the study of these rare disorders.

INTERMEDIARY METABOLISM OF THE SULFUR AMINO ACIDS

The Transsulfuration Pathway

Until 1932 cystine was considered an essential amino acid for mammals (du Vigneaud, 1952). A series of nutritional experiments in rats and humans disproved this thesis. Rose and his associates (Womack et al., 1937) demonstrated that methionine can substitute for cystine, and shortly thereafter du Vigneaud and his coworkers (1939) showed that homocysteine can also replace cystine in the diet of growing rats. Similar observations in cystinuric patients demonstrated that ingestion of methionine or homocysteine increased urinary cystine excretion (Brand et al., 1935). In 1939 Tarver and Schmidt employed ^{35}S-labeled methionine and showed that the sulfur atom of methionine is transferred to cystine. These studies established the existence of a transsulfuration pathway and defined methionine and homocysteine as precursors of cystine. They also showed that methionine is an essential amino acid except in special circumstances in which it can be replaced by homocysteine and supplementary preformed methyl groups (du Vigneaud et al., 1939).

Recent enzyme studies in vitro have defined the details of this transsulfuration pathway and have been responsible for the discovery of several important intermediates (Fig. 11–1). Methionine-activating enzyme catalyzes the formation of S-adenosyl-L-methionine, the primary methyl-group donor in mammalian metabolism (Mudd and Cantoni, 1964). Although the bulk of S-adenosyl-L-methionine (SAM) formed is utilized in transmethylation reactions yielding S-adeonsyl-L-homocysteine, SAM can also transfer its propylamine group, thereby participating in the synthesis of polyamines which may have an important role in protein synthesis (Pegg and Williams-Ashman, 1969). S-adenosyl-L-homocysteine (SAH) is cleaved enzymatically to adenosine and L-homocysteine. This reaction is reversible: in vitro SAH synthesis is favored; in vitro the equilibrium shifts to hydrolysis with removal of the reaction prod-

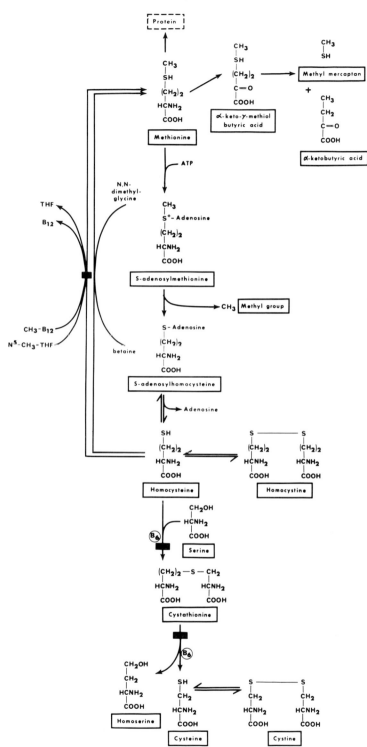

Figure 11–1 Pathways of sulfur amino acid metabolism from methionine to cysteine. Blocks shown (moving down the metabolic scheme) denote enzymatic defects in homocysteine: N^5-methyltetrahydrofolate methyltransferase, cystathionine synthase, and cystathionase, respectively. See text for details.

ucts. At least three other enzymes utilize homocysteine as substrate. Two of these reactions resynthesize methionine (Mudd and Cantoni, 1964): betaine-homocysteine methyltransferase requires the choline derivative, betaine, as the methyl donor; N^5-methyl-tetrahydrofolate methyltransferase uses N^5-methyl-tetrahydrofolate as the methyl donor in a reaction which also requires SAM and a vitamin B_{12} coenzyme. Homocysteine may be oxidized chemically or enzymatically to homocystine or catabolized to hydrogen sulfide and α-ketobutyrate. In the presence of the enzyme cystathionine synthase, homocysteine condenses with serine to form cystathionine in an irreversible reaction requiring pyridoxal phosphate. The latter thioether is cleaved to cysteine and α-ketobutyrate by the pyridoxal phosphate-dependent enzyme cystathionase. Cystathionine may also be synthesized by the latter enzyme; but in the reverse direction, homoserine is one of the cosubstrates rather than α-ketobutyrate (Wong et al., 1968).

Cysteine Metabolism

The net result of the complex reactions just described is the transfer of the sulfur atom of methionine to cysteine. The latter amino acid, like methionine and homocysteine, is metabolized in many ways (Fig. 11–2). Oxidation of cysteine to cystine occurs by enzymatic and nonenzymatic mechanisms in many tissues. Cysteine is incorporated into glutathione and virtually all protein

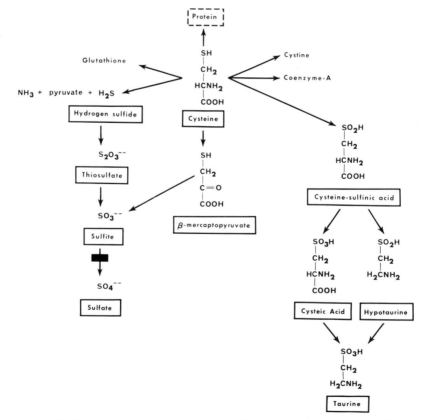

Figure 11–2 Pathways of cysteine utilization. The block shown between sulfite and sulfate denotes site of enzymatic defect in sulfite oxidase deficiency.

species. It is also a precursor for coenzyme A synthesis. In addition to these anabolic reactions, cysteine is catabolized by two general routes. One pathway involves the oxidation of the sulfhydryl group to yield cysteine-sulfinic acid, the latter compound being converted to taurine via cysteic acid or hypotaurine (Young and Maw, 1958). Taurine then condenses with cholic acid to yield the bile salt taurocholic acid, which is secreted into the gut and participates in the emulsification of fats and fat-soluble vitamins. Two other metabolites of taurine are now known. The deaminated analogue, isethionic acid, has been found in human urine. Its physiologic role is unknown, and its main site of biosynthesis is believed to be skeletal muscle (Jacobson and Smith, 1968). A guanido derivative, taurocyamine, has also been found in urine in trace amounts. Alternatively, cysteine may be transaminated to β-mercaptopyruvate or desulfhydrated to pyruvate and hydrogen sulfide (Greenberg, 1964). The latter substance is readily oxidized in mammalian tissues to thiosulfate and sulfite. Finally, sulfite is oxidized to sulfate by the enzyme sulfite oxidase. Eighty per cent of the urinary sulfur is normally excreted as inorganic sulfate, the remainder as neutral sulfur (amino acids) or "ethereal" sulfate (conjugated steroids, phenols and so forth). As noted in several reviews (Young and Maw, 1958; Greenberg, 1964; Finkelstein, 1971), many details of the biochemical sequence from methionine to sulfate and taurine remain undefined, but the scheme as presented permits a logical discussion of the inborn errors of sulfur amino acid metabolism.

Metabolic Regulation

The enzymes of the mammalian sulfur pathway respond to several regulatory stimuli (Finkelstein, 1971). In rat liver, the specific activities of methionine-activating enzyme and both methyltransferases decrease with age, while the activities of cystathionine synthase and cystathionase increase. A similar schedule exists in human tissues, with the important addition that cystathionase activity in liver and brain is not detectable throughout fetal life and for some days or weeks after birth (Gaull et al., 1972), thereby making cystine an essential amino acid for the human fetus and newborn. Dietary alterations also affect enzyme activity in rat tissues. Protein feeding leads to an increase in the specific activities of the methionine-activating enzyme, cystathionine synthase, cystathionase and betaine-homocysteine methyltransferase but to a decreased activity of the methyltetrahydrofolate methyltransferase (Finkelstein, 1971). L-Methionine reproduces these effects. Conversely, protein restriction is followed by a distinct increase in methyltetrahydrofolate methyltransferase activity, suggesting that this enzyme responds to the need for methionine resynthesis. In addition to these developmental and dietary stimuli, there appears to be a complex series of reactions whereby intermediates in the pathway affect the rate of other reactions in the sequence. The precise role that these regulatory systems play in sulfur metabolism of normal subjects or patients with inherited disorders in this pathway is under study.

THE HOMOCYSTINURIAS

"Homocystinuria" was described in 1962 independently by Carson and Neill and by Gerritsen, Vaughan and Waisman. These workers identified mentally retarded, fair-skinned, blond children who excreted large amounts of homocystine, an amino acid not normally detected in human urine. This form of homocystinuria was quickly shown to be due to a deficiency of cystathionine synthase, but it is now apparent that homocystine accumulation can be produced by either acquired or inherited blocks in the methyltetrahydrofolate-homocysteine methyltransferase reaction as well. Therefore, we can no longer refer to homocystinuria as a single disease and will, rather, classify the homocystinurias according to mechanism.

Cystathionine Synthase Deficiency

Biochemical Abnormalities

Chemically, cystathionine synthase deficiency is characterized by elevated plasma concentrations of methionine and homocystine and by the excretion of homocystine in the urine. Normally the concentration of methionine in fasting human plasma is less than 0.03 millimolar (0.45 mg per 100 ml), and homocystine is not detectable. In synthase-deficient patients, plasma methionine concentration has been reported as high as 2 millimolar (29.8 mg per 100 ml) and plasma homocystine values have reached 0.2 millimolar (5.4 mg per 100 ml) (Perry, 1967). Homocystine, not normally found in the urine, has been reported to exceed 1 mM (268 mg. per L.) in a 24-hour specimen from a patient with this form of homocystinuria, and variable amounts of methionine, methionine sulfoxide and the mixed disulfide of cysteine and homocysteine have also been reported (Perry, 1967). Many patients have also had markedly reduced concentrations or absence of cystine in plasma (Perry, 1967). In addition to these aberrations in amino acid content of body fluids, the study of amino acid concentration in tissues has also been instructive. Gerritsen (1964), Brenton (1965) and their colleagues showed that cystathionine, normally present in high concentration in human brain, was virtually absent in brain tissues from homocystinuric patients.

The Enzymatic Defect

These chemical abnormalities suggested a block in the catabolism of homocysteine, and this thesis was confirmed by enzymatic studies in vitro. As noted in Figure 11–1, homocysteine condenses with serine to yield cystathionine, this reaction being catalyzed by the enzyme cystathionine synthase. Mudd and his colleagues (1964b) postulated and demonstrated a defect in cystathionine synthesis in patients with homocystinuria. They showed that cystathionine synthase activity in the liver and brain of several homocystinuric patients was virtually absent (Mudd et al., 1964b; Laster et al., 1965b) and that this enzymatic defect was not due to an inhibitor of the enzyme in homocystinuric tissue. Other enzymes in the sulfur pathway, including methionine-activating enzyme (Mudd et al., 1964b), cystathionase (Laster et al., 1965b), betaine-homocysteine methyltransferase (Brenton et al., 1965) and glutathione-homocysteine transhydrogenase have been assayed and their activities found to be normal in the liver of such patients. Cystathionine synthase has been partially purified from rat liver (Kashiwamata et al., 1970; Kimura and Nakagawa, 1971; Brown and Gordon, 1971). It is composed of at least two subunits and requires pyridoxal phosphate as a cofactor.

Marked reduction of cystathionine synthase activity accounts for many of the biochemical abnormalities in homocystinuria. The block in the conversion of homocysteine to cystathionine leads to accumulation of homocystine and methionine, the former amino acid appearing in the urine because it exceeds the capacity of its reabsorptive system. The variable plasma concentrations of homocystine noted in different patients may depend on the activity of the alternate pathways for homocysteine utilization, such as its remethylation to methionine or its catabolism to α-ketobutyrate.

The low concentration of cystine in plasma and the absence of cystathionine in the brain indicate that the homocysteine-cystathionine-cystine pathway is either the only means by which cystathionine and cystine are made, or at least a major route of their formation. This conclusion was borne out by in vivo studies of Laster and his colleagues (1965a), who showed that two homocystinuric patients increased their urinary sulfate concentrations only minimally after oral methionine loads, compared to very substantial increments in sulfate excretion observed in normal subjects. These workers also observed that very little of the ingested methionine was excreted as homocystine by homocystinuric patients, implying that other pathways of homocysteine metabolism were operative. Perry (1967) demonstrated subsequently that homocystinurics excrete S-adenosylhomocysteine, lanthionine and 5-amino-4-imidazole-carboxamide-5'-S-homocysteinylriboside (AICHR) in the urine, and suggested that these unusual amino acids (Fig. 11–3) are formed from homocysteine and excreted because the normal pathway from homocysteine to cystathionine is blocked.

Genetics

Autosomal Recessive Inheritance.   Schimke (1967), McKusick (1971) and their colleagues have reviewed the evidence which indicates that cystathionine synthase deficiency is inherited as an autosomal recessive trait. Sex distribution

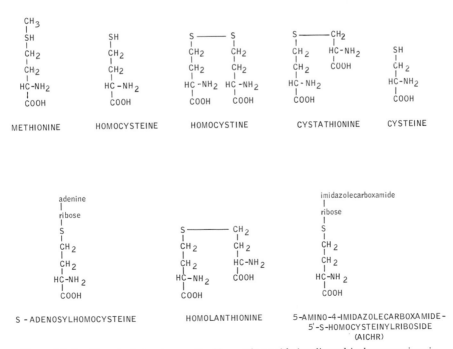

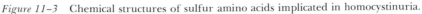

Figure 11–3   Chemical structures of sulfur amino acids implicated in homocystinuria.

has been approximately equal, and several pedigrees have shown multiple affected sibs. In six families, affected adults have normal children, and no example of generation to generation transmission has been recorded. Statistical analysis of published pedigrees is likewise consistent with recessive inheritance. The frequency of the mutant gene in the population is unknown, but the failure to find a single patient with homocystinuria among 141,000 neonates tested in Massachusetts (Levy et al., 1972) suggests that the disorder is not as frequent in the United States as anticipated from studies in Ireland (Carson and Neill, 1962).

Parents of affected children do not excrete homocystine or methionine in the urine, nor do they respond abnormally to oral methionine loading (Laster et al., 1965a). However, enzyme studies have confirmed the clinical impression of recessive inheritance. Finkelstein and coworkers (1964) showed that hepatic cystathionine synthase activity in four parents of affected children was less than half that observed in normal subjects but much greater than that seen in their affected offspring. Reduced synthase activity in obligate heterozygotes has also been demonstrated in cultured fibroblasts (Mudd, 1970) and phytohemagglutinin-stimulated lymphocytes (Goldstein et al., 1973). Thus, it seems certain that patients with homocystinuria due to cystathionine synthase deficiency are homozygous for a mutant gene and that their parents and children are heterozygous carriers for this trait. Three lines of evidence indicate that cystathionine synthase deficiency is genetically heterogeneous: marked interfamilial differences in clinical severity (McKusick et al., 1971), variable degrees of enzymatic deficiency in vitro (Mudd, 1971) and contrasting biochemical responses to vitamin B_6 supplements (see Treatment).

Signs and Symptoms

The initial descriptions of homocystinuria suggested a very characteristic clinical phenotype: mental retardation, light complexion and growth failure (Carson and Neill, 1962; Gerritsen et al., 1962). Subsequent experience has shown that these features are not constant. Nearly half of 84 patients studied by Schimke (1967), McKusick (1971) and their coworkers were tall and of normal intelligence. The skin tends to be coarse and wide-pored and becomes telangiectatic with aging. Patients often exhibit a malar flush or livedo reticularis which is accentuated by emotional upset or exertion. Homocystinuric patients tend to walk with a flat-footed, toed-out gait which has been likened to that of Charlie Chaplin. The liver is often enlarged, but hepatic function tests are within normal limits. Many affected individuals have kyphosis, scoliosis, pectus excavatum and arachnodactyly. These findings are reminiscent of Marfan's syndrome, with which homocystinuria has been confused (Schimke et al., 1965b). The skeletal abnormalities in homocystinuria are produced in part by severe, premature osteoporosis, which is not found in Marfan's syndrome.

Ectopia lentis is the most common phenotypic abnormality in homocystinuria and has been responsible for the detection of many reported cases (Schimke et al., 1965a). The ectopia lentis is not present at birth but has been described in affected patients by age two or three. Myopia, optic atrophy, glaucoma and retinal detachment are common sequelae of the lenticular dislocation. Schimke and coworkers (1965a) suggested that homocystinuria may be responsible for 5 per cent of the patients in the United States with nontraumatic dislocation of the optic lenses.

Life-threatening arterial and venous thromboses are the cardinal vascular signs in homocystinuria. Patients have died in the second or third decade from carotid and coronary occlusive disease (Schimke et al., 1967). Acute gangrene and hypertension have resulted from arterial thromboses involving the extremities and kidney, respectively. Venous thromboses have been described in the extremities and inferior vena cava as well as the pulmonary and portal circulation.

Mental retardation is not the only prominent neurological aberration. Unexplained nervousness, impairment in reasoning, seizures and schizophrenic reactions have been described repeatedly (McKusick et al., 1971; Schimke et al., 1967). Electroencephalographic abnormalities may appear even in the absence of mental retardation.

Pathology and Pathophysiology

Significant morphological findings are most prominent in the cardiovascular system (Schimke et al., 1965a, 1967; Carson et al., 1965). The media of the coronary, carotid, iliac and renal arteries tends to be thin, and the muscle fibers are separated by increased ground substance; partial or total obstruction of arteries and veins by fresh or organizing thrombi is a common autopsy finding. The zonular fibers of the lens show degenerative changes, as do fibers of the ciliary muscle. Fatty infiltration of the liver without fibrosis or regeneration is a common abnormality. Cancellous and membranous bones show no abnormalities to explain the marked osteoporosis observed during life.

The elucidation of the enzymatic defect in synthase-deficient patients has not, as yet, led to a complete understanding of the mechanism of the significant clinical abnormalities. McDonald et al. (1964) suggested that the vascular occlusive disease is caused by increased platelet adhesiveness, but this has been refuted in other laboratories (Schimke et al., 1967). McCully reported that homocysteine administration in rabbits reproduced the essential features of the vascular lesions found in synthase deficiency (McCully and Ragsdale, 1970) and that cell cultures from synthase-deficient patients produced an abnormal glycoprotein (McCully, 1972). Based on these data, he proposed that homocysteine accumulation is responsible for the vascular abnormalities by affecting the structure of blood vessel wall glycoproteins. Mental retardation could conceivably be caused by cystathionine deficiency or by competitive inhibition of transport of amino acids into the brain by the elevated concentration of methionine or homocystine in the blood. This argument, however, fails to account for affected patients who have normal intelligence. Perhaps the unusual amino acids described in the urine of homocystinuric patients (Perry, 1967) are responsible for some portion of the clinical disturbance. These and many other possible mechanisms must be explored.

Diagnosis

The urinary cyanide-nitroprusside test is a simple screening test for homocystinuria, but some patients will be missed if such screening is carried out in the first two weeks of life because they excrete too little homocystine to be detected in this way (Levy et al., 1971). The test is also positive in cystinuria, but the latter disorder can be ruled out easily by chromatographic or electrophoretic studies which separate cystine from homocystine and which demonstrate the dibasic aminoaciduria characteristic of cystinuria. Neonatal elevation of plasma methionine may be a more reliable index of synthase deficiency (Levy et al., 1971) and will distinguish synthase-deficient patients from those with homocystinuria due to defective homocysteine remethylation, in whom plasma methionine concentrations will be reduced. Marfan's syndrome is inherited as a dominant trait; hence, a careful family history and examination of the urine will exclude this possibility in patients who present with ectopia lentis, arachnodactyly and pectus excavatum. Since the clinical features of homocystinuria are so variable, all patients with nontraumatic ectopia lentis and unexplained arterial or venous occlusive disease should be tested.

Treatment

Therapeutic measures in homocystinuria due to cystathionine synthase deficiency have two aims: to eliminate potentially toxic substances accumulating proximal to the metabolic block, and to supply those substances distal to the block which may have become deficient. Since methionine is an essential amino acid and a precursor of homocystine, a low-methionine diet has been suggested to achieve the first of these aims, while cystine supplements have been suggested for the second. Several groups have shown that a low-protein, low-methionine diet can reduce the elevated plasma methionine and homocystine concentrations in affected patients. Perry (1971) and Komrower (1971) have each treated homocystinuric infants, diagnosed at birth, with diets restricted in methionine and supplemented with cystine. Perry's results have been particularly encouraging. Whereas two older, untreated, affected siblings of his patient had suffered mental retardation and repeated thrombotic accidents during the first year of life, the infant treated from birth on grew normally, was not retarded, had no evidence of thromboses and failed to develop dislocated lenses when reported at the age of 5 years. Although these results are promising, the variability in the natural history of homocystinuria and the short period of follow-up indicate the need for additional study before recommending that all children with cystathionine synthase deficiency be treated similarly. Furthermore, there are theoretical considerations which oppose the use of such a diet. Finkelstein and Mudd (1967) demonstrated that feeding rats a methionine deficient diet resulted in a decline in cystathionine synthase activity in the liver—exactly the opposite of the effect desired in homocystinuria.

In older children and adults, dietary treatment of homocystinuria raises other questions. Dietary restrictions will not reverse dislocated lenses, mental retardation or other features of the abnormal phenotype. Furthermore, a low-protein, low-methionine diet is difficult to prepare using regular foods and may lead to nutritional deficiency. Finally, some adults with homocystinuria have no disease manifestations other than ectopia lentis. Why, then, institute treatment? The only theoretical answer to this question supposes that the biochemical abnormalities responsible for the potentially lethal vascular occlusions can be lessened by dietary restriction. There are at this time no data which support or refute this rationale, and meaningful observations will be difficult to collect.

Another potentially important form of treatment has been described. Barber and Spaeth (1967) reported that three homocystinuric children in two pedigrees responded to administration of large doses of vitamin B_6 (250 to 500 mg daily) with "complete reversal" of their biochemical abnormalities. Plasma methionine fell to normal; plasma cystine rose to normal; and plasma and urinary homocystine disappeared. These findings have since been confirmed by several laboratories (Gaull et al., 1969; Hollowell et al., 1968; Hooft et al., 1967; Yoshida et al., 1968; Carson and Carré, 1969; Mudd et al., 1970a; Brenton and Cusworth, 1971; Seashore et al., 1972), thereby adding cystathionine synthase deficiency to the growing list of vitamin-responsive metabolic diseases

(Fig. 11–4). However, several facets of this form of treatment deserve additional comment. First, not all affected patients respond to vitamin B_6 (Schimke et al., 1967; Hooft et al., 1967; Carson and Carré, 1969; Brenton and Cusworth, 1971), implying that more than one mutation of the synthase molecule leads to defective catalytic activity and underscoring the need for monitored therapeutic trials before instituting long-term programs. Second, no reported patients have been treated continuously from birth to determine the long-term efficacy of such intervention. Third, the biochemical basis for such vitamin B_6-responsiveness is not clear. Some patients show small increases in synthase activity in vitro (Yoshida et al., 1968; Mudd et al., 1970a; Seashore et al., 1972), whereas other patients do not (Gaull et al., 1969; Hollowell et al., 1968; Seashore et al., 1972). Fourth, some patients may, in fact, be harmed by such vitamin therapy (Schimke et al., 1967). Despite these many questions, vitamin B_6 appears to be the simplest and, theoretically, most physiologic form of treatment of many patients with this form of homocystinuria.

Deficient Activity of N^5-Methyltetrahydrofolate Methyltransferase

As shown in Figure 11–1, the remethylation of homocysteine to methionine proceeds via two distinct enzymatic reactions: one in which the methyl group is donated by betaine, and the other in which N^5-methyltetrahydrofolate acts as the methyl donor. In the latter reaction, a coenzyme form of vitamin B_{12} is an obligate intermediate in the methylation system. Since 1969, it has been shown that inherited and acquired abnormalities in this methyltransferase system can cause homocystinuria. Thus far, three different etiologies for such homocystinuria have been identified: intestinal malabsorption of vitamin B_{12}; impaired intracellular metabolism of vitamin B_{12}; and defective formation of N^5-methyltetrahydrofolate from its precursor, methylenetetrahydrofolate.

Defective Metabolism or Absorption of Vitamin B_{12}

In 1969, Mudd et al. described a desperately ill male infant who was lethargic from the time of birth, fed poorly, failed to gain weight and died at the age of 7 weeks. This infant accumulated homocystine in blood and urine,

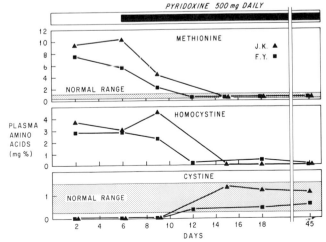

Figure 11–4 Effect of pyridoxine supplementations (500 mg daily) on sulfur amino acid concentrations in plasma of two patients (J. K. and E. Y.) with homocystinuria due to cystathionine synthase deficiency. (From Seashore et al.: Pediat. Res. 6:187–196, 1972.)

had excessive concentrations of cystathionine in blood and urine and had a very low plasma methionine concentration. Furthermore, he excreted excessive amounts of methylmalonic acid in his urine. These findings contrasted sharply with those reported in patients with homocystinuria due to cystathionine synthase deficiency and suggested a block in homocysteine remethylation. Since vitamin B_{12} in coenzyme form is required both in the remethylation of homocysteine and in the catabolism of methylmalonate, a congenital disturbance of B_{12} metabolism was proposed. Convincing evidence in support of this thesis was provided in the original and subsequent studies: tissue concentrations of sulfur amino acids mirrored those in plasma and urine (Mudd et al., 1970b); B_{12} coenzyme content of liver and kidney was markedly reduced (Mudd et al., 1969; 1970b); cultured fibroblasts showed defects in both methylmalonate oxidation and N^5-methyltetrahydrofolate methyltransferase activity which were partially or totally corrected by supplementing the growth medium with vitamin B_{12} (Mudd et al., 1970c); and conversion of labeled vitamin B_{12} to its coenzymes was markedly impaired in cell culture (Mahoney et al., 1971).

Subsequently, Goodman and his colleagues (1971b) reported two male siblings with a similar constellation of in vivo and in vitro findings, albeit in distinctly milder form. The younger of these sibs (age 2 years) was asymptomatic, whereas his older brother (age 14 years) was retarded and had significant neurologic abnormalities. Although the exact site of the metabolic block in these three boys is obscure, there is little doubt that they each suffer from a primary, inherited disturbance in intracellular metabolism of B_{12}, distinct from that proposed in children with vitamin B_{12}-responsive methylmalonicaciduria who have *no* abnormalities in sulfur amino acid metabolism (see Chapter 14).

Based on these observations, it was predicted that abnormalities in methylmalonate and sulfur amino acid metabolism might be expected in patients with typical "pernicious" anemia due to impaired intestinal absorption of vitamin B_{12}. Such abnormalities have now been reported in two B_{12}-deficient patients (Shipman et al., 1969; Hollowell et al., 1969) who had megaloblastic anemia, homocystinuria, cystathioninuria and methylmalonicaciduria — all of which disappeared when physiologic amounts of vitamin B_{12} were administered parenterally.

Decreased Methylenetetrahydrofolate Reductase Activity

A fourth cause of homocystinuria was reported in 1972 by Mudd and coworkers (1972). Three young adults from two families had homocystinuria and homocystinemia. One patient had seizures and muscle weakness; the second was schizophrenic and retarded; the third was asymptomatic. Cystathionine synthase deficiency and abnormalities in B_{12} metabolism were excluded by normal plasma methionine concentrations, normal cystathionine synthase assays and normal activities of N^5-methyltetrahydrofolate methyltransferase. Fibroblasts from each patient, however, had markedly reduced activity of methylenetetrahydrofolate reductase, the enzyme responsible for catalyzing the conversion of methylenetetrahydrofolate to N^5-methyltetrahydrofolate. Therapeutic trials with folic acid or one of its derivatives should yield interesting results.

CYSTATHIONINURIA

Cystathionine, a thioether and α-amino acid (Fig. 11–3), is a key intermediate in the transsulfuration pathway of methionine metabolism (Fig. 11–1).

It is not detectable in the blood or urine of normal humans but is excreted in considerable quantities under diverse clinical circumstances. We have discussed cystathioninemia associated with defective absorption or metabolism of vitamin B_{12}. Acquired cystathioninuria has been reported in patients with vitamin B_6 deficiency (Knox, 1958), liver disease of several kinds (Shaw et al., 1967), tumors of neural crest origin (Gjessing, 1963) and following administration of thyroxine (Gjessing, 1964). Since 1958 numerous patients have been described who excrete large amounts of cystathionine in the urine but who have none of the disorders mentioned previously. Biochemical and familial studies suggest that this group of patients suffers from an inherited defect in cystathionase activity. No reproducible clinical picture has emerged in these patients, most of whom have had a dramatic reduction in urinary cystathionine excretions following administration of large doses of vitamin B_6. The implications of these unusual findings warrant additional discussion.

Biochemical Abnormalities

Cystathionine

This complex amino acid has only one known biological function: to transfer the sulfur atom of methionine to cysteine. Although it is not found normally in body fluids, cystathionine is detectable in considerable quantities in tissue. Tallan and coworkers (1958) reported that human liver, kidney and muscle contained about 0.8 mg of cystathionine per 100 gm of tissue, but five brain specimens contained from 22.5 to 56.6 mg per 100 gm. Smaller amounts of cystathionine were detected in the brain of monkeys (12.8 mg per 100 gm), cows (1.2 to 3.9 mg per 100 gm) and chickens (0.2 to 0.6 mg per 100 gm), suggesting that cystathionine may have some role in higher integrative functions. This thesis has been refuted by findings in patients with inherited defects of sulfur amino acid metabolism. As pointed out previously (Gerritsen and Waisman, 1964; Brenton et al., 1965), cystathionine is absent from the brain of patients with homocystinuria whose intelligence may be normal or low. Examination of the brain of the first reported patient with inherited cystathioninuria revealed a very high concentration of cystathionine (Brenton et al., 1965), yet patients with this disorder may also be mentally retarded or of normal intelligence. Thus, the role of cystathionine in the central nervous system remains unclear, and its concentration may reflect differences in the activities of the enzymes responsible for its formation and catabolism (Mudd et al., 1965), rather than some purposeful evolutionary pattern.

Cystathionase

The cystathionine-cleaving enzyme, cystathionase, has been isolated and purified from rat liver (Matsuo and Greenberg, 1958a; Loiselet and Chatagner, 1965). The apoenzyme is white and has a molecular weight of about 140,000. It is inactive without pyridoxal phosphate (Matsuo and Greenberg, 1958b). The apoenzyme-coenzyme complex is yellow in color, has a molecular weight of about 200,000 and has a molar ratio of pyridoxal:apoenzyme of 4:1. The enzyme cleaves L-cystathionine to cysteine and α-ketobutyrate, but other thioethers, including L-allocystathionine lanthionine and djenkolic acid, are also attacked by the purified enzyme (Loiselet and Chatagner, 1965). Cystathionase activity has been demonstrated in the brain as well as the liver (Mudd et al., 1965) but not in leukocytes, erythrocytes or skin fibroblasts grown in tissue culture (Frimpter et al., 1967).

Chemical Abnormalities in Inherited Cystathioninuria

Plasma cystathionine has ranged from 0.01 to 0.03 millimolar (0.2 to 0.6 mg per 100 ml) in three affected patients. Frimpter (1967) reviewed urinary cystathionine excretion in six patients and noted that 24-hour values ranged from 25 mg in a two-year-old girl to 1400 mg in a 46-year-old man. Oral administration of methionine augmented cystathionine excretion markedly (Frimpter, 1967). The renal clearance of cystathionine in affected patients approximates (or even exceeds) the glomerular filtration rate, suggesting that this amino acid is poorly reabsorbed from the proximal tubule and may even be secreted. The rapid clearance of this compound by the kidney also explains the absence of prominent cystathioninemia in these patients.

In his description of the second reported case of inherited cystathioninuria, Frimpter and coworkers (1963) called attention to the fact that improvement after administration of vitamin B_6 cannot be attributed to coincidental nutritional abnormalities. Furthermore, as noted in Figure 11–5, administration of 10 gm of methionine to a cystathioninuric patient who had received pyridoxine for nine days was followed by prompt excretion of large quantities of cystathionine, an effect inconsistent with vitamin B_6 deficiency. Frimpter et al. (1963) proposed that the mutation in inherited cystathioninuria altered the cystathionase apoenzyme in such a way that its affinity for coenzyme is markedly reduced and that administration of large excesses of the coenzyme restored enzymatic activity, at least in part. This kind of vitamin *dependency*, well known in microorganisms (Bonner et al., 1960), has been confirmed by in vitro enzymatic assays.

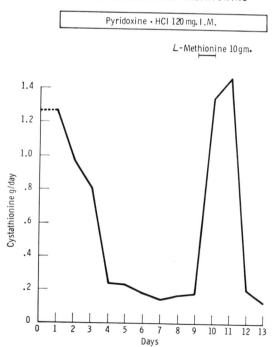

EFFECT OF PYRIDOXINE AND METHIONINE

Pyridoxine · HCl 120 mg. I.M.

L-Methionine 10 gm.

Figure 11–5 Effect of oral administration of vitamin B_6 and methionine on excretion of cystathionine in a patient with cystathioninuria. (From Frimpter, G. W.: *In* Stanbury, J. B., Wyngaarden, J. B., and Fredrickson, D. S., The Metabolic Basis of Inherited Disease, 2nd edition. McGraw-Hill, New York, 1966.)

The Enzymatic Defect

In 1965 Frimpter reported that cystathionase activity in liver homogenates from two patients with cystathioninuria was less than 10 per cent of that observed in five normal subjects and that addition of pyridoxal phosphate in vitro restored enzymatic activity toward normal. Since cystathionine cleavage was not initiated by pyridoxal phosphate in the absence of liver homogenate, a direct catabolic effect of the vitamin on cystathionine was ruled out. Finkelstein and his colleagues (1966) showed that liver from a third B_6-responsive cystathioninuric patient had reduced cystathionase activity, but they failed to demonstrate an in vitro effect of vitamin B_6. In contrast to the patient studied by Frimpter, however, this patient had been maintained on vitamin B_6 prior to biopsy.

B_6-Unresponsive Cystathionase Deficiency

In 1968 Tada et al. described an infant with cystathioninuria who did not respond to large doses of vitamin B_6. Hepatic cystathionase activity was much reduced and, in accord with the in vivo findings in this child, was not enhanced by addition of saturating concentrations of pyridoxal phosphate in vitro. They concluded that their patient had a mutation of the cystathionase molecule different from that observed in B_6-responsive patients. These findings would also appear to eliminate the theory that vitamin B_6, per se, can produce a reduction in plasma or urinary cystathionine concentrations without acting on cystathionase.

Genetics

The paucity of reported cases and the great variation in clinical and chemical findings make genetic analysis difficult. Cystathioninuria has been reported in six males and five females ranging in age from infancy to 64 years (Frimpter, 1972; Perry et al., 1967). Two affected siblings have been reported in families by Frimpter and colleagues (1963) and Perry et al. (1968). Autosomal recessive inheritance is suggested by the following observations: Harris et al. (1959) reported that a brother and a nephew of the first patient with cystathioninuria excreted about one tenth as much cystathionine as the proband did; all four children of an affected woman studied by Frimpter (1972) excreted small but definite amounts of cystathionine; Whelan and Scriver (1968) described a family in which small amounts of cystathionine were detected in the urine of five individuals in three generations, but emphasized that the quantitative excretion was far less than that reported in other affected patients; Mongeau (1966) and Perry (1968) and their colleagues failed to detect cystathionine in the urine of parents of three affected patients until they had received an oral load of methionine (0.1 g per kg). These findings imply that patients homozygous for a defect in cystathionase activity excrete large amounts of cystathionine at all times and that heterozygotes for this mutation can be detected because they excrete small amounts of cystathionine under basal conditions or after the metabolic stress of methionine loading. In vitro studies in obligate heterozygotes would strengthen the accepted hypothesis of autosomal recessive inheritance.

Signs and Symptoms

No consistent clinical pattern has emerged in inherited cystathioninuria. Five patients are severely retarded (Frimpter, 1967; Perry et al., 1967), but the other six affected individuals are of normal intelligence (Perry et al., 1968; Frimpter, 1972). Endocrinopathies of different kinds have been prominent in three patients (Frimpter, 1967; Perry et al., 1967). Other abnormalities noted in single cases include convulsions (Berlow, 1966), anemia (Perry et al., 1967), thrombocytopenia (Mongeau et al., 1966), developmental ear anomalies (Frimpter et al., 1963), phenylketonuria (Shaw et al., 1967), nephrogenic diabetes insipidus (Perry et al., 1967) and iminoglycinuria (Whelan and Scriver, 1968). Two affected siblings are in excellent health and have none of the above abnormalities (Perry et al., 1968). This clinical diversity suggests that the mutation responsible for cystathioninuria does not lead to any significant pathophysiological disturbance and that the myriad of associated abnormalities is coincidental.

Diagnosis

Since cystathionine lacks a free sulfhydryl group, it will not give a positive urinary nitroprusside test. This thioether can be detected easily by paper chromatographic or electrophoretic techniques. Quantitative estimates of cystathionine require ion exchange chromatography. A diagnosis of cystathionase deficiency cannot be made until the many other causes for this chemical disturbance are excluded: vitamin B_6 deficiency (Knox, 1958), abnormalities in B_{12} absorption (Shipman et al., 1969; Hollowell et al., 1969) or metabolism (Mudd et al., 1969), neural crest tumors (Gjessing, 1963), liver disease due to hepatoma, glycogenosis, tyrosinosis, maple syrup urine disease, galactosemia or portal vein occlusion (Shaw et al., 1967). Gjessing (1963) has suggested that cystathioninuria occurs in patients with neural crest tumors because cystathionine is rapidly synthesized by the neoplastic cells, but this has not been demonstrated. The basis for the cystathioninuria in patients with liver disease is unknown but presumably reflects a relative deficiency of cystathionase activity in the hepatic parenchymal cells.

Treatment

As pointed out previously, administration of 200 to 400 mg of pyridoxine by mouth can be expected to lead to a sharp fall in cystathionine excretion in the urine of most patients. Berlow (1966) stated that his patient with seizures and retardation improved dramatically after institution of vitamin B_6 therapy. Since it is not at all clear, however, that the cystathioninuria, per se, is responsible for any significant physiological disturbance in patients with inherited cystathionase deficiency, there is some question about the necessity for long-term pyridoxine therapy. This question will be answered by the discovery of additional patients and the characterization of the clinical phenotype associated with this disorder.

CYSTINOSIS

Cystinosis is a rare, familial disorder characterized by the widespread deposition of cystine crystals in body tissues. Electron microscopic and sucrose density gradient studies have shown that cystine accumulates within lysosomes in this disease, but the etiology of this deposition is unknown. Three forms of the disease have been identified: an infantile (nephropathic) form leading to renal insufficiency in the first decade; a juvenile (intermediate) form in which renal disease becomes manifest during the second decade; and a benign (adult) form characterized by the deposition of cystine in the cornea but not in the kidney. There appears to be a direct relationship between the amount of cystine deposited in tissues and the clinical severity of the disorder. Cystinosis is to be distinguished from cystinuria, which is characterized by the formation of cystine calculi in the renal pelvis, ureter or bladder but not by the deposition of cystine in tissues (see section on cystinuria).

Historical Introduction

In 1903 Abderhalden described a marked increase in cystine content and cystine crystals in the liver and spleen of a young child dying of "inanition." Two siblings had died of a similar disease process which Abderhalden called a "familial cystine diathesis." Twenty years later Lignac (1924) described three children with widespread deposits of cystine in their tissues. All three had progressive renal insufficiency, wasting, dwarfism and severe rickets. A sister of one of these patients was also affected, again attesting to the familial nature of the disorder. In 1937 a child with "cystine storage disease" was described by Beumer, who noted albuminuria and glycosuria as well as terminal uremia. During this same decade de Toni (1933), Debré (1934) and Fanconi (1936) each described children with rickets, dwarfism, glycosuria, albuminuria and acidosis. Fanconi pointed out that the excretion of organic acids was increased as well and established the syndrome of "nephrotic-glycosuric dwarfism with hypophosphatemic rickets" which now bears his name. Although he thought that the syndrome which he described was distinct from cystinosis, an autopsy on one of his patients demonstrated widespread cystine deposits. McCune et al. (1943) demonstrated that the organic aciduria initially described by Fanconi reflected the excretions of large quantities of free amino acids. Cystinosis was originally considered a disease restricted to infancy and early childhood. However, Cogan (1957), Lietman (1966), Aaron (1971), Hooft (1971) and their coworkers have demonstrated cystinosis in older children and adults as well.

Chemical Abnormalities

Patients with cystinosis accumulate cystine in the liver, spleen, bone marrow, peripheral leukocytes, lymph nodes, kidney and cornea. The identity of the crystals has been demonstrated by their characteristic hexagonal shape as well as by chemical and x-ray diffraction studies. Schneider and coworkers found that the cystine content of peripheral leukocytes (1967a) and cultured skin fibroblasts (1967b) was increased more than 100-fold in children with infantile cystinosis and more than 30-fold in patients with the adult form of the disease. Subsequent investigations by Patrick and Lake (1968) and by Schulman et al. (1969) demonstrated that these large quantities of intracellular cystine were confined to a membrane-bound compartment, ultimately shown to be the lysosome. This lysosomal cystine is not readily exchangeable with other pools of this amino acid. It cannot be used to sustain the growth of cells in culture, which require exogenous cystine (Schneider et al., 1968b). It is not reflected in increased plasma concentrations of either cystine or cysteine (Schneider et al., 1968b; Crawhall et al., 1968). Furthermore, it is not associated with increased intracellular concentrations of either cysteine or glutathionine (Schulman et al., 1971). Urinary cystine is increased in those patients who have the Fanconi syndrome but *not* out of proportion to the excretion of many other amino acids.

The biochemical mechanism responsible for the cystine deposition remains obscure. Worthen and Good (1961) reported that the activity of cystine reductase in the blood of cystinotic children was much reduced. They proposed that this primary defect led to the accumulation and precipitation of cystine in tissues, followed by phagocytosis and intracellular compartmentalization. This attractive hypothesis was refuted by Seegmiller and Howell (1960), who showed that cystine reductase activity in the blood of cystinotics was normal and that this enzyme played a minor role in maintaining cystine in its reduced form, cysteine. Patrick (1962) also showed that the cystine reductase activity in the liver of patients with cystinosis was not lower than that in controls. Tietze et al. (1972) studied another enzyme involved with sulfhydryl group oxidation and reduction, cystine-glutathione transhydrogenase. In cultured and peripheral leukocytes, the activity of this enzyme was comparable in controls and cystinotic patients.

Current interest now centers on the thesis that an abnormality in transcellular or intracellular transport of cystine or cysteine is responsible for the accumulation of cystine. Since in vitro studies showed that the intracellular concentration of cysteine in gut (Rosenberg et al., 1967; Crawhall and Segal, 1967) and kidney (Crawhall and Segal, 1967) from rats and humans far exceeds that of cystine, Schneider et al. (1968a) examined the transport and intracellular fate of cysteine-^{35}S in leukocytes from normal and cystinotic individuals. They demonstrated that cysteine uptake was modestly increased in cystinosis and, more significantly, that 20 times as much of the accumulated ^{35}S was present as cystine-^{35}S in the cystinotic cells than in control leukocytes. Neither these studies nor subsequent experiments by Schulman and Bradley (1970) distinguish, however, between a primary disturbance in influx of cysteine by cells, or abnormal conversion of cysteine to cystine followed by lysosomal accumulation or a primary defect in the mechanism by which cystine is transported out of lysosomes.

Pathology

The characteristic morphologic lesion of cystinosis is the deposition of cystine crystals. These crystals may be rectangular or hexagonal and are found throughout the body: in the reticuloendothelial cells of bone marrow, liver, spleen or lymph node; in peripheral leukocytes; in the medulla, cortex and glomerular mesangium of the kidney; in the rectal mucosa (Hummeler et al., 1970) and in the uvea and conjunctiva of the eye. The extent of crystal deposition varies considerably from patient to patient, depending both on the form of the disease and on the methods used to prepare pathologic specimens (Schneider and Seegmiller, 1972).

In the kidney, this deposition of cystine is apparently responsible for secondary tissue damage which leads, ultimately, to renal insufficiency in the infantile and juvenile forms of cystinosis. The kidneys are pale and shrunken, the capsule is adherent and the corticomedullary junction is obscured. Microscopically, the organization of nephrons is interrupted, glomeruli are hyalinized, connective tissue is increased and the normal epithelium at the tubules is replaced by simple cuboidal cells. Narrowing and shortening of the proximal tubule produce the so-called "swan neck deformity," now known not to be specific for cystinosis.

In the eye, patchy depigmentation of the peripheral regions of the retina have been noted in patients with the infantile and juvenile forms of the disease but not in adults with the benign form of cystinosis (Wong et al., 1967). This depigmentation reflects actual loss of continuity of the pigmented epithelium and is to be distinguished from the deposition of cystine crystals in the ocular conjunctiva or uvea.

Genetics

Cystinosis has been described with about equal frequency in males and females. Parent to child transmission has not been noted, but the occurrence of the disorder in multiple sibs has been prominent since the initial description of the disease. Schneider et al. (1967a) found that the cystine content of the leukocytes of parents of children with infantile cystinosis was significantly increased but still much lower than that observed in their affected children. This observation, confirmed subsequently in the other two forms of cystinosis (Aaron et al., 1971; Schneider et al., 1968b), adds considerable weight to the thesis that cystinosis is inherited as an autosomal recessive trait. Homozygous affected patients manifest cystine deposition in one or many tissues, while heterozygous carriers apparently have moderately elevated cystine concentrations in cells but do not develop the cystine storage diathesis. The existence of three clinical forms of cystinosis indicates genetic heterogeneity, but the nature of these different mutations must await further biochemical characterization of the disease.

Signs and Symptoms

The clinical consequences of infantile cystinosis have been discussed previously. Vitamin D-resistant rickets, chronic acidosis, polyuria and dehydration are the common presenting manifestations of the renal tubular dysfunction produced by the deposition of cystine in the kidney. Growth failure, uremia and death before the age of 10 are regular sequelae of this form of cystinosis. In contrast, adult cystinosis in three siblings (Lietman et al., 1966) was detected because of corneal cystine deposits which produced photophobia, headache and burning and itching of the eyes. No proteinuria, glycosuria, aminoaciduria or hypophosphatemia was noted. The glomerular filtration rate and intravenous pyelograms in these adults were normal. These patients ranged in age from 41 to 53 years, suggesting that adult cystinosis may have no deleterious effect on longevity. The findings in juvenile cystinosis fall between these extremes (Aaron et al., 1971; Hooft et al., 1971). These patients have both ocular and renal manifestations, but the latter do not become significant until the second decade. The kidney lesion, albeit milder than that seen in the infantile form, does lead inexorably to renal insufficiency.

Diagnosis

Cystinosis must be considered in any child with vitamin D-resistant rickets, the Fanconi syndrome or glomerular insufficiency. Cystine crystals are most easily detected in the cornea by slit lamp microscopy, in unstained preparations of peripheral blood or bone marrow or in biopsies of rectal mucosa (Hummeler et al., 1970). Urinary excretion of cystine is not a helpful diagnostic tool. Adult cystinosis will very likely be found only because of visual symptoms that lead to ophthalmologic examination. The diagnosis of cystinosis can now be confirmed by chemical determination of the cystine content of peripheral leukocytes or cultured skin fibroblasts. Prenatal detection of cystinosis has not, thus far, been achieved but should now be possible by incubating cultured aminotic fluid cells with cystine-^{35}S (Schulman et al., 1970).

Treatment

Symptomatic treatment of nephropathic cystinosis is not different from that afforded any patient with chronic renal failure: maintenance of adequate fluid intake; administration of sodium bicarbonate or sodium citrate to correct the acidosis; and ingestion of supplementary calcium and vitamin D to heal the rickets. Such measures are effective in maintaining growth, development and "well-being" in affected children and should not be neglected as more specific therapy is undertaken.

Three different forms of specific therapy for nephropathic cystinosis have been used: administration of thiol reagents; ingestion of cystine-poor diets; and renal transplantation. Thiol reagents have met with no significant success. D-Penicillamine and dimercaprol were used first by Clayton and Patrick (1961) with some encouraging results. Subsequent workers failed to note any significant clinical or chemical improvement, however, after prolonged administration of D-penicillamine (Hambraeus and Broberger, 1967). Aaron et al. (1971) showed that another sulfhydryl reagent, dithiothreitol, led to a distinct decrease in the intracellular cystine content of fibroblasts cultured from a cystinotic patient. A 10-day course of this drug was well tolerated in vivo, but it is too early to state that such therapy will yield any long-term gain.

The benefits of diet therapy have, likewise, been controversial. Several groups have reported that ingestion of low-cystine or cystine-free diets is followed by clinical improvement and accelerated growth. Other workers have noted no such benefit (Schneider and Seegmiller, 1972). All agree that the preparation and monitoring of such diets present formidable obstacles to long-term care and that no documented reduction in tissue cystine concentrations has been noted to date.

The most promising form of therapy for nephropathic cystinosis at this time appears to be renal transplantation. Since cystinosis is almost certainly caused by an intracellular abnormality, there is no theoretical reason why a kidney transplanted into such a patient should become affected. Reports on six children who have received kidney transplants have been published, with follow-ups of one to three years (Mahoney et al., 1970; Hambidge et al., 1969; Lucas et al., 1969). None of the six have developed the Fanconi syndrome since the transplantation, and all have had very substantial increases in their glomerular filtration rates. Symptomatic improvement has been regularly observed, and growth spurts have been documented in at least two patients. It is distressing, however, that cystine appears to accumulate in the donor kidneys. The source of this cystine is not known; it may reflect migration of cystine-containing cells from the recipient into the transplanted kidney as part of the expected rejection phenomenon. More prolonged follow-up of these children should define the role of this form of therapy, which is of theoretical as well as practical interest.

SULFITE OXIDASE DEFICIENCY

In 1967 Irreverre, Mudd and their colleagues described a male child with a previously unrecognized disorder of sulfur amino acid metabolism. The child had multiple neurological abnormalities at birth which progressed until he was virtually decerebrate. Bilateral ectopia lentis was described at the age of one year, and the child expired at 32 months of age. Three of seven siblings died early in infancy with a very similar disorder. The remaining four siblings and both parents appeared normal on clinical examination and demonstrated no biochemical abnormalities.

The patient's urine contained greatly increased concentrations of S-sulfo-L-cysteine, sulfite and thiosulfate but virtually *no* sulfate. Administration of cysteine to control subjects was followed by a marked increase in urinary sulfate excretion, but no increase in sulfate was noted in the patient's urine after cysteine loading. As depicted in Figure 11–2, these abnormal chemical findings suggested a deficiency of sulfite oxidase, the enzyme which catalyzes the conversion of sulfite to inorganic sulfate. Shortly after the patient's death, samples of liver, kidney and brain were assayed for sulfite oxidase and several other enzymes of the sulfur amino acid pathway (Mudd et al., 1967). No abnormalities of methionine-activating enzyme, cystathionine synthase or cystathionase were observed. Sulfite oxidase activity was readily apparent in the liver, kidney and brain of several control patients but was undetectable in all three of the patient's tissues. This enzymatic disturbance readily explains the chemical abnormalities observed. In the absence of sulfite oxidase, sulfate formation would be decreased and sulfite would accumulate behind the metabolic block. The elevated concentration of sulfite in body fluids could lead, secondarily, to the formation of abnormal amounts of S-sulfo-L-cysteine and thiosulfate by way of known reactions (Segel and Johnson, 1963; Sorbo, 1957).

Although these elegant studies do not define the substance or substances responsible for the profound neurological impairment exhibited by this patient and his siblings, they do show that enzymatic conversion of sulfite to sulfate is a vital reaction in man. Additional studies are needed to determine if sulfate deficiency leads to the central nervous system disturbances and lenticular dislocation or, conversely, if one of the sulfur compounds which accumulate because of the block is toxic. The association of ectopia lentis with two enzymatic defects of sulfur metabolism, cystathionine synthase deficiency and sulfite oxidase deficiency, demands further investigation.

β-MERCAPTOLACTATE-CYSTEINE DISULFIDURIA

Efron described a 45-year-old man, the product of a sib mating, with grand mal seizures. A positive nitroprusside test of his urine was shown not to be due to increased cystine or homocystine (Ampola et al., 1969). Subsequently, Crawhall et al. (1969) used infrared spectrophotometry to determine that the unique compound in this patient's urine was the disulfide of β-mercaptolactate and cysteine. The biological significance of this compound and its relationship to the patient's neurologic deficit remain to be ascertained.

GLUTATHIONURIA

Goodman and coworkers (1971a) described a moderately retarded 33-year-old man who excreted more than one thousand times as much glutathione as normal subjects did. Serum glutathione was also distinctly increased. Since the initial step in the degradation of glutathione (γ-glutamyl-cysteinyl-glycine) is catalyzed by the enzyme, γ-glutamyl transpeptidase, the activity of this enzyme was measured in the serum of the patient and controls. The patient's serum had less than 5 per cent of the mean control activity, leading to the proposal that the accumulation of glutathione in blood and urine was produced by a generalized deficiency of γ-glutamyl transpeptidase.

TAURINURIA

Taurine, a ubiquitous metabolite, has not yet been identified with a primary aberration of its own metabolism in man. However, it is involved secondarily in a number of metabolic disorders, and it is of quantitative importance in several tissues (Jacobson and Smith, 1968). Taurine is a β-amino compound in which the carboxyl group in the corresponding amino acid series is replaced by SO_3^-, as seen in the formula

$$^+H_3NCH_2CH_2SO_3^-.$$

As noted in Figure 11–2, taurine is an intermediate of cysteine oxidation. Taurine is found in blood plasma, urine, bile, breast milk, saliva, cerebrospinal fluid and sweat of man, and in platelets, leukocytes, muscle, brain, skin and liver; 75 per cent of the total body taurine is in striated muscle. The tissue concentration of taurine is higher in the fetus than in the adult, and blood and urine levels are higher after birth than in later life. Taurine is actively transported across the placenta to the fetus, and transport across plasma membranes is served by the β-amino-preferring system (see section on β-alanine metabolism).

The role of taurine in human tissues has not been extensively studied. Transmission of nerve impulses is known to be inhibited by taurine, and the chemical analogies between taurine and GABA invite further investigation of a neurohumoral type of function. Taurine, and its derivative isethionic acid, may regulate excitability of cardiac muscle, in particular perhaps by modifying potassium efflux from the cell. The preponderance of taurine in platelets and leukocytes suggests that it may function in platelet contractility and in leukocyte mobility and phagocytosis.

Taurine levels in blood are influenced by *age* (higher in the immediate postnatal period), *venipuncture* (transient fall after the procedure) and artifacts of sample collection (higher in serum than plasma and when leakage occurs from leukocytes and platelets during improper processing of blood samples). The normal concentration in plasma is 25 to 150 μmoles/L; higher values occur in the blood dyscrasias which augment the platelet and leukocyte fraction of formed elements in blood.

The urinary excretion of taurine is high relative to other amino acids. This finding reflects its inefficient tubular reabsorption, which is to be expected of a β-amino substance; fractional tubular reabsorption of taurine is less than 95 per cent of the normal filtered load and still lower when its plasma concentration increases. The excretion rate of taurine is considered to be abnormal when it exceeds 2500 μmoles/day in the adult and when more than 1200 μmoles/day in children under 12 years. Catabolic stimuli which produce negative nitrogen balance (burns, trauma, surgery) increase taurine excretion. High protein intake, acute liver failure and leukemia also cause hypertaurinuria. All of these conditions produce "prerenal hypertaurinuria." Disorders of renal tubular function may also cause increased taurine excretion. Vitamin B_6 deficiency impairs the synthesis of taurine from cysteine, and taurine excretion diminishes under these conditions. Taurine excretion is usually normal in the inborn errors of sulfur amino acid catabolism. Hypertaurinuria has been reported in dominantly inherited, familial camptodactyly (Nevin et al., 1966), but it is not clear whether this association is more than coincidental.

REFERENCES

Aaron, K., Goldman, H., and Scriver, C. R.: Cystinosis, new observations: 1. adolescent (type III) form. 2. correction of phenotypes in vitro with dithiothreitol. *In* Carson, N. A., and Raine, D. N., eds., Inherited Disorders of Sulphur Metabolism. Livingstone, London, pp. 150–161, 1971.

Abderhalden, E.: Familiäre cystindiathese. Z. Physiol. Chem. *38*:557–561, 1903.

Ampola, M. G., Efron, M. L., Bixby, E. M., and Meshorer, E.: Mental deficiency and a new amino-aciduria. Amer. J. Dis. Child. *117*:66–70, 1969.

Barber, G. W., and Spaeth, G. L.: Pyridoxine therapy in homocystinuria. Lancet (i), 337, 1967.

Berlow, S.: Studies in cystathioninuria. Amer. J. Dis. Child. *112*:135–142, 1966.

Beumer, H.: Über die Cystinkrankheit. Mschr. Kinderheilk. *68*:251–253, 1937.

Bonner, D. M., Suyama, Y., and Demoss, J. A.: Genetic fine structure and enzyme formation. Fed. Proc. *19*:926–930, 1960.

Brand, E., Cahill, G. F., and Block, R. J.: Cystinuria. IV. The metabolism of homocysteine and homocystine. J. Biol. Chem. *110*:399–410, 1935.

Brenton, D. P., and Cusworth, D. C.: The response of patients with cystathionine synthase deficiency to pyridoxine. *In* Carson, N. A., and Raine, D. N., eds., Inherited Disorders of Sulphur Metabolism. Livingstone, London, pp. 264–274, 1971.

Brenton, D. P., Cusworth, D. C., and Gaull, G. E.: Homocystinuria. Biochemical studies of tissues including a comparison with cystathioninuria. Pediatrics *35*:50–56, 1965.

Brown, F. C., and Gordon, P. H.: Cystathionine synthase from rat liver: Partial purification and properties. Canad. J. Biochem. *49*:484–491, 1971.

Carson, N. A., and Carré, I. J.: Treatment of homocystinuria with pyridoxine. Arch. Dis. Child. *44*:387–392, 1969.

Carson, N. A., Dent, D. E., Field, C. M. B., and Gaull, G. E.: Homocystinuria. Clinical and pathological review of ten cases. J. Pediat. *66*:565–583, 1965.

Carson, N. A., and Neill, D.: Metabolic abnormalities detected in a survey of mentally backward individuals in Northern Ireland. Arch. Dis. Child. *37*:505–513, 1962.

Challenger, F., and Walshe, J. M.: Methyl mercaptan in relation to foetor hepaticus. Biochem. J. *59*:372–375, 1955.

Clayton, B. E., and Patrick, A. D.: Use of dimercaprol or penicillamine in the treatment of cystinosis. Lancet (ii), 909–910, 1961.

Cogan, D. G., Kuwabara, T., Kinoshita, J., Sheehan, L., and Merola, L.: Cystinosis in an adult. J.A.M.A. *164*:394–396, 1957.

Crawhall, J. C., Lietman, P. S., Schneider, J. S., and Seegmiller, J. E.: Cystinosis: Plasma cystine concentrations and the effect of D-penicillamine and dietary treatment. Amer. J. Med. *44*: 330–339, 1968.

Crawhall, J. C., Parker, R., Sneddon, W., and Young, E. P.: β-mercaptolactate-cysteine disulfide in the urine of a mentally retarded patient. Amer. J. Dis. Child. *117*:71–82, 1969.

Crawhall, J. C., and Segal, S.: The intracellular ratio of cysteine and cystine in various tissues. Biochem. J. *105*:891–896, 1967.

Debré, R., Marie, J., Cleret, F., and Messimy, R.: Rachitism tardif coexistent avec un enéphriti chronique et une glycosurie. Arch. Med. Enf. *37*:597–606, 1934.

de Toni, G.: Remarks on the relations between renal rickets (renal dwarfism) and renal diabetes. Acta Paediat. *16*:479–484, 1933.

du Vigneaud, V.: A Trail of Research in Sulfur Chemistry. Cornell University Press, Ithaca, 1952.

du Vigneaud, V.. The significance of labile methyl groups in the diet and their relation to transmethylation. Harvey Lect. *38*:39–62, 1942–43.

du Vigneaud, C., Chandler, J. P., Moyer, A. W., and Keppel, D. M.: The effect of choline on the ability of homocystine to replace methionine in the diet. J. Biol. Chem. *131*:57–76, 1939.

Fanconi, G.: Der nephrotisch-glykosurische Zwergwuchs mit hypophosphatämischer Rachitis. Dtsch. Med. Wschr. *62*:1169–1171, 1936.

Finkelstein, J. D.: Methionine metabolism in mammals. *In* Carson, N. A., and Raine, D. N., eds., Inherited Disorders of Sulphur Metabolism. Livingstone, London, pp. 1–13, 1971.

Finkelstein, J. D., and Mudd, S. H.: Trans-sulfuration in mammals. J. Biol. Chem. *242*:873–880, 1967.

Finkelstein, J. D., Mudd, S. H., Irreverre, F., and Laster, L.: Deficiencies of cystathionase and homoserine dehydratase activities in cystathioninuria. Proc. Nat. Acad. Sci. U.S.A. *55*: 865–872, 1966.

Finkelstein, J. D., Mudd, S. H., Irreverre, F., and Laster, L.: Homocystinuria due to cystathionine synthetase deficiency. The mode of inheritance. Science *146*:785–787, 1964.

Frimpter, G. W.: Cystathioninuria. *In* Nyhan, W. L., ed., Amino Acid Metabolism and Genetic Variation. McGraw-Hill, New York, pp. 315–323, 1967.

Frimpter, G. W.: Cystathioninuria: Nature of the defect. Science *149*:1095–1096, 1965.

Frimpter, G. W.: Cystathioninuria, sulfite oxidase deficiency, and "β-mercaptolactate-cysteine disulfiduria." *In* Stanbury, J. B., Wyngaarden, J. B., and Fredrickson, D. S., eds., The Metabolic Basis of Inherited Disease, 3rd edition. McGraw-Hill, New York, pp. 413–425, 1972.

Frimpter, G. W., Greenberg, A. J., Hilgartner, M., and Fuchs, F.: Cystathioninuria: Management. Amer. J. Dis. Child. *113*:115–118, 1967.

Frimpter, G. W., Haymovitz, A., and Horwith, M.: Cystathioninuria. New Eng. J. Med. *268*:333–339, 1963.

Gaull, G., Rassin, D. K., and Sturman, J. A.: Enzymatic and metabolic studies of homocystinuria: Effects of pyridoxine. Neuropediatrie *1*:199–226, 1969.

Gaull, G., Sturman, J. A., and Raiha, N. C. R.: Development of mammalian sulfur metabolism: Absence of cystathionase in human fetal tissues. Pediat. Res. *6*:538–547, 1972.

Gerritsen, T., Vaughn, J. G., and Waisman, H. A.: The identification of homocystine in the urine. Biochem. Biophys. Res. Commun. *9*:493–496, 1962.

Gerritsen, T., and Waisman, H. A.: Homocystinuria: Absence of cystathionine in the brain. Science *145*:588, 1964.

Gjessing, L. R.: Cystathioninuria and vanillacticaciduria in neuroblastoma and argentaffinoma. Lancet (ii), 1281–1282, 1963.

Gjessing, L. R.: Cystathioninuria during a load of thyroxine. Scand. J. Clin. Lab. Invest. *16*:680–681, 1964.

Goldstein, J. L., Campbell, B. K., and Gartler, S. M.: Homocystinuria: Heterozygote detection using phytohemagglutinin-stimulated lymphocytes. J. Clin. Invest. *52*:218–221, 1973.

Goodman, S. I., Mace, J. W., and Pollak, S.: Serum gamma-glutamyl transpeptidase deficiency. Lancet (i), 234–235, 1971a.

Goodman, S. I., Moe, P. G., Hammond, K. B., Mudd, S. H., and Uhlendorf, B. W.: Homocystinuria with methylmalonicaciduria: Two cases in a sibship. Biochem. Med. *4*:500–515, 1971b.

Greenberg, D. M.: Amino acid metabolism. Ann. Rev. Biochem. *33*:633–666, 1964.

Hambidge, K. M., Goodman, S. I., Walravens, P. A., Maner, S. M., Brettschneider, L., Penni, I., and Starzl, T. E.: Accumulation of cystine following renal homotransplantation for cystinosis. Pediat. Res. *3*:364–365, 1969.

Hambraeus, L., and Broberger, O.: Penicillamine treatment of cystinosis. Acta Paediat. Scand. *56*:243–248, 1967.

Harris, H., Penrose, L. S., and Thomas, D. H. H.: Cystathioninuria. Ann. Hum. Genet. *23*:442–453, 1959.

Hollowell, J. G., Coryell, M. E., Hall, W. K., Findley, J. K., and Thevaos, T. G.: Homocystinuria as affected by pyridoxine, folic acid and vitamin B_{12}. Proc. Soc. Exp. Biol. Med. *129*:327–333, 1968.

Hollowell, J. G., Jr., Hall, W. K., Coryell, M. E., McPherson, J., Jr., and Hahn, D. A.: Homocystinuria and organic aciduria in a patient with vitamin B_{12} deficiency. Lancet (ii), 1428, 1969.

Hooft, C., Carton, D., deSchrijver, F., Delbeke, M. J., Samyn, W., and Kint, J.: Juvenile cystinosis in two siblings. *In* Carson, N. A., and Raine, D. N., eds., Inherited Disorders of Sulphur Metabolism. Livingstone, London, pp. 141–149, 1971.

Hooft, C., Carton, D., and Samyn, W.: Pyridoxine treatment in homocystinuria. Lancet (i), 1384, 1967.

Hummeler, K., Zajac, B. A., Genel, M., Holtzapple, P. G., and Segal, S.: Human cystinosis: Intracellular deposition of cystine. Science *168*:859–860, 1970.

Irreverre, F., Mudd, S. H., Heizer, W. D., and Laster, L.: Sulfite oxidase deficiency: Studies of a patient with mental retardation, dislocated ocular lenses and abnormal urinary excretion of S-sulfo-L-cysteine, sulfite and thiosulfate. Biochem. Med. *1*:187–217, 1967.

Jacobson, J. G., and Smith, L. H., Jr.: Biochemistry and physiology of taurine and taurine derivatives. Physiol. Rev. *48*:424–511, 1968.

Kashiwamata, S., Kotake, Y., and Greenberg, D. M.: Studies of cystathionine synthetase of rat liver: Dissociation into two components by sodium dodecyl sulfate disc electrophoresis. Biochim. Biophys. Acta *212*:501–503, 1970.

Kimura, H., and Nakagawa, H.: Studies on cystathionine synthase characteristics of purified rat liver enzyme. J. Biochem. *69*:711–723, 1971.

Knox, W. E.: Adaptive enzymes in the regulation of animal metabolism. *In* Prosser, C. L., ed., Physiological Adaptation. American Physiological Society, Washington, D.C., pp. 107–125, 1958.

Komrower, G. M., and Sardharwalla, I. B.: The dietary treatment of homocystinuria. *In* Carson, N. A., and Raine, D. N., eds., Inherited Disorders of Sulphur Metabolism. Livingstone, London, pp. 254–263, 1971.

Laster, L., Mudd, S. H., Finkelstein, J. D., and Irreverre, F.: Homocystinuria due to cystathionine synthase deficiency: The metabolism of L-methionine. J. Clin. Invest. *44*:1708–1719, 1965a.

Laster, L., Spaeth, G. L., Mudd, H. S., and Finkelstein, J. D.: Homocystinuria due to cystathionine synthase deficiency. Ann. Intern. Med. *63*:1117–1142, 1965b.

Levy, H. J., Shih, V. E., and MacCready, R. A.: Massachusetts metabolic disorders screening program. *In* Harris, M., ed., Early Diagnosis of Human Genetic Defects. U. S. Government Printing Office, Washington, D.C., pp. 47–66, 1972.

Levy, H. L., Shih, V. E., and MacCready, R. A.: Screening for homocystinuria in the newborn and mentally retarded population. *In* Carson, N. A., and Raine, D. N., eds., Inherited Disorders of Sulfur Metabolism. Livingstone, London, pp. 235–244, 1971.

Lietman, P. S., Frazier, P. D., Wong, V. G., Shotton, D., and Seegmiller, J. E.: Adult cystinosis—a benign disorder. Amer. J. Med. *40*:511–517, 1966.

Lignac, G. O. E.: Über störung des Cystinstoffwechsels bei Kindern. Dtsch. Arch. Klin. Med. *145*:139–150, 1924.

Loiselet, J., and Chatagner, F.: Purification et étude de quelques propriétés de la cystéine désulfurase "soluble" (cystathionase) du foie de rat. Bull. Soc. Chim. Biol. *47*:33–46, 1965.

Lucas, Z. J., Kempson, R. L., Palmer, J., Korn, D., and Cohn, R. B.: Renal allotransplantation in man. II. Transplantation in cystinosis, a metabolic disease. Amer. J. Surg. *118*:158–168, 1969.

Mahoney, C. P., Striker, G. E., Hickman, R. O., Manning, G. B., and Marchioro, T. L.: Renal transplantation for childhood cystinosis. New Eng. J. Med. *283*:397–402, 1970.

Mahoney, M. J., Rosenberg, L. E., Mudd, S. H., and Uhlendorf, B. W.: Defective metabolism of vitamin B_{12} in fibroblasts from children with methylmalonicaciduria. Biochem. Biophys. Res. Commun. *44*:375–381, 1971.

Matsuo, Y., and Greenberg, D. M.: A crystalline enzyme that cleaves homoserine and cystathionine. I. Isolation procedure and some physicochemical properties. J. Biol. Chem. *230*:545–560, 1958a.

Matsuo, Y., and Greenberg, D. M.: A crystalline enzyme that cleaves homoserine and cystathionine. II. Prosthetic group. J. Biol. Chem. *230*:561–571, 1958b.

McCully, K. S.: Macromolecular basis for homocysteine-induced changes in proteoglycan structure in growth and arteriosclerosis. Amer. J. Path. *66*:83–92, 1972.

McCully, K. S., and Ragsdale, B. D.: Production of arteriosclerosis by homocysteinemia. Amer. J. Path. *61*:1–8, 1970.

McCune, D. J., Mason, H. H., and Clarke, H. T.: Intractable hypophosphatemic rickets with renal glycosuria and acidosis (the Fanconi syndrome). Amer. J. Dis. Child. *65*:81–146, 1943.

McDonald, L., Bray, C., Field, C., Love, F., and Davies, B.: Homocystinuria, thrombosis, and the blood-platelets. Lancet (i), 745–746, 1964.

McKusick, V. A., Hall, J. G., and Char, F.: The clinical and genetic characteristics of homocystinuria. *In* Carson, N. A., and Raine, D. N., eds., Inherited Disorders of Sulphur Metabolism. Livingstone, London, pp. 179–203, 1971.

Mongeau, J.-G., Hilgartner, M., Worthen, H. G., and Frimpter, G. W.: Cystathioninuria: Study of infant with normal mentality, thrombocytopenia, and renal calculi. J. Pediat. *69*:1113–1120, 1966.

Mörner, C. T.: On present knowledge of cystinuria. Uppsala Läk.-fören. Förh. *31*:171, 1925.

Mudd, S. H.: Errors of sulfur metabolism. *In* Muth, O. H., and Oldfield, J. E., eds., Sulphur in Nutrition. AVI Publishers, Westport, Conn., p. 222, 1970.

Mudd, S. H.: Homocystinuria: The known causes. *In* Carson, N. A., and Raine, D. N., eds., Inherited Disorders of Sulphur Metabolism. Livingstone, London, pp. 204–220, 1971.

Mudd, S. H., and Cantoni, G. L.: Biological transmethylation, methyl-group neogenesis and other "one-carbon" metabolic reactions dependent upon tetrahydrofolic acid. *In* Florkin, M., and Stotz, E. H., eds., Comprehensive Biochemistry. Elsevier, Amsterdam, pp. 1–47, 1964a.

Mudd, S. H., Edwards, W. A., Loeb, P. M., Brown, M. S., and Laster, L.: Homocystinuria due to cystathionine synthase deficiency: The effect of pyridoxine. J. Clin. Invest. *49*:1762–1773, 1970a.

Mudd, S. H., Finkelstein, J. D., Irreverre, F., and Laster, L.: Homocystinuria: An enzymatic defect. Science *143*:1443–1445, 1964b.

Mudd, S. H., Finkelstein, J. D., Irreverre, F., and Laster, L.: Transsulfuration in mammals. J. Biol. Chem. *240*:4382–4392, 1965.

Mudd, S. H., Irreverre, F., and Laster, L.: Sulfite oxidase deficiency in man: Demonstration of the enzymatic defect. Science *156*:1599–1601, 1967.

Mudd, S. H., Levy, H. L., and Abeles, R. H.: A derangement in B_{12} metabolism leading to homocystinuria, cystathioninemia and methylmalonicaciduria. Biochem. Biophys. Res. Commun. *35*:121–126, 1969.

Mudd, S. H., Levy, H. L., and Morrow, G., III: Deranged B_{12} metabolism: Effects on sulfur amino acid metabolism. Biochem. Med. *4*:193–214, 1970b.

Mudd, S. H., Uhlendorf, B. W., Freeman, J. M., Finkelstein, J. D., and Shih, V. E.: Homocystinuria associated with decreased methylenetetrahydrofolate reductase activity. Biochem. Biophys. Res. Commun. *46*:905–912, 1972.

Mudd, S. H., Uhlendorf, B. W., Hinds, K. R., and Levy, H. L.: Deranged B_{12} metabolism: Studies of fibroblasts grown in tissue culture. Biochem. Med. *4*:215–239, 1970c.

Nevin, N. C., Hurwitz, L. J., and Neill, D. W.: Familial camptodactyly with taurinuria. J. Med. Genet. *3*:265–268, 1966.

Patrick, A. D.: The degradative metabolism of L-cysteine and L-cystine in vitro by liver in cystinosis. Biochem. J. *83*:248–256, 1962.

Patrick, A. D., and Lake, B. D.: Cystinosis: Electron microscopic evidence of lysosomal storage of cystine in lymph node. J. Clin. Path. *21*:571–575, 1968.

Pegg, A. E., and Williams-Ashman, A. G.: On the role of 5-adenosyl-L-methionine in the biosynthesis of spermidine by rat prostate. J. Biol. Chem. *244*:682–693, 1969.

Perry, T. L.: Treatment of homocystinuria with a low methionine diet and supplemented by L-cystine. *In* Carson, N. A., and Raine, D. N., eds., Inherited Disorders of Sulphur Metabolism. Livingstone, London, pp. 245–253, 1971.

Perry, T. L.: Unsolved problems in homocystinuria. *In* Nyhan, W. L., ed., Amino Acid Metabolism and Genetic Variation. McGraw-Hill, New York, pp. 279–296, 1967.

Perry, T. L., Hardwick, D. F., Hansen, S., Love, D. L., and Israels, S.: Cystathioninuria in two healthy siblings. New Eng. J. Med. *278*:590–592, 1968.

Perry, T. L., Robinson, G. C., Teasdale, J. M., and Hansen, S.: Concurrence of cystathioninuria, nephrogenic diabetes insipidus and severe anemia. New Eng. J. Med. *276*:721–725, 1967.

Rosenberg, L. E., Crawhall, J. L., and Segal, S.: Intestinal transport of cystine and cysteine in man: Evidence for separate mechanisms. J. Clin. Invest. *46*:30–34, 1967.

Schimke, R. N., McKusick, V. A., Huang, T., and Pollack, A. D.: Homocystinuria. J.A.M.A. *193*: 711–719, 1965a.

Schimke, R. N., McKusick, V. A., and Pollack, A. D.: Homocystinuria simulating the Marfan syndrome. Trans. Ass. Amer. Physicians *78*:60–72, 1965b.

Schimke, R. N., McKusick, V. A., and Weilbaecher, R. G.: Homocystinuria. *In* Nyhan, W. L., ed., Amino Acid Metabolism and Genetic Variation. McGraw-Hill, New York, pp. 297–313, 1967.

Schneider, J. A., Bradley, K., and Seegmiller, J. E.: Increased cystine in leukocytes from individuals homozygous and heterozygous for cystinosis. Science *157*:1321–1322, 1967a.

Schneider, J. A., Bradley, K. H., and Seegmiller, J. E.: Transport and intracellular fate of cystine-^{35}S in leukocytes from normal subjects and patients with cystinosis. Pediat. Res. *2*:441–450, 1968a.

Schneider, J. A., Rosenbloom, F. M., Bradley, K. H., and Seegmiller, J. E.: Increased free cystine content of fibroblasts cultured from patients with cystinosis. Biochem. Biophys. Res. Commun. *29*:527–531, 1967b.

Schneider, J. A., and Seegmiller, J. E.: Cystinosis and the Fanconi syndrome. *In* Stanbury, J. B., Wyngaarden, J. B., and Fredrickson, D. S., eds., The Metabolic Basis of Inherited Disease, 3rd edition. McGraw-Hill, New York, pp. 1581–1604, 1972.

Schneider, J. A., Wong, V., Bradley, K. H., and Seegmiller, J. E.: Biochemical comparisons of the adult and childhood forms of cystinosis. New Eng. J. Med. *279*:1253–1257, 1968b.

Schulman, J. D., and Bradley, K. H.: Cystinosis: Selective induction of vacuolation in fibroblasts by L-cysteine-D-penicillamine disulfide. Science *169*:595–597, 1970.

Schulman, J. D., Bradley, K. H., and Seegmiller, J. E.: Cystine: Compartmentalization within lysosomes in cystinotic leukocytes. Science *166*:1152–1154, 1969.

Schulman, J. D., Fujimoto, W. Y., Bradley, K. H., and Seegmiller, J. E.: Identification of heterozygous genotype for cystinosis in utero by a new pulse-labeling technique: Preliminary report. J. Pediat. *77*:468–470, 1970.

Schulman, J. D., Schneider, J. H., Bradley, K. H., and Seegmiller, J. E.: Cystine, cysteine and glutathione metabolism in normal and cystinotic fibroblasts in vitro and in cultured normal amniotic fluid cells. Clin. Chim. Acta *35*:383–388, 1971.

Seashore, M. R., Durant, J. L., and Rosenberg, L. E.: Studies of the mechanism of pyridoxine-responsive homocystinuria. Pediat. Res. *6*:187–196, 1972.

Seegmiller, J. E., and Howell, R.: Cystine metabolism in de Toni-Franconi syndrome with cystinosis. Clin. Res. *9*:189, 1960.

Segel, I. H., and Johnson, M. J.: Synthesis and characterization of sodium cysteine-S-sulfate monohydrate. Anal. Biochem. *5*:330–337, 1963.

Shaw, K. N. F., Lieberman, E., Koch, R., and Donnell, G. N.: Cystathioninuria. Amer. J. Dis. Child. *113*:119–127, 1967.

Shipman, R. J., Townley, R. R. W., and Danks, D. M.: Homocystinuria, Addisonian pernicious anemia and partial deletion of a G chromosome. Lancet (ii), 693–694, 1969.

Sorbo, B.: Enzymic transfer of sulfur from mercaptopyruvate to sulfite or sulfinates. Biochim. Biopshys. Acta *24*:324–329, 1957.

Tada, K., Yoshida, T., Yokoyama, Y., Sato, T., Nakagawa, H., and Arakawa, T.: Cystathioninuria not associated with vitamin B$_6$ dependency: A probable new type of cystathioninuria. Tohoku J. Exp. Med. *95*:235–242, 1968.

Tallan, H. H., Moore, S., and Stein, W. H.: L-Cystathionine in human brain. J. Biol. Chem. *230*: 707–716, 1958.

Tarver, H., and Schmidt, C. L. A.: The conversion of methionine to cystine: Experiments with radioactive sulfur. J. Biol. Chem. *130*:67–80, 1939.

Tietze, F., Bradley, K. H., and Schulman, J. D.: Enzymatic reduction of cystine by subcellular fractions of cultured and peripheral leukocytes from normal and cystinotic individuals. Pediat. Res. *6*:649–658, 1972.

Whelan, T., and Scriver, C. R.: Cystathioninuria and renal iminoglycinuria in a pedigree. New Eng. J. Med. *278*:924–927, 1968.

Womach, M., Kemmerer, K. S., and Rose, W. C.: The relation of cystine and methionine to growth. J. Biol. Chem. *121*:403–410, 1937.

Wong, P. W. K., Schwarz, V., and Lomrower, C. H.: The biosynthesis of cystathionine in patients with homocystinuria. Pediat. Res. *2*:149–160, 1968.

Wong, V. G., Lietman, P. S., and Seegmiller, J. E.: Alterations in pigment epithelium in cystinosis. Arch. Ophthal. *77*:361–369, 1967.

Worthen, H. G., and Good, R. A.: The pathogenesis of cystinosis. Amer. J. Dis. Child. *102*:494–495, 1961.

Yoshida, T., Tada, K., Yokoyama, Y., and Arakawa, T.: Homocystinuria of vitamin B_6 dependent type. Tohoku J. Exp. Med. *96*:235–242, 1968.

Young, L., and Maw, G. A.: The Metabolism of Sulfur Compounds. Methuen & Co., London, 1958.

Chapter Twelve

UREA CYCLE AND AMMONIA

The amino nitrogen of amino acids is in a state of dynamic equilibrium in mammalian organisms. Schoenheimer and his associates (1942) showed that amino acids are continually being removed from and returned to the amino acid pool during the synthesis and degradation of proteins. Transamination, deamination and reamination reactions lead to a constant shifting of amino acid nitrogen from one amino acid to another. The deamination of amino acids also forms large quantities of ammonia which, if allowed to accumulate, would be highly toxic. Ammonia is disposed of in several ways. It may be reutilized in the synthesis of amino acids by reversal of deamination reactions. It participates in the synthesis of purines, pyrimidines and porphyrins indirectly after its incorporation into glutamine, aspartate, carbamyl phosphate and glycine. Glutamine is synthesized in many tissues from glutamic acid and ammonia, a reaction dependent on ATP. In the kidney, glutamine is also hydrolyzed to glutamic acid and ammonia by the enzyme glutaminase, and ammonia is then secreted into the renal tubule and excreted in the urine. This hydrolysis of glutamine accounts for about 60 per cent of the ammonia found in the urine, but its total contribution to ammonia removal is small. The detoxication of ammonia is achieved by conversion to urea in mammals, whereas in birds and reptiles uric acid is the end product of ammonia removal. The general scheme of urea synthesis has been known for 30 years, but its relevance to the study of human inherited disease has been apparent for only the past decade.

THE UREA CYCLE

Site of Urea Formation

In 1924 Bollman et al. demonstrated that the liver is the major site of urea synthesis in mammals. They measured the blood urea in dogs after removal of the liver or the kidneys or both. If the kidneys alone were removed, urea excretion ceased and the blood urea rose rapidly. If the liver alone was removed, the blood urea fell; but if both the liver and the kidneys were removed, blood urea remained constant since urea was neither being formed nor being excreted. In vitro studies have also demonstrated that the liver predominates in the conversion of ammonia to urea, but recent findings indicate that small amounts of urea are also formed in the brain and perhaps in other tissues.

Krebs and Henseleit (1932) incubated liver slices with ammonium salts, bicarbonate (as a source of carbon dioxide) and lactate (as a source of energy) and demonstrated that urea was formed in vitro. They found that the addition of ornithine or citrulline greatly increased the rate of urea formation and that arginine was an intermediate product of the reaction sequence. Balance experiments showed that the sum of the concentrations of ornithine and arginine did not change during urea synthesis, while the quantity of ammonia removal was approximately equal to the amount of urea formed. On the basis of these studies, Krebs and Henseleit proposed a cyclic mechanism for urea synthesis, involving ammonia, carbon dioxide, ornithine, citrulline and arginine (Fig. 12–1). Two molecules of ammonia and one molecule of carbon dioxide are converted to a molecule of urea for each turn of the cycle, and ornithine is regenerated.

The Enzymatic Pathway

The overall process of urea synthesis just outlined has been confirmed by many additional experiments in vitro which have defined the biochemical complexities of the Krebs-Henseleit cycle. Cohen et al. have shown that the first step in the synthesis of urea is the formation of carbamyl phosphate from ATP, carbon dioxide and ammonia. The mitochondrial enzyme, carbamyl phosphate synthetase, catalyzes a two-step reaction leading to the formation of this high energy compound (Cohen and Brown, 1960). Magnesium and acetylglutamate are cofactors producing an allosteric change in the synthetase enzyme which allows binding of two molecules of ATP (Marshall et al., 1961; Fahien and Cohen, 1964). Citrulline is formed from carbamyl phosphate and ornithine by the action of ornithine transcarbamylase, a reaction which is irreversible and involves binding of the two substrates at different sites on the enzyme (Joseph et al., 1963). Ornithine transcarbamylase, a mitochondrial enzyme, has been isolated and purified from *Streptococcus faecalis* and bovine liver (Marshall and Cohen, 1972). In liver it is a trimer with a total molecular weight of 108,000.

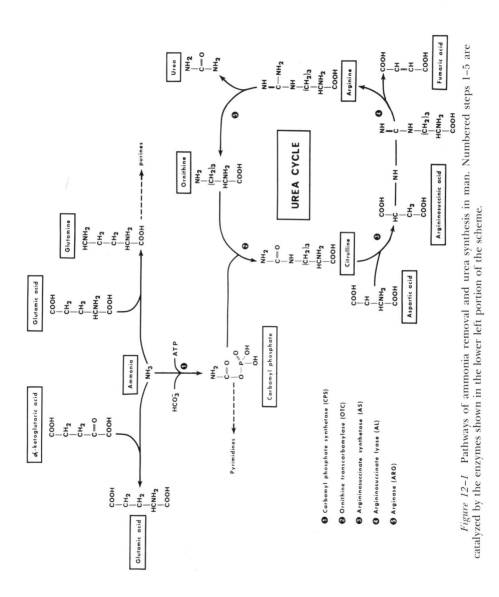

Figure 12-1 Pathways of ammonia removal and urea synthesis in man. Numbered steps 1–5 are catalyzed by the enzymes shown in the lower left portion of the scheme.

Arginine is formed from citrulline by two sequential reactions. The first involves the formation of argininosuccinic acid from citrulline and aspartate, a reaction catalyzed by argininosuccinic acid synthetase (Ratner et al., 1953b). The second reaction, catalyzed by argininosuccinic acid lyase (formerly called argininosuccinase), cleaves argininosuccinic acid to arginine and fumarate (Ratner et al., 1953a). Finally, arginine is hydrolyzed to ornithine and urea by the enzyme arginase. It can be seen that one of the two nitrogen atoms in urea is derived from ammonia through carbamyl phosphate and the other from aspartic acid through argininosuccinic acid. It is of note that argininosuccinic acid synthetase, argininosuccinic acid lyase and arginase are all found in the soluble portion of the cell rather in the mitochondrion, where the first two enzymes required for urea synthesis reside.

Brown and Cohen (1959) demonstrated that the activity of the five enzymes which catalyze urea synthesis can be studied in a single homogenate of human liver. The relative activity of these enzymes is shown in Table 12–1. Argininosuccinic acid synthetase is the rate-limiting enzyme, followed in order of increasing activity by argininosuccinic acid lyase and carbamyl phosphate synthetase. Arginase and ornithine transcarbamylase activities are more than 100 times as great as that of argininosuccinic acid synthetase, an observation which may be of importance in the subsequent discussion of the inherited disorders of the urea cycle. It should be emphasized, however, that these relative enzymatic activities were determined under optimal conditions in vitro and do not necessarily reflect the situation in the intact liver.

Extrahepatic Urea Synthesis

Certain of the enzymes involved in urea biosynthesis have been demonstrated in tissues other than liver. Ratner and Petrack (1953) showed that kidney tissue contains argininosuccinic acid synthetase, argininosuccinate lyase and arginase. Reichard (1960) demonstrated that ornithine transcarbamylase was also detectable in the kidney, but its activity was only one hundred thousandth that of liver. Thus, urea synthesis in the kidney is probably dependent upon citrulline supplied from plasma and is further limited by the low activity of arginase which converts arginine to urea (Ratner and Petrack, 1953). Sporn and his colleagues (1959) noted that arginine was converted to urea in rat brain in vivo, an observation supported by enzymatic studies which have demonstrated that ornithine transcarbamylase, argininosuccinic acid synthetase, argininosuccinate lyase and arginase are present in this tissue (Reichard, 1960; Ratner et al., 1960). Detectable activities of ornithine transcarbamylase (Reichard,

Table 12–1 Relative Activity of Urea Cycle Enzymes in Normal Human Liver*

Enzyme	μM product/mg protein/hr	Relative Activity
Carbamyl phosphate synthetase	3.1	4.5
Ornithine transcarbamylase	111	163
Argininosuccinic acid synthetase	0.8	1
Argininosuccinic acid lyase	2.7	3.3
Arginase	108	149

*From two healthy adults. Source: Kennan and Cohen, 1961.

1960) and argininosuccinate lyase (Soriano et al., 1967) have also been found in many other tissues, including skeletal muscle, heart, intestine, spleen, pancreas, gallbladder, testis and circulating blood cells. Finally, Tedesco and Mellman (1967) reported that normal human fibroblasts grown in tissue culture converted citrulline to urea, indicating that this tissue preparation contains argininosuccinate synthetase, argininosuccinate lyase and arginase. These observations demonstrate that tissues other than liver can synthesize urea. However, the very low enzymatic activities relative to those found in hepatic cells suggest that the physiological contribution of extrahepatic urea synthesis is very small.

Regulation of Blood Ammonia

In addition to the endogenous synthesis of ammonia from protein and amino acid catabolism, ammonia is also formed in the mammalian intestinal tract by microbial deaminases and ureases which cleave amino acids and urea, respectively. The ammonia thus formed is absorbed from the gut and contributes significantly to the total body burden of this potentially toxic substance. Normally, the blood ammonia concentration in man is less than 150 μg per 100 ml. In patients with severe acquired liver disease, whether acute or chronic, the blood ammonia may rise to values as high as 500 μg per 100 ml. This acquired hyperammonemia is caused by hepatocellular failure and by portal-systemic vascular shunts which divert ammonia from the portal to the systemic circulation. There is considerable evidence that hyperammonemia contributes significantly to the encephalopathy characteristic of hepatic failure, but the specific enzymatic dysfunction responsible for the hyperammonemia of acquired liver disease is not known.

Since 1958 many patients have been described who exhibit hyperammonemia which cannot be explained by acquired hepatic disease. Some of these patients suffer from specific inherited defects of one of the enzymes catalyzing the conversion of ammonia to urea. Five distinct disorders have been defined thus far: hyperammonemia due to carbamyl phosphate synthetase deficiency; hyperammonemia due to ornithine transcarbamylase deficiency; citrullinemia due to a defect in argininosuccinic acid synthetase activity; argininosuccinic aciduria due to argininosuccinate lyase deficiency; and argininemia due to arginase deficiency. Each of these disorders is characterized by hyperammonemia which, as expected, is most severe in patients with deficiencies of carbamyl phosphate synthetase and ornithine transcarbamylase but which may also produce serious, and even lethal, consequences in citrullinemia and argininosuccinicaciduria. In addition to these primary disorders of the urea cycle, hyperammonemia has been described in patients with other inherited disorders, including lysine dehydrogenase deficiency (Bürgi et al., 1966), hyperglycinemia (Wada et al., 1972; Soriano et al., 1967), propionicacidemia (Hsia and Walker, 1973), methylmalonicaciduria (Hsia and Walker, 1973), defective intestinal and renal transport of dibasic amino acids (Perheentupa and Visakorpi, 1965; Kekkomaki et al., 1967) and hyperornithinemia (Shih et al., 1969). The latter condition will be discussed with the primary hyperammonemias, although a specific enzymatic defect has not been defined. Lysine dehydrogenase deficiency, the hyperglycinemias, propionicacidemia, methylmalonicaciduria and the familial dibasic amino acid transport defect are considered elsewhere in this volume.

CARBAMYL PHOSPHATE SYNTHETASE DEFICIENCY

Two patients, presumed to have primary carbamyl phosphate synthetase (CPS) deficiency, were reported between 1960 and 1970. Freeman et al. (1970)

detected blood ammonia concentrations as high as 480 μg per 100 ml in a female infant with episodic vomiting, lethargy, ketoacidosis and dehydration. The clinical attacks and the hyperammonemia were precipitated by a high-protein diet. Elevated plasma glycine values were also recorded, but these bore no relationship to the clinical course. The patient's blood urea nitrogen (BUN) concentration was 12 mg% when she was fed a regular diet but fell to 2 to 4 mg% when protein was restricted. At the age of 5 months, following an open liver biopsy, she developed intractable ketoacidosis and expired. Postmortem examination revealed only a fatty liver. Hepatic assay of each of the urea cycle enzymes revealed a selective reduction of CPS activity to about 20 per cent of normal. Her family history is remarkable: two sibs died in infancy with a clinical picture like that of the proband; three other pregnancies of the mother ended in spontaneous abortion; and a maternal aunt and great-aunt died in the neonatal period with convulsions.

Hommes and coworkers (1969) also described a female infant who succumbed at 7 months of age after an illness characterized by poor feeding, lethargy, irregular eye movements and convulsions. In contrast to the patient described by Freeman et al., she had a mild metabolic alkalosis, normal blood ammonia values and normal plasma glycine concentrations. Her liver, too, showed CPS activity about 30 per cent of that in controls, without abnormality of other urea cycle enzymes. Two sibs, one male and one female, had died with a similar clinical picture at the age of 4 weeks.

It is difficult to reconcile the disparate clinical and chemical findings in these two children with their apparently similar enzymatic deficiency, particularly when it is becoming clear that patients with primary abnormalities of propionate, methylmalonate or glycine metabolism may also demonstrate some reduction in activity of one or more of the urea cycle enzymes.

More convincing evidence for primary mitochondrial CPS deficiency has recently been provided by Gelehrter and Snodgrass (1973). These workers described two infant males in a single sibship who died on the fourth day of life. The second child had a blood ammonia of 1480 μg% on the day of his death. Postmortem analysis of urea cycle enzyme activity in his liver revealed virtually complete absence of mitochondrial CPS activity, though cytoplasmic CPS activity remained detectable.

ORNITHINE TRANSCARBAMYLASE DEFICIENCY

In 1962 Russell and coworkers described two female first cousins with attacks of episodic vomiting and screaming followed by lethargy and stupor, severe developmental retardation and cerebral cortical atrophy. In both patients blood ammonia (980 and 480 μg/100 ml) and cerebrospinal fluid concentrations of ammonia (360 and 320 μg/100 ml) exceeded even the toxic levels found in patients with hepatic coma. Glutamine was increased in the urine and cerebrospinal fluid, but plasma citrulline and ornithine were normal, as were the concentrations of other amino acids in blood and urine (Levin and Russell, 1967). The urea cycle enzymes were assayed in a liver biopsy from one patient and in a necropsy specimen from the second (Russell et al., 1962; Levin and Russell, 1967). Ornithine transcarbamylase (OTC) activity was less than 10 per cent of that noted in controls, while argininosuccinic acid synthetase and argininosuccinic acid lyase activities were normal. In the ensuing decade, 13 additional children with ammonia intoxication due to partial deficiency of OTC have been described (Hopkins et al., 1969; Levin et al., 1969a, 1969b; Corbeel et al., 1969; Nagayama et al., 1970; Matsuda et al., 1971; MacLeod et al., 1972; Sunshine et al., 1972; Short et al., 1973). All but two of these patients are females. In addition to this group with *partial* OTC deficiency, four male infants with virtually *complete* absence of hepatic OTC activity have been reported by Campbell (1971; 1973), Short (1973) and their colleagues. These males, whose clinical and enzymologic findings contrast sharply with those reported in children with partial OTC deficiency, also provided the clue that OTC deficiency is almost certainly inherited as an X-linked dominant trait.

Biochemical Findings

Hyperammonemia has been the only constant chemical abnormality noted in patients with OTC deficiency. The blood ammonia has been as low as 200 μg% and as high as 1200 μg% in children with partial OTC deficiency, whereas it has ranged consistently between 1000 and 2000 μg% in those infants with complete OTC deficiency. Plasma and urinary glutamine have been increased in several patients, presumably because of condensation of the increased ammonia load with glutamic acid (Fig. 12–1). The BUN has been in the normal or low normal range, even in patients with complete OTC deficiency, thereby demonstrating that urea synthesis continues despite an essentially totally blocked urea cycle.

Enzymatic Defects

Hepatic OTC activity has ranged from less than 0.5 per cent of normal in males with "complete" OTC deficiency to 40 per cent of normal in patients with partial deficiency. Reduced activity of OTC has also been documented in the jejunal mucosa (Levin et al., 1969a; Campbell et al., 1973) and kidney (Campbell et al., 1973) of affected patients, the degree of deficiency in these tissues mirroring that noted in liver. Kinetic analyses of residual OTC activity have been carried out only in a few patients and have provided variable, interesting data. Levin et al. (1969b) reported that the "variant" OTC in a male with partial OTC deficiency had an abnormal pH optimum but normal affinities for carbamyl phosphate and ornithine. Matsuda and coworkers (1971) found that the mutant OTC activity in their female patient had a reduced affinity for carbamyl phosphate but a normal pH optimum and affinity for ornithine. Campbell et al. (1973) found no abnormalities in pH optimum or affinity for either substrate in the remaining, minuscule hepatic OTC activity from their male patient. These findings suggest that several different mutations of the OTC molecule may render it catalytically defective, but additional studies with purified enzyme are required to confirm this thesis.

Clinical Findings

All of the reported males with complete OTC deficiency have succumbed by 10 days of age with a reproducible clinical picture characterized by failure to feed, vomiting, lethargy, coma, seizures and respiratory alkalosis (Campbell et al., 1973). Even ingestion of tiny amounts of essential amino acids provoked clinical deterioration and a concomitant sharp rise in blood ammonia. In contrast, none of the patients with partial OTC deficiency presented during the first week of life. Their signs and symptoms, temporally well correlated with blood ammonia concentrations, also consisted of vomiting, lethargy, seizures and coma. Several of these children have died in infancy or childhood, but others are living and well provided their dietary protein is markedly restricted.

Diagnosis

The definitive diagnosis of OTC deficiency can only be made by assay of urea cycle enzymes in liver or other tissues. Since hyperammonemia is found in patients with each of the inherited defects of the urea cycle, in children with disorders of glycine, propionate and methylmalonate metabolism, as well as in patients with other forms of inherited or acquired liver disease, the blood ammonia can only be used as the initial screening test for this condition. Plasma and urinary amino acid and organic acid analyses will aid considerably in the differential diagnosis, but only a high degree of suspicion will enable the neonatologist and the pediatrician to differentiate OTC deficiency from other conditions, such as intracranial hemorrhage or sepsis, which produce vomiting, lethargy and coma in the neonatal period. The presence of orotic aciduria (MacLeod et al., 1972) is a valuable clue (see Figure 12–1).

Treatment

The report by Campbell et al. (1973) suggests that complete OTC deficiency is an absolutely lethal disorder. Their patients failed to respond to protein restriction, peritoneal dialysis, exchange transfusion or administration of neomycin or lactulose. This dreadful prognosis, however, should not be extended to patients with partial OTC deficiency, who respond very favorably to dietary protein restriction (1.0–1.5 g protein/kg/day). It is clear that the magnitude of the OTC deficiency must dictate the degree of dietary restriction, but the findings of several groups suggest that even 10 per cent of normal OTC activity is compatible with normal growth and mental development provided that dietary protein is decreased enough to prevent episodic hyperammonemia with its resultant central nervous system toxicity. Theoretically, induction of OTC activity by glucocorticoid hormones or glucagon may offer a possible lifesaving form of therapy for patients with complete or nearly complete OTC deficiency, but this form of treatment has not yet been evaluated in patients.

Genetics

In the first reported pedigree (Russell et al., 1962), each of the mothers of two affected female first cousins with partial OTC deficiency had an abnormal ammonium chloride tolerance test, while the one father studied was normal. In 1969 Levin et al. (1969a) reported a girl with partial hepatic OTC deficiency. Her mother's OTC activity was also reduced, but her father's value was normal. These results, plus the impressive preponderance of affected females with partial OTC deficiency (13/15) led to the proposal that OTC deficiency was inherited as an autosomal dominant, sex-limited trait. Recently, however, the reports of Campbell (1971), Short (1973) and their colleagues provide convincing evidence that OTC is coded for by a gene on the X chromosome. In their most telling pedigree (Fig. 12–2), these workers found a female proband with a mother and a maternal aunt with *partial* OTC deficiency; three maternal uncles and two male siblings of the proband who had died in the neonatal period, one of whom had proven *complete* deficiency of hepatic OTC activity; and a father who had normal OTC activity. In a second family three male infants died in the neonatal period with documented complete deficiency of OTC activity. Their father had normal OTC activity, but their mother had ammonia

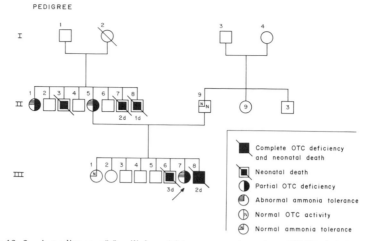

Figure 12-2   A pedigree of familial ornithine transcarbamylase (OTC) deficiency which supports the theory of X-linked dominant inheritance of this disorder. Note the neonatal male deaths in generations II and III, the documented complete OTC deficiency in a male in generation III and the partial OTC deficiency in females in generations II and III. (From Short, E. M., et al.: New Eng. J. Med. *288*:7–12, 1973.)

intolerance. Furthermore, review of published reports of partial OTC deficiency reveals several families in which male siblings or maternal uncles of affected female probands died of unexplained cause in the neonatal period. These pedigree data, plus finding the expected ratio of affected and unaffected females and males in all reported pedigrees (Short et al., 1973), provide strong support for the thesis that OTC deficiency is inherited as an X-linked dominant trait leading to lethal neonatal hyperammonemia in affected hemizygous males and partial enzyme deficiency with variable severity of hyperammonemia in affected heterozygous females. This hypothesis must be tested in other families by appropriate enzymatic and linkage analyses and by attempting to identify two clones of liver cells in presumed heterozygous females. If corroborated, knowledge of the mode of inheritance should lead to more rational genetic counseling than has been available to affected families heretofore.

HYPERORNITHINEMIA

Shih, Efron and Moser (1969) described a three-year-old boy with another apparently distinct disorder of the urea cycle in which the clinical manifestations appear to be related to hyperammonemia. The patient was the first child of unrelated, healthy parents. From early infancy he was irritable and disliked his formula. Growth and development were apparently normal until about nine months of age, when he seemed to lose interest in physical activity. At age 13 months he was hospitalized because of vomiting, constipation, screaming and apparent abdominal pain. When next seen at 16 months of age, he was unable to speak or walk and exhibited myoclonic spasms during the neurological examination. Routine laboratory tests were normal except for a slightly elevated serum glutamic-oxalacetic transaminase value. Plasma ornithine concentration was 10 to 15 times normal (12–14 mg/100 ml), and the blood ammonia was distinctly increased as well (150 μg/100 ml). Urinary amino acids were unremarkable except for prominent homocitrullinuria. On a low-protein diet (1.5 gm/kg/

day) the plasma ornithine and ammonia fell toward normal and the child's clinical course improved markedly. The metabolic basis for this syndrome is obscure. Hepatic enzyme studies have not been carried out, but serum ornithine transcarbamylase activity was repeatedly elevated, suggesting that hepatic ornithine transcarbamylase deficiency is unlikely. The homocitrullinuria, presumably of endogenous origin, is likewise unexplained. Both parents responded to oral loads of ornithine normally, and the patient's only sibling is well.

CITRULLINEMIA

Since 1962, children with citrullinemia and neurological dysfunction have been described by McMurray et al. (1963), Mohyuddin et al. (1967), Morrow (1967), Wick (1970), Scott-Emuakpor (1972), Van der Zee (1971) and their colleagues. The clinical and biochemical features of the illness in the early cases (Mohyuddin et al., 1967; Morrow, 1967) were similar, these patients presenting with mental retardation and neurologic deficit during the first year of life. In contrast, the patients described by Wick (1970), Van der Zee (1971) and their colleagues had a lethal neonatal course.

Biochemical Abnormalities

Plasma and urinary and cerebrospinal fluid concentrations of citrulline were elevated markedly in all patients. The normal daily urinary excretion of citrulline is less than 1 mg, but these patients excreted between 1.3 and 1.7 g per day. No reproducible abnormalities of other plasma or urinary amino acids were noted. Blood ammonia was not elevated during the fasting state but rose to abnormal values after a high-protein meal. The postprandial blood ammonia in the patient reported by McMurray and his associates (1963) reached nearly 1000 μg per 100 ml. Morrow found a postprandial blood ammonia of 180 to 270 μg per 100 ml.

The blood urea nitrogen was persistently normal in McMurray's patient but was low in the patient studied by Morrow. A normal blood urea nitrogen value has been observed in most patients with inherited defects of the urea cycle. This has led to considerable speculation regarding alternate pathways for urea synthesis and isozymic variants in different tissues (Efron, 1966). There are, however, two reasonable explanations for the normal blood urea nitrogen concentrations which do not depend on such new biochemical pathways: the enzymatic defects, albeit severe, may be incomplete and thus allow for the synthesis of sufficient urea to maintain the blood urea nitrogen concentration within the normal range; or the metabolic blocks may be bypassed by supplying sufficient arginine from dietary sources to sustain its hydrolysis to urea and ornithine.

The Enzymatic Defect

A defect in argininosuccinic acid synthetase activity has been found in these patients. The activity of this enzyme was reduced to less than 5 per cent of normal in a liver biopsy from the patient studied by McMurray (1963). Tedesco and Mellman (1967) cultured skin fibroblasts from Morrow's patient and from controls and studied urea synthesis in these cells. They found that argininosuccinic acid synthetase activity in the cells of the patient with citrullinemia was normal when the concentration of citrulline in the incubation mixture was high, but was much depressed when the citrulline concentration was lowered. Michaelis-Menten analysis revealed that the K_m for argininosuccinic acid synthetase in the cells from the citrullinemic patient was 25 times that of control cells, indicating that the affinity of the mutant enzyme for its substrate was markedly reduced. As anticipated from her fulminant clinical course, the liver of the patient studied by Van der Zee et al. (1971) had no detectable argininosuccinate synthetase activity.

Genetics

The patient described by McMurray and associates was the offspring of a consanguineous mating. Neither parent had citrullinemia or citrullinuria. Both parents and two sibs of the patient reported by Wick et al. (1970) had modestly elevated plasma citrulline values. The paucity of cases precludes definitive genetic analysis, but the findings to date suggest that citrullinemia is inherited as an autosomal recessive trait.

Clinical Considerations

Both patients described by McMurray et al. (1963) and Morrow (1967) appeared to do well for the first six to nine months of life and then seemed to plateau in their growth and development. Vomiting, irritability, seizures and mental deterioration appeared subsequently and led to hospitalization and diagnosis. The massive amounts of citrulline excreted in the urine made identification by chromatography relatively easy. Identification of this amino acid was confirmed by staining with Ehrlich's aldehyde reagent, which gives a yellow or pink color with citrulline. Homocitrulline may be excreted by infants ingesting an artificial milk formula but can be differentiated from citrulline easily by column chromatographic techniques.

Institution of a low-protein diet was followed by a fall in urinary citrulline and blood ammonia and by cessation of vomiting and seizures. Unfortunately, protein restriction failed to reverse the mental retardation, which was severe in both patients. Dietary arginine supplements have not influenced the biochemical findings or clinical course of the disease. Thyroid extract, known to induce argininosuccinic acid synthetase activity in developing tadpoles (Metzenberg et al., 1961), appeared to improve one of the two patients (McMurray et al., 1963) but was completely ineffective in the second. These findings suggest that patients with citrullinemia must be diagnosed in the neonatal period if dietary protein restriction is to have any chance of preventing the central nervous sequelae produced by the hyperammonemia, the elevated citrulline value, the reduced tissue concentrations of argininosuccinic acid or other still undescribed biochemical disturbances which might result from such a metabolic block. As appears to be the case with complete OTC deficiency, complete argininosuccinate synthetase deficiency probably represents an untreatable disorder.

ARGININOSUCCINICACIDURIA

Allan and his colleagues, in 1958, and Westall, in 1960, found that two severely mentally retarded siblings excreted very large amounts of argininosuccinic acid (ASA) in the urine. This urea cycle intermediate has since been found in the urine of many other patients, all but one of whom have been mentally retarded. Postprandial hyperammonemia has been demonstrated in a few of these patients, suggesting that an elevated blood ammonia may play some role in the central nervous system dysfunction in argininosuccinicaciduria, as it does in patients with citrullinemia, hyperornithinemia and deficiencies of ornithine transcarbamylase or carbamyl phosphate synthetase. A lethal, neonatal variant of this urea cycle defect has been described in two patients (Baumgartner et al., 1968; Carton et al., 1969). In vitro studies have defined the enzymatic defect and the mode of inheritance of this disorder.

Accumulation of ASA in Blood, Urine and Cerebrospinal Fluid

No traces of ASA have been found in normal plasma, urine or cerebrospinal fluid (Westall, 1955), nor has it been detected in extracts of rat liver, brain or kidney (Ratner et al., 1960). As described previously, ASA is synthesized from citrulline and aspartic acid and is broken down to arginine and fumarate (Fig. 12–1). All the patients with argininosuccinicaciduria have excreted enormous quantities of ASA in the urine (2 to 9 g per 24 hr). In addition to ASA, Westall (1960) found other unusual ninhydrin-positive compounds in the urine which were subsequently shown to represent five-membered and six-membered ring anhydrides of ASA. ASA accumulates in the plasma and cerebrospinal fluid as well. Interestingly, the concentration of ASA in cerebrospinal fluid has been two to four times that noted in plasma (Efron, 1966; Moser et al., 1967), suggesting that most, if not all, of the ASA in the spinal fluid is formed in the brain. The fasting blood ammonia concentration in these patients has been normal, but postprandial hyperammonemia (250 μg/100 ml) has been documented in three patients (Moser et al., 1967).

Determinations of other amino acids in plasma, urine and cerebrospinal fluid have yielded normal results except for distinct citrullinemia, described in two siblings by Moser and his colleagues (1967). As has been noted in other patients with primary disturbances of the urea cycle, blood urea concentrations have been normal. The accumulation of ASA (and citrulline) suggested a defect in argininosuccinate lyase activity, and subsequent in vitro observations by Tomlinson and Westall (1964) confirmed this hypothesis.

The Enzymatic Defect

As mentioned previously, argininosuccinate lyase activity is present in many tissues, including the liver and brain (Soriano et al., 1967). Tomlinson and Westall (1960) found that all regions of the brain, spinal cord and meninges had measurable lyase activity. They also demonstrated that hemolysates of circulating erythrocytes from 54 normal humans had measurable lyase activity, but they found no detectable activity of this enzyme in hemolysates from three patients with argininosuccinicaciduria. This observation was confirmed subsequently in three others affected (Moser et al., 1967; Ziter et al., 1968). Levin (1967) reported that argininosuccinate lyase activity was also absent in a liver biopsy of one patient with this disorder. Argininosuccinic acid synthetase activity was elevated in the liver of this patient, but the activity of the other urea cycle enzymes was normal. If, as these in vitro studies suggest, argininosuccinate lyase is completely or virtually completely inactive in all tissues in this disorder, the normal blood urea nitrogen can be explained by postulating either that sufficient arginine is provided in the diet to be converted to urea by the last enzyme in the cycle, arginase, or that another pathway for urea synthesis exists in man. There is no evidence for the latter thesis.

Genetics

Several findings suggest that argininosuccinicaciduria is inherited as an autosomal recessive trait: Two affected siblings have been reported in four of the eight families studied; four of the affected patients are males and seven are females; parental consanguinity has been described in one family; no instance of parent to child transmission has been recorded; and presumed carriers for the trait can be detected by urinary studies or enzymatic assays.

ASA has not been found in the urine of all obligate heterozygotes, but small amounts of this amino acid have been noted in at least four parents of affected children (Efron, 1966). In three families studied, argininosuccinate lyase activity in red cell hemolysates of both parents of affected children was significantly lower than that noted in controls but far higher than that found in their affected children (Efron, 1966; Tomlinson and Westall, 1964). These observations indicate that patients homozygous for argininosuccinate lyase deficiency excrete large amounts of ASA in the urine and develop the clinical manifestations of the disease, whereas heterozygous carriers for this enzyme defect are clinically well but may excrete very small amounts of ASA in the urine.

Signs and Symptoms

The clinical features of argininosuccinicaciduria have been reviewed recently by Efron (1966) and Moser et al. (1967). Patients have ranged in age from 4 days to 18 years. Severe mental retardation has been the clinical hallmark of the disorder. Only one of 11 patients reviewed had an IQ above 67, and most of the reported patients have required institutionalization. Seizures, ataxia and an abnormal electroencephalogram have been noted in about half the affected patients, as has trichorexis nodosa, an abnormality of the hair characterized by friability and the formation of small nodes along the hair shaft. Hepatomegaly has been described in three patients and liver function tests have been mildly abnormal in four. These clinical manifestations could be produced by the accumulation of ASA, the hyperammonemia or by arginine deficiency. The latter possibility, however, seems unlikely in the face of normal plasma and cerebrospinal fluid concentrations of arginine. The recent observations of Baumgartner (1968), Carton (1969) and their colleagues indicate that some patients with argininosuccinicaciduria have a much more severe clinical course but there is no enzymatic evidence to date which differentiates these patients from the larger group with milder manifestations.

Diagnosis

Argininosuccinicaciduria should be easy to detect because of the enormous excretion of ASA in the urine. Paper chromatography or electrophoresis may show three abnormal spots due to the presence of ASA and its two anhydrides. Since ASA is quite unstable compared to the anhydrides, quantitation of ASA may be facilitated by boiling the urine to convert ASA to its anhydride forms and then quantitating the latter by column chromatography (Armstrong et al., 1964). The diagnosis of argininosuccinicaciduria must be entertained in any patient with hyperammonemia, particularly in the younger age group.

Treatment

No successful treatment for this disorder has been defined to date. As expected, a high-protein diet or the administration of ornithine and citrulline augments the urinary excretion of ASA (Westall, 1960), and a low-protein diet reduces the excretion of this amino acid (Levin, 1967). Arginine supplements have been administered without notable success (Efron, 1966), but patients treated in this way were already severely retarded. This approach seems worth trying in infants who are diagnosed prior to the appearance of central nervous system damage. A diet containing just enough protein to sustain normal growth might be expected to control the hyperammonemia, particularly if administered in several small feedings rather than a few large ones. Effective therapy almost surely depends on diagnosis in the neonatal period, before brain injury has been produced by the metabolic disturbances so characteristic of this disease.

ARGININEMIA

Two sisters, ages 18 months and 5 years, with spastic diplegia, seizures and severe retardation were reported by Terheggen and colleagues (1969). Their parents were related by blood. Plasma and CSF concentrations of arginine in these sisters were distinctly increased, while erythrocyte arginase activity was much lower than in controls. Their parents appeared to have plasma arginine and red cell arginase values between those noted in controls and in the affected girls. Blood ammonia was increased in both patients as was urinary excretion of dibasic amino acids and cystine. Ingestion of a low-protein diet resulted in a lowering of the blood ammonia. These findings suggest that arginase deficiency is inherited as an autosomal recessive trait. The dibasicaminoaciduria and cystinuria almost surely reflect competitive inhibition of renal tubular reabsorption of lysine, ornithine and cystine by the elevated filtered load of arginine.

REFERENCES

Allan, J. K., Cusworth, D. C., Dent, C. E., and Wilson, V. K.: A disease, probably hereditary, characterised by severe mental deficiency and a gross abnormality of amino acid metabolism. Lancet (i), 182–187, 1958.

Armstrong, M. D., Yates, K. N., and Stemmermann, M. G.: An occurrence of argininosuccinic aciduria. Pediatrics *33*:280–283, 1964.

Baumgartner, R., Sheidegger, S., Stalder, G., and Hottinger, A.: Argininbernsteinsäure – Krankheit der Neugeborenen mit letalem verlauf. Helv. Pediat. Acta *23*:77–106, 1968.

Bollman, J. L., Mann, F. C., and Magath, T. B.: Studies on the physiology of the liver. VIII. Effect of total removal of the liver on the formation of urea. Amer. J. Physiol. *64*:371–392, 1924.

Brown, G. W., Jr., and Cohen, P. P.: Comparative biochemistry of urea synthesis. J. Biol. Chem. *234*:1769–1777, 1959.

Bürgi, W., Richterich, R., and Colombo, J. P.: L-Lysine dehydrogenase deficiency in a patient with congenital lysine intolerance. Nature (London) *211*:854–855, 1966.

Campbell, A. G. M., Rosenberg, L. E., Snodgrass, P. J., and Nuzum, C. T.: Lethal neonatal hyperammonemia due to complete ornithine transcarbamylase deficiency. Lancet (ii), 217, 1971.

Campbell, A. G. M., Rosenberg, L. E., Snodgrass, P. J., and Nuzum, C. T.: Ornithine transcarbamylase deficiency: A cause of lethal neonatal hyperammonemia in males. New Eng. J. Med. *288*:1–6, 1973.

Carton, D., deSchrijver, F., Kint, J., VanDurme, J., and Hooft, C.: Argininosuccinicaciduria. Neonatal variant with rapid fatal course. Acta Paediat. Scand. *58*:528–534, 1969.

Cohen, P. P., and Brown, G. W.: Ammonia metabolism and urea biosynthesis. *In* Florkin, M., and Mason, H. S., eds., Comparative Biochemistry, Vol. 2. Academic Press, New York, pp. 161–244, 1960.

Corbeel, L. M., Colombo, J. P., Van Sande, M., and Weber, A.: Periodic attacks of lethargy in a baby with ammonia intoxication due to a congenital defect in ureogenesis. Arch. Dis. Child. *44*:681–687, 1969.

Efron, M. L.: Diseases of the urea cycle. *In* Stanbury, J. B., Wyngaarden, J. B., and Fredrickson, D. S., eds., The Metabolic Basis of Inherited Disease. McGraw-Hill, New York, pp. 393–408, 1966.

Fahien, L., and Cohen, P. P.: A kinetic study of carbamyl phosphate synthetase. J. Biol. Chem. *239*:1925–1934, 1964.

Freeman, J. M., Nicholson, J. F., Schimke, R. T., Rowland, L. P., and Carter, S.: Congenital hyperammonemia: Association with hyperglycinemia and decreased levels of carbamyl phosphate synthetase. Arch. Neurol. *23*:430–437, 1970.

Gelehrter, T. D., and Snodgrass, P. J.: Lethal neonatal hyperammonemia secondary to carbamyl phosphate synthetase deficiency. (Abstract.) Annual Meeting of the American Pediatric Society, San Francisco, May 1973.

Hommes, F. A., DeGroot, C. J., Wilmink, C. W., and Jonxis, J. H. P.: Carbamylphosphate synthetase deficiency in an infant with severe cerebral damage. Arch. Dis. Child. *44*:688–693, 1969.

Hopkins, I. J., Connelly, J. F., Dawson, A. G., Hird, F. J. R., and Maddison, T. G.: Hyperammonemia due to ornithine transcarbamylase deficiency. Arch. Dis. Child. *44*:143–148, 1969.

Hsia, Y. E., and Walker, F.: Personal communication, 1973.

Joseph, R. L., Baldwin, E., and Watts, D. C.: Studies on carbamoyl phosphate-L-ornithine carbamoyltransferase from ox liver. Biochem. J. *87*:409–416, 1963.

Kekkomaki, M., Visakorpi, J. K., Perheentupa, J., and Saxen, L.: Familial protein intolerance with deficient transport of basic amino acids. An analysis of ten patients. Acta Paediat. Scand. *56*:617–630, 1967.

Kennan, A. L., and Cohen, P. P.: Ammonia detoxication in liver from humans. Proc. Soc. Exp. Biol. Med. *106*:170–173, 1961.

Krebs, H. A., and Henseleit, K.: Untersuchungen über die Harnstoffbildung in tierkörper. Z. Physiol. Chem. *210*:33–66, 1932.

Levin, B.: Argininosuccinic aciduria. Amer. J. Dis. Child. *113*:162–165, 1967.

Levin, B., Abraham, J. M., Oberholzer, V. G., and Burgess, E. A.: Hyperammonemia: A deficiency of liver ornithine transcarbamylase. Occurrence in mother and child. Arch. Dis. Child. *44*: 152–161, 1969a.

Levin, B., Dobbs, R. H., Burgess, E. A., and Palmer, T.: Hyperammonemia. A variant type of deficiency of liver ornithine transcarbamylase. Arch. Dis. Child. *44*:162–169, 1969b.

Levin, B., and Russell, A.: Treatment of hyperammonemia. Amer. J. Dis. Child. *113*:142–145, 1967.

MacLeod, P., Mackenzie, S., and Scriver, C. R.: Partial ornithine carbamyl transferase deficiency: An inborn error of the urea cycle presenting as orotic aciduria in a male infant. Canad. Med. Ass. J. *107*:405–408, 1972.

Marshall, M., and Cohen, P. P.: Ornithine transcarbamylase from streptococcus faecolis and bovine liver. I. Isolation and subunit structure. J. Biol. Chem. *247*:1641–1653, 1972.

Marshall, M., Metzenberg, R. L., and Cohen, P. P.: Physical and kinetic properties of carbamyl phosphate synthetase from frog liver. J. Biol. Chem. *236*:2229–2237, 1961.

Matsuda, I., Arashima, S., Nambu, J., Takekoshi, Y., Anakura, M.: Hyperammonemia due to a mutant enzyme of ornithine transcarbamylase. Pediatrics *48*:595–600, 1971.

McCormick, D. B., and Snell, E. E.: Pyridoxal phosphokinase. II. Effects of inhibitors. J. Biol. Chem. *236*:2085–2088, 1961.

McMurray, W. C., Rathbun, J. C., Mohyuddin, F., and Koegler, S. J.: Citrullinuria. Pediatrics *32*:347–357, 1963.

Metzenberg, R. L., Marshall, M., Paik, W. K., and Cohen, P. P.: The synthesis of carbamyl phosphate synthetase in thyroxin-treated tadpoles. J. Biol. Chem. *236*:162–165, 1961.

Mohyuddin, F., Rathbun, J. C., and McMurray, W. C.: Studies on amino acid metabolism in citrullinuria. Amer. J. Dis. Child. *113*:152–156, 1967.

Morrow, G.: Citrullinemia. Amer. J. Dis. Child. *113*:157–159, 1967.

Moser, H. W., Efron, M. L., Brown, H., Diamond, R., and Neumann, C. G.: Argininosuccinicaciduria: Report of two new cases and demonstration of intermittent elevation of blood ammonia. Amer. J. Med. *42*:9–26, 1967.

Nagayama, E., Kitayama, T., Oguchi, H., Ogata, K., Tamura, E., and Onisawa, J.: Hyperammonemia: A deficiency of liver ornithine transcarbamylase. Pediatria Univ. Tokyo *18*:167–173, 1970.

Perheentupa, J., and Visakorpi, J. K.: Protein intolerance with deficient transport of basic amino acids: Another inborn error of metabolism. Lancet (ii), 813–816, 1965.

Ratner, S., Anslow, W. P., Jr., and Petrack, B.: Biosynthesis of urea. VI. Enzymatic cleavage of argininosuccinic acid to arginin and fumaric acid. J. Biol. Chem. *204*:115–125, 1953a.

Ratner, S., Morell, H., and Carvalho, E.: Enzymes of arginine metabolism in brain. Arch. Biochem. Biophys. *91*:280–289, 1960.

Ratner, S., and Petrack, B.: The mechanism of arginine synthesis from citrulline in kidney. J. Biol. Chem. *200*:175–185, 1953.

Ratner, S., Petrack, B., and Rochovansky, O.: Biosynthesis of urea. V. Isolation and properties of argininosuccinic acid. J. Biol. Chem. *204*:95–113, 1953b.

Reichard, H.: Ornithine carbamyl transferase activity in human tissue homogenates. J. Lab. Clin. Med. *56*:218–221, 1960.

Russell, A., Levin, B., Oberholzer, V. G., and Sinclair, L.: Hyperammonaemia. A new instance of an inborn enzymatic defect of the biosynthesis of urea. Lancet (ii), 699–700, 1962.

Schoenheimer, R.: The Dynamic State of Body Constituents. Harvard University Press, Cambridge, Mass., 1942.

Scott-Emuakpor, A., Higgins, J. V., and Kohrman, A. F.: Citrullinemia: A new case with implications concerning adaptation to defective urea synthesis. Pediat. Res. *6*:626–633, 1972.

Shih, V. E., Efron, M. L., and Moser, H. W.: Hyperornithinemia and homocitrullinuria with ammonia intoxication, myoclonic seizures and mental retardation. Amer. J. Dis. Child. *117*: 83–92, 1969.

Short, E. M., Conn, H. O., Snodgrass, P. J., Campbell, A. G. M., and Rosenberg, L. E.: Evidence for X-linked dominant inheritance of ornithine transcarbamylase deficiency. New Eng. J. Med. *288*:7–12, 1973.

Soriano, J. R., Teitz, L. S., Finberg, L., and Edelmann, C. M., Jr.: Hyperglycinemia with ketoacidosis and leukopenia. Pediatrics *39*:818–828, 1967.

Sporn, M. B., Dingman, W., Defalco, A., and Davies, R. K.: The synthesis of urea in the living rat brain. J. Neurochem. *6*:62–67, 1959.

Sunshine, P., Lindenbaum, J. E., and Levy, H. L.: Hyperammonemia due to a defect in hepatic ornithine transcarbamylase. Pediatrics, *50*:100–111, 1972.

Tedesco, T. A., and Mellman, W. J.: Argininosuccinate synthetase activity and citrulline metabolism in cells cultured from a citrullinemic subject. Proc. Nat. Acad. Sci. U.S.A. *57*:829–834, 1967.

Terheggen, H. G., Schwenk, A., Lowenthal, A., Van Sande, M., and Colombo, J. P.: Argininemia with arginase deficiency. Lancet (ii), 748–749, 1969.

Tomlinson, S., and Westall, R. G.: Argininosuccinic aciduria, argininosuccinase and arginase in human blood cells. Clin. Sci. *26*:261–269, 1964.

Tomlinson, S., and Westall, R. G.: Argininosuccinase activity in brain tissue. Nature (London) *188*:235–236, 1960.

Van der Zee, S. P. M., Trijbels, J. M. F., Monnens, L. A. H., Hommes, F. A., and Schretlen, E. D. A. M.: Citrullinemia with rapidly fatal neonatal course. Arch. Dis. Child. *46*:847–851, 1971.

Wada, Y., Tada, K., Takada, G., Omura, K., Yoshida, T., Kuniya, T., Auyama, T., Hakui, T., and Harada, S.: Hyperglycinemia associated with hyperammonemia: in vitro glycine cleavage in liver. Pediat. Res. *6*:622–625, 1972.

Westall, R. G.: Argininosuccinic aciduria: Identification and reactions of the abnormal metabolite in a newly described form of mental disease, with some preliminary metabolic studies. Biochem. J. *77*:135–144, 1960.

Westall, R. G.: The amino acids and other ampholytes of urine. Biochem. J. *60*:247–255, 1955.

Wick, H., Brechbuhler, T., and Girard, J.: Citrullinemia: Elevated serum citrulline levels in healthy siblings. Experientia *26*:823–824, 1970.

Ziter, F. A., Bray, P. F., Madsen, J. A., and Nyhan, W. L.: The clinical findings in a patient with nonketotic hyperglycinemia. Pediat. Res. *2*:250–253, 1968.

Chapter Thirteen

LYSINE

Lysine is an essential, dibasic amino acid in man. Its metabolism is unique in that it is the only amino acid which cannot be reaminated from the cellular ammonia pool (Schoenheimer and Rittenberg, 1940). The catabolic pathways for lysine are less well defined than those for most other amino acids, despite its importance in many human diseases. Defects in renal and intestinal transport of lysine exist in cystinuria, in the syndrome of familial protein intolerance and in dibasicaminoaciduria. In recent years several patients have been described with markedly increased concentrations of lysine in the blood and urine. Clinical and biochemical data indicate that at least two different mutations underlie these abnormalities in lysine metabolism, but our understanding of these disorders is far from complete.

INTERMEDIARY METABOLISM OF LYSINE

Current evidence suggests that lysine is catabolized via several routes in mammalian organisms (Fig. 13–1). Lysine is converted to homocitrulline and homoarginine by rats and humans (Ryan and Wells, 1964), but the enzymatic steps involved are unknown, and these compounds appear to be quantitatively unimportant in lysine catabolism. Paik and Benoiten (1963) isolated ϵ-lysine acylase from rat and hog kidney and demonstrated its ability to deacetylate α-keto-ϵ-acetamidocaproic acid, a derivative of ϵ-N-acetyl lysine. These workers proposed that the latter compound may be the first metabolite in the pathway of lysine catabolism, which leads to pipecolic acid and ultimately to α-amino-adipic-δ-semialdehyde. Subsequent to the demonstration that saccharopine (ϵ-N-(L-glutaryl-2)-L-lysine) is a precursor of lysine biosynthesis in yeast (Darling and Olesen-Larsen, 1968), Higashino et al. (1965) showed that rat liver mitochondria catalyzed the condensation of lysine and α-ketoglutarate to saccharopine. No other cellular organelles appeared to support this reaction. These workers proposed that a major pathway for lysine catabolism involved the formation of saccharopine, which is then cleaved to α-aminoadipic-δ-semialdehyde. Subsequent studies by Ghadimi and Zischka (1967) and Hutzler and Dancis (1968) confirmed this impression in human tissues. The oxidation of

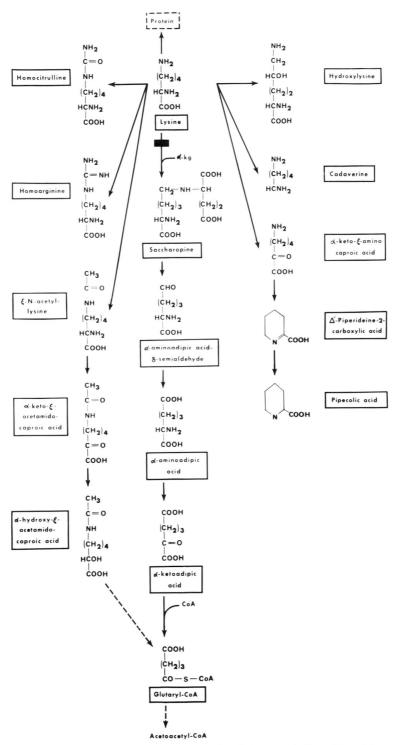

Figure 13–1 Metabolic pathways of mammalian lysine metabolism. Dotted lines represent intermediate or undefined steps in reaction sequence. Block between lysine and saccharopine denotes site of enzymatic defect (lysine:α-ketoglutarate reductase) responsible for one form of persistent hyperlysinemia.

α-aminoadipic-δ-semialdehyde to α-aminoadipic acid followed by deamination to α-ketoadipic acid has previously been described in mammalian tissues (Borsook et al., 1948). Ultimately, the complete degradation of lysine yields acetyl-CoA.

THE HYPERLYSINEMIAS

Since 1963 several patients have been described with moderately or markedly elevated concentrations of lysine in plasma (Ghadimi, 1972). The clinical and biochemical abnormalities in these patients have varied greatly and there is no convincing evidence that the hyperlysinemia is responsible for any pathophysiological disturbance. In one group of patients, hyperammonemia accompanies the hyperlysinemia. In the other group, this does not appear to be the case.

Periodic Hyperlysinemia and Hyperammonemia

In 1964 Colombo and his colleagues described a three-month-old girl with neonatal vomiting, seizures and episodic coma. Blood ammonia was only slightly increased on a low-protein diet (1.5 g/kg/day), and she did well on this restricted formula. However, when dietary protein was increased to 3 g/kg/day, hyperammonemia (500 to 600 μg/100 ml), hyperlysinemia (6.8 mg/100 ml) and hyperargininemia (6.2 mg/100 ml) were noted. Urinary lysine was also increased, but no other metabolites of lysine were described in blood or urine. The activities of all the urea cycle enzymes in a liver biopsy from this patient were normal, suggesting that a defect in lysine metabolism might be the primary metabolic derangement. This thesis was supported by in vivo and in vitro observations. An oral load of lysine was followed by distinct hyperammonemia and only a slow rise in blood urea nitrogen. Since lysine is a potent competitive inhibitor of arginase, these findings suggested that the elevated plasma lysine concentration found after a high-protein meal or lysine loading inhibited arginase activity and thus produced both hyperammonemia and impaired urea synthesis. Hyperammonemia has not been detected in several other patients whose plasma lysine concentrations were distinctly higher than those noted in this patient, suggesting that other mechanisms may contribute to the hyperammonemia. In a liver biopsy from this patient, the activity of L-lysine dehydrogenase, an enzyme which converts lysine to α-keto-ε-aminocaproic acid, was reduced to about 25 per cent of that found in control samples (Bürgi et al., 1966).

Persistent Hyperlysinemia

Since 1964 six patients with idiopathic hyperlysinemia have been reported by Ghadimi (1965), Woody (1964, 1966, 1967), Armstrong (1967) and their colleagues. Elevated plasma and urinary concentrations of lysine have been the only consistent features among these patients, who almost surely suffer from several different metabolic disorders.

Both patients studied by Ghadimi (males age 26 and two years) were severely mentally retarded and had muscular hypotonia and lax ligaments. Their plasma lysine concentrations ranged from 4 to 8 mg per 100 ml (two to four times normal). Cerebrospinal fluid concentrations of lysine were increased in both patients, as was urinary lysine. After oral lysine loads, plasma lysine rose far more than in controls and remained elevated for much longer intervals. One of these patients was given lysine-^{14}C intravenously, after which collections were made of his expired air, blood and urine. $^{14}CO_2$ evolution by the patient did not differ significantly from that observed in two controls. Homoarginine and homocitrulline were found in the urine of both patients, but pipecolic acid was not demonstrated despite repeated attempts to identify this proposed intermediate. These studies indicated a defect in lysine catabolism but failed to define the blocked pathway. One of these patients was the product of a father-daughter mating.

Mental retardation was observed in one of three affected girls in a single family studied by Woody. However, a sibling and cousin with hyperlysinemia were clinically well, suggesting that the hyperlysinemia was not responsible for the mental retardation in this patient. Plasma lysine concentrations in all three affected patients were distinctly higher than those reported by Ghadimi (10 to 22 mg per 100 ml). In addition to exhibiting hyperlysinuria, these patients excreted excessive amounts of ornithine, ethanolamine and α-aminobutyric acid in the urine, but the mechanism for this aminoaciduria was not defined. Two of these patients were given lysine-^{14}C parenterally, and their response was distinctly different from controls. Less than 1 per cent of the administered lysine was found as $^{14}CO_2$ in the expired air after six hours, while controls excreted 5 to 8 per cent of lysine-^{14}C as $^{14}CO_2$. These differences were not due to dilution of the labeled precursor in an enlarged lysine pool. Pipecolic acid, α-aminoadipic acid, homoarginine, homocitrulline and ϵ-N-acetyl lysine were present in the urine of all three patients, suggesting that several of the known catabolic pathways for lysine were open. Dancis et al. (1969) found that the activity of lysine: α-ketoglutarate reductase, the enzyme responsible for catalyzing saccharopine formation, was markedly reduced in fibroblast extracts from two of these patients. The occurrence of the same metabolic abnormality in three members of the same family and the presence of consanguinity among the parents of the affected sibs suggests that this reductase defect is inherited as a recessive trait and that it is the primary aberration which leads to the observed hyperlysinemia. These results also demonstrate that the pathway by which saccharopine is formed from lysine is a major one in man.

Hyperlysinemia with Saccharopinuria

During the routine screening of mentally retarded persons in Ireland, Carson and colleagues (1968) described a 22-year-old girl of short stature who excreted large quantities of lysine and citrulline. Homocitrulline and α-aminoadipic acid were also present in the urine. Serum concentrations of lysine and citrulline were four to five times normal. Of special interest, saccharopine was detected in both the urine and the serum of this patient. As noted in Figure 13-1, saccharopinuria could result from a block in the catabolism of this intermediate or from augmentation of its synthesis due to a block in some pathway of lysine degradation. The elevated concentrations of citrulline as well as lysine are of interest but are unexplained. Enzymatic studies in this patient and others with hyperlysinemia will be awaited with interest.

HYDROXYLYSINEMIA AND HYDROXYLYSINURIA

The δ-hydroxylated amino acid hydroxylysine is found in mammals almost exclusively in collagen (Hamilton and Anderson, 1955) and collagen-like proteins (Spiro, 1967). Peptide-bound hydroxyline is not incorporated into these proteins as such but rather derives from the hydroxylation of already incorporated lysine residues (Diez and Likins, 1957; Sinex et al., 1959). The hydroxylysine released during the turnover of collagen and collagen-like proteins cannot be incorporated into other protein molecules. Most of it appears to be excreted in the urine in the form of small hydroxylysyl-glycosides, the quantity of such peptides mirroring the rate of collagen turnover as does the excretion of hydroxyprolyl-peptides (Segrest and Cunningham, 1970). Free hydroxyproline is barely detectable in normal human plasma and is found in only trace amounts in normal urine.

There is evidence in the rat and monkey that free hydroxylysine is phosphorylated to O-phosphohydroxylysine, this reaction being catalyzed by a GTP-requiring kinase (Hiles et al., 1970; Hiles and Henderson, 1972). O-phosphohydroxylysine is then converted to α-aminoadipic acid by a phospholyase enzyme. This phospholyase has also been noted in human liver, suggesting that a similar metabolic pathway for hydroxylysine metabolism may exist in man.

Since 1969, free hydroxylysinemia or hydroxylysinuria or both have been noted in six patients. Benson et al. (1969) described a severely retarded brother and sister who excreted 10 to 12 mg of free hydroxylysine per 24 hour urine. A year later, Parker et al. (1970) and Hoefnagel and Pomeroy (1970) described three additional retarded children with hydroxylysinuria, and the sixth affected patient has recently been reported by Goodman and his colleagues (1972). The amount of urinary hydroxylysine has varied widely between patients (10 to 80 mg/g creatinine). Hydroxylysine has been found in the serum of two of these patients (Parker et al., 1970; Goodman et al., 1972) but not in the other four. Peptide-bound hydroxylysine excretion has been normal in all patients in whom it was measured.

The basis for this metabolic disturbance is unclear. Goodman et al. (1972) noted delayed plasma disappearance of hydroxylysine after an oral load of this compound and suggested that this finding plus the hydroxylysinemia were best explained by a defect in free hydroxylysine degradation. No in vitro studies of the nature of this proposed defect have been forthcoming as yet.

Even though all of the reported patients have been severely mentally retarded, we cannot conclude that the hydroxylysinemia and central nervous system disease are causally related, for these patients have been identified by screening retarded children for abnormal metabolites. It should be noted in this regard that two other siblings of the first reported affected patients were also severely retarded but had *no* detectable hydroxylysine in blood or urine. Surveys of unselected neonates and children will surely provide an answer to this question.

REFERENCES

Armstrong, M. D., and Robinow, M.: A case of hyperlysinemia: biochemical and clinical observations. Pediatrics *39*:546–554, 1967.
Benson, P. F., Swift, P. N., and Young, V. K.: Hydroxylysinuria. (Abstract.) Arch. Dis. Child. *44*:134–135, 1969.
Borsook, H., Deasy, C. L., Haagen-Smit, A. J., Keighley, G., and Lowy, P. H.: α-Aminoadipic acid: A product of lysine metabolism. J. Biol. Chem. *173*:423–424, 1948.
Bürgi, W., Richterich, R., and Colombo, J. P.: L-Lysine dehydrogenase deficiency in a patient with congenital lysine intolerance. Nature (London) *211*:854–855, 1966.
Carson, N. A. J., Scally, B. G., Neill, D. W., and Carre, I. J.: Saccharopinuria: A new inborn error of lysine metabolism. Nature (London) *218*:679, 1968.
Colombo, J. P., Richterich, R., Donath, A., Spahr, A., and Rossi, E.: Congenital lysine intolerance with periodic ammonia intoxication. Lancet (i), 1014–1015, 1964.
Dancis, J., Hutzler, J., Cox, R. P., and Woody, N. L.: Familial hyperlysinemia with lysine-ketoglutarate reductase deficiency. J. Clin. Invest. *48*:1447–1452, 1969.

Darling, S., and Olesen-Larsen, P.: Saccharopine, a new amino acid in baker's and brewer's yeast. Acta Chem. Scand. *15*:743–749, 750–759, 1968.

Ghadimi, H.: The hyperlysinemias. *In* Stanbury, J. B., Wyngaarden, J. B., and Fredrickson, D. S., eds., The Metabolic Basis of Inherited Disease, 3rd edition. McGraw-Hill, New York, pp. 393–403, 1972.

Ghadimi, H., Binnington, V. I., and Pecora, P.: Hyperlysinemia associated with retardation. New Eng. J. Med. *273*:723–729, 1965.

Ghadimi, H., and Zischka, R.: Hyperlysinemia and lysine metabolism. *In* Nyhan, W. L., ed., Amino Acid Metabolism and Genetic Variation. McGraw-Hill, New York, p. 227, 1967.

Goodman, S. I., Browder, J. A., Hiles, R. A., and Miles, B. S.: Hydroxylysinemia—a disorder due to a defect in the metabolism of free hydroxylysine. Biochem. Med. *6*:344–354, 1972.

Hamilton, P. B., and Anderson, R. A.: Hydroxylysine in proteins. J. Amer. Chem. Soc. *77*:2892–2893, 1955.

Higashino, K., Tsukada, K., and Lieberman, I.: Saccharopine, a product of lysine breakdown by mammalian liver. Biochem. Biophys. Res. Commun. *20*:285–290, 1965.

Hiles, R. A., and Henderson, L. M.: The partial purification and properties of hydroxylysine kinase from rat liver. J. Biol. Chem. *247*:646–651, 1972.

Hiles, R. A., Triebwasser, K. C., and Henderson, L. M.: The degradation of hydroxy-L-lysine in liver via its phosphate ester. Biochem. Biophys. Res. Commun. *41*:662–668, 1970.

Hoefnagel, D., and Pomeroy, J.: Hydroxylysinuria. Lancet (i), 1342–1343, 1970.

Hutzler, J., and Dancis, J.: Conversion of lysine to saccharopine by human tissues. Biochim. Biophys. Acta *158*:62–69, 1968.

Paik, W. K., and Benoiten, L.: Purification and properties of hog kidney ε-lysine acylase. Canad. J. Biochem. *41*:1643–1654, 1963.

Parker, C. E., Shaw, K. N. F., Jacobs, E. E., and Butenstein, M.: Hydroxylysinuria. Lancet (i), 1119–1120, 1970.

Piez, K. A., and Likins, R. C.: The conversion of lysine to hydroxylysine and its relation to the biosynthesis of collagen in several tissues of the rat. J. Biol. Chem. *299*:101–109, 1957.

Ryan, W. L., and Wells, I. C.: Homocitrulline and monoarginine synthesis from lysine. Science *144*:1122–1127, 1964.

Schoenheimer, R., and Rittenberg, D.: The study of intermediary metabolism of animals with the aid of isotopes. Physiol. Rev. *20*:218–248, 1940.

Segrest, J. P., and Cunningham, L. W.: Variations in human urinary O-hydroxylysyl glycoside levels and their relationship to collagen metabolism. J. Clin. Invest. *49*:1497–1509, 1970.

Sinex, F. M., Van Slyke, D. D., and Christman, D. R.: The source and state of the hydroxylysine of collagen. II. Failure of free hydroxylysine to serve as a source of the hydroxylysine or lysine of collagen. J. Biol. Chem. *234*:918–921, 1959.

Spiro, R. G.: Studies on the renal glomerular basement membrane. J. Biol. Chem. *242*:1915–1922, 1967.

Woody, N. C.: Hyperlysinemia. Amer. J. Dis. Child. *108*:543–553, 1964.

Woody, N. C., Hutzler, J., and Dancis, J.: Further studies of hyperlysinemia. Amer. J. Dis. Child. *112*:577–580, 1966.

Woody, N. C., and Ong, E. B.: Paths of lysine degradation in patients with hyperlysinemia. Pediatrics *40*:986–992, 1967.

Chapter Fourteen

BRANCHED-CHAIN AMINO ACIDS

Irreversible steps in their degradative metabolism make the branched-chain compounds (leucine, isoleucine and valine) essential amino acids. All three amino acids are oxidized by similar steps initially, after which they form three series of interesting organic acids. Not all the carbon atoms of the branched-chain amino acids enter the tricarboxylic acid cycle, since some are lost as CO_2 during catabolism. New carbons are also taken in by CO_2 fixation. Eventually, leucine yields one molecule each of acetoacetyl-CoA and acetyl-CoA; isoleucine yields one molecule each of acetyl-CoA and succinyl-CoA (via propionyl-CoA); and valine yields succinyl-CoA via methylmalonyl-CoA. The isomerization of methylmalonyl-CoA to succinyl-CoA requires vitamin B_{12}.

There are at least 14 disorders of the various steps in branched-chain amino acid oxidation (Fig. 14–1). Those which involve reactions prior to oxidative decarboxylation cause accumulation of the ninhydrin-positive free amino acid and may be detected by amino acid analytical methods. Those affecting later steps of oxidation require special methods of detection, of which gas chromatography has proved to be the most useful.

METABOLIC SCHEME OF BRANCHED-CHAIN AMINO ACID CATABOLISM

Branched-chain amino acids are so designated because each contains a methyl group divergent from the main aliphatic carbon chain. The degradative metabolism of these three amino acids is complex. Only after loss of their amino

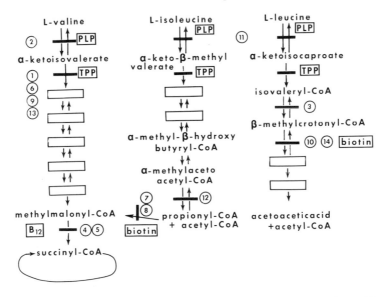

Figure 14–1   The sites of the known disorders of branched-chain amino acid metabolism in man. The circled numbers indicate the chronological order in which the diseases were reported in the literature; the first was reported in 1959.

Heavy black bars indicate the proposed sites of the defects. Compounds accumulating behind the block in catabolism are named in the boxes. Empty boxes indicate the other steps of branched-chain amino acid catabolism not yet known to be affected by an inborn error of metabolism.

The 14 known diseases are as follows: *1, 6, 9* and *13*, four different types of maple syrup urine disease; *2*, hypervalinemia; *3*, isovalericacidemia; *4* and *5*, B_{12}-unresponsive and B_{12}-responsive methylmalonicaciduria (the latter is further subdivided into two different traits responsive to B_{12}); *7* and *8*, propionicacidemia (formerly "ketotic hyperglycinemia"), of which there are biotin-responsive and biotin-unresponsive types; *10* and *14*, β-methylcrotonicaciduria of biotin-responsive and biotin-unresponsive forms; *11*, hyperleucine-isoleucinemia, a disease of transamination; *12*, α-methylacetoaceticaciduria.

Each of these diseases is discussed in the appropriate section of this chapter.

and carboxyl groups are the resulting acylcoenzyme-A compounds modified to short-chain fragments, which serve either energy metabolism or metabolic syntheses. Loss of the amino group in the first step of catabolism (Fig. 14–2) is accomplished by transamination (Coon, 1955). The amino group is transferred to α-ketoglutarate when the respective keto acids are formed (Meister, 1955); pyridoxal phosphate is the coenzyme for the transamination reaction. A certain degree of substrate specificity has been claimed for the branched-chain amino transferases (Aki et al., 1967); this proposal gains added support from the existence of two different disorders of branched-chain transamination (Fig. 14–2), one of which affects the 6-carbon compounds, and the other, the 5-carbon amino acid.

Alloisoleucine has been found in human plasma and urine (Norton et al., 1962). Alloisoleucine has two asymmetric carbons (Fig. 14–3) and consequently

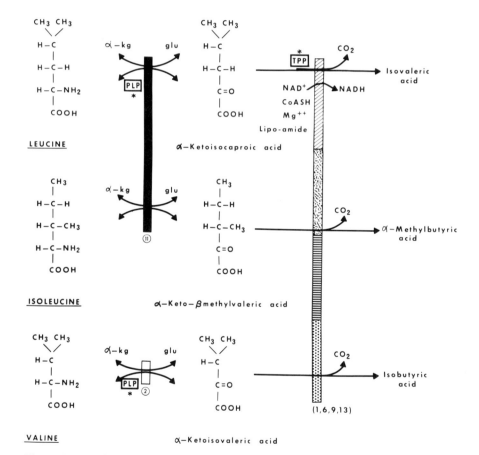

Figure 14–2 The initial steps in branched-chain amino acid catabolism. The first involves transamination to form the keto acid analogue. There are apparently two transamination functions, one serving the two 6-carbon amino acids and the other the 5-carbon amino acids. Oxidative decarboxylation of the keto acid occurs at the second step. This reaction is irreversible in man, so that the keto acid and amino acid analogues are then essential nutrients. At least two decarboxylase functions have been identified serving the 6-carbon keto acids and the 5-carbon substrate. Coenzyme and cofactors for the transamination and decarboxylation reactions are indicated in the diagram. The different types of shading for the bars indicate that six different enzyme deficiencies, each probably inherited, are known to affect the first two steps of branched-chain amino acid catabolism (see also Figure 14–1).

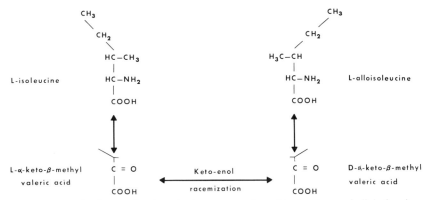

Figure 14–3   A scheme showing the interconversion of isoleucine and alloisoleucine.

has two pairs of stereoisomers. Racemization of α-keto-β-methylvaleric acid can explain the in vivo formation of alloisoleucine; the natural substance has the L-configuration with inversion at the β-carbon (Halpern and Pollock, 1970).

Alloisoleucine appears in plasma after injection of L-isoleucine into subjects in whom branched-chain keto acid oxidation is blocked. The plasma concentration of alloisoleucine is directly proportional to that of isoleucine when a threshold concentration of the latter has been achieved (Fig. 14–4). The un-

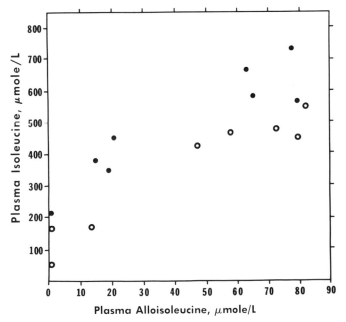

Figure 14–4   The relationship of alloisoleucine to isoleucine in the plasma of a patient with impaired branched-chain keto acid oxidation (maple syrup urine disease, thiamine-responsive variant [Scriver et al., 1971]). The normal isoleucine concentration is <62 μM/L; alloisoleucine is formed when the plasma isoleucine is about three times above normal. Both substances accumulate because the isomers of α-keto-β-methylvalerate (see Figure 14–3) accumulate and form the corresponding amino acid by reverse transamination. Open circles on figure indicate A.M. samples; closed circles are P.M. samples. A circadian variation of branched-chain amino acid concentration in plasma is apparent.

usual amino acid persists in the fluids of the body for many days, indicating that its reverse transamination is probably very slow and that its renal tubular absorption is very efficient.

Oxidative decarboxylation of the keto acids is believed to be accomplished by a very complex reaction (Goedde and Keller, 1967; Connelly et al., 1968; Bowden and Connelly, 1968). A multienzyme complex (Fig. 14–5) analogous to the dehydrogenases for pyruvic and α-ketoglutaric acids (Reed and Cox, 1966) is believed to carry out a similar reaction for oxidation of branched-chain keto acids (Goedde and Keller, 1967). Three different apoenzymes are apparently involved. First, an "active acetaldehyde" is formed when the keto acid is decarboxylated by a reaction between the substrate and thiamine pyrophosphate; this is catalyzed by a thiamine-dependent decarboxylase (E.C. 1.2.4.1). Second, the active acetaldehyde is converted to acetyldihydrolipoic acid and acetyl-CoA by the enzyme lipoate reductase transacetylase (E.C. 1.2.4.2). Finally, the enzyme lipoamide oxidoreductase (E.C. 1.6.4.3) reoxidizes reduced lipoate in the presence of NAD^+. If the system for branched-chain keto acid decarboxylation and oxidation is comparable to pyruvate oxidase, it will be a three-dimensional structure comprising 16 decarboxylase units, 64 lipoate reductase transacetylase components, and 8 lipoamide oxidoreductases; the latter components form the core of the polyhedron (Fernandez-Moran et al., 1964).

It was initially assumed that the oxidative decarboxylation system for branched-chain amino acids was common to its three substrates, thus explaining the accumulation of all three keto acids in a defect of oxidative decarboxylation such as maple syrup urine disease (Dancis, 1971). This view has been questioned, and there is now considerable evidence against a "unitarian" concept. Goedde and Keller (1967) found evidence for substrate specificity, specific pH optima, distinctive coenzyme utilization and important qualitative differences in the modes of inhibition when the "common" enzyme was exposed to the three substrates. The differences observed with the three substrates were sufficient to convince the German team that more than one, and perhaps three, oxidative decarboxylation reactions served the conversion of the three branched-chain keto acids. Connelly, Danner and Bowden (1968) and Bowden and Con-

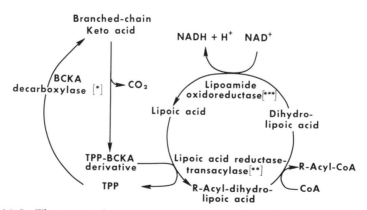

Figure 14–5   The proposed sequence of reactions for the oxidation of branched-chain keto acids to the corresponding acyl-CoA derivative, by a multienzyme complex analogous to the pyruvate oxidase system (Reed and Cox, 1966). Three enzymes are believed to be involved: one responsible for decarboxylation [*]; a second with transacylating activity [**]; and a third responsible for regeneration of lipoic acid [***]. (Modified from Goedde, H. W., and Keller, W.: *In* Nyhan, W. L., ed., Amino Acid Metabolism and Genetic Variation. McGraw-Hill, New York, p. 194, 1967.)

nelly (1968) studied a soluble dehydrogenase complex from bovine liver which oxidatively decarboxylated the two 6-carbon acids α-ketoisocaproate and α-keto-β-methylvalerate. Upon isolation and partial purification of the enzyme complex, these authors were able to show that two enzymes with considerable substrate specificity must perform decarboxylation of the three branched-chain keto acids. One semispecific enzyme complex converted the two 6-carbon acids, but, since this enzyme was not active toward the 5-carbon substrate (α-keto-isovalerate), another enzyme must be required for its oxidation.

Transamination and oxidative decarboxylation reactions for branched-chain amino acids were first studied in human leukocytes by Dancis, Hutzler and Levitz (1960, 1963b) and in cultured skin fibroblasts by Dancis, Jansen, Hutzler and Levitz (1963). Dancis, Hutzler and Cox (1969) demonstrated clearly that the mutation in maple syrup urine disease affects all three decarboxylation reactions in cultured fibroblasts. This rules out the possibility that the keto acid for one type of decarboxylase accumulates and inhibits the other type(s) of decarboxylase. The mutant allele perhaps expresses itself in a gene product common to the different branched-chain keto acid decarboxylases.

The steps in branched-chain amino acid oxidation after decarboxylation were of interest primarily to biochemists (Meister, 1965) until a number of "new" diseases of these catabolic pathways came to the attention of physicians and investigators. New technology, such as gas chromatography, helped to document these disorders, which often presented under the guise of severe metabolic acidosis. The generic term "organic acidoses" has become popular to classify this group of conditions.

For the purpose of discussion, we have grouped these inborn errors of metabolism into two sections. The first includes disorders which affect branched-chain amino acid oxidation prior to decarboxylation; accumulation of the free amino acid occurs in this group. The second group comprises diseases of oxidation of the carbon chain in which there is no diagnostic accumulation of amino acid, because the defect lies after the irreversible decarboxylation step. The latter group is subdivided into the diseases involving the common pathway propionate→methylmalonate→succinate and the diseases involving the earlier steps in oxidation of all three branched-chain organic acids.

DISORDERS OF BRANCHED-CHAIN AMINO ACID OXIDATION CAUSING ACCUMULATION OF FREE AMINO ACID

There are several diseases in which the oxidation of branched-chain amino acids is blocked at or prior to the oxidative decarboxylation step (Fig. 14–2). If it is the transaminase which is deficient, free amino acid alone will accumulate; if the decarboxylase is defective, the keto acid analogue may revert to the amino acid by reverse transamination, and both metabolites will accumulate. Consequently, these disorders of branched-chain amino acid metabolism may be identified by simple partition chromatography and a ninhydrin location reagent. All of the diseases described in the following section were initially discovered by such simple screening techniques.

Disorders of Transamination

Hypervalinemia

A single Japanese infant with hypervalinemia has been described by Wada and coworkers (1963). The infant was discovered at two months of age with symptoms of vomiting, lethargy and failure to thrive which began soon after birth. Retardation of mental and motor development and nystagmus were observed. The patient did *not* have an unusual odor.

The concentration of valine, but not of other amino acids, was increased in urine and in plasma; there was no excess of α-ketoisovalerate in the patient's urine. These findings were sufficient to suspect the diagnosis of defective valine transamination.

L-Valine is metabolized poorly in this condition (Wada, 1965), whereas the corresponding keto acid is cleared from plasma normally. No abnormality is found when branched-chain oxidation is challenged with leucine or isoleucine. During valine loading in the patient, the EEG tracing became abnormal, suggesting that valine accumulation is the "toxic" event, and that defective valine transamination initiates the clinical phenotype.

Dancis, Hutzler, Tada et al. (1967) identified a defect in valine transamination in the peripheral leukocytes of the patient, while transamination of leucine, isoleucine, methionine and phenylalanine were all normal. This finding implies that there is substrate specificity in branched-chain amino acid transamination. On the other hand, Aki and colleagues (1967) and Taylor and Jenkins (1968) believe that a single amino transferase serves the branched-chain amino acids. The genetic evidence suggests either that more than one type of amino transferase may exist or that more than one reactive site is present on a single apotransaminase.

Amino acid transamination requires vitamin B_6 coenzyme. Tada et al. (1967) found no evidence for pyridoxine deficiency in the hypervalinemic patient, nor were they able to stimulate transamination and reduce valine accumulation with dietary pyridoxine supplements 50 to 100 times greater than the recommended daily allowance for this vitamin.

Clinical symptoms in the patient subsided after initiation of a low-valine diet and correction of hypervalinemia (Tada et al., 1967). The valine intake required to control biochemical imbalance and support growth in this patient was equivalent to earlier estimates of the minimum valine requirement for human infants of similar age (Holt et al., 1960; Snyderman et al., 1959). This important observation implies that the block in valine transamination in the patient is probably complete. Any intake of valine in excess of the minimal requirement for protein synthesis is apparently disposed of by the oxidation pathway.

Hypervalinemia is likely to be an inherited trait, but this has not been proved. The parents of the Japanese patient were not consanguineous, and loading tests to demonstrate the heterozygous phenotype were unsuccessful (Wada, 1965).

Hyperleucine-isoleucinemia

Jeune and coauthors (1970) reported two sibs (male and female) with a disorder of leucine and isoleucine catabolism associated with Type II hyperprolinemia (see pedigree L described in Table 20–1, p. 418). The clinical symptoms included failure to thrive, mental retardation, convulsions, retinal degeneration and apparent nerve deafness. The male sib died in coma at $3\frac{1}{2}$ years of age; the other sib was alive at $2\frac{1}{2}$ years.

The concentrations of leucine and isoleucine in plasma were two to three times the upper limit of normal; their urinary excretion was normal, in keeping with their efficient tubular reabsorption. Valine concentration in plasma was normal. Alloisoleucine was not detected in plasma. Loading by mouth with leucine (250 mg/kg; isomer not stated) augmented plasma leucine, but did *not* induce the expected fall in plasma isoleucine which occurs when isoleucine catabolism is normal (Phansalkar et al., 1970).* The post-load fall in plasma leucine was slower in the patient than in a control subject, and leucine excretion in urine increased during the 24-hour period after loading in the former but not in the latter. Restriction of dietary protein to about 2 g/kg/day or selective restriction of leucine and isoleucine both reduced the plasma amino acid levels to normal.

A simplified assay of branched-chain transamination and decarboxylation was performed in leukocytes with the three amino acids. A partial but specific defect of leucine and isoleucine transamination was found in both affected sibs. The residual aminotransferase activity was about half normal at substrate concentrations apparently not greater than about 0.25 mM. The stimulative effect of pyridoxal phosphate was not examined in vitro, but an augmented dietary intake of pyridoxine (250 mg daily for two weeks) had no effect on amino acid accumulation in vivo.

The parents were not consanguineously related. Their plasma amino acid levels were normal, and there was no significant deficiency of leukocyte enzyme activity in vitro.

These interesting observations complement those from the hypervalinemic infant and suggest that C-5 and C-6 branched-chain amino acid transaminations occur on different enzymes or at least on distinctive binding sites which are under separate genetic control.

Disorders of Oxidative Decarboxylation

There are at least four conditions known as maple syrup urine disease (MSUD). Each is associated with deficient decarboxylation of the branched-chain keto acids (BCKA), and in each, all three keto acids are affected. There are sufficient clinical and biochemical differences between the traits to allow a tentative classification (Table 14–1).

The combined frequency of these traits is about 1 per 250,000 live births, yet interest in such rare diseases is high, probably because they illustrate many of the classical theses of human biochemical genetics. Because of the complex nature of oxidative decarboxylation, one anticipates heterogeneity of its mutant genotypes and phenotypes. The rarity of heterozygotes (about one in 250 persons) and the pan-ethnic appearance of homozygotes throughout the world make it likely, in genetic terms, that more than one mutation causing branched-chain decarboxylase deficiency should occur in the human species (Scriver et al., 1971). So-called homozygotes will be "genetic compounds" should they inherit two different forms of these rare mutant alleles, and this is more likely to be the case if their parents are not consanguineous. Under such circumstances we should anticipate that each new propositus with MSUD may have a form of the trait which is different from previously reported cases, particularly when the patient is a member of a pedigree or deme where there were no previous cases of MSUD.

---

*No explanation for this interesting observation has yet been published. The possibility that substrate induction with leucine of an aminotransferase common to the C-6 amino acids is worth consideration. The unresponsiveness of plasma isoleucine in the leucine-isoleucine transaminase deficiency state is compatible with this interpretation.

Table 14-1 Tentative Classification of Disorders of Branched-Chain Keto Acid Decarboxylation

Name of Disorder	Principal Clinical Features	Usual Concentration of BCAA* in Plasma	Ketoaciduria	Keto Acid Decarboxylase Activity (Per Cent of Normal)**	Type of Treatment Required to Lower Plasma Amino Acids
"Classical" maple syrup urine disease (MSUD)	Onset soon after birth; convulsions, severe mental retardation, acidosis, coma; death in half the patients	>10 × Normal	Constant	<5	Specific and strict restriction of BCAA intake. Peritoneal dialysis during postnatal period and during acute illness
"Intermittent" MSUD	Intermittent severe symptoms provoked by intercurrent illness; can be fatal. Well between attacks. Mild mental retardation in some patients	Normal except during episodes, when >10 × normal	Intermittent	10–20 (Between episodes)	Peritoneal dialysis during acute episodes, and substrate restriction. Low-protein diet for precaution between episodes
"Mild" MSUD	Moderately retarded mental development	5–15 × Normal	Constant	<25	BCAA restriction or low-protein diet alone (possibly)
Thiamine-responsive MSUD	Mild developmental retardation	3 × Normal	Variable	Partial 20% at physiological substrate conc.; normal, at elevated substrate conc.	Thiamine therapy (10 mg/day) and reduced protein intake (2 g/kg/day).

*BCAA = Branched-chain amino acids: leucine, isoleucine and valine.
**Compared to control cells (leukocytes or fibroblasts) analyzed under comparable conditions.

Classical Branched-Chain Ketoaciduria
(BCKA or Maple Syrup Urine Disease*)

Clinical Features. In 1954, Menkes, Hurst and Craig described the clinical features of what was then an unnamed disease affecting four sibs. Dancis and colleagues formally published in 1959 the results of their preliminary study (Westall et al., 1957) of a single North American patient. At the same time, Mackenzie and Woolf (1959) described two English patients with a similar disease. Both groups had identified an apparently congenital disorder of branched-chain keto acid oxidation and had observed the odor of maple syrup. In such patients, feeding difficulties, vomiting, hypertonicity, and a shrill cry are observed in the first week of life. Flaccidity and apnea (perhaps due to hypoglycemia) may intervene. The Moro reflex is then lost, and deep tendon reflexes are suppressed; convulsions are frequent, and death may occur in early infancy. Untreated children who survive usually have severe retardation of mental and motor development. The odor, which is the clinical hallmark of the condition (Cone, 1968), is detectable in the urine and on the body of the patient. It has been known to appear as early as the fifth day of life. The disease is pan-ethnic, having been described in Japanese (Tada et al., 1963), in Negroes (Woody et al., 1963) as well as in many patients of Western European origin.

The autopsy findings of BCKA reveal changes in the brains of patients who live long enough to develop mental retardation (Crome et al., 1961; Silberman et al., 1961). Status spongiosus of white matter, defective myelinization, gliosis and edema occur. The myelin changes suggest that the biochemical insult does not appear before birth. Total lipid, proteolipid and cerebroside content is diminished in the brains of untreated patients (Prensky et al., 1966, 1968). Lipid abnormalities are not found in patients in whom dietary treatment began early in life and was continued for a long period (Menkes and Solcher, 1967; Prensky et al., 1968; Gaull, 1969). However, normalization of brain lipids does not assure normal mental development; one patient treated from the age of 35 days was severely retarded yet had normal brain lipids at death in the fourth year of life (Prensky et al., 1968).

Metabolic Features

The branched-chain keto acids are the metabolites immediately proximal to the deficient enzyme. The significance of ketoaciduria and ketoacidemia was recognized early in the history of this disease (Dancis et al., 1959; Mackenzie and Woolf, 1959; Menkes, 1959a, 1959b; Dancis et al., 1960). The concentration of the keto acids is also increased in the cerebrospinal fluid. Their excretion into urine is rapid, and the concentration there is great, relative to plasma (Dent and Westall, 1961). The keto acids can be readily identified by thin-layer chromatography (Dancis et al., 1963a); α-ketoisocaproic acid is the predominant keto acid. Hydroxy derivatives of the keto acids are formed to a small extent (Dancis et al., 1960; Mackenzie and Woolf, 1959), probably by reduction of the keto acid analogue.

Because of reverse transamination from the keto acids, the branched-chain

---

*The correct term should be "maple syrup"; maple sugar, the name sometimes used in error, has no odor. The terms "curry-like odor" and "burnt sugar smell" also appear in the literature. Since not all persons are fortunate enough to have smelled or tasted maple syrup, while others dislike curry and burnt sugar, the term "branched-chain ketoaciduria" offers a better if less piquant description.

amino acids (including alloisoleucine) are greatly elevated in plasma. Their concentration is also increased in urine, but since these amino acids are efficiently absorbed by kidney, the altered amino acid pattern is most easily seen in plasma (Dent and Westall, 1961); leucine accumulates to the greatest extent. Alloisoleucine, which elutes at the methionine position in some ion-exchange column chromatographic systems (Norton et al., 1962), may not be identified unless this artifact is remembered when interpreting the chromatogram.

Branched-chain amino acids have been measured in abnormal amounts in other body fluids and tissues, including cerebrospinal fluid (Mackenzie and Woolf, 1959; Snyderman et al., 1964), red blood cells (Snyderman et al., 1964; Snyderman, 1967) and saliva (Mackenzie and Woolf, 1959).

The Enzymatic Defect. Transamination of branched-chain amino acids is normal (Dancis et al., 1960; Dancis, Jansen et al., 1963; Dancis, Hutzler and Levitz, 1963b), and accumulation of free amino acids in body fluid reflects the normal reverse transamination of keto acids.

Release of $^{14}CO_2$ from the labeled keto acid is greatly impaired, whereas the rate of oxidation of labeled isovalerate, the normal product of the decarboxylation step for leucine, is normal in BCKA cells. These findings indicate a block in the oxidative decarboxylation of branched-chain keto acids. The block affects all three keto acids equally (Dancis, Hutzler, and Cox, 1969).

Dent and Westall (1961) gave large amounts of the cofactors required for the decarboxylation reaction to their patient without effect on the metabolic block in vivo; this observation has since been confirmed in other patients (Wong et al., 1971). Most investigators believe that the mutation in BCKA affects the decarboxylase portion of the multienzyme complex, since other keto acid substrates, which also undergo oxidation by analogous enzymes requiring the same cofactors, are not affected in the disease. There is no comprehensive explanation of why a single pair of mutant alleles can affect more than one branched-chain decarboxylase.

Goedde's group (Rüdiger et al., 1972) has now had the opportunity to examine enzyme kinetics in the liver of a patient with classical branched-chain keto acid oxidase deficiency and to compare the results with activity in normal human liver and kidney. They found two normal components with *decarboxylase* activity, one with high affinity for keto acid substrate and another with lower affinity; this was true whether a 6-carbon or a 5-carbon keto acid was used to assay decarboxylation. Only low-affinity decarboxylase activity was found in the patient's tissue. These studies are the first to demonstrate functional heterogeneity in the normal decarboxylase component of the multienzyme complex and the first to pinpoint the enzyme defect in classical maple syrup urine disease specifically as a component of the decarboxylase enzyme in the overall reaction. Goedde rightly points out, however, that probands from different pedigrees with this disease may well reveal different abnormal enzyme kinetics in vitro. The simplest interpretation assumes that each decarboxylase has an apoprotein subunit in common, and that it is affected by the mutation.

Phenotypic Mechanisms. The relationship between the enzyme defect and the clinical phenotype is largely unknown. Waisman and colleagues (1962) reported that force-feeding of infant monkeys with the three branched-chain amino acids caused retarded mental development and a biochemical "model" of maple syrup urine disease. This observation, if valid, suggests that accumulation of metabolites, rather than deficiency of the enzyme itself, may be the source of harm to the central nervous system. Unfortunately, the problem of nutrition and appropriate controls in such experiments makes their interpretation difficult. Tashian (1961) reported, in an often-quoted paper, that branched-chain amino acids inhibited brain glutamic acid decarboxylase, thus presumably compromising energy metabolism and γ-aminobutyric acid synthesis in brain. However, the substrate concentrations used in this experiment were many times greater than those present in plasma of patients, and the in vitro findings may have little relevance to the situation in vivo. Bowden and colleagues (1970) reviewed previous work and showed that 1 mM α-ketoisocaproic acid inhibits rat liver pyruvate and α-ketoglutarate dehydrogenases; they argued that there might be impairment of energy metabolism in brain and inhibition of myelin formation. Dreyfus and Prensky (1967) found the concentration of branched-chain keto acids to be about 0.8 mM in gray matter and 2 mM in plasma in vivo for the clinical disease. These concentrations produce significant inhibition of pyruvate decarboxylase activity in vitro. Valine and α-ketoisocaproic acid inhibit respiration of brain slices (Howell and Lee, 1963), and the latter substance is hypoglycemic in vivo (Cochrane et al., 1956). High plasma levels of branched-chain amino acids perturb brain amino acid pools (Carver, 1969) and may perturb protein synthesis in neurons (Appel, 1966). Serotonin levels are also depressed by leucine elevation (Yuwiler and Geller, 1965).

Diagnosis. The diagnosis can often be made from the patient's odor. A number of simple chemical tests on urine will also indicate the diagnosis, which can then be confirmed by more specific analysis. The ferric chloride reaction may yield a gray-blue color in the presence of branched-chain keto acids. The addition to urine of an equivalent volume of 2,4-dinitrophenylhydrazine (0.5% in 2N HCl) will produce a heavy yellow precipitate with these substances within a few minutes. Detailed descriptions for the preparation and identification of branched-chain keto acids are given in the paper by Dent and Westall (1961). Other methods are described in the review by Dancis and Levitz (1971). Partition chromatography on filter paper of amino acids in urine or plasma (Dent, 1949; Smith, 1960) will demonstrate the specific accumulation of branched-chain amino acids.

Genetics. Inheritance of the "classical" trait is consistent with an autosomal recessive pattern. The frequency at birth of the homozygous form, according to recent estimates (Levy et al., 1971), is about 1 in a quarter-million live births. The corresponding frequency for the heterozygote is about 1 per 250 persons, but this phenotype cannot be identified with complete reliability despite much work on this facet of the trait (Langenbeck et al., 1971). Lonsdale and colleagues (1963) found evidence for discrimination of heterozygotes from normal subjects by means of a leucine-loading test, but Snyderman (1967) could not confirm their observation. Dancis et al. (1965) were not able to classify the *individual* heterozygote with any statistical confidence by studying leucine disappearance in vivo after loading with α-ketoisocaproate. On the other hand, a peripheral leukocyte assay in vitro, modified to discriminate impairment of decarboxylation with maximum efficiency, allowed the same authors to identify the male obligate heterozygote reliably but not the female. Goedde's group (Langenbeck et al., 1971) found that lymphocytes gave better discrimination than mixed leukocytes, but despite all efforts to improve discrimination, these workers and others still find it impossible to segregate normal and heterozygous subjects with absolute certainty. Fibroblast cultures do not clarify the issue.

Treatment. Classical branched-chain ketoaciduria cannot be treated effectively unless there is stringent withdrawal of branched-chain amino acids from the diet from very early postnatal life. The constraints must be sufficient to prevent any abnormal accumulation of metabolites in the body fluids and yet lenient enough to support somatic growth and protein synthesis. Since all proteins with good biological value contain branched-chain amino acids, a semi-synthetic diet must be used (Lowe et al., 1967; Goodman et al., 1969; Smith and Waisman, 1971). Preparation and supply of a diet that is restricted in branched-chain amino acids yet nutritionally adequate is a difficult, tedious and expensive challenge (Westall, 1963; Snyderman et al., 1964). Westall achieved this goal with a gelatin-based diet to which were added other amino acids and constituents to meet nutritional needs; the efficacy of this diet, which was begun at six days of age in one patient, is evident in the normal, successful performance of the patient, who consumed the diet for five years (Westall, 1967). Later follow-up on the same patient (Hatcher, 1968) indicated continued normal physical and mental growth at $6\frac{1}{2}$ years. Bilateral small lenticular opacities, which may be attributable to periods of biochemical imbalance, appear to be the only stigmata of the diet.

Snyderman's group (1964, 1967) has discussed carefully their approach to therapy. They use a totally synthetic amino acid component of the diet, to which are added the other nutrients. A painstaking study carried out over several years indicates that this careful approach to treatment can achieve excellent biochemical control. These workers and others (Dickinson et al., 1969; Gaull, 1969) also showed that it is necessary to begin the diet within the first week of life if permanent neurological damage is to be prevented.

Under such conditions, screening in the neonatal period assumes an important dimension if the maximum benefit is to be gained from treatment. Whether mass screening for such a rare condition is practical and feasible is a matter still under surveillance. Of course, high-risk persons (subsequent sibs of known cases) should be screened carefully at birth, preferably by enzyme assay of leukocytes.

The infant is at maximum risk during the immediate postnatal period. Until dietary therapy has been successfully established, it may be necessary to undertake other forms of aggressive treatment. Peritoneal dialysis can remove amino acids from body pools (Gaull, 1969; Sallan and Cotton, 1969; Rey et al., 1969; Harris, 1971), and this technique is useful to control abrupt branched-chain amino acid accumulation and to initiate treatment in the newborn. Protein intake can be eliminated completely for a short period. However, it is important not to stimulate tissue catabolism by prolonged, excessive over-restriction of protein and calories, since tissue catabolism will cause accumulation of the endogenously released branched-chain amino acids (see Figure 2 in Snyderman et al., 1964). Acute intercurrent infections, common to later infancy, can cause temporary accumulation of metabolites and provoke grave illness. Therefore, very close and continuous monitoring of the patient is probably mandatory, and treatment is likely to be necessary throughout childhood and longer if the toxic aspect of the illness is to be avoided. Death has been reported in the ninth year of life of one patient who developed an infection and was not controlled effectively (Dancis and Levitz, 1971).

Hypoglycemia has been described in a number of untreated patients (Donnell et al., 1967). The finding is of interest because of the well-known hypoglycemic response to dietary loading with L-leucine (Cochrane et al., 1956), but it should not be a problem in the well-treated patient.

Variants of Maple Syrup Urine Disease

Three variants of branched-chain ketoaciduria, each associated with a deficiency of keto acid decarboxylation, are known at present (Table 14–1; Fig. 14–2). The future discovery of more variants is virtually certain.

"Intermittent" (Late-Manifesting) Branched-Chain Ketoaciduria

In this condition, the patient may not come to medical attention until late infancy or childhood, usually during the course of an intercurrent illness. Although the general well-being of the patient is much greater than in the "classical" trait, illness can be as severe during the intermittent episodes of the late-manifesting form. The characteristic odor, lethargy, vomiting and neurological signs can appear suddenly when acute catabolic stimuli or an abrupt increase in protein intake precipitate the appearance of the typical metabolic abnormalities with striking accumulation of branched-chain amino acids and keto acids. Of the seven or eight reported patients who presumably have had the trait (Morris et al., 1961; Morris et al., 1966; Lonsdale et al., 1963; Kiil and Rokkones, 1964; Van der Horst and Wadman, 1971; Irwin et al., 1971), at least two have died during an acute episode. One child, mentally retarded at seven months of age, improved markedly with dietary treatment (Van der Horst and Wadman, 1971).

Dancis, Hutzler and Rokkones (1967) and Goedde et al. (1970) examined branched-chain keto acid oxidation in mixed peripheral leukocytes of Scandinavian and American patients. Both groups identified a small but significant amount of decarboxylase activity, as shown in Figure 14–6A. Whether this partial activity is retained during the acute episodes of illness is unknown. Dancis (1967) drew attention to the fact that this minimal enzyme activity apparently made the difference between the good general health of patients with the intermittent trait and the usually devastating progression of the classical trait. (The clinical importance of modest differences in mutant enzyme activity will certainly receive increasing general attention in the future.)

A point of unusual interest about the heterozygous phenotype in this trait has been found by Dancis, Hutzler and Rokkones (1971) and confirmed by Goedde et al. (1970) in three pedigrees. Only one of the obligate heterozygotes (parents) with the intermittent trait showed the expected partial deficiency of keto acid decarboxylation in leukocytes; the other parent had normal enzyme activity. This finding suggests, within the limits of heterozygote identification, that the intermittent trait may be genetically heterogeneous and that symptomatic probands may be "double heterozygotes" with two different mutant alleles. When inherited together, the alleles produce a mutant form of branched-chain keto acid decarboxylase complex with low native activity that is perhaps susceptible to further inhibition under certain conditions.

"Mild" Branched-Chain Ketoaciduria

Schulman and collaborators (1970) described a 20-month-old female infant with mental retardation associated with an unusually mild form of MSUD. Clinical and birth histories and family history were otherwise unremarkable; the major finding was persistent evidence of defective branched-chain keto acid oxidation with the expected metabolic aberrations. Plasma levels of the three branched-chain amino acids and alloisoleucine were *continuously* elevated (5 to 15 times normal); the corresponding keto acids were also present in plasma and urine. Dietary loading with branched-chain amino acids exaggerated the biochemical imbalance and produced mild clinical symptoms (irritability and vomiting). Hyperuricemia was recorded when the keto acids were formed in large amounts.

Treatment with a low-protein diet alone did not correct the biochemical phenotype, and a semisynthetic diet specifically restricted in branched-chain

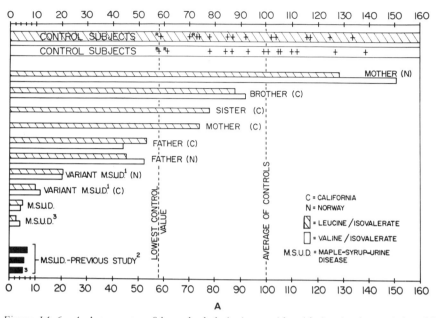

Figure 14–6   A. A measure of branched-chain keto acid oxidation in the peripheral blood leukocytes of normal subjects and patients with intermittent and classical forms of maple syrup urine disease (MSUD). The index of enzyme activity is expressed as a value relative to the rate of CO_2 formation from the decarboxylation reaction in normal cells. The average normal value is 100. Leukocytes from homozygotes with the "classical" MSUD trait have less than 5 per cent of the normal oxidation rate. The "intermittent" variant of MSUD has significantly higher activity than cells from classical MSUD patients.

[1] = average of two determinations
[2] = ^{14}C-α-keto isocaproic
[3] = determinations on same subject
(Figure from Dancis, J., Hutzler, J., and Rokkones, T.: New Eng. J. Med. *276*:84–89, 1967.)

amino acids was required. The subsequent clinical course of the patient has not yet been reported.

Decarboxylation of all three branched-chain keto acids was deficient in leukocytes and fibroblasts of the patient; the residual activity was 15 to 25 per cent of normal. Decarboxylase activity in cells from both parents was normal. No kinetic studies have been described which might elucidate why the residual enzyme activity, which is greater than that in the intermittent trait, is associated with a persistent metabolic abnormality and retarded development.

Fischer and Gerritsen (1971) have reported a healthy adolescent girl with an I.Q. of 76, but no previous history of illness, who may have a similar type of branched-chain ketoaciduria. Accumulation of branched-chain amino acids in plasma was only two to three times normal but could be increased by amino acid loading. The residual keto acid decarboxylase activity in leukocytes and fibroblasts was about 2 to 5 per cent of normal; the concentration of substrate used in the experiment was not specified and kinetic studies were not described. Thiamine administration was apparently not attempted either in vivo or in vitro.

Comment.   It is not yet clear upon what grounds the distinction between "intermittent" and "mild" branched-chain ketoaciduria should be made. A clinical distinction is likely to be invalid because environmental conditions may

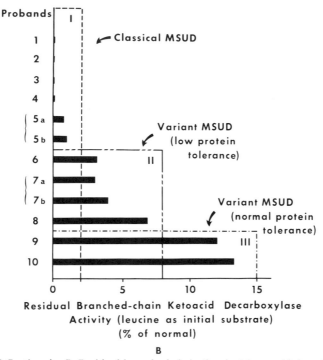

Figure 14–6 Continued. B. Residual branched-chain (leucine) keto acid decarboxylase activity in cultured skin fibroblasts obtained from patients with classical and variant types of maple syrup urine disease (MSUD). Classical patients have less than 2 per cent of the normal decarboxylase activity. When residual activity is between 2 and 8 per cent of normal, the trait is milder, and protein tolerance is about 1.5 to 2 g/kg/day during infancy and childhood and in the absence of infection. When residual activity exceeds 8 per cent (but is less than 15 per cent of normal) a normal tolerance for protein is observed. The two variant enzymic phenotypes do not necessarily correlate with the "intermittent" and "mild" MSUD terminologies which are used for *clinical* phenotypes. (Residual decarboxylase activities for isoleucine and valine are similar to that for leucine but for the sake of simplicity are not shown.) (Adapted from Dancis et al., 1972.)

be the major determinant of the clinical phenotype. Classification in terms of enzyme activity is more promising. Dancis et al. (1972) have observed that residual activity of the branched-chain oxidative decarboxylase in cultured fibroblasts from patients with "classical" maple syrup urine disease have less than 2 per cent of normal activity (Type I MSUD, Dancis classification, Fig. 14–6B). Cells derived from subjects with the intermittent trait or with mild forms of maple syrup urine disease have abnormally low activity (<15 per cent of normal) but significantly more activity than in the classical disease. Patients with about 2 to 8 per cent of normal enzyme activity (Type II MSUD) tolerate more dietary latitude and under most conditions of daily life can handle a protein intake of 2 g/kg/day in later infancy and childhood. When residual enzyme activity is between 8 and 15 per cent of normal, dietary control under usual conditions is unnecessary (Type III MSUD). Infection, abrupt change in protein intake, and tissue catabolism in the latter two types of MSUD provoke acute episodes of ataxia, lethargy and branched-chain ketoaciduria. The distinction between "mild" and "intermittent" MSUD may therefore be determined more by environmental than by enzymic conditions. Important but subtle differences in enzyme activity and stability are probably awaiting discovery in these latter traits.

Thiamine-Responsive Branched-Chain Ketoaciduria

The above-mentioned forms of MSUD are not responsive to thiamine, at least in those patients to whom the vitamin was specifically given in larger than normal doses. Thiamine, as thiamine pyrophosphate, is required for the decarboxylation step in the branched-chain keto acid dehydrogenation reaction.

Thiamine was given in large doses (10 mg/day, or about 10 times the recommended intake) to an infant who presented with modestly retarded development at 11 months of age and who was subsequently shown to have a thiamine-responsive partial deficiency of branched-chain keto acid decarboxylation (Scriver et al., 1971); thiamine corrected the associated metabolic abnormality in vivo. The patient had a small but abnormal accumulation of leucine, isoleucine, valine and alloisoleucine (two to three times normal) at the time of diagnosis. Intercurrent illness and infection provoked amino acid accumulation in plasma up to 10 times normal. Thiamine administration produced a dramatic amelioration of this biochemical phenotype (Fig. 14–7), and withdrawal of the vitamin supplement was followed by a return of branched-chain amino acids to abnormal levels. Studies of the branched-chain keto acid decarboxylation reaction, using labeled amino acid substrates in leukocytes and cultured skin fibroblasts from the patient, showed low activity (20 per cent of normal) in the physiological range of branched-chain amino acid concentrations, and near normal activity at 5 to 10 times the normal concentration. These kinetics were unaltered by thiamine administration in vivo or in vitro. Further studies are needed to interpret the clinical and biochemical significance of these observations (see also Chapter 22, Vitamin-Responsive Aminoacidopathies).

The patient has now been followed for 15 months while on thiamine treatment and a restricted protein intake (2 g/kg/day). Steady improvement in mental development has occurred, and the performance level is now almost normal for age, whereas at the time of diagnosis, it was estimated by two observers to be half of normal. Genetic studies were not possible because the child is adopted.

It is possible that another patient classified as having the intermittent trait and reported by Steen-Johnsen and colleagues (1970) also has a thiamine-responsive form of MSUD, but further investigation would be required to confirm our interpretation of the authors' report.

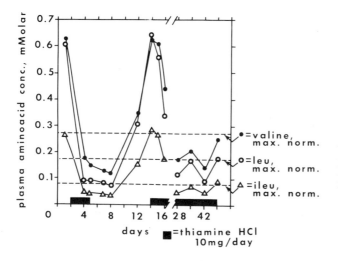

Figure 14–7 Effect of thiamine hydrochloride (10 mg/day by mouth) on the concentration of branched-chain amino acids in the plasma of a patient with thiamine-responsive MSUD. The response of alloisoleucine paralleled that of isoleucine. (Adapted from Scriver et al.: Lancet (i), 310–312, 1971.)

DISORDERS OF BRANCHED-CHAIN AMINO ACID OXIDATION
WITHOUT ACCUMULATION OF FREE AMINO ACID

Keto acid decarboxylation is an irreversible step in the oxidation of the branched-chain amino acids. Blocks in catabolism below this step will not cause accumulation of keto acid or the corresponding amino acid. Oxidation of the valine and isoleucine keto acid equivalent is initially analogous to β-oxidation of short-chain fatty acids (Robinson et al., 1956); leucine undergoes carboxylation instead of hydration at the third step. After formation of a CoA thiol ester, and addition of a carboxyl group or water, catabolism of the carbon chains yields acetyl-CoA, propionyl-CoA or methylmalonyl-CoA. These relationships are shown in Figure 14–8.

Increasing clinical use of gas chromatography (Perry et al., 1970), often coupled to mass spectrometry (Horning and Horning, 1969; Jellum et al., 1971; Mamer et al., 1971), has helped to identify several "new" disorders of branched-chain amino acid catabolism. A characteristic clinical feature common to most of the patients afflicted with these diseases is "organic acidosis." An unexplained, severe recurrent metabolic acidosis is often the first clinical indication; if perusal of the anion-cation balance in plasma reveals a significant "anion gap" (e.g., >20 mEq/L) during an acidotic episode, the possibility of a disorder of branched-chain amino acid catabolism should be considered and the offending organic acid should be sought by appropriate methods. How these diseases produce clinical signs and symptoms is unknown. Analogous short-chain fatty acid accumulation causes loss of respiratory control in cells and uncoupling of oxidative phosphorylation (Hird and Weidemann, 1966).

The disorders can be grouped for convenience into those affecting the oxidation of short-chain acids and those which affect the metabolism of propionate and methylmalonate (see Figure 14–11). Although study of the inborn errors described in the following pages has been a great boon to the elucidation of the details of branched-chain amino acid catabolism in man, it will be readily apparent that many of the interrelationships are still not clear and are, in fact, contradictory and confusing at times.

Disorders of Oxidation of Short-Chain Acids

Isovalericacidemia

This disorder of leucine catabolism was first described in 1966 by Tanaka and coworkers. Two sibs were affected in the original pedigree (Budd et al., 1967; Efron, 1967), and at least 13 patients in seven additional pedigrees are known (Ulstrom, 1966; Newman et al., 1967; Sidbury et al., 1967; Ando et al., 1971; Allen et al., 1969; Ando et al., 1973; Lott et al., 1972). The condition appears to be autosomal recessive, and approximately equal numbers of male and female patients have been reported.

Clinical signs may appear in early infancy, or when tissue catabolism occurs. Severe metabolic acidosis and ketosis ensue, causing lethargy, neurological symptoms and even death. About half the known patients have died in the first month of life. Some mental retardation is a likely sequela in surviving patients not treated from birth.

An offensive odor is usually present, although one patient has been said not to have this finding (Ando et al., 1971). In this patient, the major

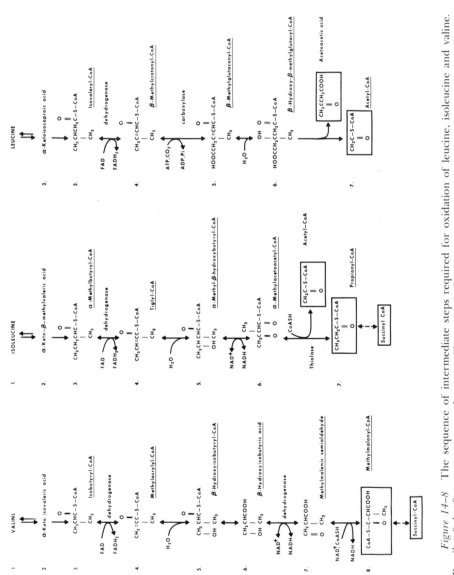

Figure 14–8 The sequence of intermediate steps required for oxidation of leucine, isoleucine and valine. Details of the first two steps are shown on Figure 14–2. Coenzymes are necessary at certain stages of oxidation.

metabolite was isovalerylglycine, a non-odorous conjugate of isovalerate. The odor, which is pungent like sweat, attracted the attention of the clinicians and others in the vicinity of the patients (Budd et al., 1967). Its origin in isovaleric acid was initially identified by two gentlemen (L. B. Sjostrim and D. T. Kendall) from the Arthur D. Little Company of Cambridge, Massachusetts, who used only the ancient art of olfaction. Tanaka et al. (1966) confirmed their impression and demonstrated striking isovalericacidemia by methods of modern technology including gas chromatography (Fig. 14–9) and mass spectrometry.

The biochemical features of isovalericacidemia include elevation of isovaleric acid to 5 to 500 times the normal amounts in serum (<3 μmoles) and urine (<25 μmoles/24 hr). Under conditions of extreme free isovalerate accumulation, there is formation and excretion in urine of N-isovalerylglycine (Tanaka and Isselbacher, 1967), sometimes in great amounts (up to about 3 g/day, normal 2 mg/day) and of free β-hydroxyisovaleric acid, formed apparently by direct hydroxylation of isovaleric acid (Tanaka and Isselbacher, 1968). The quantity of free isovaleric acid may not be impressive if it is excreted as the conjugate (Ando et al., 1971); conjugation may have a protective effect for the patient (Tanaka et al., 1972). Other short-chain fatty acids, including isobutyric,

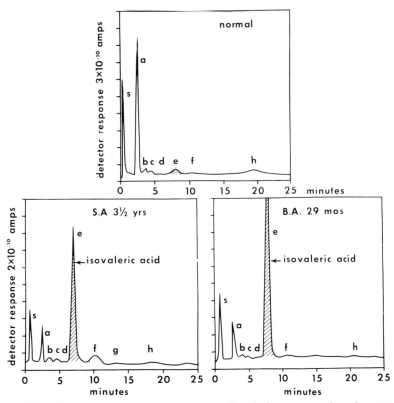

Figure 14–9 Chromatograms produced by gas-liquid chromatography of serum samples from a normal subject and the two original siblings with isovalericacidemia. This was the first disorder of branched-chain amino acid metabolism to be identified specifically by gas chromatography. The large peak (e) observed in both patients is isovaleric acid. Other peaks are acetic (a), propionic (b), isovaleric (c), butyric (d), *n*-valeric (f), β-methylcrotonic (g), *n*-caproic (h) and solvents (s). (After Tanaka et al.: Proc. Nat. Acad. Sci. U.S.A. *56*:236–242, 1966; and Budd et al.: New Eng. J. Med. *277*:321–327, 1967.)

n-butyric and *n*-hexanoic acids, do not accumulate. Plasma amino acids are usually normal, although hyperglycinemia may occur for reasons which are unclear (Ando et al., 1971). β-Methylcrotonic acid, the next substance formed from isovalerate, is not present in abnormal amounts. L-Leucine loading causes isovalerate, its conjugate, and the β-hydroxy derivative to accumulate. The possibility that the latter substance is formed "exogenously" in the intestine, then reabsorbed and excreted in urine has not been ruled out.

The enzyme defect in tissues has been demonstrated indirectly (Tanaka et al., 1966). Mixed peripheral leukocytes oxidize $1\text{-}^{14}\text{C}$-isovalerate to $^{14}\text{CO}_2$ with only about 15 per cent efficiency compared to normal cells. During acidosis, isovalerate oxidation is further inhibited to about 5 per cent of normal. Glycine metabolism is normal in leukocytes (Ando et al., 1971), and a specific partial defect of isovaleryl-CoA dehydrogenase is implied by these findings. The human disease indicates that isovaleryl-CoA dehydrogenase is distinct from the green acyl dehydrogenase which oxidizes other short-chain fatty acids (Green et al., 1954). This interpretation has subsequently received strong support from studies with hypoglycin A, a metabolite of which is an inhibitor of isovaleryl-CoA dehydrogenase. Exposure to hypoglycin A causes isovalericacidemia in man (Tanaka et al., 1971; Tanaka et al., 1972).

Urine may be screened for diagnostic purposes by a simple extraction method and analyzed for isovaleryl glycine by thin-layer chromatography (Ando and Nyhan, 1970). Confirmation of the diagnosis should be made by formal analytic method and evaluation of enzyme activity, but odor may lead one to the diagnosis. For example, a child with a strong smell of "sweaty feet" was originally reported by Sidbury et al. (1967) to have a "new" syndrome accompanied by hexanoic and butyric acid excretion, perhaps related to a deficiency of green acyl dehydrogenase. Reinvestigation of this proband by Ando et al. (1972) has shown that the patient actually has isovalericacidemia.

Treatment consists of careful management of intermittent acidosis and control of acute catabolic stimuli; during the latter periods, strict control of leucine intake is warranted (Lott et al., 1972). A low-protein diet employing amounts of protein just sufficient to maintain normal growth, according to the age-specific recommended daily allowances, may be effective in preventing impaired neurological development (Lott et al., 1972).

β-Methylcrotonylglycine, β-Hydroxyisovalericaciduria

Two forms of this condition have been described, one of which is biotin-responsive. The block involves a biotin-dependent carboxylase in the pathway of leucine catabolism.

Eldjarn and associates (1970) and Stokke et al. (1972) from Norway described a $4\frac{1}{2}$-month-old female, born to first-cousin parents, who came to attention because of retarded motor development with muscular hypotonia and atrophy. There was also an odor like cat's urine. Gas chromatography and mass spectrometry identified β-methylcrotonylglycine (100 mg/day) and β-hydroxyisovaleric acid (400 mg/day) in the patient's urine. The plasma level of both compounds was lower than the detection limits (0.5 mg/100 ml). Both parents excreted slightly increased amounts of the two compounds in their urine (15 to 40 mg/day).

The findings indicate a block in the metabolism of β-methylcrotonyl-CoA at the carboxylase step. The presumed relationships between the three metabolites are shown in Figure 14–10. Note that β-hydroxyisovaleric acid, in this situation, will be formed from β-methylcrotonate, in contrast to its presumed route of formation in isovalericacidemia.

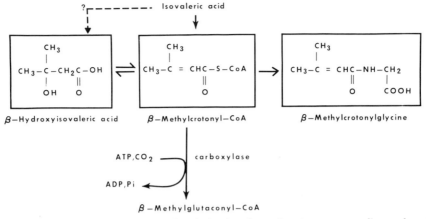

Figure 14–10 Relationships of leucine derivatives formed at the step preceding carboxylation of β-methylcrotonyl-CoA. β-Hydroxyisovaleric acid can be formed endogenously from β-methylcrotonyl-CoA. Formation from isovaleric acid has also been proposed by Tanaka and Isselbacher (1968); the latter reaction may occur exogenously in the intestinal lumen. One or more of these metabolites accumulate in isovaleric acidemia and in β-methylcrotonyl-CoA carboxylase deficiency (biotin-responsive and biotin-unresponsive forms).

Dietary treatment with leucine intake restricted to 150 mg/kg/day (the average requirement) caused excretion of β-hydroxyisovaleric acid to drop eightfold in the Norwegian patient (Eldjarn et al., 1970), while excretion of the glycine conjugate remained unchanged. This suggests that conjugation of β-methylcrotonyl-CoA occurs in preference to its reduction to β-hydroxyisovaleric acid. The original patient died soon after the investigations described above were completed.

Another patient with somewhat similar findings has been reported by Gompertz and colleagues (1971). However, it is quite likely on clinical and biochemical evidence that the second patient has a disease which is different from that of the first patient. The second child was 5 months old when he presented with vomiting, irritability, a rash and severe metabolic acidosis. β-Methylcrotonylglycine was excreted in amounts up to 250 mg/day; no β-hydroxyisovaleric acid was identified. Tiglylglycine was found in the urine, but, as this is a derivative of isoleucine, its presence is peculiar and unexplained in a disorder of leucine catabolism. Either an error in identification of the tiglyl derivative or inhibition of isoleucine oxidation by the leucine metabolite comes to mind as a possible explanation for the finding. The important difference between this patient and the patient reported by Eldjarn and coworkers (1970) is the responsiveness to biotin in the former. A dose of 10 mg/day (100 times the usual intake) had a dramatic effect on the clinical and biochemical aspects of the disease (Fig. 14–11). Whether the patient was truly "biotin-dependent" cannot be determined from the authors' report. Moreover, it should be noted that rats deficient in biotin excrete β-hydroxyisovalerate (Tanaka and Isselbacher, 1970); β-methylcrotonylglycine was not excreted by the biotin-deficient rat, but formation of this compound may require a conjugation system that is present in man but not in rat. β-Methylcrotonyl-CoA carboxylase activity is depressed by biotin deficiency, as expected, since carboxylation reactions are biotin-dependent. Metabolite accumulation is not as impressive in the deficiency model as in the patients, but species and dietary differences may influence this observation.

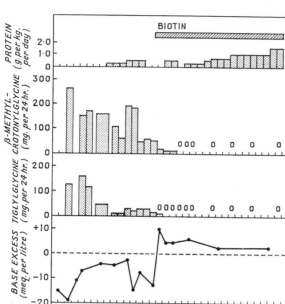

Figure 14–11 Effect of biotin administration on β-methylcrotonylglycine excretion in urine and the degree of metabolic acidosis in patient with β-methylcrotonyl-β-hydroxyisovalericacidemia. The defect in leucine metabolism is biotin-responsive; the enzyme defect is believed to involve the biotin-dependent carboxylase. Acidosis was corrected completely with biotin treatment. Intravenous bicarbonate shown by stippled bars in bottom portion of graph. (After Gompertz et al.: Lancet (ii), 22–24, 1971.)

α-Methylacetoacetic α-Methyl-β-hydroxybutyricaciduria

This abnormality of isoleucine catabolism, with its uncomfortable name, has been reported in a family by Daum et al. (1971) and identified in a second pedigree by the same authors (Daum et al., 1973). Late-onset, intermittent metabolic acidosis without apparent cause again characterizes the clinical presentation. There is no unusual odor to aid clinical diagnosis. Gas chromatography and mass spectrometry will identify the large amounts of α-methyl-β-hydroxybutyric acid, α-methylacetoacetic acid and n-butanone which are present in the urine. The excretion of these compounds is augmented when the intake of protein or isoleucine is increased. Metabolic acidosis is effectively controlled by a low-protein (2 g/kg/day), high-calorie diet and aggressive management of intercurrent illnesses.

A partial defect in the latter stages of isoleucine oxidation has been demonstrated in fibroblasts which is presumed to affect the formation of propionyl-CoA and acetyl-CoA by the thiolase enzyme. Propionate levels in blood and urine are normal (<3 μmoles in blood) in this disease, as are the levels of isoleucine itself.

The condition is apparently inherited as an autosomal recessive trait, since the parents of probands excrete abnormal amounts of α-methyl-β-hydroxybutyrate in the urine. The disease is again a cause for concern; one child, presumably affected in the second sibship, died during an episode of acidosis and vomiting.

Disorders in the Conversion of Propionate to Succinate

Isoleucine and valine eventually yield succinyl-CoA (Figs. 14–8, 14–12), the former via propionyl-CoA and methylmalonyl-CoA and the latter via methyl-malonyl-CoA only. Other substances also enter the tricarboxylic acid cycle through these steps, as shown in Figure 14–12. Virtually all of the propionate in man is derived from the oxidation of protein and lipid. One mole of pro-pionyl-CoA is formed during β-oxidation of each mole of odd-chain fatty acids; the same is true for the three amino acids shown in Figure 14–12. The side chain of cholesterol contributes very little to propionate synthesis. The principal sources of methylmalonyl-CoA are propionyl-CoA and valine; thymine is a minor source of methylmalonate (see Chapter 18).

Rosenberg (1971) has reviewed the important general aspects of propionate and methylmalonate metabolism. Of particular clinical interest are the biotin requirement of propionyl-CoA carboxylase, a CO_2-fixing reaction, and the vitamin-B_{12} requirement of L-methylmalonyl-CoA mutase, a deoxyadenosyl-cobamide-dependent reaction. Four molecules of biotin are utilized by the carboxylase apoprotein, which consists of four subunits with molecular weights of about 175,000 (Kaziro et al., 1961). Isomerization of methylmalonyl-CoA to succinyl-CoA involves a shift of the CoA-carboxyl group; deoxyadenosylcobal-amin participates in this reaction in a manner as yet undisclosed. The K_m for vitamin B_{12} coenzyme binding is $10^{-8}M$, or about 1000 times greater than for the methylmalonyl-CoA substrate. The mutase comprises two subunits of equal

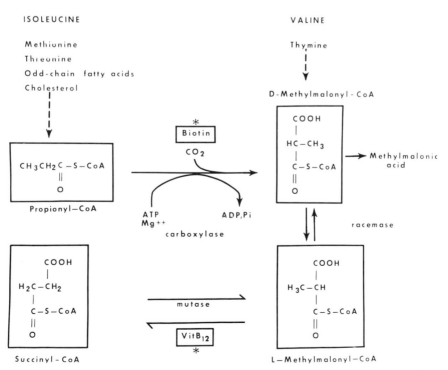

Figure 14–12 Oxidation of propionyl-CoA to succinyl-CoA. The carboxylase and mutase apoenzymes are dependent on biotin and deoxyadenosylcobalamin coenzyme (*), respectively.

size and the coenzyme, the total molecular weight being about 165,000 (Cannata et al., 1965).

There are at least four hereditary disorders of this pathway in man. All produce profound metabolic acidosis, long-chain ketonuria and clinical illness, sometimes of sufficient gravity to cause death. Early diagnosis and careful clinical management may be compatible with satisfactory growth and development in these patients. Two of the traits respond to massive doses of vitamin coenzyme.

Propionyl-CoA Carboxylase Deficiency (Biotin-Unresponsive and Biotin-Responsive Forms)

Over the years, three different groups (Childs et al., 1961; Childs and Nyhan, 1964; Nyhan et al., 1961; Nyhan et al., 1967; Hommes et al., 1968; Hsia et al., 1969) have disclosed the nature of a puzzling disease first reported as "ketotic hyperglycinemia"* (Childs et al., 1961; Nyhan et al., 1961).

Clinical Aspects. Recurrent attacks of ketoacidosis and neutropenia, aggravated by infections or high protein intake and ameliorated by dietary control, characterize the disease. The range of clinical expression varies from death in early infancy (Hommes et al., 1968) to a relatively mild course with developmental retardation as the major clinical finding (Rosenberg, 1971; Hsia et al., 1969, 1971).

Investigators at first focused on the factors which precipitated ketoacidosis (Childs et al., 1961; Nyhan et al., 1961). It was observed that isoleucine, threonine and methionine induced ketosis and hyperglycinemia; leucine, valine and a high protein intake also had the same effect. The pathogenesis of the hyperglycinemia still remains obscure, but it became apparent why some of the above-mentioned amino acids provoked ketoacidosis when a block in propionate metabolism was discovered. The first three amino acids form propionyl-CoA during their own oxidation. Leucine, which does not participate in this oxidative pathway, will stimulate oxidation of isoleucine and can therefore increase endogenous propionate formation (Phansalkar et al., 1970). Valine may have a similar effect.

The striking long-chain ketonuria comprises butanone, pentanone and hexanone (Menkes, 1966); this finding reflects the conversion of propionate and its precursor, α-methylacetoacetate, to the ketones during isoleucine oxidation. Propionate levels in serum exceed 3 μmoles and may be many times greater than that (Ando et al., 1971).

The site of the enzyme defect in ketotic hyperglycinemia was deduced by Hsia and colleagues (1970, 1971) from the clinical and metabolic data. Leukocytes and cultured skin fibroblasts were obtained from a surviving sibling in the original pedigree reported by Childs and colleagues (1961) and were used to demonstrate an almost complete deficiency of propionyl-CoA carboxylase activity. It was also possible to demonstrate a partial deficiency of this enzyme in fibroblast cultures from both parents of the proband (Fig. 14–13), thus revealing the apparent autosomal recessive nature of the trait.

Gompertz and coworkers (1970) were able to correlate the biochemical findings in vivo (propionicacidemia, hyperglycinemia, accumulation of odd-chain fatty acids and butanonuria) with markedly deficient propionyl-CoA carboxylase activity in vitro. The latter evidence was obtained from liver tissue

---

*Nonketotic hyperglycinuria is a different disease; see Chapter 19.

Figure 14–13 Propionyl-CoA carboxylase activity in fibroblast extracts obtained from control subjects, a proband with ketotic hyperglycinemia and her parents. The rate of conversion of propionate to succinate is severely impaired in the proband, who is presumably homozygous for the mutant allele; it is about half of normal in the parents, who are presumably obligate heterozygotes. This autosomal recessive trait was formerly known as "ketotic hyperglycinemia" but has been reclassified as propionicacidemia. (From Hsia et al.: J. Clin. Invest. *50*:127–130, 1971.)

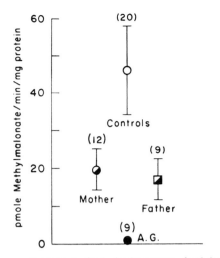

Propionyl-CoA Carboxylase Activity

at death on the eighth day of life. This study provides an effective link between the reports of Hommes et al. (1968) and Ando et al. (1971), which describe propionicacidemia and other biochemical abnormalities in vivo, and the report of Hsia et al. (1970, 1971), which focused on the enzyme defect in vitro but did not document the presumed propionicacidemia.

The demonstration of propionyl-CoA carboxylase deficiency explains many of the once-puzzling clinical features of "ketotic hyperglycinemia." However, some features are not yet clarified — for example, the pathogenesis of hyperglycinemia and the mechanism of acidemia whose intensity exceeds the contribution from propionate alone.

Diagnosis. Diagnosis requires clinical suspicion and a search for propionic acid accumulation in plasma or urine (Ando et al., 1971). Propionicacidemia is a more reliable metabolic index of the trait than is hyperglycinemia (Ando et al., 1971), but it should not be relied upon as a specific index, since propionate will also accumulate in methylmalonicaciduria (see subsequent text). Propionate does not accumulate in nonketotic hyperglycinemia (Nyhan et al., 1967), indicating the different pathogenesis of this disorder compared to ketotic hyperglycinemia.

It is interesting that no patient with propionicacidemia has had plasma or urine analyzed by gas chromatography for α-methylacetoacetate. This compound precedes propionate in the pathway of isoleucine oxidation (Fig. 14–8), and since the thiolase reaction is apparently reversible in human tissues, its accumulation will be evident (butanone, a derivative of α-methylacetoacetate, is present in propionicacidemia). This point is of some importance if the disease α-methylacetoaceticaciduria, which does not have propionicacidemia (Daum et al., 1970), is to be distinguished from propionicacidemia. Specific diagnosis of propionicacidemia requires assay of the carboxylase in leukocytes (Hsia et al., 1970) or in cultured skin fibroblasts (Hsia et al., 1971).

Treatment. Effective treatment of propionicacidemia may be possible by protein restriction and careful attention to the management of acute intercurrent illnesses. However, the critical location of the metabolic block imposes serious constraints on the options for treatment, and we suspect that a complete block may be incompatible with life.

BIOTIN-RESPONSIVE PROPIONIC ACIDEMIA. A new outlook on treatment (and diagnosis) was introduced by Barnes and colleagues (1970), who reported one patient with propionicacidemia and "ketotic hyperglycinemia" in whom the biochemical phenotype disappeared after treatment with biotin (10 mg/day for 5 days). This patient is believed to have a biotin-responsive plasma propionate level which, during a period free of overt acidosis, was 100 times normal. Two sibs of the propositus had died four days after birth with unexplained "respiratory distress." It is unlikely that the biotin-responsive proband was deficient in biotin.

The findings in this patient illustrate the importance of attempting coenzyme treatment each time the opportunity presents itself. It should be noted that two other patients with propionyl-CoA carboxylase deficiency were specifically investigated and found to be unresponsive to biotin (Gompertz et al., 1970; Hsia et al., 1971). This means that at least two forms of propionicacidemia exist, both of which are associated with carboxylase deficiency.

Methylmalonicaciduria (B_{12}-Unresponsive and B_{12}-Responsive Forms)

Methylmalonyl-CoA is formed as an intermediate during the conversion of propionate, or valine and thymine, to succinyl-CoA (Fig. 14–12). Methylmalonate exists in two isomers; the D-form is racemized to the L-form; and the latter is the immediate precursor of succinyl-CoA. Conversion of L-methylmalonyl-CoA to succinate by the mutase enzyme requires 5'-deoxyadenosylcobalamin, a monovalent coenzyme of vitamin B_{12}. Synthesis of the coenzyme is a complex reaction which will be discussed later (see Chapter 22).

Abnormal methylmalonicaciduria was first identified in humans as a consequence of vitamin-B_{12} deficiency (Cox and White, 1963; Barness et al., 1963). A hereditary form of methylmalonicaciduria associated with methylmalonyl-CoA mutase deficiency was subsequently reported, and at least 13 patients with this condition have been identified (reviewed by Rosenberg, 1971). Two forms of hereditary methylmalonicaciduria due to mutase deficiency have been described. One is *not* vitamin B_{12}-responsive (Stokke et al., 1967; Oberholzer et al., 1967); it is a disorder of the carbonylmutase apoenzyme (Morrow, Barness et al., 1969). The other is a specific disorder of deoxyadenosylcobalamin biosynthesis, which secondarily impairs mutase activity (Morrow, Barness et al., 1969; Rosenberg et al., 1969). The frequencies of the traits seem to be similar. Both diseases cause similar clinical and biochemical abnormalities. Methylmalonicaciduria also occurs in a disease associated with abnormal methionine metabolism; this condition is another disorder of vitamin B_{12} coenzyme biosynthesis (Mahoney and Rosenberg, 1970; Levy et al., 1970).

Clinical Findings. The major clinical findings of methylmalonicaciduria include severe metabolic ketoacidosis appearing soon after birth or during infancy. Neutropenia is evident during acidemia. Death has occurred in about half the patients; the clinical course is generally milder in those who are vitamin B_{12}-responsive. None of the patients had megaloblastic anemia, and the vitamin B_{12} concentration in blood is not decreased.

Biochemical Findings. The important biochemical findings are accumulation of methylmalonic acid in urine (up to 5 g/day, normal <5 mg/day), in plasma (up to 34 mg/100 ml; normally undetectable) and in cerebrospinal fluid, where it is present in amounts equivalent to the plasma concentration. Methylmalonate also accumulates in cultured fibroblasts with the mutant phenotype (Morrow, Mellman et al., 1969b). Long-chain ketones and propionic acid are also present in abnormal amounts, and there are hyperglycinemia and hypoglycemia, particularly during ketosis.

Rosenberg's group (1968a) and Hsia et al. (1970) showed that dietary loading with amino acid precursors of propionate and methylmalonate enhanced excretion of the dicarboxylic acid. Stokke and coworkers (1967) showed that the isotopic label of valine-^{14}C appeared in the methylmalonate excreted by their patient. Morrow, Mellman and colleagues (1969b) showed that the ^{14}C label of propionate accumulated in methylmalonate in fibroblast cultures carrying the mutant allele. A block in the conversion of methylmalonyl-CoA to succinyl-CoA is implied by these findings.

The presence of a defect in methylmalonyl-CoA mutase was first demonstrated conclusively by Morrow et al. (1969a) in cell-free liver extracts from patients dying with the disease. Two types of mutase deficiency were identified. In one form (three of the patients studied by Morrow and colleagues), mutase activity was less than 1 per cent of control. Addition of the deoxyadenosyl form of B_{12}-coenzyme did not enhance the residual activity. In the second form (one patient) the residual mutase activity was 10 per cent of control tissue, and addition of B_{12} coenzyme restored activity to the level of control tissue similarly treated. This important study demonstrates unequivocally that two forms of methylmalonicaciduria occur in man. Morrow and colleagues (1969b) were also able to demonstrate the defect in propionate oxidation to succinate with methylmalonate accumulation in cultured skin fibroblasts obtained from a living patient. Oberholzer et al. (1967) and Rosenberg et al. (1968b) demonstrated the appropriate deficiency of oxidation in leukocytes.

Rosenberg and colleagues (1968b) were the first to demonstrate vitamin B_{12}-responsiveness in a living patient. When the vitamin was given in doses 1000 times greater than the daily requirement, methylmalonate metabolism improved greatly in their patient (Fig. 14–14). Accumulation of the dicarboxylic acid diminished, and its oxidation by leukocytes improved during cycles of vitamin therapy; the metabolic derangement reappeared after withdrawal of the vitamin supplement. The response to the vitamin is not easily demonstrated in vitro in isolated cells (leukocytes and fibroblasts) (Hsia et al., 1970), presumably because the in vitro system does not allow efficient vitamin-B_{12} transport in the cells. Subsequent studies (Rosenberg et al., 1969; Mahoney and Rosenberg, 1970) have shown that biosynthesis of deoxyadenosylcobalamin is defective in the B_{12}-responsive trait. The cellular concentration of the active coenzyme form is depressed but can be restored in the presence of sufficient precursor vitamin B_{12}. These findings complement those of Morrow et al. (1969a),

Figure 14–14 Suppression of methylmalonicaciduria and enhancement of methylmalonate conversion to succinate in leukocytes after vitamin B_{12} administration (1,000 μg/day) to a patient with methylmalonicaciduria. The deficiency of methylmalonyl-CoA mutase activity is due to a defect of cobamide coenzyme formation; a specific adenosylated form of vitamin B_{12} is required by the mutase. After withdrawal of the B_{12} supplement, methylmalonate oxidation is again inhibited and its excretion in urine increases. (Rosenberg et al., 1968b.)

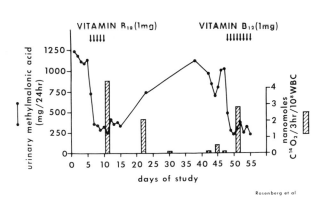

who showed that carbonyl mutase apoenzyme is present in the tissues of the patient with B_{12}-responsive methylmalonicaciduria.

Diagnosis. Diagnosis again demands a high order of clinical suspicion from the physician faced with unexplained ketoacidosis. Methylmalonicaciduria may be detected by a relatively simple urine screening test. Unfortunately, the test is not very sensitive, since the methylmalonate concentration in urine must exceed 1 mg/ml to give a positive result (Giorgio and Luhby, 1969). More sensitive and specific methods should be used to confirm the screening test or to detect the modest dicarboxylicaciduria which occurs in patients with the B_{12}-responsive trait; the methods of choice are gas chromatography (Sprinkle et al., 1969) and thin-layer chromatography (Rosenberg et al., 1968a). Methylmalonate is said to be excreted in the urine of the mother carrying an affected fetus (Morrow et al., 1970).

The possibility of vitamin B_{12} deficiency should be eliminated, and deficient mutase activity should be confirmed, before the diagnosis of primary methylmalonicaciduria is accepted.

Methylmalonicaciduria occurs in another specific disorder of B_{12} coenzyme biosynthesis in which methionine metabolism is also impaired (Levy et al., 1970). The occurrence of homocystinuria and hypomethioninemia with modest methylmalonicaciduria gives the clue to this condition (see section on methionine metabolism, pp. 218–219, and Chapter 22).

Genetics. Methylmalonicaciduria (mutase-deficient and vitamin B_{12}-responsive forms) is probably inherited.

The trait affects male and female patients equally; its occurrence in sibs suggests that the trait is likely to be autosomal recessive. Methylmalonicaciduria has occurred in many different ethnic groups, suggesting that the mutant alleles affecting its metabolism are widely distributed in the human species.

It has not been possible to demonstrate deficient methylmalonic oxidation in leukocytes or cultured skin fibroblasts of the parents of patients with methylmalonicaciduria. Dicarboxylic acid excretion is also normal in these subjects. A specific assay of mutase activity will probably be required to elucidate the heterozygous phenotype.

Pathogenesis and Treatment. Methylmalonicaciduria can be a devastating illness, but the pathogenesis of its clinical signs is still unclear. It is known that methylmalonyl-CoA in excessive amounts inhibits fatty acid synthesis and is incorporated in place of malonyl-CoA into fatty acids (Cardinale et al., 1970). These events may contribute to abnormal lipid turnover and ketosis. Methylmalonyl-CoA is also an inhibitor of pyruvate carboxylase (Utter et al., 1964) and of the dicarboxylate carrier in liver mitochondria (Halperin et al., 1971). In the presence of ketosis, hypoglycemia could occur during methylmalonate accumulation. Methylmalonate accumulation itself is insufficient to account for the degree of acidosis. Treatment should attempt to control methylmalonyl-CoA accumulation by reducing the dietary intake of precursors and by preventing tissue catabolism and acidosis. Vitamin B_{12} should be given by injection in large doses for several days (1000 μg/day) to discern whether the patient has the B_{12}-responsive trait. Since the unresponsive form runs a more violent clinical course, it may be the wish of parents not to give birth to children with this disease. In that case, amniocentesis could provide fetal skin fibroblasts from which cultures could be developed to discern in the early mid-trimester whether the fetus has the disease or not. This approach is preferable to monitoring maternal urine excretion for methylmalonicaciduria as an index of an affected fetus (Morrow et al., 1970).

REFERENCES

Aki, K., Ogawa, K., Shirai, A., and Ichihara, A.: Transaminase of branched-chain amino acids. III. Purification and properties of the mitochondrial enzyme from hog heart and comparison with the supernatant enzyme. J. Biochem. (Tokyo) 62:610–617, 1967.

Allen, D., Necheles, T. F., Rieker, R., and Senior, B.: Reversible neonatal pancytopenia due to isovalericacidemia. (Abstract.) Proceedings of the Society for Pediatric Research, 39th Annual Meeting, Atlantic City, N.J., p. 156, 1969.

Ando, T., Klingsberg, W. D., Ward, A. N., Rasmussen, K., and Nyhan, W. L.: Isovaleric acidemia presenting with altered metabolism of glycine. Pediat. Res. 5:478–486, 1971.

Ando, T., and Nyhan, W. L.: A simple screening method for detecting isovaleryl glycine in urine of patients with isovaleric acidemia. Clin. Chem. 16:420–422, 1970.

Ando, T., Nyhan, W. L., Bachmann, C., Rasmussen, K., Scott, R., and Smith, E. K.: Isovaleric acidemia. Identification of isovalerate, isovalerylglycine, and 3-hydroxyisovalerate in urine of a patient previously reported as butyric and hexanoic acidemia. J. Pediat. 82:243–248, 1973.

Ando, T., Rasmussen, K., Nyhan, W. L., Donnell, G. N., and Barnes, N. D.: Propionic acidemia in patients with ketotic hyperglycinemia. J. Pediat. 78:827–832, 1971.

Appel, S. H.: Inhibition of brain protein synthesis: An approach to the biochemical basis of neurological dysfunction in the amino-acidurias. Trans. N.Y. Acad. Sci. 29:63–70, 1966.

Barnes, N. D., Hull, D., Balgobin, L., and Gompertz, D.: Biotin-responsive propionic acidemia. Lancet (ii), 244–245, 1970.

Barness, L. A., Young, D., Mellman, W. J., Kahn, S. B., and Williams, W. J.: Methylmalonate excretion in a patient with pernicious anemia. New Eng. J. Med. 268:144–146, 1963.

Bowden, J. A., Brestel, E. P., Cope, W. T., McArthur, C. I., III, Westfall, D. N., and Fried, M.: α-Keto-isocaproic acid inhibition of pyruvate and α-ketoglutarate oxidative decarboxylation in rat liver slices. Biochem. Med. 4:69–76, 1970.

Bowden, J. A., and Connelly, J. L.: Branched-chain α-keto acid metabolism. II. Evidence for the common identity of α-keto-isocaproic acid and α-keto-β-methylvaleric acid dehydrogenases. J. Biol. Chem. 243:3526–3531, 1968.

Budd, M. A., Tanaka, K., Holmes, L. D., Efron, M. L., Crawford, J. D., and Isselbacher, K. J.: Clinical features of a new genetic defect of leucine metabolism. New Eng. J. Med. 277:321–327, 1967.

Cannata, J. J. B., Focesi, A., Jr., Mazumder, R., Warner, R. C., and Ochoa, S.: Metabolism of propionic acid in animal tissues. XII. Properties of mammalian methylmalonyl coenzyme A mutase. J. Biol. Chem. 240:3249–3257, 1965.

Cardinale, G. J., Carty, T. J., and Abeles, R. H.: Effect of methylmalonyl coenzyme A, a metabolite which accumulates in vitamin B_{12} deficiency, on fatty acid synthesis. J. Biol. Chem. 245:3771–3775, 1970.

Carver, M. J.: Free amino acids of fetal brain. Influence of branched-chain amino acid. J. Neurochem. 16:113–116, 1969.

Childs, B., and Nyhan, W. L.: Further observations of a patient with hyperglycinemia. Pediatrics 33:403–412, 1964.

Childs, B., Nyhan, W. L., Borden, M., Bard, L., and Cooke, R. E.: Idiopathic hyperglycinemia and hyperglycinuria: A new disorder of amino acid metabolism I. Pediatrics 27:522–538, 1961.

Cochran, W. A., Payne, W. W., Simphiss, M. J., and Woolf, L. I.: Familial hypoglycemia precipitated by amino acids. J. Clin. Invest. 35:411–422, 1956.

Cone, T. E., Jr.: Diagnosis and treatment: Some diseases, syndromes and conditions associated with an unusual odor. Pediatrics 41:993–995, 1968.

Connelly, J. L., Danner, D. J., and Bowden, J. A.: Branched-chain α-keto acid metabolism. I. Isolation, purification and partial characterization of bovine liver α-ketoisocaproic: α-keto-β-methylvaleric acid dehydrogenase. J. Biol. Chem. 243:1198–1203, 1968.

Coon, M. J., Robinson, W. G., and Bachhawat, B. K.: Enzymatic studies on the biological degradation of the branched-chain amino acids. In McElroy, W. D., and Glass, B., eds., Amino Acid Metabolism. Johns Hopkins Press, Baltimore, Md., pp. 431–441, 1955.

Cox, E. V., and White, A. M.: Methylmalonic acid excretion: Index of vitamin-B_{12} deficiency. Lancet (ii), 853–856, 1962.

Crome, L., Dutton, G., and Ross, C. F.: Maple syrup urine disease. J. Path. Bact. 81:379–384, 1961.

Dancis, J.: Intermittent branched-chain ketonuria. In Nyhan, W. L., ed., Amino Acid Metabolism and Genetic Variation. McGraw-Hill, New York, pp. 185–189, 1967.

Dancis, J., Hutzler, J., and Cox, R. P.: Enzyme defect in skin fibroblasts in intermittent branched-chain ketonuria and in maple syrup urine disease. Biochem. Med. 2:407–411, 1969.

Dancis, J., Hutzler, J., and Levitz, M.: Metabolism of the white blood cells in maple syrup urine disease. Biochim. Biophys. Acta 43:342–343, 1960.

Dancis, J., Hutzler, J., and Levitz, M.: Thin-layer chromatography and spectrophotometry of α-keto acid hydrazones. Biochim. Biophys. Acta 78:85–90, 1963a.

Dancis, J., Hutzler, J., and Levitz, M.: The diagnosis of maple syrup urine disease (branched chain ketoaciduria) by the in vitro study of the peripheral leukocyte. Pediatrics 32:234–238, 1963b.

Dancis, J., Hutzler, J., and Levitz, M.: Detection of the heterozygote in maple syrup urine disease. J. Pediat. 66:595–603, 1965.

Dancis, J., Hutzler, J., and Rokkones, T.: Intermittent branched-chain ketonuria: Variant of maple syrup urine disease. New Eng. J. Med. 276:84–89, 1967a.

Dancis, J., Hutzler, J., Snyderman, S. E., and Cox, R. P.: Enzyme activity in classical and variant forms of maple syrup urine disease. J. Pediat. 81:312–320, 1972.

Dancis, J., Hutzler, J., Tada, K., Waday, Y., Morikawa, T., and Arakawa, T.: Hypervalinemia. A defect in valine transamination. Pediatrics 39:813–817, 1967b.

Dancis, J., Jansen, V., Hutzler, J., and Levitz, M.: The metabolism of leucine in tissue culture of skin fibroblasts of maple syrup urine disease. Biochim. Biophys. Acta 77:523–524, 1963.

Dancis, J., and Levitz, M.: Abnormalities of branched-chain amino acid metabolism. In Stanbury, J. B., Wyngaarden, J. B., and Fredrickson, D. S., eds., The Metabolic Basis of Inherited Disease, 3rd edition. McGraw-Hill, New York, pp. 426–439, 1972.

Dancis, J., Levitz, M., Miller, S., and Westall, R. G.: Maple syrup urine disease. Brit. Med. J. (i), 91–93, 1959.

Dancis, J., Levitz, M., and Westall, R. G.: Maple syrup urine disease: branched-chain ketoaciduria. Pediatrics 25:72–79, 1960.

Daum, R. S., Lamm, P. H., Mamer, O. A., and Scriver, C. R.: A "new" disorder of isoleucine catabolism. Lancet (ii), 1289–1290, 1971.

Daum, R. S., Scriver, C. R., Mamer, O. A., Delvin, E., Lamm, P. H., and Goldman, H.: An inherited disorder of isoleucine catabolism causing accumulation of α-methylacetoacetate and α-methyl-β-hydroxybutyrate, and intermittent metabolic acidosis. Pediat. Res. 7:149–160, 1973.

Dent, C. E.: A study of the behaviour of some sixty amino acids and other ninhydrin reacting substances on phenol-"collidine" filter paper chromatograms with notes as to the occurrence of some of them in biological fluids. Biochem. J. 43:169–180, 1948.

Dent, C. E., and Westall, R. G.: Studies in maple syrup urine disease. Arch. Dis. Child. 36:259–268, 1961.

Dickinson, J. P., Holton, J. B., Lewis, G. M., Littlewood, J. M., and Steel, A. E.: Maple syrup urine disease. Four years' experience with dietary treatment of a case. Acta Paed. Scand. 58:341–351, 1969.

Donnell, G. M., Lieberman, E., Shaw, K. N. F., and Koch, R.: Hypoglycemia in maple syrup urine disease. Amer. J. Dis. Child. 113:60–63, 1967.

Dreyfus, P. M., and Prensky, A. L.: Further observations on the biochemical lesion in Maple Syrup Urine disease. Nature 214:276, 1967.

Efron, M. L.: Isovaleric acidemia. Amer. J. Dis. Child. 113:74–76, 1967.

Eldjarn, L., Jellum, E., Stokke, O., Pande, H., and Waaler, P. E.: β-Hydroxyisovaleric aciduria and β-methylcrotonylglycinuria: A new inborn error of metabolism. Lancet (ii), 521–522, 1970.

Fernandez-Moran, A., Reed, L. J., Koike, M., and Willms, C. R.: Electron microscopic and biochemical studies of pyruvate dehydrogenase complex of Escherichia coli. Science 145:930–932, 1964.

Fischer, M. H., and Gerritsen, T.: Biochemical studies on a variant of branched-chain ketoaciduria in a 19-year-old female. Pediatrics 48:795–801, 1971.

Gaull, G. E.: Pathogenesis of maple syrup urine disease: Observations during dietary management and treatment of coma by peritoneal dialysis. Biochem. Med. 3:130–149, 1969.

Giorgio, A. J., and Luhby, A. L.: A rapid screening test for the detection of congenital methylmalonic aciduria in infancy. Amer. J. Clin. Path. 52:374–379, 1969.

Goedde, H. W., and Keller, W.: Metabolic pathways in maple syrup urine disease. In Nyhan, W. L., ed., Amino Acid Metabolism and Genetic Variation. McGraw-Hill, New York, pp. 191–214, 1967.

Goedde, H. W., Langenbeck, U., Brackertz, D., Keller, W., Rokkones, T., Halvorsen, S., Kiil, R., and Morton, B.: Clinical and biochemical genetic aspects of intermittent branched-chain ketoaciduria. Acta Paediat. Scand. 59:83–87, 1970.

Gompertz, D., Bau, D. C. K., Storrs, C. N., Peters, T. J., and Hughes, E. A.: Localisation of enzymic defect in propionicacidaemia. Lancet (i), 1140–1143, 1970.

Gompertz, D., Draffan, G. H., Watts, J. L., and Hull, D.: Biotin responsive β-methyl crotonylglycinuria. Lancet (ii), 22–24, 1971.

Goodman, S. I., Pollak, S., Miles, B., and O'Brien, D.: The treatment of maple syrup urine disease. J. Pediat. 75:485–488, 1969.

Green, D. E., Mii, S., Mahler, H. R., and Bock, R. M.: Studies on the fatty acid oxidizing system of animal tissues. III. Butyryl coenzyme A dehydrogenase. J. Biol. Chem. 206:1–12, 1954.

Halperin, M. L., Schiller, C. M., and Fritz, I. B.: The inhibition by methylmalonic acid of malate transport by the dicarboxylate carrier in rat liver mitochondria. J. Clin. Invest. 50:2276–2282, 1971.

Halpern, B., and Pollock, G. E.: The configuration of the alloisoleucine present in maple syrup urine disease. Biochem. Med. 4:352–354, 1970.

Harris, R. J.: Infection in maple-syrup-urine disease. Lancet (ii), 813–814, 1971.

Hatcher, G. W.: Case demonstration: Maple syrup urine disease. Proc. Roy. Soc. Med. *61*:287, 1968.

Hird, F. J. R., and Weidemann, M. J.: Oxidative phosphorylation accompanying oxidation of short-chain fatty acids by rat-liver mitochondria. Biochem. J. *98*:378–388, 1966.

Holt, L. E., Jr., Gyorgy, P., Pratt, E. L., Snyderman, S. E., and Wallace, W. M.: Protein and amino acid requirements in early life. New York University Press, New York, 1960.

Hommes, F. A., Kuipers, J. R. G., Elema, J. D., Jansen, J. F., and Jonxis, J. H. P.: Propionicacidemia, a new inborn error of metabolism. Pediat. Res. *2*:519–524, 1968.

Horning, E. C., and Horning, M. G.: Human metabolic profiles obtained by GC and GC/MS. J. Chrom. Sci. *9*:129–140, 1971.

Howell, R. K., and Lee, M.: Influence of α-ketoacids on the respiration of brain in vitro. Proc. Soc. Exp. Biol. Med. *113*:660–663, 1963.

Hsia, Y. E., Scully, K. J., and Rosenberg, L. E.: Defective propionate carboxylation in ketotic hyperglycinaemia. Lancet (i), 757–758, 1969.

Hsia, Y. E., Scully, K. J., Lilljeqvist, A. C., and Rosenberg, L. E.: Vitamin-B_{12} dependent methylmalonicaciduria. Pediatrics *46*:497–505, 1970.

Hsia, Y. E., Scully, K. J., and Rosenberg, L. E.: Inherited propionyl-CoA carboxylase deficiency in "ketotic hyperglycinemia." J. Clin. Invest. *50*:127–130, 1971.

Irwin, W. C., Martel, S. B., and Galuboff, N.: Intermittent branched-chain ketonuria (variant of maple syrup urine disease). Clin. Biochem. *4*:52–58, 1971.

Jellum, E., Stokke, O., and Eldjarn, L.: Screening for metabolic disorders using gas-liquid chromatography, mass spectrometry and computer technique. Scand. J. Clin. Lab. Invest. *27*:273–285, 1971.

Jeune, M., Collombel, C., Michel, M., David, M., Guibault, P., Guerrier, G., and Albert, J.: Hyperleucinisoleucinemie par défaut partiel de transamination associée à une hyperprolinemie de Type 2. Observation familiale d'une double aminoacidopathie. La Semaine des Hôpitaux (Ann. Pediat. [Paris]) *17*:85–99, 1970.

Kaziro, Y., Ochoa, S., Warner, R. C., and Chen, J.: Metabolism of propionic acid in animal tissues. VIII. Crystalline propionyl carboxylase. J. Biol. Chem. *236*:1917–1923, 1961.

Kiil, R., and Rokkones, T.: Late manifesting variant of branched-chain ketoaciduria (maple syrup urine disease). Acta Paediat. Scand. *53*:346–364, 1964.

Langenbeck, U., Rüdiger, H. W., Schulze-Schencking, M., Keller, W., Brackertz, D., and Goedde, H. W.: Evaluation of a heterozygote test for maple syrup urine disease in leukocytes and cultured fibroblasts. Humangenetik *11*:304–315, 1971.

Levy, H. L., Mudd, S. H., Schulman, J. D., Dreyfus, P. M., and Abeles, R. H.: A derangement of B_{12} metabolism associated with homocystinemia, cystathioninemia, hypomethioninemia and methylmalonic aciduria. Amer. J. Med. *48*:390–397, 1970.

Levy, H. L., Shih, V. E., and MacCready, R. A.: Inborn errors of metabolism and transport: Prenatal and neonatal diagnosis. Proceedings of the Eighth International Congress of Pediatrics *V-1*: 1–16, 1971.

Lonsdale, D., Mercer, R. D., and Faulkner, W. R.: Maple syrup urine disease. Amer. J. Dis. Child. *106*:258–266, 1963.

Lott, I. T., Erickson, A. M., and Levy, H. L.: Dietary treatment of an infant with isovaleric acidemia. Pediatrics *49*:616–618, 1972.

Lowe, C. U., et al.: Committee on Nutrition, American Academy of Pediatrics: Nutritional management in hereditary metabolic disease. Pediatrics *40*:289–304, 1967.

Mackenzie, D. Y., and Woolf, L. I.: Maple syrup urine disease. An inborn error of the metabolism of valine, leucine and isoleucine associated with gross mental deficiency. Brit. Med. J. (i), 90–91, 1959.

Mahoney, M. J., and Rosenberg, L. E.: Inherited defects of B_{12} metabolism. Amer. J. Med. *48*: 584–593, 1970.

Mamer, O. A., Crawhall, J. C., and Tjoa, S. S.: The identification of urinary acid by coupled gas chromatography-mass spectrometry. Clin. Chim. Acta *32*:171–184, 1971.

Meister, A.: Transamination. Advances Enzymol. *16*:185–246, 1955.

Meister, A.: Valine, isoleucine and leucine. *In* Meister, A., ed., Biochemistry of the Amino Acids, Vol. II. pp. 729–757, 1965.

Menkes, J. H.: Idiopathic hyperglycinemia: Isolation and identification of three previously undescribed urinary ketones. J. Pediat. *69*:413–431, 1966.

Menkes, J. H.: Maple syrup disease: Isolation and identification of organic acids in the urine. Pediatrics *23*:348–353, 1959.

Menkes, J. H.: Maple syrup disease: Investigations into the metabolic disease. Neurology *9*:826–835, 1959.

Menkes, J. H., Hurst, P. L., and Craig, J. M.: A new syndrome: Progressive familial infantile cerebral dysfunction associated with an unusual urinary substance. Pediatrics *14*:462–466, 1954.

Menkes, J. H., and Solcher, H.: Maple syrup urine disease: effects of diet therapy on cerebral lipids. Arch. Neurol. *16*:486–491, 1967.

Morris, M. D., Fisher, D. A., and Fiser, R.: Late-onset branched-chain ketoaciduria (maple syrup urine disease). Lancet *86*:149–152, 1966.

Morris, M. D., Lewis, B. D., Doolan, P. D., and Harper, H. A.: Clinical and biochemical observations on an apparently nonfatal variant of branched-chain ketoaciduria (maple syrup urine disease). Pediatrics *28*:918–923, 1961.

Morrow, G., III, Barness, L. A., Cardinale, G. J., Abeles, R. H., and Flaks, J. G.: Congenital methylmalonic acidemia: Enzymatic evidence for two forms of the disease. Proc. Nat. Acad. Sci. U.S.A. *63*:191–197, 1969.

Morrow, G., III, Mellman, W. J., Barness, L. A., and Dimitrov, N. V.: Propionate metabolism in cells cultured from a patient with methylmalonic acidemia. Pediat. Res. *3*:217–219, 1969.

Morrow, G., III, Schwarz, R. H., Hallock, J. A., and Barness, L. A.: Prenatal detection of methylmalonic acidemia. J. Pediat. *77*:120–123, 1970.

Newman, C. G. H., Wilson, B. D. R., Callaghan, P., and Young, L.: Neonatal death associated with isovalericacidemia. Lancet (ii), 439–442, 1967.

Norton, P. M., Roitman, E., Snyderman, S. E., and Holt, L. E., Jr.: A new finding in maple syrup urine disease. Lancet (i), 26–27, 1962.

Nyhan, W. L., Borden, M., and Childs, B.: Idiopathic hyperglycinemia: a new disorder of amino acid metabolism. II. The concentrations of other amino acids in the plasma and their modification by the administration of leucine. Pediatrics *27*:539–550, 1961.

Oberholzer, V. G., Levin, B., Burgess, E. A., and Young, W. F.: Methylmalonic aciduria. An inborn error of metabolism leading to chronic metabolic acidosis. Arch. Dis. Child. *42*:492–504, 1967.

Perry, T. L., Hansen, S., Diamond, S., Bullis, B., Mok, C., and Malancon, S.: Volatile fatty acids in normal human physiological fluids. Clin. Chim. Acta *29*:369–374, 1970.

Phansalkar, S. V., Norton, P. M., Holt, L. E., Jr., and Snyderman, J. E.: Amino acid relationships: The effect of a load of leucine on the metabolism of isoleucine. Proc. Soc. Exp. Biol. Med. *134*:262–263, 1970.

Prensky, A. L., Carr, S., and Moser, H. W.: Development of myelin in inherited disorders of amino acid metabolism. Arch. Neurol. *19*:552–558, 1968.

Prensky, A. L., and Moser, H. W.: Brain lipids, proteolipids, and free amino acids in maple syrup urine disease. J. Neurochem. *13*:863–874, 1966.

Reed, L. J., and Cox, D. J.: Macromolecular organization of enzyme systems. Ann. Rev. Biochem. *35*:57–84, 1966.

Rey, F., Rey, J., Cloup, M., Feron, J. F., Dore, F., Labrune, B., and Fiezal, J.: Traitement d'urgence d'une forme alguë de leucinose par dialyse péritonéale. Arch. Franc. Pediat. *26*:133–137, 1969.

Robinson, W. G., Bachhawat, B. K., and Coon, M. J.: Tiglyl-coenzyme A and α-methylacetoacetyl coenzyme A, intermediates in the enzymatic degradation of isoleucine. J. Biol. Chem. *218*: 391–400, 1956.

Rosenberg, L. E.: Disorders of propionate, methylmalonate, and vitamin B_{12} metabolism. *In* Stanbury, J. B., Wyngaarden, J. B., and Fredrickson, D. S., eds., The Metabolic Basis of Inherited Disease, 3rd edition. McGraw-Hill, New York, pp. 440–458, 1972.

Rosenberg, L. E., Lilljeqvist, A. C., and Hsia, Y. E.: Methylmalonic aciduria: An inborn error leading to metabolic acidosis, long-chain ketonuria, and intermittent hyperglycinemia. New Eng. J. Med. *278*:1319–1322, 1968a.

Rosenberg, L. E., Lilljeqvist, A. C., and Hsia, Y. E.: Methylmalonic aciduria: metabolic block localization and vitamin B_{12} dependency. Science *162*:805–807, 1968b.

Rosenberg, L. E., Lilljeqvist. A. C., Hsia, Y. E., and Rosenbloom, F. M.: Vitamin B_{12} dependent methylmalonic aciduria: Defective B_{12} metabolism in cultured fibroblasts. Biochem. Biophys. Res. Commun. *37*:607–614, 1969.

Rüdiger, H. W., Langenbeck, U., Schulze-Schencking, M., Goedde, H. W., and Schuchmann, L.: Defective decarboxylase in branched-chain keto acid oxidase multi-enzyme complex in classic type of maple syrup urine disease. Humangenetik *14*:257–267, 1972.

Sallan, S. E., and Cottom, D.: Peritoneal dialysis in maple syrup urine disease. Lancet (ii), 1423–1424, 1969.

Schulman, J. D., Lustberg, T. J., Kennedy, J. L., Museles, M., and Seegmiller, J. E.: A new variant of maple syrup urine disease (branched-chain ketoaciduria). Amer. J. Med. *49*:118–124, 1970.

Scriver, C. R., Mackenzie, S., Clow, C. L., and Delvin, E.: Thiamine-responsive maple syrup urine disease. Lancet (i), 310–312, 1971.

Seegmiller, J. E., and Westall, R. G.: The enzyme defect in maple syrup urine disease (branched-chain ketoaciduria). J. Ment. Defic. Res. *11*:288–294, 1967.

Sidbury, J. B., Smith, E. K., and Harlan, W.: Inborn error of short-chain fatty acid metabolism. J. Pediat. *70*:8–15, 1967.

Silberman, J., Dancis, J., and Feigin, I. H.: Neuropathological observations in maple syrup urine disease (branched-chain ketoaciduria). Arch. Neurol. *5*:351–363, 1961.

Smith, B. A., and Waisman, H. A.: Leucine equivalency system in managing branched-chain keto-aciduria. J. Amer. Diet. Ass. 59:342–346, 1971.

Smith, I.: Chromatographic and Electrophoretic Techniques, Vol. I, 2nd edition. William Heinemann, Ltd., London, p. 269, 1960.

Snyderman, S. E.: Maple syrup urine disease. In Nyhan, W. L., ed., Amino Acid Metabolism and Genetic Variation. McGraw-Hill, New York, pp. 171–183, 1967.

Snyderman, S. E., Holt, L. E., Jr., Smellie, F., Boyer, A., and Westall, R. G.: The essential amino acid requirements of infants: Valine. Amer. J. Dis. Child. 97:186–191, 1959.

Snyderman, S. E., Norton, P. M., Roitman, E., and Holt, L. E., Jr.: Maple syrup urine disease, with particular reference to dietotherapy. Pediatrics 34:454–472, 1964.

Sprinkle, T. J., Proter, A. H., Greer, M., and Williams, C. M.: A simple method for the determination of methylmalonic acid by gas chromatography. Clin. Chim. Acta 24:476–478, 1969.

Steen-Johnsen, J., Vellan, E. J., and Gjessing, L. R.: Maple syrup urine disease variant—amino acid pattern and problems of treatment during acute attacks. Acta Paediat. Scand. 59:71–73, 1970.

Stokke, O., Eldjarn, L., Jellum, E., Pande, H., and Waaler, P. E.: Beta-methylcrotonyl-CoA carboxylase deficiency: A new metabolic error in leucine degradation. Pediatrics 49:726–735, 1972.

Stokke, O., Eldjarn, L., Norum, K. R., Steen-Johnsen, J., and Halvorsen, S.: Methylmalonic acidemia: A new inborn error of metabolism which may cause fatal acidosis in the neonatal period. Scand. J. Clin. Lab. Invest. 20:313–328, 1967.

Tada, K., Wada, Y., and Arakawa, T.: Hypervalinemia. Amer. J. Dis. Child. 113:64–67, 1967.

Tanaka, K., Budd, M. A., Efron, M. L., and Isselbacher, K. J.: Isovalericacidemia: a new genetic defect of leucine metabolism. Proc. Nat. Acad. Sci. U.S.A. 56:236–242, 1966.

Tanaka, K., and Isselbacher, K. J.: Experimental β-hydroxyisovaleric acidemias induced by biotin deficiency. Lancet (ii), 930–931, 1970.

Tanaka, K., and Isselbacher, K. J.: The isolation and identification of N-isovalerylglycine from urine of patient with isovaleric acidemia. J. Biol. Chem. 242:2966–2972, 1967.

Tanaka, K., Isselbacher, K. J., and Shih, V.: Isolvaleric and α-methylbutyric acidemias induced by hypoglycin A: Mechanism of Jamaican vomiting sickness. Science 175:69–71, 1972.

Tanaka, K., Miller, E. M., and Isselbacher, K. J.: Hypoglycin A: A specific inhibitor of isovaleryl-CoA dehydrogenase. Proc. Nat. Acad. Sci. U.S.A. 68:20–24, 1971.

Tanaka, K., Orr, J. C., and Isselbacher, K. J.: Identification of β-hydroxyisovaleric acid in the urine of a patient with isovaleric acidemia. Biochim. Biophys. Acta 152:638–641, 1968.

Tashian, R. E.: Inhibition of brain glutamic acid decarboxylase by phenylalanine, valine and leucine derivatives: A suggestion concerning the etiology of the neurological defect in phenylketonuria and branched-chain ketonuria. Metabolism 10:393–402, 1961.

Taylor, R. T., and Jenkins, W. T.: Leucine aminotransferase. II. Purification and characterization. J. Biol. Chem. 241:4396–4405, 1966.

Ulstrom, R. A.: Commentary on paper by Holmes, L. B., et al., Isovalericacidemia: a new genetic defect of leucine metabolism. J. Pediat. 69:961–962, 1966.

Utter, M. F., Keech, D. B., and Scrutten, M. L.: A possible role of acetyl-CoA in the control of gluconeogenesis. In Weber, G., ed., Advances in Enzyme Regulation, Vol. 2. Pergamon Press, New York, p. 49, 1964.

Van der Horst, J. L., and Wadman, S. K.: A variant form of branched-chain ketoaciduria. Acta Paediat. Scand. 60:594–599, 1971.

Wada, Y.: Idiopathic hypervalinemia: Valine and alpha ketoacids in blood following an oral dose of valine. Tohoku J. Exp. Med. 87:322–331, 1965.

Wada, Y., Tada, K., Minagawa, A., Yoshida, T., Morikawa, T., and Okamura, T.: Idiopathic valinemia: Probably a new entity of inborn error of valine metabolism. Tohoku J. Exp. Med. 81:46–55, 1963.

Waisman, H. A., Gerritsen, T., Boggs, D. E., Polidora, V. J., and Harlow, H. R.: Mental retardation in monkeys. II. Branched-chain aminoaciduria and ketoaciduria. Amer. J. Dis. Child. 104:488–489, 1962.

Westall, R. G.: Dietary therapy of a child with maple syrup urine disease: branched-chain ketoaciduria. Arch. Dis. Child. 38:485–491, 1963.

Westall, R. G.: Dietary treatment of maple syrup urine disease. Amer. J. Dis. Child. 113:58–59, 1967.

Westall, R. G., Dancis, J., and Miller, S.: Maple sugar urine disease. Amer. J. Dis. Child. 94:571–572, 1957.

Wong, P. W. N., Justice, P., Smith, G. F., and Hsia, D. Y. Y.: A case of classical maple syrup urine disease thiamine-non-responsive. Clin. Genet. 3:27–33, 1972.

Woody, N. C., Woody, H. B., and Tilden, T. D.: Maple syrup urine disease in a Negro infant. Amer. J. Dis. Child. 105:381–386, 1963.

Yuwiler, A., and Geller, E.: Serotonin depletion by dietary leucine. Nature (London) 208:83–84, 1965.

Chapter Fifteen

PHENYLALANINE

Følling (1934) stimulated interest in aberrations of phenylalanine metabolism in man when he discovered phenylpyruvic acid in excess in the urine of mentally retarded patients with a peculiar odor. Penrose and Quastel (1937) gave to this condition the name phenylketonuria, by which it has been known ever since. However, it is no longer possible to confine a discussion of phenylalanine metabolism and its abnormalities to phenylketonuria, since numerous disorders of phenylalanine metabolism in man can now be recognized. Mass screening of the newborn infant is largely responsible for the new awareness of these variants, and from this perspective, interest in the chemistry of phenylalanine hydroxylation and in its genetic control has become extremely relevant.

As a position paper of its times, the Conference on Phenylketonuria and Allied Diseases (Anderson and Swaiman, 1968) is still an informative document which bridges the gap between the earlier work and present-day concern about phenylalanine metabolism. A more recent conference report (Bickel, Hudson and Woolf, 1971) continues to update information on research on the genetic and enzymic nature of phenylketonuria. The impact of mass screening and treatment on the expression of the phenylketonuric gene is also described in detail in the same 1971 Symposium, in a manner that shows why this disease has become the prototype for the application of Garrodian principles to inborn errors of metabolism in general.

METABOLISM OF PHENYLALANINE

L-Phenylalanine is an essential amino acid for man. Observations on phenylalanine requirements in patients with classical phenylketonuria reveal that less than 50 per cent of the normal dietary intake of L-phenylalanine consumed by the growing child can be used for protein synthesis, while the remainder must be oxidized primarily to tyrosine and, to a much lesser extent, to other metabolites. The fraction of phenylalanine intake which is disposed of by specific hydroxylation to form tyrosine increases as the growth rate declines. When hydroxylation is impaired, the rate of metabolism along the minor pathways is greatly augmented. It is the accumulation of these normal metabolites in abnormal amounts which has usually first attracted attention to the disorders of phenylalanine metabolism.

The Hydroxylase Reaction

The major chemical conversion of L-phenylalanine in human tissues involves para-hydroxylation to form L-tyrosine. This reaction was first postulated by Neubauer in 1909 and was tentatively demonstrated by Embden and Baldes in 1913 by means of liver perfusion experiments. The validity of the reaction was eventually confirmed (Moss and Schoenheimer, 1940) by using rat liver and deuterium-labeled phenylalanine. The irreversibility of phenylalanine hydroxylation was shown by Grau and Steele (1954). Udenfriend and Cooper (1952) demonstrated that phenylalanine hydroxylation occurs primarily in the soluble fraction of liver homogenates in several mammalian species. The available methodology also indicated that the reaction was absent from muscle, lung, brain and kidney. New methods of assay have shown that, in the mouse at least, there is appreciable phenylalanine hydroxylase activity in pancreas and kidney as well as in the liver (Tourian et al., 1969). The relative specific activities of pancreas and kidney are about one third and one half, respectively, of that in liver, but because of the differences in organ weight, most of the total body hydroxylating activity is confined to liver.

The hydroxylation reaction requires molecular oxygen and a pyridine nucleotide. Mitoma (1956) fractionated rat liver phenylalanine hydroxylase into two protein components, one of which was labile (phenylalanine hydroxylase) and the other a more stabile fraction (dihydropteridine reductase) which is present in many tissues other than liver. Kaufman (1957) was the first to characterize the hydroxylation process in detail, and he subsequently showed (Kaufman, 1958) that an oxidized pteridine, derived from tetrahydropteridine, is required as cofactor for the reaction. The structure of the *natural* cofactor was eventually shown by Kaufman (1963) to be an unconjugated pteridine, dihydrobiopterin or 7,8-dihydro-2-amino-4-hydroxy-6-[1,2-dihydroxypropyl-(L-erythro)]-pteridine (Fig. 15–1).

The cofactor is not active until it has been reduced to the tetrahydro form by the enzyme dihydrofolate reductase. This enzyme is sensitive to antifolate drugs, such as aminopterin. The pteridine transformation occurs according to the scheme shown in Figure 15–2, where 7,8-XH_2 is the oxidized biopterin and XH_4 is the reduced tetrahydropteridine.

The nature of the phenylalanine hydroxylation could not be studied until the coenzyme requirement and the constituent components of the reaction had been identified. Development of suitable assays employing saturating amounts of reduced *synthetic* cofactor (LaDu, 1967; Kaufman, 1968; Bublitz, 1969) has helped greatly to study the reaction in vitro. Kaufman (1971), in a review of the phenylalanine hydroxylating reaction in mammalian liver, mentions that literally thousands of assays were done in his laboratory to elucidate the reaction, and even now some controversy over its real nature still exists.

The substrate specificity of phenylalanine hydroxylation is known. A *reduced pterin* must participate in the reaction. Several types of tetrahydropterin can participate but, as shown in Table 15–1, it is the *natural* cofactor, tetrahydrobiopterin, which has the lowest K_m value (highest affinity) for the reaction. This feature insures saturation of the hydroxylating enzyme even at low concentrations of cofactor in vivo, an important compensation for the relatively low V_{max} with tetrahydrobiopterin. The cofactor plays a role as electron donor in the system. The *amino acid substrate* must have an unmodified alanine side chain at position 4 of the aromatic ring; the L-isomer is essential. Modification of the ring structure is apparently less important, since L-phenylalanine, L-tryptophan, β-2-thienylalanine and various methyl, chloro and fluoro phenylalanines are all acted upon by the hydroxylase. The third substrate is an *oxygen* atom which originates from atmospheric oxygen and not from water (clearly shown from studies with $H_2{}^{18}O$ and ${}^{16}O_2$).

The mechanism of hydroxylation has been of great interest because the conversion of phenylalanine to tyrosine is very complex. It involves the transfer of an oxygen atom from O_2 and a hydrogen atom from the cofactor to the para position of the phenolic ring of phenylalanine. The available evidence suggests that no intermediates are formed other than a quaternary complex of enzyme, cofactor, oxygen and phenylalanine. The important ordering of the reaction sequence is controversial. Kaufman believes that no product is released until

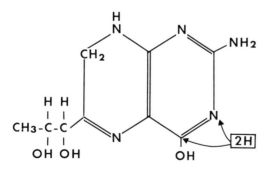

DIHYDROBIOPTERIN

& TETRAHYDROBIOPTERIN

Figure 15–1 The natural cofactor for phenylalanine hydroxylase. The molecule dihydrobiopterin (7,8-dihydro-2-amino-4-hydroxy-6-[1,2-dihydroxypropyl-(L-erythro)]-pteridine) is reduced by the addition of 2H to form tetrahydrobiopterin. Two accessory enzyme systems provide and maintain the reduced coenzyme (see Figure 15–2).

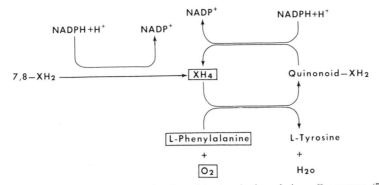

Figure 15–2 Scheme for enzymatic phenylalanine hydroxylation. Coenzyme (7,8-XH_2) is first reduced by a TPNH-dependent reductase (so-called "sheep liver enzyme," which is equivalent to *dihydrofolate reductase*). Coenzyme then participates with L-phenylalanine and O_2 in the hydroxylation reaction. So-called "rat liver enzyme" or *phenylalanine hydroxylase* catalyzes this conversion to tyrosine. Expended (oxidized) coenzyme (Quinonoid-XH_2) is regenerated by a third enzyme *(dihydropteridine reductase)* for reutilization in the hydroxylation reaction.

the three substrates have combined randomly with the enzyme. On the other hand, LaDu and coworkers (Zannoni and Moraru, 1970; LaDu, 1967; Zannoni et al., 1967) suggest that the reaction is ordered, involving a sequential addition and removal of substrates and products as depicted in Figure 15–3. The latter type of reaction exhibits "ping-pong" kinetics, the general features of which were formally described by Cleland (1963). Kaufman (1971) notes that the studies from his laboratory are at variance with those from LaDu's group. He concludes that the kinetics of hydroxylation clearly favor a random, rapid equilibrium type of reaction—that is, one which is unordered in terms of sequential addition and removal of substrates and products. The discrepancy between the two interpretations may reside in the different approaches used by the two groups of investigators. LaDu and colleagues performed their studies at ranges of substrate concentrations which were narrow but in the usual physiological range, particularly for phenylalanine. Kaufman chose a wider range of substrate concentration, reaching well beyond physiological limits. Under such conditions, Kaufman noted that the hydroxylase protein cannot be reduced by synthetic cofactor in the absence of oxygen *and* phenylalanine.

Table 15–1   Kinetic Constants of Various Cofactors for the Phenylalanine Hydroxylation Reaction in Rat Liver[1]

Tetrahydropterin Species	V_{max}[2]	K_m *(mM)*
6,7, dimethyl	1.0	0.070
6, methyl	3.0	0.045
7, methyl	0.8	0.060
Pterin	0.4	—
Biopterin[3]	0.3	0.0045

[1]From Kaufman, 1971.

[2]Expressed as the *relative* rate of NADPH oxidation (see Figure 15–2).

[3]The preferred substrate for the in vivo reaction and the naturally occurring form of cofactor in rat liver.

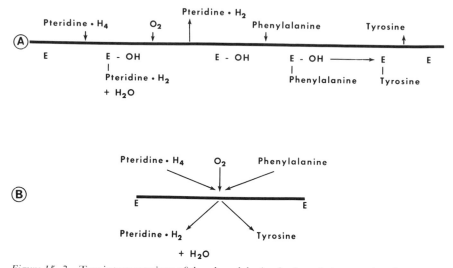

Figure 15-3 Two interpretations of the phenylalanine hydroxylation reaction shown in Figure 15-2. In the upper section an *ordered reaction* is shown, involving sequential addition and removal of substrates and products as proposed by LaDu (1967). The kinetics of this type of reaction are "ping-pong" (Cleland, 1963); the sequence of events is not necessarily as shown. The lower figure depicts the formation of a quaternary relationship between the three substrates and the enzyme as proposed by Kaufman (1971). This proposed mechanism is of the rapid-equilibrium, random type (Cleland, 1963). The experiments supporting the "ping-pong" type of mechanism were performed over a narrow concentration range of substrate concentration, while the random mechanism was deduced from experiments carried out over a wide range of reactant concentration.

There is evidence that the *physical state of the enzyme* itself influences the efficiency with which electron transfer from the coenzyme is coupled to hydroxylation of the phenylalanine substrate. At least two forms of hydroxylase apparently exist in mammalian liver (Kaufman, 1971). One identified at low enzyme concentration is characterized by less efficiency in coupling cofactor oxidation (enzyme reduction) to substrate hydroxylation. The other form is found at high concentrations of enzyme and is characterized by very high efficiency in coupling the components of the overall reaction. Temperature also affects coupling: raising the temperature reduces efficiency. Association or conformational states of enzyme subunits, influenced by the protein concentration and temperature, are evident from such observations. If mutation by one means or another should significantly lower or raise the effective concentration of enzyme in the cell, this might modify the reaction kinetics sufficiently to affect phenylalanine metabolism in vivo.

Kaufman (1971) found evidence that rat liver phenylalanine hydroxylase exists as two isozymes which differ in charge but not in molecular weight. The isozymes can each exist in three forms, as monomer (MW about 55,000), dimer (MW, 110,000) or tetramer (MW 210,000). Tourian (1971) showed that phenylalanine activates the rat liver hydroxylation reaction in the presence of synthetic cofactor. An initial "burst" of activity is apparent when phenylalanine is added to the reaction *before* the tetrahydrobiopterin cofactor (but not when added *after* the cofactor). An activating site, independent of the hydroxylating site, was proposed by Tourian (1971), who noted that activation shifts the equilibrium of liver enzyme from the dimer conformation to the tetramer. Activation is not dependent on enzyme concentration. The apparent K_m for phenylalanine of the activated rat liver enzyme at pH 7 and at 25°C is about 1.75 mM (Tourian, 1971).

Phenylalanine Hydroxylation in Human Liver

Kaufman (1968) has studied phenylalanine hydroxylase in human liver. The characteristics of the reaction are similar to those found for rat liver. Dependence on reduced pteridine cofactor is evident. Human liver apparently also contains a dihydropteridine reductase-like activity. The apparent K_m value of the hydroxylating enzyme for phenylalanine is about 1 mM (similar to rat liver), and for the synthetic cofactor it is 0.057 mM (again similar to rat liver).

Ontogeny of Phenylalanine Hydroxylase

Hepatic phenylalanine hydroxylase activity changes with age during fetal development and perinatally in rat and man (Kretchmer et al., 1956). Friedman and Kaufman (1971) found different developmental patterns in different species. In the rat, there is no appreciable activity until the last day of fetal life. In the guinea pig and in man, activity is apparent from the mid trimester in both species, and the activity at birth is equivalent to that of adult liver. Fetal and adult human phenylalanine hydroxylase activities apparently have similar K_m values for phenylalanine and synthetic cofactor. Jacubovic (1971) confirmed that hepatic hydroxylase activity appears in the early mid trimester (11th to 12th week) of the human fetus. The kinetics of hydroxylation were also examined by Jacubovic in fetal human liver. He found the apparent K_m value for phenylalanine in this system to be about 0.4 mM; values at various fetal ages were comparable. The K_m value for the cofactor was 10 times less. These findings reveal that phenylalanine hydroxylase activities of both rat and human fetal and adult livers are quite similar in their catalytic properties.

A recent paper from Bessman's group (Barranger et al., 1972) indicates that measurement of catalytic activity does not tell the whole story about the ontogeny of phenylalanine hydroxylase. These investigators report two isozymes in human fetal (19th to 20th week) liver, both of which are similar in chemical properties but which differ in charge and can be separated on calcium phosphate gels. The estimated molecular weight of these enzymes is 200,000. Fetal rat liver contains three such enzymes. The findings by this group corroborate Kaufman's data on the physical nature of the hydroxylase and indicate that the complexity of the quaternary structure is a feature of fetal development and adult life.

Berry and colleagues (1972) and Murthy and Berry (1971) have reported developmental patterns similar to that already described, not only in the rat and guinea pig but also in mouse and monkey. The ontogeny of hydroxylation apparent in liver is also found in kidney. However, the latter has a specificity which suggests that the kidney enzyme is different from that present in liver. Evidence for hydroxylase activity in human kidney has not yet been reported or denied.

Regulation of Phenylalanine Hydroxylase Activity

We have indicated earlier in this discussion that the hydroxylation reaction is complex, involves cosubstrates and protein subunits and is subject to a developmental pattern which may involve isozymes. The possibility of more than one type of catalytic function seems likely, given these conditions. Kaufman (1971)

presents evidence that the catalytic function for hydroxylation is not homogeneous in the presence of synthetic cofactor (Fig. 15–4). At concentrations of
phenylalanine below 0.03 mM (the lower limit of the usual phenylalanine content
in the intracellular and extracellular fluids of mammals), and in the presence
of the *natural* cofactor (tetrahydrobiopterin), the enzyme has a low apparent K_m
value for phenylalanine (about 0.04 mM), and a low V_{max} value. At higher concentrations of substrate, the hydroxylase reaction exhibits the characteristic
high K_m value (around 1 mM) and a high V_{max}, as reported in earlier work.
The findings *may* indicate multiple forms of the enzyme, but they may also reflect
conformational changes which occur as the protein undergoes saturation with
its substrate(s). Certainly, the observed phenomenon needs further study.
Biphasic catalysis is not apparent with respect to the two other substrates (the
cofactor and oxygen) which participate in the hydroxylation reaction.

   In the presence of the *natural* cofactor (tetrahydrobiopterin), oxygen above
4 per cent concentration is inhibitory to the hydroxylation reaction (Fig. 15–5A),
and at 21 per cent oxygen concentration there is 25 per cent inhibition; under
hyperbaric conditions, inhibition would be even greater. Phenylalanine excess
also inhibits the hydroxylase in the presence of its *natural* cofactor (Fig. 15–5B).
Inhibition is more pronounced at low enzyme concentrations, suggesting that
the substrate effect is related to enzyme dissociation. It should be noted that
biphasic hydroxylation kinetics and inhibition by substrates are observed only
when the *natural* cofactor is used. Molecular heterogeneity of the hydroxylase
may account for these findings.

   Less stringent evidence of the regulation of phenylalanine hydroxylase
activity has been known for many years. Sex determines its activity to a certain
extent. Male adult rats have about 25 per cent more specific activity in liver
than do females (Brenneman and Kaufman, 1965). The relative sex-dependent
specific activity in the liver of newborn rat and man has not yet been reported,
but in view of the recent evidence for a sex ratio in the frequency with which

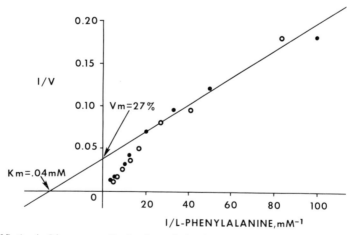

Figure 15–4 A Lineweaver-Burk plot of the initial rate of phenylalanine concentration
in the presence of a fixed concentration of tetrahydrobiopterin (the natural cofactor) at varying
concentrations of L-phenylalanine. The biphasic plot indicates at least two different forms of the
enzyme serving hydroxylation below and above 0.03 mM phenylalanine. The low-K_m constant is
about 0.04 mM and the high K_m value is in the vicinity of 1mM. The V_{max} of the low-K_m component
in the unresolved plot (which does not assign proportional rates to two independent components) is
about 27 per cent of the total velocity. (Redrawn from Kaufman, S.: Advances Enzym. *35*:245–
319, 1971.)

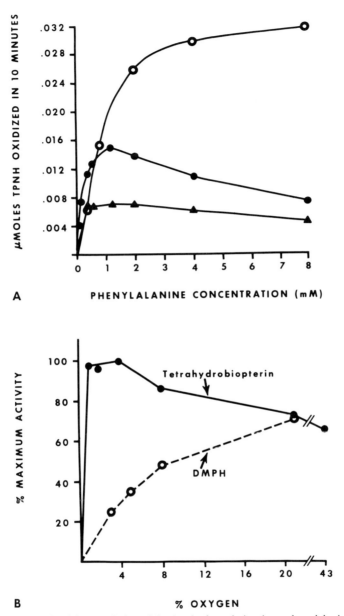

Figure 15–5 The initial rate of phenylalanine hydroxylation by L-phenylalanine hydroxylase in the presence of tetrahydrobiopterin as a function of phenylalanine concentration (*A*) and oxygen (*B*).

A. Increasing the phenylalanine concentration in the presence of *natural* cofactor inhibits hydroxylation (triangles), a finding not present with *synthetic* cofactor, dimethyl tetrahydropterin (open circles). Phenylalanine hydroxylation is augmented by a *stimulator* (closed circles), which is a heat-labile protein (MW 50,000 to 60,000) that may prevent association of the hydroxylase to a form with lower activity. However, the dissociated form of the enzyme is more sensitive to inhibition at high concentrations of substrate. These findings may be relevant to some forms of human hyperphenylalaninemia.

B. The *natural* cofactor renders the hydroxylase susceptible to inhibition by oxygen at concentrations of the latter above 4 per cent. Twenty-one per cent O_2 (physiological) produces 25 per cent inhibition of the maximal hydroxylation rate; the K_m for O_2 is about 0.35 per cent oxygen concentration in solution. O_2 does not inhibit in the presence of synthetic cofactor ($DMPH_4$). (Redrawn from Kaufman, S.: Advances Enzym. *35*:245–319, 1971.)

postnatal hyperphenylalaninemia is recognized in the human newborn (see next section), this aspect of hydroxylase regulation deserves special attention.

Auerbach et al. (1958) reported that rats fed a high phenylalanine diet had severely deficient hepatic phenylalanine hydroxylase activity. Later reports (cited in Kaufman, 1971) were more modest in their claims about "deficient" activity; the question remains unresolved at present. The findings are relevant to the role of diet in the hyperphenylalaninemic states in man.

Phenylalanine Hydroxylase Activity in Hyperphenylalaninemic States in Man

Phenylketonuria, the prototypical form of hyperphenylalaninemia, is apparently associated with a complete deficiency of hepatic phenylalanine hydroxylase activity in man (Jervis, 1953; Mitoma et al., 1957; Wallace et al., 1957; Kaufman, 1958b). These findings have been recently confirmed by Justice and colleagues (1967), who took advantage of the newer assay systems employing synthetic cofactor at saturating levels. The most recent study (Friedman et al., 1973) using the natural cofactor, tetrahydrobiopterin, lysolecithin (a stimulator of activity) and antiserum raised to rat liver enzyme has shown that residual hepatic phenylalanine hydroxylase activity in one patient with phenylketonuria was 0.27 per cent of normal. Substrate inhibition was absent, lysolecithin stimulation was impaired and antiserum inhibition was 30 per cent of normal; the K_m for phenylalanine was normal. The data indicate that phenylketonuria is probably the result of a structural gene mutation at the specific hydroxylase locus.

Several types of hyperphenylalaninemia are known (see following section) in which the degree of phenylalanine accumulation in body fluids is less than in classical phenylketonuria. In vitro assay of hepatic phenylalanine hydroxylase activity in liver biopsy material obtained from a few such patients has revealed low but detectable levels of residual activity (Justice et al., 1967; Kang et al., 1970). This activity can be augmented significantly by the addition of *synthetic* cofactor in vitro; this response is not observed during assay of the mutant enzyme in phenylketonuric liver. This is an important observation, for it implies that, should the hyperphenylalaninemia in vivo be sustained to any extent by phenylalanine inhibition of the mutant hydroxylase in the presence of the *natural* cofactor, it is possible that use of the *synthetic* cofactor in vivo might be able to activate the mutant enzyme and correct the hyperphenylalaninemia.

ALTERNATIVE ROUTES OF PHENYLALANINE METABOLISM

Phenylalanine can be metabolized by minor pathways which form products other than tyrosine (Fig. 15–6). Transamination to form *phenylpyruvic acid* is the best-known initial step; the cosubstrate for the specific amino transferase is pyruvate. The enzyme is apparently inducible by its substrate, but, at least in the rat, it is not inducible by the coenzyme (pyridoxal phosphate) or by steroid hormones (Lin and Knox, 1958). The enzyme is not sex- or hormone-dependent, but its activity increases in the postnatal period (Lin et al., 1959; Armstrong and Low, 1957). Delayed postnatal augmentation impairs the synthesis of phenylpyruvic acid, and this factor is of critical importance to the interpretation of urine testing for phenylpyruvic acid in the newborn. For this reason, a negative ferric chloride test in the newborn period does not exclude the presence of hyperphenylalaninemia. Moreover, the phenylalanine concentration in

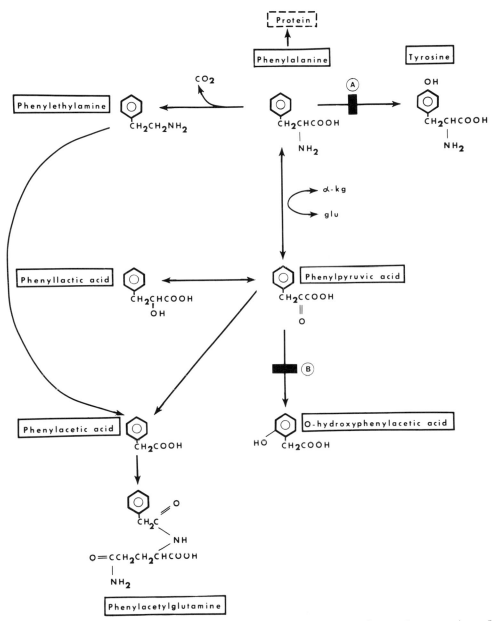

Figure 15–6 Metabolism of phenylalanine by normal *minor* pathways. Incorporation of phenylalanine accounts for less than 50 per cent of the disposal of phenylalanine entering the free pool, even at time of maximum growth. Site of block in phenylketonuria is shown at Ⓐ ; oxidation of phenylpyruvic acid is blocked in disorders of *p*HPPA oxidase at Ⓑ (see Chapter 16).

plasma must be above about 0.5 mM (Armstrong and Low, 1957; Berry et al., 1958) before sufficient phenylpyruvic acid is formed and excreted in urine when the transaminase is normally active. The 2,4-dinitrophenylhydrazine and ferric chloride reactions both detect phenylpyruvic acid; the former is the more sensitive test.

Phenylpyruvic acid can be converted to *phenylacetic* and *phenyllactic acids*. Phenylacetic acid is responsible for the "mousy" odor of the phenylketonuric patient, which first attracted Følling's attention in his investigation of the trait (Følling, 1934). Man and other primates conjugate most of their phenylacetic acid with glutamine before it is excreted into urine (Ambrose et al., 1933), whereas lower mammals use glycine to form the conjugate. *Phenylacetylglutamine* is excreted by renal tubular secretion. Phenylpyruvic acid is converted to its lactate derivative primarily by an aromatic α-keto acid reductase and not by lactate dehydrogenase (Weber and Zannoni, 1966). The keto acid can also be orthohydroxylated by p-hydroxyphenylpyruvic acid oxidase (see Chapter 16), and the product o-hydroxyphenylacetic acid is an important constituent of phenylketonuric urine (Armstrong et al., 1955). In phenylketonuria, its excretion is increased 300 to 400 times above the normal limit of 1 mg/g creatinine.

Another normal pathway for phenylalanine degradation is initiated by decarboxylation of the amino acid. The product of this reaction is phenylethylamine, a pharmacologically potent amine (Oates et al., 1963). An amine oxidase converts phenylethylamine to phenylacetic acid. Udenfriend (1967) has suggested that the amine is more likely to be of significance in the development of the cerebral phenotype in phenylketonuria than those derivatives initiated by transamination.

The above-mentioned reactions can also be performed by the microorganisms which colonize the intestinal tract. Accumulation of phenylalanine in the intestinal lumen may therefore cause formation of the various derivatives, which in this case have an exogenous origin.

DISTRIBUTION IN BODY FLUIDS

The concentration of phenylalanine in plasma is normally held within narrow limits (approximately 0.030 to 0.120 mM), and there is only modest circadian variation in its concentration. The plasma concentration of phenylalanine is slightly lower in the child than in the adult—a reflection, presumably, of the effect of growth upon the distribution of this essential amino acid between intracellular and extracellular compartments. The plasma concentration of phenylalanine is transiently higher in the perinatal period of life. Recognition of this feature is important when trying to discriminate between abnormal hyperphenylalaninemia and the normal postnatal variation which may be detected in mass screening programs.

Phenylalanine is filtered from plasma into the glomerular filtrate and is then reabsorbed efficiently by the renal tubule. The blocked catabolic mutant phenotype of phenylketonuria is associated with very high phenylalanine concentrations in the glomerular filtrate and presumably in renal tissue as well. Brodehl and colleagues (1969) and Scriver (1969) have shown that phenylalanine reabsorption is not impaired under these conditions, indicating that its transport occurs independently from its catabolism in kidney and other tissues. The maximum rate of tubular absorption (Tm_{phe}) has never been clearly determined, but is probably well in excess of 300 μmoles/min/1.73 m^2 (Brodehl et al., 1969).

Phenylalanine is avidly transported by tissues other than kidney. The characteristics of its transport have been discussed in detail (Scriver, 1967). Membrane transport may have some bearing on the phenylketonuric phenotype; and competitive inhibition during transport between phenylalanine and other amino acids, particularly tyrosine and tryptophan, probably accounts for some of the phenotypic features of phenylketonuria (Yarbro and Anderson, 1966).

Phenylpyruvic acid is scarcely detectable in plasma, and over 90 per cent of that which is present is protein-bound (Vink and Kroes, 1961). Lin and co-workers (1962) showed that tissues do not transport the keto acid actively. Renal excretion of phenylpyruvic acid is apparently achieved by net tubular secretion (Vink and Kroes, 1961), the process being susceptible to inhibition by probenecid [p-(di-n-propylsulfamoyl)benzoic acid]. Since alkalinization does not influence the renal excretion of this organic acid, excretion by nonionic diffusion is unlikely (Milne et al., 1958), and active secretion is probable. Phenylacetylglutamine is probably also secreted by kidney into the tubular fluid.

PHENOTYPIC MECHANISMS IN HYPERPHENYLALANINEMIC TRAITS

Animal Models

Limitations in the knowledge of phenylalanine hydroxylation in human tissues, and the lack of a precise understanding of the sequence of events causing the complex clinical phenotype which is associated with hyperphenylalaninemia in man, have led to the search for animal models of hyperphenylalaninemia (Waisman, 1967). The need for such studies is made more acute by the current lack of cultured human cell lines in which phenylalanine hydroxylation can be examined in normal and mutant states.

The objective of hyperphenylalaninemic animal models is to create the biochemical and behavioral analogue of human phenylketonuria. Much work has been done over the years with such models to examine the biochemical facets of the human phenotype.

Considerable hope was placed initially in the homozygous dilute lethal (d^l/d^l) phenotype in the mouse. The homozygote has dilute coat color and a progressive neurological disorder culminating in convulsions and death between three and four weeks after birth. Phenylalanine hydroxylase activity in liver is lower than normal in d^l/d^l mice prior to death (Coleman, 1960), and the K_m values for phenylalanine and cofactor are apparently abnormal (Zannoni and Moraru, 1970). However, the deficiency of activity is not sufficient to cause hyperphenylalaninemia when a normal diet is offered (Zannoni et al., 1966; Woolf et al., 1970), and reinvestigation of the trait (Woolf et al., 1970) has not confirmed the initial impression of a modified K_m value for the phenylalanine hydroxylase of d^l/d^l mice. In fact, there is no evidence that the d^l gene determines any aspect of the phenylalanine hydroxylation reaction. Woolf and colleagues worked with d^l/d^l mice which were younger than those used by previous investigators, and they found that deficient hydroxylation was an artifact of starvation and the terminal illness in these animals. Although the d^l/d^l phenotype may be a valuable model for a gene affecting the nervous system, it is *not* a biochemical model for phenylalanine hydroxylase deficiency causing hyperphenylalaninemia and brain dysfunction.

Natural analogues of phenylketonuria have not yet been found in non-human vertebrates (Lush, 1967). However, Jones and colleagues (1971), by testing the tolerance to intravenous phenylalanine infusion in a colony of 174 primates, have identified one male *Macaca cyclopis* (Taiwan macaque) with an abnormal response resembling the heterozygous phenotype for phenylalanine hydroxylase deficiency. It is hoped that further screening will discover a similar female so that selective breeding may eventually yield a primate offspring with a "homozygous" defect in the oxidation of phenylalanine to tyrosine.

The induction in nonhuman vertebrates of hyperphenylalaninemia with the associated excretion of phenylketones and impaired development of the nervous system has been a difficult challenge, and work in this area has proceeded erratically. Errors are often inadvertently introduced into the experimental protocol to produce "phenylketonuria"; these errors divert the model from anything resembling the human disease. Loading with L-phenylalanine has been used most often, but this procedure also causes a rise in plasma tyrosine so that the high ratio of phenylalanine to tyrosine that is characteristic of human phenylketonuria is not achieved. Because tyrosine accumulation itself may influence brain metabolism (Guroff and Udenfriend, 1962), this model may not be valid. Addition of *p*-chlorophenylalanine to the loading protocol establishes a more realistic model of hyperphenylalaninemia without the equivalent hypertyrosinemia, because the phenylalanine analogue is an inhibitor of phenylalanine hydroxylase (Lipton et al., 1967; Guroff, 1969). However, *p*-chlorophenylalanine is also an inhibitor of tryptophan hydroxylase (Koe and Weissman, 1966), which causes serotonin depletion, and it has not yet been shown whether the analogue produces its effect on cognitive and behavioral development through a serotonin-dependent or a phenylalanine-dependent mechanism or both.

The timing of the induction of hyperphenylalaninemia is important. The procedure must be carried out to affect the brain during the phase of rapid development. Moreover, the effect of the loading technique itself (by injection or gastric intubation) and possible nutritional amino acid imbalance resulting from an excess of phenylalanine (Leung et al., 1968) must be controlled to be sure that it is only the hyperphenylalaninemia which is responsible for abnormal behavior. Longenecker et al. (1970) developed a technique to produce hyperphenylalaninemia in rat pups, and Kerr and Waisman (1967) also studied the induction of long-term postnatal hyperphenylalaninemia in the rat. Any experiments done at a later age would be of little value. Kerr and Waisman (1968) also examined a prenatal induction model in the monkey, which may be of value for the interpretation of human maternal phenylketonuria.

The third area of doubt about animal models concerns the timing and design of the tests for impaired behavior. How does one assess a retarded rat or chimpanzee? The animals should be tested only after the induction procedure has terminated, and there should be pair-fed controls to exclude a nutritional effect of the protocol upon brain development. Polidora et al. (1968) noted that a behavioral deficit associated with induced hyperphenylalaninemia in the rat was reversible, when testing was repeated several weeks after termination of the phenylalanine treatment. Perry and colleagues (1965) had also shown previously that delayed testing found no learning deficits in rats made hyperphenylalaninemic by dietary methods in the postnatal period. It is now believed that the initial deficits in test performance in such experiments were a function of impaired movement and somatic coordination, being artifacts of the protocol rather than effects of the induced hyperphenylalaninemia. A wide range of tests should also be used, since human phenylketonuria impairs many aspects of development and behavior. Earlier experiments which depended on one or two behavioral tests may have missed deficits detectable by other methods.

Two promising models have recently been developed in the rat. Butcher (1970) and Berry and Butcher (1972) have chosen prenatal induction of hyperphenylalaninemia using phenylalanine loading and p-chlorophenylalanine. Pair-fed controls are employed, and multiple testing parameters are used to assess the behavioral deficit during development and at maturity of the offspring. Chemical and neurohistological assessments are also made. This protocol is actually a model more of maternal phenylketonuria than of classical phenylketonuria. Andersen and Guroff (1972) used postnatal induction with p-chlorophenylalanine and phenylalanine injections. The procedure was continued until weaning. Behavioral testing was delayed until six months later. A large number of tests were used, and brain histological correlations were made. This particular experimental design has achieved the closest model of human phenylketonuria so far. Unfortunately, the published report did not give any plasma amino acid data for these particular experiments, and a possible toxic effect of p-chlorophenylalanine itself was not excluded. Also, the model did not produce the myelin deficit in rat brain which is characteristic of the human disease. Despite these reservations, the experiment of Andersen and Guroff and the reporting of it are models for other workers to emulate.

Biochemical Models

The mechanism whereby phenylalanine accumulation may impair brain growth and development of cognitive function has been examined by Aoki and Siegel (1970). They observed that polyribosome structure in cell-free preparations from developing rat brain is disrupted by concentrations of phenylalanine in vitro equivalent to those found in the plasma in phenylketonuria (>1 mM). The disruptive effect is to some extent dependent on tryptophan depletion in vitro. Lindroos and Oja (1971) found that in vivo induction of hyperphenylalaninemia also impaired cerebral protein synthesis in the rat. The phenomenon in vivo is probably part of a generalized perturbation of amino acid transport and distribution in brain in hyperphenylalaninemic states (McKean et al., 1968; Lowden and LaRamee, 1969). Grumer et al. (1971) have studied the effect of L-benzylamine (L-2-amino-4-phenylbutyric acid), a compound which resembles phenylalanine chemically and metabolically, and they have shown that its accumulation in brain also causes amino acid depletion in that tissue. Chase and O'Brien (1970) showed that the protein and DNA content of rat cerebrum and cerebellum is reduced after repeated phenylalanine injection subcutaneously during the first 18 days of postnatal life.

Sulfatide in rat brain (Chase and O'Brien, 1970) and cerebroside in monkey brain (O'Brien and Ibbot, 1966) are both decreased in vivo after prolonged exposure to hyperphenylalaninemia. These findings are relevant to the well documented abnormal lipid content of the brain in human phenylketonuria (Menkes, 1967, 1968). Although the origin of the defect in cerebral lipid metabolism remains unknown, three lines of current investigation hold some promise to explain this important abnormality. Shah and colleagues (1970) found that deaminated metabolites of phenylalanine were potent inhibitors of glucose incorporation into the total lipid fraction of developing brain, which may explain the hypomyelinization characteristic of phenylketonuric brain (Shah et al., 1972). Several workers have shown that phenylalanine and its metabolites, particularly phenylpyruvic acid, inhibit glucose metabolism and oxidative phosphorylation in brain. Very high concentrations of phenylalanine competitively inhibit brain pyruvate kinase, and phenylpyruvate inhibits brain hexokinase (Weber, 1969); immature brain may be especially susceptible to this type of inhibition. However, it should be noted that the concentration of inhibitor used in these experiments bears little resemblance to the equivalent concentration found in the phenylketonuric patient. Swaiman and Lemieux (1969) showed that the ability of rabbit brain slices to utilize glucose to support respiration in vitro was not inhibited by phenylpyruvate, whereas Gallagher (1969) found inhibition with a mitochondrial preparation of rat brain. Bowden and McArthur (1972) found phenylpyruvate to be a strong competitive inhibitor of pyruvate decarboxylation in vitro.

Studies of this type suggest that any impairment of pyruvate availability and oxidation to acetyl-CoA may compromise the synthesis of fatty acids and cholesterol and the yield of ATP from glycolysis, and might account for the depression of myelin synthesis and deposition which accompanies the mental retardation of phenylketonuria. However, myelin deficiency may not be the primary cause for mental retardation. This particular "guilt by association" has not withstood critical analysis in the case of the branched-chain aminoacidopathies, in which mental retardation and myelin defects occur together but clearly not in a consistent cause-and-effect relationship. Moreover, the real significance of any of these experimental data should be questioned as long as there are so few measurements of phenylpyruvic acid in blood and tissues in phenylketonuria. The published evidence suggests that the keto acid content is only about 0.1 mM — that is, much lower than the concentrations used in the in vitro experiments. Careful measurement of the phenylpyruvate content in relation to the phenylalanine concentration must be performed in tissues and in serum of human subjects and in the hyperphenylalaninemic models if we are to be allowed to extrapolate from in vitro models to the in vivo situation.

Only one attempt has been made, to our knowledge, to examine the effects of high concentrations of phenylalanine at a physicochemical level. Because water plays a major role in biological systems and has its own physical chemistry (Grant, 1965), it was suggested that phenylalanine, with its bulky, apolar side chain, might act to disrupt normal water structure in biological systems and thereby disrupt electron conductance (Scriver, 1967). This hypothesis has been tested by Neal (1971), who found that phenylalanine, at the concentrations present in phenylketonuria, does not alter the structure of water.

In summary, although there are many interpretations of the brain disorders in phenylketonuria, it is unlikely that any single event explains this outcome. A combination of events, perhaps related to polymorphic variation in the disposal of phenylalanine metabolites and in target points of many metabolic pathways, is more likely to account for the basic phenotype and the natural variation of the expression of the phenylketonuric allele.

PHENYLKETONURIA

At one time, *phenylketonuria* was believed to be the only primary abnormality of phenylalanine metabolism. However, within the first decade of mass screening for *hyperphenylalaninemia*, it became clear that there were several abnormalities of phenylalanine metabolism in man, each apparently inherited or related to an alteration in the ontogeny of the hydroxylation reaction, and each with its own distinctive phenotype (Table 15–2); like any other inborn error of metabolism, the hyperphenylalaninemic trait is phenotypically and genetically hetero-

Table 15–2 The Hyperphenylalaninemic Traits of Man

Trait Identified	Enzyme Defect	Urine Tests	Clinical Features
1. "Classical" phenylketonuria	Trace of phenylalanine hydroxylase activity[a]	FeCl$_3$, (+)[d] (not always in newborn period)	Mental retardation and other signs; preventable by early treatment. Phe tolerance 250–500 mg/day.
2. Phenylketonuria ("mild" variant with relaxed phenylalanine tolerance)	Unknown[b]	FeCl$_3$, (+) (not always in newborn period)	Mental retardation without early treatment; high tolerance for dietary phenylalanine during treatment (>500 mg/day).
3. Phenylketonuria ("transient" variant)	Partial phenylalanine hydroxylase deficiency[b]	FeCl$_3$ (+)/(−) (not always (+) in newborn period)	Mental retardation without early treatment; changing status affects treatment need (<500 mg/day → normal tolerance).
4. Hyperphenylalaninemia (without phenylketone excretion)	Partial phenylalanine hydroxylase deficiency	Negative	Plasma phenylalanine is consistently less than 1 mM. Asymptomatic trait.
5. Neonatal hyperphenylalaninemia	Presumed phenylalanine hydroxylase deficiency[c]	Usually negative	Often associated with hypertyrosinemia; normal adaptive phenomenon, predominantly in prematures.
6. Offspring of maternal phenylketonuria	No significant deficiency in (heterozygous) offspring	Expected to be negative after birth	Transient falling postnatal hyperphenylalaninemia. Congenital malformation, somatic and cognitive development impaired.

[a]Irreversible, virtually complete deficiency of hepatic phenylalanine hydroxylase in vitro. (Reviewed by Justice et al., 1967; Kaufman, 1971.)

[b]Correlation of "enzyme" phenotype with "clinical" phenotype is difficult. Partially deficient activity in type 4 phenotype responds to cofactor in vitro (Justice et al., 1967; Kang et al., 1970).

[c]The precise nature of the apparent partial enzyme deficiency is unknown; an abnormality in the cofactor system or in the ontogeny of phenylalanine hydroxylase is possible (Kaufman, 1971).

[d]The phenylketone phenylpyruvic acid is responsible for the green color of the positive ferric chloride test. The 2,4-DNPH reaction is said to be more sensitive (Armstrong et al., 1955). Ortho-hydroxyphenylacetic acid is also excreted when there is phenylketonuria.

geneous. Patients with persistent "phenylketonuria" probably have hyperphenylalaninemia; however, it is not true that patients with hyperphenylalaninemia necessarily have the disease phenylketonuria. This disease is described first; the variants are discussed in the section on the genetics of hyperphenylalaninemia.

Classical Phenylketonuria

The mentally retarded, phenylketonuric patient with eczema, pigment dilution and seizures is likely to become a historical oddity, described at length only in out-of-date medical textbooks and rarely encountered in the population. In theory, nearly all patients with homozygous phenylketonuria can be detected by mass screening in the neonatal period; and if the appropriate treatment is administered, the proband should never express the classical phenylketonuric phenotype.

Clinical Features

The clinical features of untreated homozygous classical phenylketonuria are described in detail in reviews by Paine (1957), Partington (1961a), Pitt (1971) and Knox (1972). The sex ratio of untreated patients is not different from that of the non-phenylketonuric population. However, an abnormal sex ratio which favors males exists in the treated group of patients who have been identified in the past decade by mass screening at birth. The great majority of untreated patients have an IQ below 20, and the remainder are usually below 50. The mean value (and standard error) of IQ for untreated patients older than three years of age is 40.2 ($\pm$3.2); less than four per cent of all untreated phenylketonurics apparently have IQ values above 60.

The severe penalty exacted by phenylketonuria on mental development is reflected in the educational distribution of patients. The prevalence ratio of patients in California in the educable retarded group is only 1:750. The ratio rises to 1:175 for trainable retardates; and it is 1:100 in the state institutions for the retarded (Williamson et al., 1968). These figures are probably representative of a worldwide experience with phenylketonuria (Partington, 1961b; Pitt, 1971). Kleinman and colleagues (1964) questioned whether the low intellectual achievement of phenylketonuric patients reflected their mode of ascertainment. However, specific evaluation of this question (Brown and Waisman, 1967; Levy et al., 1970) indicates that untreated phenylketonurics are rarely found outside the mentally retarded population in the community, and it is safe to conclude that untreated phenylketonuria causes severe mental retardation in 96 per cent or more of homozygotes. Therefore, any change in the intellectual phenotype of phenylketonuria which follows the initiation of a program for early diagnosis and treatment can be attributed to this intervention.

The life expectancy of untreated patients is reduced, probably because of the hazards of institutional life. Three quarters of the patients die by 30 years of age. Nothing is yet known about the life expectancy of treated phenylketonuric patients reared at home, although experience up to now shows that current treatment practice is not associated with any excessive risk to life (Knox, 1970). The pattern and frequency of morbidity through intercurrent illness in untreated (and treated) patients is not different from comparable control groups.

It has been customary to believe that the phenylketonuric patient is normal at birth. Saugstad (1972) studied the birth weights of 86 sibs of 53 Norwegian children with classical phenylketonuria. The affected probands, as a group, were 500 g lighter than the control population corrected for gestational age, whereas the unaffected sibs were 300 g heavier. This finding, and a prevalence of preterm births and perinatal difficulties which was higher than normal, may contribute to impaired performance of phenylketonuric children in later life. These important observations clearly need further study and a prospective evaluation by cohort analysis.

A variety of neurological and behavioral manifestations are apparent in later life in the majority of untreated patients. Sixty per cent are agitated, aggressive and hyperactive, and muscular hypertonicity tremor and hyperkinesis affect their gait movement and posture. Microcephaly is also found in about

70 per cent of untreated patients. Electroencephalographic abnormalities are present in 80 per cent, and a characteristic finding can be elicited by photic stimulation (Watson et al., 1968). About 25 per cent of patients have a convulsive disorder, including infantile spasms.

Pigment dilution of hair, skin and irides occurs in untreated patients, who will be more lightly colored than expected for the family, ethnic or racial norm. Eczema is a frequent but not universal finding. Its origin is obscure. The finding should not be confused with a dermatitis which is observed in treated patients who develop hypophenylalaninemia because of insufficient phenylalanine intake.

The untreated patient may have a characteristic odor. As mentioned earlier, Følling's interest in the disease is said to have arisen because of the musty or "mousy" odor of patients he met. The smell is attributed to phenylacetic acid in urine and sweat, but it may be absent if the majority of the acid is excreted as the glutamine conjugate.

The signs and symptoms of phenylketonuria (with the exception of the mental retardation) largely disappear or improve at any age when the hyperphenylalaninemia and attendant biochemical abnormalities are brought under control. Bruhl (1966) documented considerable improvement in the behavior of many retarded phenylketonurics when they were placed on low-phenylalanine diets. However, once mental retardation is established, it can rarely, if ever, be improved by the introduction of a low-phenylalanine diet (Knox, 1960, 1972). Treatment must begin early in life if mental retardation is to be avoided. The IQ penalty for delay in diagnosis and treatment is depicted in Figure 15-7,

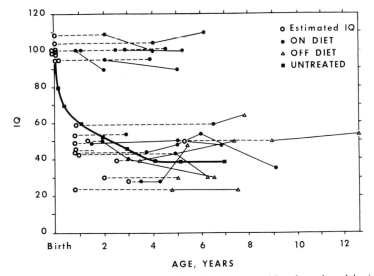

Figure 15-7 The effect of early diagnosis and treatment with a low-phenylalanine diet that prevents hyperphenylalaninemia in classical phenylketonuria. Early-treated patients maintain IQ levels appropriate for family of proband; late-treated probands suffer serious deficits in cognitive development (unpublished data from Clow and Scriver, findings very similar to those reported by Knox, 1972). The heavy line joining the squares (■———■) indicates the mean IQ of patients diagnosed at later and later intervals after birth. Several hundred patients are represented in this graph, which includes the data of Baumeister (1969), Scriver, Katz and Clow (1968) and Knox (1972). It is apparent that early diagnosis and intervention can prevent mental retardation in phenylketonuria. (○ − − − indicates apparent IQ at time of diagnosis; ●———● IQ estimates with patient on treatment; △———△ IQ estimates with patient off treatment.)

which summarizes the data compiled by Baumeister (1967), Scriver et al. (1968), Rosenberg and Scriver (1969) and Knox (1972).

The pathology of phenylketonuria reveals that the brain is the organ which is critically affected (Poser and Van Bogaert, 1959; Crome and Pare, 1960; Crome et al., 1962; Menkes, 1967). Brain weight is less than normal, and myelinization is deficient. The presumed biochemical origins of this outcome were discussed in the preceding section of this chapter.

Biochemical Features

There is abnormal accumulation of phenylalanine in body fluids so that the plasma concentration typically exceeds 1 mM (16.5 mg per cent); if it does not, and if the patient is consuming a normal amount of protein (2 to 3 g/kg per day), then the diagnosis of "classical" phenylketonuria should be questioned and a variant of the trait considered. The concentrations of many other amino acids in plasma are usually significantly decreased (Linneweh and Ehrlich, 1960, 1962; Efron et al., 1969). This finding is not a function of renal loss or of the altered dietary habits in mental retardation, and it probably reflects a complex interaction of phenylalanine with other amino acids in tissue pools

Many of the *normal minor metabolites* of phenylalanine are excreted in greater than normal amounts in phenylketonuria. This response reflects substrate accumulation in phenylalanine hydroxylase deficiency and subsequent deviation of phenylalanine to normally dormant catabolic pathways (Fig. 15–6). The majority of these compounds are most easily detected in the urine, but their accumulation may also occur in blood and sweat (Knox, 1972). Phenylpyruvic acid, phenyllactic acid, phenylacetic acid and its glutamine conjugate and *o*-hydroxyphenylacetic acid are each excreted in large amounts into urine in phenylketonuria. The rate of phenylacetylglutamine synthesis by phenylketonuric liver is much greater than normal (Meister, 1958), suggesting an adaptive increase of this conversion reaction in phenylketonuria. The pharmacologically active compound phenylethylamine is also excreted in increased amounts in phenylketonuria (Oates et al., 1963), and it may be of significance in the pathogenesis of mental deficiency (Udenfriend, 1967). Derivatives of phenylalanine, co-dependent on the availability of pyridoxine, have also been found in phenylketonuric urine (Loo and Ritman, 1964).

All of the minor metabolites are excreted in proportion to the plasma concentration of phenylalanine. In turn, the phenylalanine concentration in plasma is partly related to the amount of phenylalanine released from protein in the diet and from turnover of endogenous protein pools. The plasma concentration of phenylalanine required for the formation of phenylpyruvic acid and its derivatives (threshold value) is at least 0.5 mM (about 8 mg per cent). A detailed analysis by Knox (1970b) of 545 ferric chloride tests in 301 patients showed that a positive test indicating phenylpyruvate excretion was present in only 50 per cent of patients in whom the plasma phenylalanine was 1 mM. The substrate concentration required to yield positive tests in all patients was about 1.8 mM (about 30 mg per cent).

No correlation has been established between the degree of hyperphenylalaninemia above 1 mM and the final IQ level in untreated phenylketonuric patients. Prospective studies indicate that restraint of phenylalanine accumulation to less than 1 mM in plasma is compatible with normal mental development (see following text).

There are many secondary biochemical abnormalities in phenylketonuria which appear to be related to the accumulation of phenylalanine and its metabolites (Table 15–3). The depression of blood serotonin concentration attracted attention long ago (Pare et al., 1957, 1958, 1959), and it has been proposed that serotonin depletion is responsible for the pathogenesis of mental retardation in phenylketonuria (Woolley and Van der Hoeven, 1964a, 1964b; Wooley, 1966).

The excretion of indole (tryptophan) derivatives is increased in phenylketonuria. These metabolites are mainly of intestinal origin, being absorbed after formation by bacterial action on nonabsorbed tryptophan. The absorption of tryptophan is inhibited by phenylalanine (Linneweh et al., 1963; Drummond et al., 1966; Yarbro and Anderson, 1966; Scriver, 1967; Vassella et al., 1968); phenylalanine accumulation in plasma will equilibrate with the intestinal lumen (Christensen et al., 1962) so that the concentration of inhibitor (phenylalanine) will be raised in the lumen and will impair substrate (tryptophan) absorption.

Tyrosine metabolism is altered in phenylketonuria. Catecholamine synthesis may be impaired in the disease, and pressor amines in plasma are decreased in some patients. However, this finding is also true of other causes of mental deficiency (Weil-Malherbe, 1955), and the catecholamine content of the phenylketonuric adrenal gland at autopsy is apparently normal (Fellman and Devlin,

Table 15–3 Effects of Phenylalanine and Its Derivatives on Biochemical Events Which May Be of Potential Significance in Phenylketonuria*

Metabolite	Event or Reaction Affected	Results
Phenylalanine	Amino acid distribution in plasma, tissues, and intestine	Perturbed amino acid transport and protein synthesis in brain
	Tryptophan hydroxylase. Transport of 5-hydroxytryptophan (serotonin, 5HT). 5HT decarboxylase	Serotonin synthesis ↓
	Tyrosinase	Melanin synthesis ↓ Epinephrine synthesis ↓
	(Pyruvate kinase) (Hexokinase)	(Glycolysis) ↓
Phenylpyruvic acid	DOPA decarboxylase	Epinephrine synthesis ↓
	(Pyruvate carboxylase) Pyruvate dehydrogenase	Gluconeogenesis ↓ Acetyl-CoA synthesis ↓
	(Pyruvate kinase) (Hexokinase)	Glycolysis ↓
	Cerebral diglycinase	Peptide cleavage ↓
o-Hydroxyphenylacetic acid	(L-Glutamic acid decarboxylase)	(GABA synthesis) ↓

*Adapted from various sources (Knox, 1972; Bowden and MacArthur, 1972; Weber, 1969; Menkes, 1967). Reactions and results in brackets () are unlikely to occur in vivo in phenylketonuria where concentrations of metabolites are not equivalent to those required to achieve the effect in vitro.

1958). Melanin synthesis is also impaired by excess phenylalanine, and this is the cause of pigment dilution; the latter is reversible when the phenylalanine concentration of plasma is lowered to the normal range (Armstrong and Tyler, 1955). Boylen and Quastel (1962) confirmed that the usual extracellular concentration of phenylalanine found in the patients with phenylketonuria was sufficient to inhibit the tyrosinase system in vitro.

Various workers have suggested that phenylalanine may impair glucose metabolism in brain (see page 304). Amino acids and insulin release are interrelated, but Heffernan (1971) showed that plasma values for glucose and insulin are not abnormal in phenylketonuria.

Chronic glutamine deficiency in body fluids and, by inference, in brain has been advocated by Perry and colleagues (1970) as an important determinant of the mental retardation in phenylketonuria. Their proposal was based upon the discovery of two untreated adult phenylketonuric individuals without mental retardation and in whom the plasma glutamine levels were normal. Taken in perspective with the known depression of plasma glutamine in most untreated patients (Efron, 1969) and the effect of high plasma phenylalanine concentration on brain amino acids in animals (McKean et al., 1968), the presence of normal plasma glutamine in phenylketonuria seemed to be an important finding. It was argued at the time (Scriver, 1970) that the relationship was probably not as simple as it seemed and that a cause-and-effect relationship for phenylalanine and glutamine in brain parallel to that proposed in plasma did not necessarily exist.

Following the publication by Perry and associates, three replies appeared in the literature. Wong et al. (1971) reported briefly that they could find no significant difference between the plasma glutamine content of eight untreated phenylketonuric patients with mental retardation and four similar patients without serious mental retardation. Colombo (1971) found no correlation between IQ and plasma glutamine in two phenylketonuric sibs with borderline normal IQ levels. The major challenge to the glutamine hypothesis came from McKean and Peterson (1970), who measured glutamine in the plasma, cerebrospinal fluid and cerebral gray and white matter of mentally retarded phenylketonuric patients and of retarded patients without phenylketonuria. Plasma glutamine was decreased, whereas glutamine was elevated in the cerebrospinal fluid of phenylketonuric individuals as compared with the control patients, and brain glutamine was also increased in the former. A disturbance of influx or efflux of amino acids into brain was implied, but glutamine depletion as the major cause of mental retardation could not be supported by this evidence. The study of McKean and Peterson is important because it assures the clinician that glutamine feeding will not be a substitute for a low-phenylalanine diet as a treatment mechanism to prevent mental retardation in phenylketonuria.

Heterozygosity for phenylketonuria has been claimed to predispose to mental illness and behavioral abnormalities in later life. Perry (1966) studied 1268 relatives of 34 unrelated phenylketonuric patients and found no greater frequency of mental illness in this group than in a control population of equivalent size composed of the relatives of 34 patients with Down's syndrome.

There remains a large deficit in our knowledge about the cause of mental retardation in phenylketonuria (Kleinman, 1964), and none of the studies in vitro or in vivo, in animals or in man, have yet solved the riddle. Menkes (1967) spoke for most students of the disease when he said, "It is likely that no single answer will be found, but rather that cerebral malfunction is the outcome of a number of chemical abnormalities occurring within the brain as a consequence of a deranged internal milieu present during a critical phase of development."

The Enzymatic Defect

Jervis (1953) was the first to demonstrate a defect in the hepatic conversion of phenylalanine to tyrosine in phenylketonuria, confirming earlier hypotheses about the probable nature of the disease. Mitoma et al. (1957), Wallace et al. (1957) and Kaufman (1958) confirmed this finding with the assays available at that time. Each group showed that the deficient activity involved the labile hepatic enzyme (hydroxylase) and not the cofactor system. Evidence of severe hydroxylase deficiency has been found with the newer assay methods using saturating concentrations of cofactor (Justice et al., 1967; Friedman et al., 1973). Supplementation of the diet with folic and folinic acids has been attempted without effect on phenylalanine accumulation in the disease (Copenhaver et al., 1965). There are no reports of the effect of synthetic cofactor on phenylalanine metabolism in the classical trait. Negative results are expected, but this may not be so in the variant forms of phenylketonuria.

Diagnosis

The infant with phenylketonuria or any other form of postnatal hyperphenylalaninemia is born with a normal level of phenylalanine in the plasma (Hsia et al., 1964) if, under usual conditions, transplacental exchange is normal and the maternal liver disposes of fetal phenylalanine (Fig. 15–8). Plasma phenylalanine rises in the neonate because the exogenous and endogenous loads of free phenylalanine cannot be oxidized normally and because less than half of the free phenylalanine can be incorporated in peptide linkage, even during this period of rapid somatic growth. Therefore, the trait can be detected in the newborn either by screening for hyperphenylalaninemia or by detection of phenylalanine metabolites in abnormal amounts in urine.

The excretion of phenylpyruvic acid and its derivatives (Fig. 15–6) is one of the hallmarks of phenylketonuria. However, the diagnosis of one quarter to one half of infants with phenylketonuria is missed in the neonatal period, when *urine testing* for phenylpyruvic acid and its derivatives is used as the basis for screening (Medical Research Council, 1968). Two factors account for this poor record. One is the instability of phenylpyruvic acid in solution or on the diaper; ferric chloride testing will be negative if the target compound has disappeared by the time the test is performed. The other factor is the likelihood that phenylpyruvic acid may not be formed because of transient phenylalanine aminotransferase deficiency in the newborn period; ferric chloride testing of urine will be negative if this compound is not excreted by the newborn infant.

It is recommended that *blood screening* be performed to detect the hyperphenylalaninemic state (Medical Research Council, 1968; WHO, 1967; American Academy of Pediatrics, 1966). The relative merits of a bacterial inhibition assay, fluorimetric methods and partition chromatographic methods applied to blood collected on filter paper or in heparinized capillary tubes have been discussed in these reports. Experience with several million tests now indicates that each method has its own merits. Fluorimetric and inhibition assays applied to dried blood spots on filter paper have logistical advantages and sufficient sensitivity to detect hyperphenylalaninemia greater than 4 mg per cent (Holton and West, 1970). This value is equivalent to +3 SD above the mean value for Caucasian full-term infants during the first week of life. One-dimensional chromatography also meets the criteria for accurate screening of hyperphenylalaninemia (Partington, 1968). This method is of greatest value when amino acids other than phenylalanine are also of interest for disease detection. The need for constant internal monitoring of the screening method is now well

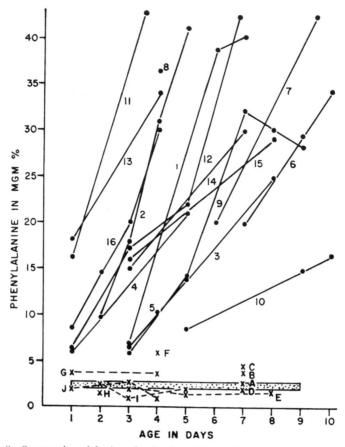

Figure 15–8   Serum phenylalanine after birth and change in relation to age in phenylketonuric probands (●━━●) and their non-phenylketonuric sibs (**X**). The normal mean ±1 SD for serum phenylalanine is indicated by shaded area. All probands had early hyperphenylalaninemia and a rapid further rise in concentration with age. Sex of probands not specified. (Data of Hsia, Berman, and Slatis [1964], used with permission.)

recognized. This need is well illustrated by the study of Hill (1969), who found a seasonal, humidity-dependent variation in the mean value for the phenylalanine content determined by fluorimetric assay of filter paper blood samples collected from newborn infants.

The rate of rise in plasma phenylalanine after birth (Fig. 15–8) in the hyperphenylalaninemic trait is partly dependent on phenylalanine intake. Therefore, the age at which the test is performed will influence the degree of hyperphenylalaninemia observed. It has been discovered that the rate of rise of phenylalanine in plasma after birth may also be sex-dependent (Hsia and Dobson, 1970). The sex ratio in hyperphenylalaninemic states has been found to favor males among the population (Hsia, 1971) ascertained through newborn screening (Table 15–4), whereas (as mentioned earlier) the ratio is unity among classical phenylketonuric patients ascertained by mental retardation. The finding implies that there is a deficit in the detection, by screening in the newborn period, of female patients with the hyperphenylalaninemic trait. Of the 13 known patients who were missed by the initial screening test but were found in later life to have classical phenylketonuria, 10 are female (Hsia, 1971). These

Table 15–4 Sex Ratio in Patients With Hyperphenylalaninemic Traits
Classified According to Diagnosis and Method of Ascertainment[a]

Diagnosis	Method of Ascertainment	Males	Females	Total	M/F ratio
Classical phenylketonuria	1) By mental retardation	385	373	758	1.03 (NS)[b]
	2) By mental retardation and screening	314	312	626	1.01 (NS)
	3) By *a priori* newborn screening alone	151	95	246	1.58 (**)
Non-phenylketonuric hyperphenylalaninemia	1) By *a priori* newborn screening alone	98	72	170	1.37 (*)

[a] Adapted from Hsia (1971)
[b] Probability that observed ratio is different from the expected ratio: **, $p < .001$; *, $p < .05$;
NS, not significant

findings suggest that there is a sex-dependent factor which retards the rise of phenylalanine in the female infant; the nature of this factor is unknown. Clearly, it is desirable to screen for hyperphenylalaninemia as late as possible after birth, yet before mental retardation begins. Scriver et al. (1968) and Kang et al. (1970), among others, have shown that treatment should be started before the end of the first month of life if the full potential of treatment is to be achieved (Fig. 15–7). The latitude for testing is therefore somewhere between the latter part of the first week and the fourth week of life. Economic factors indicate that the ideal schedule for screening can probably never be achieved.

It is now evident that hyperphenylalaninemia is not synonymous with classical phenylketonuria (see further discussion under genetics of hyper-phenylalaninemia). There is a phenylketonuric trait (plasma phenylalanine >1 mM) usually associated with mental retardation in the absence of treatment; and there is a simple hyperphenylalaninemic trait without phenyl-ketonuria (plasma phenylalanine <1 mM), which is *not* usually associated with mental retardation in the absence of treatment. Both types of hyperphenylala-ninemia are apparently more common in Caucasians than in the other races of man, but this opinion may change as there is broader coverage by mass screen-ing (WHO, 1967). The current estimates for the pan-ethnic frequency and dis-tribution of hyperphenylalaninemia in man are given in Table 15–5, which has been compiled from the data of Levy (1972) and others.

To summarize current opinion, the diagnosis of classical phenylketonuria in early life must entertain several criteria, the details of which have been dis-cussed by others (for example: Berry et al., 1966; Castells and Brandt, 1968; Hsia, 1970). The broad principles of diagnosis include the following:

(i) There should be evidence of sustained hyperphenylalaninemia (>1 mM) when the dietary intake of phenylalanine is normal.

(ii) Plasma tyrosine should not rise after a challenge with phenylalanine.

(iii) Formation of phenylpyruvic acid and derivatives should be expected when phenylalanine aminotransferase activity is adequate. This enzyme is substrate inducible, and exposure to substrate for several hours may be neces-sary before formation of the keto acid occurs in vivo in amounts sufficient to appear in urine.

(iv) Plasma phenylalanine concentration should fall to near-normal values when phenylalanine intake in the diet is restricted to about 250 to 500 mg/day.

Table 15–5   Frequency (per 100,000 live births) and Regional
Distribution of Patients with Phenylketonuria (PKU) and
Non-Phenylketonuric Hyperphenylalaninemia[a]

Geographical Region	Number Screened	Approximate frequency (per 100,000 live births)	
		PKU	Hyperphenylalaninemia
Australia	514, 421	11.1	2.9
Austria	362,776	9.1	2.8
Belgium	160,942	16.6	1.8
Canada	435,889	6.4*	2.1
Czechoslovakia	45,504	14.2	4.3
Denmark	195,000	7.1	3.0
France	672,276	7.7	9.1
Germany (West)	1,325,730	16.6	—
Great Britain			
England	395,046	12.0	1.25
N. Ireland	20,919	10.0	—
Scotland	252,821	16.6*	2.8
Eire	62,856	22.2*	—
Israel	315,476	5.3*	—
Japan	35,755	5.5	—
New Zealand	162,223	6.2	1.3
Poland	619,231	12.5	0.5
Switzerland	334,958	5.5	3.7
United States	7,706,643	7.1*	—
Yugoslavia	100,000	7.7	—
TOTAL	12,412,716 AVERAGE	8.5	3.3

[a]Adapted from Levy (1972) and other sources.
*Frequency variation recognizable in samples. For example, frequency of phenylketonuria in French Canadians appears to be about ½ of Canadian national average; the frequency of phenylketonuria in American Negroes and Indians is much lower than the national (US) average, while in the Scots and Irish, it is higher; phenylketonuria in Israel is limited almost exclusively to non-Ashkenazic Jews and Arabs.

The dietary tolerance for phenylalanine should remain in this range throughout infancy and early childhood.

(v) Parents should display partial impairment of phenylalanine conversion to tyrosine compatible with the heterozygous phenotype.

(vi) The apparent diagnosis should be monitored continuously to avoid misdiagnosis of a variant trait.

Treatment

Replacement of the deficient enzyme, or induction of residual activity, is not yet feasible in phenylketonuria. Liver transplantation from a non-phenylketonuric donor could provide a source of enzyme and, if transplantation becomes less difficult, a "permanent" treatment of phenylketonuria could be provided to the patient of the future. In the meantime, the only practical mode of therapy is restriction of phenylalanine in the diet.

Bickel, Gerrard and Hickman (1953, 1954) were the first to use a protein hydrolysate, from which most of the phenylalanine had been removed, for treatment of phenylketonuria. Armstrong and Tyler (1955) soon confirmed that biochemical control of phenylalanine accumulation in phenylketonuria could be achieved by dietary means, and later reports (Blainey and Gulliford, 1956; Woolf et al., 1958; Brimblecombe et al., 1959) maintained the enthusiasm generated by the first published results. Knox reviewed the experience with diet up to 1960 on a small series of patients, and he concluded that dietary treatment definitely held promise for the patient with phenylketonuria. It then became apparent that there were a few phenylketonuric patients who achieved near-normal intelligence without the benefit of any treatment whatsoever; and when retarded somatic growth, rashes, bone changes, unexpectedly low IQ attainment and even death began to be reported, serious doubts about the safety and value of the dietary treatment were raised (Bessman, 1966; Birch and Tissard, 1967; Bessman, 1968). This skepticism made it apparent to all that treatment of classical phenylketonuria is a serious undertaking which requires careful supervision to achieve the desired benefits.

The beneficial effects which derive from *appropriate* dietary treatment have been well documented. The Medical Research Council of Great Britain (1963) reported a favorable outcome in 20 of 25 patients in whom treatment began before three months of age. This collaborative report and many subsequent studies have shown that a delay in the initiation of treatment after birth impairs later cognitive development (see, for example, Baumeister, 1967; Dobson et al., 1968; Scriver et al., 1968; McBean et al., 1968; Knox, 1972), which shows that mental development with early diagnosis and treatment is clearly better than the performance which follows late diagnosis and treatment. It can be concluded from such results that early treatment with low-phenylalanine diet in classical phenylketonuria prevents the characteristic impairment of mental development (Fig. 15–7).

The benefit of early treatment in phenylketonuria can also be illustrated by comparing the performance of early-treated patients and their late-treated or untreated phenylketonuric sibs. A survey of such sib pairs in eastern Canada revealed that early-treated sibs perform better than the less well-treated sibs (Table 15–6). Similar data by Berman et al. (1969) and Hanley et al. (1971) on 46 sib pairs confirm that the average IQ for early-treated patients approaches the normal range and is much higher than the mean value for the late-treated and untreated sibs. Hudson et al. (1970) and O'Grady et al. (1971) also demonstrated that the IQ of treated sibs approached the intrafamilial IQ of parents and unaffected sibs.

It is customary to think of the beneficial effects of low phenylalanine intake in phenylketonuria mainly in terms of the IQ. However, dietary treatment can also ameliorate behavior abnormalities in the retarded older phenylketonuric patient. Bruhl (1966) recorded improved behavior after administering a low-phenylalanine diet to adult phenylketonuric patients, and McKean (1971) found evidence of improved behavior during a six-month period of low-phenylalanine diet treatment in four retarded adolescent phenylketonurics. Behavioral improvements were most apparent when the plasma phenylalanine concentration remained below 0.75 mM. On the other hand, Hambraeus and colleagues (1971) could not see any benefit from short-term dietary treatment in the behavior of retarded adult phenylketonurics despite biochemical improvement. These studies imply that a long exposure to treatment may be required to observe improvement in the hyperactive and aggressive behavior of retarded phenylketonuric patients.

Table 15–6   Comparison of Cognitive Development in Sib Pairs
Diagnosed at Different Ages, but Treated Similarly with
Low-Phenylalanine Diet for Classical Phenylketonuria*

Sib Pair	IQ Achieved After 2 Years of Age	
	Late-treated Sib[a]	Early-treated Sib[b]
1	45	93
2	22	113
3	75	92
4	27	100
5	75	100
6	37	70
7	65	88
8	69	86
9	51	94
10	54	96
Mean IQ	53.0	93.2[c]

[a]Mean age at onset of treatment in late-treated group is 11.7 months.
[b]Mean age at onset of treatment in early-treated group is 18 days.
[c]Significance of difference by Student's t test: $p<.001$.
*Unpublished data from study of Scriver, Katz, and Clow (1968).

The quality of treatment is clearly an important determinant of the outcome, and numerous complications of inadequate treatment have been observed. Fisch et al. (1969) found growth retardation in many treated patients, and Rouse (1966) documented signs of simple phenylalanine deficiency in other patients on low-phenylalanine diets. Hackney et al. (1968) found behavioral and learning problems with poorer school progress than anticipated in treated patients with adequate IQ attainment. Berman and Ford (1970) noted that phenylketonuric children treated from early infancy may still function below the intellectual levels expected of them, and Fuller and Shuman (1969, 1971) discovered similar discrepancies between expectation and attainment of IQ in another group of treated patients. There is a certain likelihood that some treated phenylketonuric children underachieve because of perinatal difficulties. This was documented by Scriver et al. (1968) and Hanley and colleagues (1971).

Several groups with much practical experience in the treatment of phenylketonuria have found that relentless attention to the details of treatment are essential for a good outcome. Hanley et al. (1970) published an important paper reporting that too much stringency in the treatment regimen can be harmful. Over-restriction of phenylalanine intake causes chronic hypophenylalaninemia, which may impair cognitive and behavioral development during the formative years. Umbarger and colleagues (1965), Koch and coworkers (1970) and Clow et al. (1971) have published valuable reports which describe how frequent monitoring of blood phenylalanine levels during treatment, careful attention to caloric and total phenylalanine intake and continuous supervision of the patient in all aspects of health care can insure normal somatic growth, prevent phenylalanine deficiency and yield cognitive and behavioral development equivalent to expectations. Berry and colleagues (1965) published descriptions of procedures for monitoring treatment sufficiently long ago that some of the pitfalls of treatment could have been avoided if their warnings had been heeded; and Berry and Wright (1967) summarized the recommendations of a conference on treatment at which these concerns were discussed in depth.

The amount of phenylalanine required to maintain the plasma phenylalanine level between the normal range and about 0.75 mM is more or less constant throughout childhood. Kennedy et al. (1967) determined that between 250 and 500 milligrams of L-phenylalanine per day is satisfactory. However, there is new evidence (Scriver and Clow, unpublished; McKean, 1971) that an intake of phenylalanine that is higher by about one third than the intake in early life can be tolerated by phenylketonuric patients during later childhood and adolescence.

The diet used for treatment comprises natural foods with low phenylalanine compositions and a semisynthetic component derived from protein foods and treated to remove a substantial amount of the phenylalanine. This semisynthetic component is available commercially in North America, Europe and the Far East under various labels. Bentovim and colleagues (1970) described ways to improve the monotony of these diets and to overcome the unpleasant flavor of the protein hydrolysate. Hunt and colleagues (1971) and Boisse et al. (1971) report in detail how one can assure an adequate intake of essential amino acids and other important nutrients, while restraining the intake of phenylalanine, through the use of semisynthetic components in the diet. McCarthy et al. (1969) published a most useful article on the phenylalanine and tyrosine content of a wide variety of fruits and vegetables—information which the doctor rarely has but which the mother needs in order to feed her phenylketonuric child.

Whereas the low-phenylalanine diet is the mainstay of treatment for phenylketonuria at present, other potential approaches to treatment should not be ignored. Woolley and Van der Hoeven (1964a, 1964b) and McKean et al. (1967) proposed that serotonin congeners of L-tryptophan could offset the effects of hyperphenylalaninemia upon the nervous system. Their experiments showed a benefit of this chemical approach in animals exposed to phenylalanine loading in a model system. However, there has been no comparable study in man, and there probably will not be one as long as other modes of treatment are effective. Lines and Waisman (1970) suggested that β-2-thienylalanine, which is a competitor for phenylalanine uptake by the cell, might block phenylalanine transport in the intestine, but controlled studies have not been performed in animals to indicate whether such an approach to treatment could be either safe or beneficial for a human patient.

Untoward effects of the semisynthetic diet have been observed. For example, Arakawa et al. (1965) reported folic acid deficiency during the use of a low-phenylalanine diet which was deficient in this vitamin. This report and others in a similar vein draw attention to the fact that when a semisynthetic diet is the major source of nutrients for a growing infant, it *must* be nutritionally adequate to prevent harm.

The question of when to terminate the diet has not been resolved. Horner et al. (1962) recommend termination of treatment in the preschool period, at which time brain growth is virtually complete. Vanderman (1963) expressed a similar opinion, and the theme was heard again from Solomon and colleagues in 1966. Nonetheless, caution of this opinion is advisable because it is not known whether phenylalanine accumulation can perturb the chemical basis of learning in *later* childhood. If suboptimal treatment causes behavioral disorders and learning deficits, then perhaps termination of treatment too early in a child's development may also be undesirable. At present, there seems to be no real justification for termination of diet in the preschool child except for the social convenience of this action. Controlled prospective studies are required to

compare cognitive function in adolescent phenylketonuric patients treated
continuously through childhood and adolescence with cognitive function in
those who experienced termination of treatment upon entering the school years.

Genetics of Hyperphenylalaninemia (Phenylketonuria)

Persistent postnatal hyperphenylalaninemia is no longer sufficient evidence by itself for the diagnosis of phenylketonuria (Auerbach et al., 1967;
Allen et al., 1967; Berman et al., 1969; Hsia, 1970; Woolf, 1970). It is now very
apparent that the trait is genetically heterogeneous. Many types of hyperphenylalaninemia are known, some of which may be "homozygous" phenotypes, while
others may be "double heterozygotes" for mutant alleles at a common or at different gene loci controlling phenylalanine hydroxylation. When assays of phenylalanine hydroxylase can be performed easily, there will be a better opportunity
for interpretation and classification of hyperphenylalaninemic probands. In
the meantime, clinical and metabolic features must be used to distinguish the
different traits.

Classical Phenylketonuria

This condition has long been recognized as an autosomal recessive trait
(Jervis, 1964), the frequency of which was originally estimated by Jervis (1954),
using indirect methods of ascertainment, to be about 1:25,000 in the general
population. However, since the advent of mass screening, the frequency estimates from direct ascertainment at birth have proven to be about twice as high
(see Table 15–5). The latter finding suggests that, in the past, classical phenylketonuric homozygotes were either missed because ascertainment at birth and
thereafter was incomplete or that current estimates include probands who do not
have classical phenylketonuria. It is quite likely that both alternatives are true.

When the prevalence of phenylketonuric homozygotes (q^2) is about 0.0001,
the frequency of heterozygotes ($2\,pq$) will be about 0.02 according to the Hardy-
Weinberg equation, and identification of the heterozygote can be of value under
certain conditions for counseling, case-finding and confirmation of diagnosis.
However, the procedures required to confirm the heterozygous state are often
cumbersome or even unreliable (Knox, 1972).

Detection of heterozygotes has usually relied on one of two primary approaches. Either a phenylalanine loading test is performed to challenge the
reduced capacity for phenylalanine hydroxylation in the heterozygote, or steady-
state levels of phenylalanine and tyrosine in plasma are measured under carefully controlled conditions. Some form of discriminatory analysis is usually
applied to improve classification of the heterozygote. Bremer and Neumann
(1966) and Woolf and colleagues (1967a) showed that rapid intravenous infusion
of L-phenylalanine allowed accurate measurement of the phenylalanine clearance rate from plasma. By plotting the rate of plasma amino acid disappearance
on a semilogarithmic graph, it was possible to segregate heterozygotes from normal subjects with considerable reliability. Unfortunately, the results of Bremer's
and Woolf's studies cannot be compared directly, because each investigator
used a different infusion protocol.

Rampini and colleagues (1969) re-examined the more conventional oral
loading test for heterozygote detection. They recognized that while intravenous
loading overcomes the perturbing effect of intestinal absorption upon the
plasma phenylalanine response, the challenge of preparing and infusing the
phenylalanine solution limits the use of an intravenous loading protocol.

Rampini's studies were done in the morning after an overnight fast and employed L-phenylalanine (100 mg/kg body weight) administered in a drink. Blood was drawn five times, at 0, 1, 2, 3 and 4 hours during the period of amino acid loading. The blood samples were then analyzed for phenylalanine and tyrosine by a rapid-elution chromatographic method on ion exchange resin. The values for the hourly phenylalanine increments above the pre-load baseline, and for the corresponding phe/tyr ratios, were summed and various discriminant functions calculated. It was then possible to identify heterozygotes with great accuracy. The discriminant index derived by Rampini and colleagues was better than any of the corresponding indices which they calculated from the data published by 10 other groups of investigators. The only exception was a study of female heterozygotes investigated with the intravenous loading method by Woolf et al. (1967a). However, the work involved with an oral loading test carried out over several hours, and the demands that were placed on the subject by the test procedure are sufficient to compromise the usefulness of even this approach.

A very simple test was proposed by Perry et al. (1967a, 1967b) and by Rosenblatt and Scriver (1968). Both groups utilized a single blood sample, subsequently analyzed for phenylalanine and tyrosine by rapid-elution chromatography on modified ion exchange resin columns. The rapid-column chromatographic methods (Shih et al., 1967; Perry et al., 1967b; Scriver et al., 1968) have a number of advantages; Levy and colleagues (1971) have shown that filter-paper blood spots can be used for analysis by these techniques. Rosenblatt and Scriver (1968) examined the circadian variations in plasma concentration of the two amino acids and selected noon (before lunch) as the preferred time to draw the sample, after a normal breakfast. Perry's group examined a morning blood sample obtained after an overnight fast. Both groups noted that the ratio of phenylalanine in tyrosine (phe/tyr ratio) in blood plasma or serum gave rather better discrimination between heterozygotes and normal subjects than did direct comparison of the phenylalanine or tyrosine concentrations in the two populations. Discrimination was further improved when the plasma phenylalanine concentration was plotted against the phe/tyr ratio (Rosenblatt and Scriver, 1968), and a division between normal and heterozygous populations was found in both planes of the graph (Fig. 15–8). The reliability of this approach was subsequently affirmed by Jackson et al. (1971), who estimated that the chances of misdiagnosis with the method were less than 5 per cent. The graphic approach to discriminatory analysis was re-examined by Gold, Maag, Neal and Scriver (unpublished data), and a bivariate analysis using a Bayesian combination of density functions was employed to develop a map of probabilities (also shown in Figure 15–9). Statistical boundaries between normal and heterozygous populations could be defined with this method, and they will provide the counselor with an estimate of the probability that a given individual is, or is not, a carrier of the phenylketonuric gene. The reliability of this method seems to be as good as any other approach published so far; and good discrimination can now be achieved on the basis of a *single* blood specimen. For those individuals whose values are outside the 0.01 probability boundary in Figure 15–9, yet close to that line, the counselor can recommend more stringent studies with intravenous or oral loading techniques. In this way, it should be possible to "screen" for carriers of the phenylketonuric gene with reasonable accuracy and efficiency.

An important and interesting artifact has been identified which may influence the classification of females. Pregnancy is often associated with a slightly raised phenylalanine concentration and phe/tyr ratio in plasma (Kang

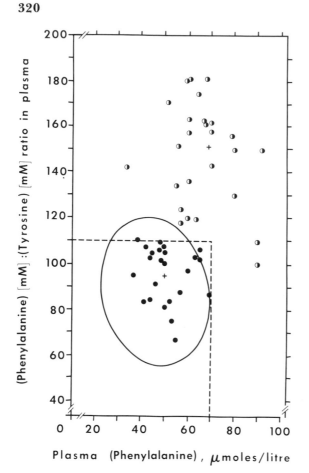

Figure 15–9 The relationship of the millimolar phenylalanine:tyrosine ratio in plasma to the concentration (millimolar) of phenylalanine in obligate heterozygotes for classical phenylketonuria (half-shaded circles) and (presumed) homozygous normal subjects (shaded circles). A single sample of blood was drawn at 12 noon, before a meal. The dotted rectangle indicates the upper range of "normal" values in the original study reported by Rosenblatt and Scriver (1968). The ellipse is the contour for a probability of 0.01. The probability is greater than 0.01 that values inside the contour indicate the homozygous normal phenotype; the same is true for values outside the contour when referring to heterozygotes, assuming the a priori frequency of heterozygotes in the random population to be 0.02. The "counseling ellipse" is derived from bivariate analysis of Bayesian density functions for the two populations of genotypes according to the method of Gold et al. (1973).

et al., 1963). It has also been reported by Jackson and colleagues (1971) that the "pseudopregnancy" associated with oral contraceptives may raise the fasting phe/tyr ratio above the normal range. The latter investigators claimed that the corresponding levels of phenylalanine and tyrosine were lower than usual, a point which may be in dispute according to our own observations. Nonetheless, it would be appropriate to use caution when interpreting an abnormal test for heterozygosity in women of fertile age. In this respect, it is of interest that the discriminant function for women in the study of Woolf et al. (1967) was much higher (i.e., more indicative of heterozygosity) than for the male subjects in the same study. An artifact related to hormonal effects may explain this finding, particularly if the obligate heterozygotes studied by Woolf et al. were taking oral contraceptives subsequent to the birth of phenylketonuric offspring.

Variant Forms of Hyperphenylalaninemia

A division of the variants into two subgroups can be proposed to include traits with associated phenylpyruvate excretion and traits without phenylketonuria. The difference between the two groups probably reflects the intensity of hyperphenylalaninemia. Patients with phenylketone excretion usually have plasma phenylalanine levels above 1 mM (16.5 mg per cent), while those without it generally have a degree of hyperphenylalaninemia below 1 mM.

The phenotypic and genetic heterogeneity of the hyperphenylalaninemias has caused much confusion. Some of the turmoil lies in terminology. Hsia's review (1970) mentions articles describing "persistent hyperphenylalaninemia," "mild phenylketonuria," "transient hyperphenylalaninemia," "hyperphenylalaninemia without phenylketonuria" and "normal phenylketonuria," among other terms. Scriver (1967) suggested that the term *transient newborn hyperphenylalaninemia* could be reserved for a normal postnatal adaptive phenomenon without disease significance. The general term *hyperphenylalaninemia* should be reserved for harmless traits without phenylketonuria whose greatest hazard lies in misdiagnosis for phenylketonuria. The remainder of the hyperphenylalaninemic disorders include phenylketonuria and are hence classified as *phenylketonurias*; these are important because they can cause mental retardation. The enzymatic basis for most of the hyperphenylalaninemic variants has only rarely been defined (Table 15–7) or correlated with the corresponding clinical and biochemical phenotype.

Nonclassical Phenylketonuria. Phenotypic classification on the basis of the day-to-day levels of phenylalanine in plasma and the tolerance for phenylalanine in the diet reveals two proband groups in addition to the group of classical phenylketonurics (Figs. 15–10 and 15–11).

PHENYLKETONURIA WITH RELAXED TOLERANCE FOR DIETARY PHENYLALANINE. In order to maintain the plasma phenylalanine level well below 1 mM in classical phenylketonuria, the usual dietary tolerance for L-phenylalanine is between 250 mg and 500 mg per day (Kennedy et al., 1967). However, some phenyl-

Table 15–7 Hepatic Phenylalanine Hydroxylase Activity in Controls and Patients with Classical Phenylketonuria (PKU) and Variant Forms of Hyperphenylalaninemia

Reference	Subject or Trait (n)	Age (Yr.)	Phenylalanine Hydroxylase Activity[a] (μmoles tyrosine formed/g protein/hr)	
			Without Synthetic Cofactor	With Pteridine[b]
Kang et al. (1970)	Controls (3)	10–86	0–1.70	58.8–96.0
Justice et al. (1970) and Hsia (1970)	Controls (5)	20–60	3.0 ± 1.6	57.0 ± 10.0
Justice et al. (1970)	Classical PKU	19	0	0
	PKU with increased tolerance for phe	$1\frac{6}{12}$	0	0
	Transient PKU	$1\frac{10}{12}$	0.6	6.0
	Hyperphenylalaninemia	35	1.6	24.7
Kang et al. (1970)	Hyperphenylalaninemia (double heterozygote)	$\frac{3}{12}$	1.3	4.7
Hsia (1970)	Hyperphenylalaninemia	$\frac{3}{12}$	0.7	6.3

[a]Measured as described in cited references. Fresh liver obtained by open or percutaneous needle biopsy, and homogenized for assay.

[b]Synthetic cofactor (dimethyltetrahydropterin) at saturating concentration.

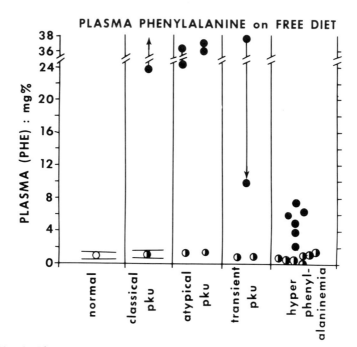

Figure 15–10 Plasma phenylalanine under free diet conditions in affected probands with three phenylketonuric phenotypes, in a hyperphenylalaninemic subject without phenylketonuria and in normal homozygotes. ● = probands who are presumed homozygotes or perhaps double heterozygotes for two mutant alleles or genes; ◑ = obligate heterozygotes for the trait. (Unpublished data of Scriver et al.)

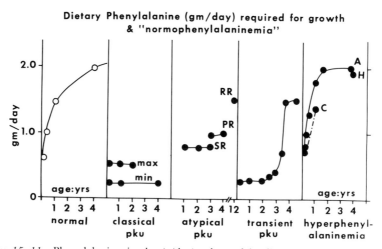

Figure 15–11 Phenylalanine intake (g/day) tolerated in diet by normal subjects, probands with three different types of phenylketonuria and probands with hyperphenylalaninemia without phenylketonuria. (See Figure 15–10 for symbol legends.)

ketonuric patients can tolerate a higher phenylalanine intake, and the post-natal rise in plasma phenylalanine in these patients is slower than in the classical phenylketonurics (Kennedy et al., 1967). At one time, it was believed that these patients filled a portion of the spectrum for the expression of classical phenyl-ketonuria (Hsia, 1967), but continuing observation suggests that they represent an independent genetic variant of the phenylketonuric trait.

Klein, Scriver and colleagues (unpublished data) have followed a pedigree for eight years in which three sibs with this form of phenylketonuria were found in a sibship of eight. Two of these patients are mentally retarded; the third was diagnosed at birth and was treated with a low-phenylalanine diet which resulted in normal intelligence in this proband. The phenylalanine in-take which can be tolerated by these three sibs without causing severe hyper-phenylalaninemia varies between 750 mg/day in the youngest and 1500 mg/day in the oldest (Fig. 15–11). The latter patient was carefully studied with regard to his phenylalanine tolerance and his ability to form phenylpyruvic acid and its derivatives, and the results are shown in Figure 15–12. Over 2 g of phenyl-alanine per day was tolerated before marked hyperphenylalaninemia and phenylpyruvic acid excretion appeared. When phenylketone excretion was restrained by a reduction of the phenylalanine intake, the plasma phenylalanine could then be raised abruptly by oral loading with phenylalanine (100 mg/kg). However, phenylpyruvate was not formed under these conditions; and further-more, tyrosine rose in plasma—a response not found in classical phenylketo-nuria. The failure to excrete phenylpyruvate might be wrongly interpreted as a deficiency of phenylalanine-pyruvate aminotransferase activity (Auerbach et al., 1967), when in fact it is probably the normal behavior of an inducible enzyme which must be exposed to its substrate (phenylalanine) for a period of time in excess of a few hours before the product (phenylpyruvate) can be formed.

The mechanism for the relaxed dietary tolerance of phenylalanine in this type of phenylketonuria is unknown. It does not appear to be the result of

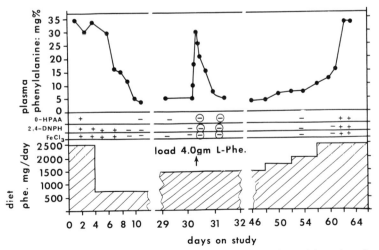

Figure 15–12 Biochemical phenotype of a 12-year-old patient with variant form of phenyl-ketonuria characterized by relaxed tolerance for dietary phenylalanine. Note failure to form phenylpyruvic acid and derivatives after phenylalanine loading. The transaminase which allows for-mation of these metabolites was apparently not induced under transient loading conditions, although it is sufficiently active in this patient when persistent hyperphenylalaninemia is present. (Un-published data of Scriver et al.)

intestinal or renal wastage of phenylalanine secondary to a specific impairment of membrane transport. Lines and Waisman (1971) published evidence which they believed supported the wastage hypothesis, but recalculation of their data shows no abnormality of phenylalanine clearance by kidney in the atypical patients. Incomplete loss of phenylalanine hydroxylating activity or retention of a normal isozyme of phenylalanine hydroxylase in hepatic or other tissues may explain this condition.

The parents of probands with this form of phenylketonuria exhibit a heterozygous phenotype typical of the classical trait (Rosenblatt and Scriver, 1968), and the variant is apparently autosomal recessive.

TRANSIENT PHENYLKETONURIA.   This variant has been reported by O'Flynn et al. (1967), Castells et al. (1968), Cohn et al. (1968) and Komrower (cited in Hsia, 1970). We also have observed probands with the trait, and its occurrence is probably not exceptionally rare among individuals with phenylketonuria. The course of a patient with transient phenylketonuria which declared itself in the *fourth* year of life is seen in Figures 15–10 and 15–11. Probands in other pedigrees have usually exhibited a transition in phenylalanine tolerance at an earlier age.

The transient condition is of special interest for two reasons. First, it must be recognized at birth and treated with a low-phenylalanine diet, as if it were classical phenylketonuria, in order to avoid mental retardation. Second, the patient must be followed carefully: otherwise, when the transition in phenylalanine tolerance occurs, a state of phenylalanine deficiency might develop should the restricted phenylalanine intake be continued. An example of this complication is cited by Hsia (1970).

The available evidence suggests that this trait is inherited as an autosomal recessive and that the parents of probands exhibit the "heterozygous" phenotype for conversion of phenylalanine to tyrosine. The mutant allele is unlikely to be the same as that which causes the classical trait, but a mixture of two different mutant alleles, either at the same locus or at two loci controlling different components of the hydroxylase reaction, provides two possible explanations for this trait.

The mechanism of hyperphenylalaninemia has not been well studied. However, Justice et al. (1970) have examined phenylalanine hydroxylase activity in a liver biopsy specimen obtained from one infant (patient 4 in their report) who may have had the transient trait. They found low residual hydroxylase activity (20 per cent of normal) in untreated liver homogenates. This residual activity could be augmented tenfold with saturating concentrations of synthetic cofactor in vitro.

Hyperphenylalaninemia Without Phenylketonuria

The data in Table 15–5 show that about one quarter of all patients with hyperphenylalaninemia have a "mild" or "benign" type of hyperphenylalaninemia without coexistent phenylketonuria. At first the trait was most often recognized in North Americans of Mediterranean origin; this association encouraged the eponym "Mediterranean hyperphenylalaninemia" (Scriver, 1967), a practice which can be abandoned now that the trait is known to occur widely in Anglo-Saxons (particularly the Scots), Central Europeans, Arabs and Jews (both Ashkenazim, among whom classical phenylketonuria is very rare, and non-Ashkenazim).

The postnatal rise in plasma phenylalanine is usually slower than in classical phenylketonuria, and the plateau reached is *below* 1 mM, even when the dietary intake of phenylalanine is unrestricted (Figs. 15–10 and 15–11). Phenylpyruvate and its derivatives are not formed in significant amounts. Normal development of cognitive functions in probands, in the absence of treatment, is the most important clinical feature of this type of hyperphenylalaninemia (Berman and Ford, 1969; Levy et al., 1971). Phenylalanine loading tests reveal clearance of phenylalanine from plasma which is slower than normal in the probands, yet faster than in homozygotes with classical phenylketonuria (Blaskovics et al., 1968). Plasma tyrosine rises in the hyperphenylalaninemic proband after a phenylalanine load (Kang et al., 1970), whereas it does not in the proband with the classical trait.

The enzymatic mechanism of hyperphenylalaninemia has now been examined in several probands (Justice et al., 1967; Tada et al., 1969; Kang et al., 1970). In each case, significant residual phenylalanine hydroxylation activity was found in the liver biopsy material. This residual activity, which was about 10 to 20 per cent of normal, could be increased at least threefold by the addition of synthetic cofactor (dimethyltetrahydropterin) to the incubation mixture. Kaufman (1971) has speculated that the substrate (phenylalanine) could inhibit a mutant form of the enzyme (see Fig. 15–5) in the presence of the *natural* coenzyme in vivo and that this inhibition could perhaps be alleviated by the therapeutic use of *synthetic* cofactor.

The genetic basis of hyperphenylalaninemia is likely to be very complex. Affected siblings of propositi in six pedigrees with non-phenylketonuric hyperphenylalaninemia all had an identical trait (Hsia, 1970). On the other hand, there were four families in which hyperphenylalaninemic and phenylketonuric sibs were found, among 33 families in which the classical mutant allele appeared. The possibility that such probands might be heteroallelic for two different mutant genes has been proposed by Kang et al. (1970) on the basis of their careful examination of a pedigree with the hyperphenylalaninemic trait.

Cunningham et al. (1969) and Klein et al. (1969) gained little satisfaction from phenylalanine loading as a method for discriminating presumed heterozygotes for the hyperphenylalaninemic trait from heterozygotes for classical phenylketonuria, a finding which may support Kaufman's proposal for substrate inhibition of the mutant enzyme. Woolf et al. (1967b, 1968) used intravenous phenylalanine infusions to show a peculiar delay in the rate of phenylalanine clearance from plasma in the mothers of two different hyperphenylalaninemic probands (Fig. 15–13). On the other hand, the fathers of these two patients displayed the "classical" heterozygous phenotype under similar conditions. The mutant gene in the maternal parent appeared to allow augmented inhibition in the conversion of phenylalanine to tyrosine when the phenylalanine concentration was abruptly increased. There is no statement as to whether the mothers were on contraceptive hormone medication, and this important study was unfortunately not confirmed with in vitro assays of the liver enzyme. But the available evidence indicates that heteroallelism may exist for the hyperphenylalaninemic trait, with two different mutant alleles controlling phenylalanine hydroxylase activity in the probands.

Transient Neonatal Hyperphenylalaninemia (with Hypertyrosinemia)

Hyperphenylalaninemia is a normal common transient phenomenon in the newborn infant, and it usually occurs in association with hypertryrosinemia (La Du et al., 1963; Menkes and Avery, 1963). Its frequency for all live births is about 0.2 per cent, and there is a direct correlation between the accumulation

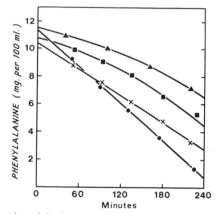

Figure 15–13 Plasma phenylalanine (semilogarithmic plot) after intravenous loading with L-phenylalanine (80 mg/kg in fasting state). Normal subjects ●———●: obligate heterozygote for classical phenylketonuria ×———×; ▲———▲ and ■———■ indicate two female parents of two probands with non-phenylketonuric hyperphenylalaninemia. An unusual form of phenylalanine hydroxylase with high affinity for phenylalanine and inhibited conversion to tyrosine at high phenylalanine concentrations was suggested to interpret the finding. It is not known whether the two mothers were receiving contraceptive hormones. (From Woolf, L. I., et al.: Lancet (i), 114–117, 1968.)

of the two amino acids in plasma in the early postnatal period (Fig. 15–14). The degree of tyrosinemia is usually greater than the corresponding level of hyperphenylalaninemia, the latter being defined as a value more than +3 SD above the mean value for the population under surveillance. The condition is seen most often in the premature infant, but it also occurs in the full-term infant, and it is believed to result from concomitant functional immaturity of the phenylalanine hydroxylating and tyrosine oxidizing enzymes. Human liver has phenylalanine hydroxylating activity prior to 40 weeks gestation (Friedman and Kaufman, 1969; Jakubovic, 1971; Barranger et al., 1971), but the basis for the apparently impaired hydroxylation as the cause of neonatal hyper-phenylalaninemia has not been revealed, although a reduced amount of enzyme may exist as suggested by the data of Jakubovic (1971). On the other hand, the kinetics of the perinatal enzyme resemble those of the adult liver enzyme complex (Friedman and Kaufman, 1969); and the isozymic nature of the fetal adult enzyme (Barranger et al., 1972) may permit different regulation of its activity at birth, particularly in the presence of the relatively high protein and phenylalanine intake of protein which characterizes the diet of young infants who are not breast-fed. Premature infants who are fed human milk, which is low in protein compared to cow's milk, have a lower prevalence of hyper-phenylalaninemia (Hambraeus and Wranne, 1968).

Neonatal hyperphenylalaninemia appears to be a benign condition. It is significant only because of its relatively high frequency compared to other forms of hyperphenylalaninemia and because follow-up investigation is required to distinguish it from the persistent and potentially harmful hyperphenyl-alaninemias.

MATERNAL HYPERPHENYLALANINEMIA

Jervis (1954), Richards (1964), Denniston (1963), and Mabry et al. (1963) were among the first to draw attention to maternal phenylketonuria and the

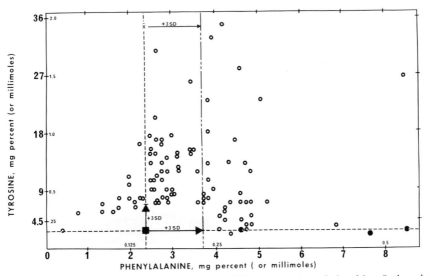

Figure 15-14 Neonatal transient hyperphenylalaninemia: the relationship of phenylalanine to tyrosine concentration in dried blood spots collected from 4065 newborn infants (open circles) in Quebec province between 2 and 10 days of age and regardless of gestational age or birth weight. Analyses were performed by automated fluorimetric methods. The shaded area represents the distribution of values for the majority of infants; abnormal values are those which exceed ±3 SD beyond the mean as indicated on the graph. The perimeter of the shaded area joins all values for clusters of five or more subjects. The graph was generated by a computer print-out from data collected by the Central Screening Laboratory at the Centre Hôpitalier de l'Université Laval in the Quebec Network of Genetic Medicine; it is used here with permission (Laberge, Scriver et al., 1971, unpublished data). The filled circles represent the comparable initial values for three subjects who upon follow-up were found to have the persistent hyperphenylalaninemic trait without phenylketonuria.

occurrence of mental retardation in the non-phenylketonuric (heterozygous) offspring of such mothers. The report by Mabry et al. (1966) was the first to describe the full significance of "maternal phenylketonuria." There are now at least 121 reported offspring of 33 phenylketonuric mothers (Howell and Stevenson, 1971), and these progeny clearly indicate that intrauterine hyperphenylalaninemia is harmful to cognitive and somatic development of the child.

A fetal:maternal plasma gradient for phenylalanine exists across the placenta. The average transplacental gradient in man is about 1.8, in favor of the fetus. Kerr and associates (1966, 1968) studied the effect of maternal hyperphenylalaninemia during pregnancy in the monkey, and they found that as the maternal blood level of phenylalanine rose, a constant fetal:maternal gradient was maintained. Thus, fetal hyperphenylalaninemia will occur and will be proportional to the maternal hyperphenylalaninemia in the presence of a normal placental circulation. Similar characteristics have been observed with respect to the rat transplacental gradient (Lines and Waisman, 1971b).

The normal transplacental gradient for phenylalanine is of little significance for the infant born to a phenylketonuric *heterozygote*. Kang and Paine (1963) found that pregnant heterozygotes have a slight elevation of plasma phenylalanine (at most, 150 per cent of the homozygous normal level during pregnancy), and this slight maternal elevation yields an average cord-blood phenylalanine of 0.14 mM in the offspring (that is, about 115 per cent of the normal mean value for newborn infants). The plasma phenylalanine concentration rises steeply after birth only if the offspring is deficient in phenylalanine hydroxylase activity (Fig. 15–8). On the other hand, the infant exposed to intrauterine hyperphenylalaninemia is hyperphenylalaninemic *at birth* and exhibits the usual fetal: maternal gradient of about 1.8 (Howell and Stevenson, 1971). Plasma phenylalanine in the infant then falls if the capacity to metabolize phenylalanine is not impaired.

It should be noted that plasma phenylalanine may not fall to the normal level if the newborn infant is breast-fed by a hyperphenylalaninemic mother, because the breast milk of such mothers contains a great excess of free phenylalanine (Fisch et al., 1967).

Postnatal phenylketonuria is associated with brain damage, and therefore it is of interest to know what harm intrauterine hyperphenylalaninemia does to the offspring. Most of the known progeny of hyperphenylalaninemic women (79 patients reviewed by Hsia [1970] and 42 additional patients reviewed by Howell and Stevenson [1971]) have congenital malformations, impaired physical development and blunted cognitive development; these manifestations may now be considered as the almost universal sequel to maternal phenylketonuria. The outcome in the offspring appears to be related to the degree of hyperphenylalaninemia in the mother. Therefore, the discussion will be divided to consider first the effect of maternal *phenylketonuria* and then the effect of *maternal non-phenylketonuric hyperphenylalaninemia* on the offspring.

Offspring in Maternal Phenylketonuria

Congenital Anomalies.   One quarter of the offspring reviewed by Hsia (1970) had congenital anomalies, and there were an equivalent number of spontaneous abortions. No particular class of anomaly was observed in the surviving children; and skeletal, cardiac, vascular, intestinal, ocular, hematopoietic and pulmonary systems were randomly affected (Stevenson and Huntley, 1967; Fisch et al., 1969).

Growth Retardation.   All offspring have some manifestation of intrauterine growth retardation. The infants have a low birth-weight for gestational age, and microcephaly (occipitofrontal circumference) has been systematically recorded by several authors (Stevenson and Huntley, 1967; Frankenburg et al., 1968; Fisch et al., 1969). Small physical stature is characteristic throughout infancy and childhood, suggesting that a state of intrauterine malnutrition determines the poor somatic growth in later life.

Mental Retardation.   Over 90 per cent of non-phenylketonuric offspring from mothers with phenylketonuria are definitely retarded in their cognitive development. Chance matings between homozygous phenylketonuric mothers and heterozygous fathers have also been recorded, the results of which were seven homozygous phenylketonuric offspring; as expected, all are severely retarded.

Mental retardation caused by intrauterine hyperphenylalaninemia resembles the retardation of classical phenylketonuria. The nervous system undergoes maturation during the latter half of intrauterine life, and it is therefore not surprising that Menkes and Aeberhard (1969) found abnormalities of cerebral lipids and fatty acids and of myelin glycolipids in the brain of a retarded heterozygous offspring of a phenylketonuric mother which resembled those abnormalities found in classical phenylketonuria.

Offspring in Non-phenylketonuric Maternal Hyperphenylalaninemia

At least 16 non-phenylketonuric offspring have been born to women whose hyperphenylalaninemia does not exceed 1 mM. Hsia (1970) reviewed the outcome of these infants. None had detectable congenital anomalies, and all but one were not retarded in somatic or mental development. The single mentally retarded child had an abnormal perinatal history. These important observations suggest that it is the intensity of intrauterine fetal hyperphenylalaninemia, which is dependent on transplacental gradient and will therefore be proportional to the maternal plasma phenylalanine level, that influences the outcome of the pregnancy.

Management of Maternal Hyperphenylalaninemia

There is only limited experience with treatment of hyperphenylalaninemia during pregnancy. Allan and Brown (1968) prescribed a low-phenylalanine diet for a phenylketonuric mother during the latter half of her pregnancy and the offspring was said to be doing well at eight months of age. Arthur and Hulme (1970) treated another phenylketonuric mother (plasma phenylalanine 0.75 mM; phenylpyruvic acid in the urine) from the 22nd week of pregnancy. A normal infant was delivered at 38 weeks who was considered to be normal in mental and physical development two years later. A third (unsuccessful) attempt at antepartum treatment has been reported (Huntley and Stevenson, 1969).

Half of all the hyperphenylalaninemic probands are female, and about one in every 10,000 births in the white race is a proband with this trait. Consequently, mass screening programs which are in wide use throughout the world are now finding many patients who in the future will impose the risk of intrauterine hyperphenylalaninemia on their offspring. These women will need special attention during their pregnancies. A continuing effort to counsel such individuals prospectively and to provide a mode of treatment which is safe to use during pregnancy should demand a high priority. The students of hereditary disorders of phenylalanine metabolism do not lack important challenges.

REFERENCES

Allan, J. D., and Brown, J. K.: Maternal phenylketonuria and foetal brain damage. An attempt at prevention by dietary control. *In* Holt, K. S., and Coffey, V. P., eds., Some Recent Advances in Inborn Errors of Metabolism. Livingston, Edinburgh, 1968, pp. 14–38.

Allen, R. J., Fleming, L., and Spirito, R.: Variations in hyperphenylalaninemia. *In* Nyhan, W. L., ed., Amino Acid Metabolism and Genetic Variation. McGraw-Hill, New York, 1967, pp. 69–96.

Ambrose, A. M., Power, F. W., and Sherwin, C. P.: Further studies on the detoxication of phenylacetic acid. J. Biol. Chem. *101*:669–675, 1933.

Anderson, A. E., and Guroff, G.: Enduring behavioral changes in rats with experimental phenylketonuria. Proc. Nat. Acad. Sci. *69*:863–867, 1972.

Anderson, J. A., and Swaiman, K. F., eds.: Proceedings of a Conference on Phenylketonuria and Allied Metabolic Diseases. U.S. Department of Health, Education and Welfare, Social and Rehabilitation Service Children's Bureau, 1967. U.S. Govt. Printing Office, 1967-0-282-371.

American Academy of Pediatrics: Committee Statement on Screening of Newborn Infants for Metabolic Disease. Pediatrics *35*:499–501, 1965.

Aoki, K., and Siegel, F. L.: Hyperphenylalaninemia: Disaggregation of brain polysomes in young rats. Science *168*:129–130, 1970.

Arakawa, T., Hirata, K., Ohara, K., Fujii, M., Takahashi, Y., and Kato, H.: Folic acid deficiency due to a low-phenylalanine diet. Tohoku J. Exp. Med. *87*:296–300, 1965.

Armstrong, M. D., and Low, N. L.: Phenylketonuria VIII. Relation between age, serum phenylalanine level, and phenylpyruvic acid excretion. Proc. Soc. Exp. Biol. Med. *94*:142–146, 1957.

Armstrong, M. D., Shaw, K. N. F., and Robinson, K. S.: Studies on phenylketonuria. II. The excretion of *o*-hydroxyphenylacetic acid in phenylketonuria. J. Biol. Chem. *213*:797–804, 1955.

Armstrong, M. D., and Tyler, F. H.: Studies on phenylketonuria. I. Restricted phenylalanine intake in phenylketonuria. J. Clin. Invest. *34*:565–580, 1955.

Arthur, L. J. H., and Hulme, J. D.: Intelligent small-for-dates baby born to oligophrenic phenylketonuric mother after low phenylalanine diet during pregnancy. Pediatrics *46*:235–239, 1970.

Auerbach, V. H., DiGeorge, A. M., Carpenter, G. G., and Wood, P.: Phenylalaninemia. *In* Nyhan, W. L., ed., Amino Acid Metabolism and Genetic Variation. McGraw-Hill, New York, pp. 11–68, 1967.

Auerbach, V. H., Waisman, H. A., and Wyckof, L. B., Jr.: Phenylketonuria in the rat associated with decreased temporal discriminational learning. Nature (London) *182*:871–872, 1959.

Barranger, J. A., Geiger, P. J., Huzino, A., and Bessman, S. P.: Isozymes of phenylalanine hydroxylase. Science *175*:903–905, 1972.

Baumeister, A. A.: The effects of dietary control on intelligence in phenylketonuria. Amer. J. Ment. Defic. *71*:840–847, 1967.

Bentovim, A., Clayton, B. E., Francis, D. E. M., Shepherd, J., and Wolff, O. H.: Use of amino acid mixture in the treatment of phenylketonuria. Arch. Dis. Child. *45*:640–650, 1970.

Berman, J. L., Cunningham, G. C., Day, R. W., Ford, R., and Hsia, D. Y. Y.: Causes for high phenylalanine with normal tyrosine. Amer. J. Dis. Child. *117*:54–65, 1965.

Berman, J. L., and Ford, R.: Intelligence quotients and intelligence loss in patients with phenylketonuria and some variant states. J. Pediat. *77*:764–770, 1970.

Berry, H. K., and Butcher, R.: Personal communication, 1971.

Berry, H. K., Cripps, R., Nicholls, K., McCandless, D., and Harper, C.: Development of phenylalanine hydroxylase activity in guinea pig liver. Biochim. Biophys. Acta *261*:315–320, 1972.

Berry, H. K., Sutherland, B. S., Guest, G. M., and Umbarger, B.: Chemical and clinical observation during treatment of children with phenylketonuria. Pediatrics *21*:929–940, 1958.

Berry, H. K., Sutherland, B. S., and Umbarger, B.: Diagnosis and treatment: Interpretation of results of blood screening studies for detection of phenylketonuria. Pediatrics *37*:102–106, 1966.

Berry, H. K., Umbarger, B., and Sutherland, B. S.: Procedures for monitoring the low phenylalanine diet in treatment of phenylketonuria. J. Pediat. *67*:609–616, 1965.

Berry, H. K., and Wright, S.: Conference on treatment of phenylketonuria. J. Pediat. *70*:142–147, 1967.

Bessman, S. P.: Legislation and advances in medical knowledge. Acceleration or inhibition. J. Pediat. *69*:334–338, 1966.

Bessman, S. P.: Guest editorial: PKU—Some skepticism. New Eng. J. Med. *278*:1176–1177, 1968.

Bickel, H., Gerrard, A. J., and Hickman, E. M.: Influence of phenylalanine intake on phenylketonuria. Lancet (ii), 812, 1953.

Bickel, H., Gerrard, J., and Hickman, E. M.: Influence of phenylalanine intake on the chemistry and behavior of a phenylketonuric child. Acta Paediat. *43*:64–77, 1954.

Bickel, H., Hudson, F. P., and Woolf, L. I., eds.: Phenylketonuria and some other inborn errors of amino acid metabolism. Biochemistry, Genetics, Diagnosis, Therapy. Thieme Edition, Geórg Thieme Verlag, Stuttgart, 1971.

Birch, H. G., and Tizard, J.: The dietary treatment of phenylketonuria: not proven? Develop. Med. Child. Neurol. *9*:9–12, 1967.

Blainey, J. D., and Gulliford, R.: Phenylalanine-restricted diets in the treatment of phenylketonuria. Arch. Dis. Child. *31*:452–466, 1956.

Blaskovics, M. E., Shaw, K. N. F., Donnel, G. N., and Koch, R.: Phenylketonuria: extended phenylalanine loading studies (Abstract.) Soc. Ped. Res. Program, 158, Atlantic City, 1968.

Boisse, J., Sandubray, J. M., Caty, T., and Mozziconacci, P.: Le traitement de la phénylcétonurie. Ann. Pediat. *18*:109–117, 1971.

Bowden, J. A., and McArthur, C. L., III: Possible biochemical model of phenylketonuria. Nature (London) *235*:230, 1972.

Boylen, J. B., and Quastel, J. H.: Effects of L-phenylalanine and sodium phenylpyruvate on the formation of melanin from L-tyrosine in melanoma. Nature (London) *193*:376–377, 1962.

Bremer, H. J., and Neumann, W.: Tolerance of phenylalanine after intravenous administration in phenylketonurics, heterozygous carriers and normal adults. Nature *209*:1148–1149, 1966.

Brenneman, A. R., and Kaufman, S.: Characteristics of the hepatic phenylalanine-hydroxylating system in newborn rats. J. Biol. Chem. *240*:3617–3622, 1965.

Brimblecombe, F. S. W., Stoneman, M. E. R., and Maliphant, R.: Dietary treatment of an infant with phenylketonuria. Lancet (i), 609–611, 1959.

Brodehl, J., Gellissen, K., and Kaas, W. P.: The renal transport of amino acids in untreated infants with phenylketonuria. Acta Paediat. Scand. *59*:241–248, 1970.

Brown, E. S., and Waisman, H. A.: Intelligence of the unidentified phenylketonuric child. Pediatrics *40*:247–249, 1967.

Bruhl, H. H.: Dietary treatment in older PKU patients. *In* Proceedings of a Conference on Nutrition and the Inherited Diseases of Man as Related to Public Health. Minneapolis, pp. 73–86, 1966.

Bublitz, C.: A direct assay for liver phenylalanine hydroxylase. Biochim. Biophys. Acta *191*:249–256, 1969.

Butcher, R. E.: Learning impairment associated with maternal PKU in rats. Nature (London) *226*:555–556, 1970.

Castells, S., and Brandt, I. K.: Phenylketonuria: evaluation of therapy and verification of diagnosis. J. Pediat. *72*:34–40, 1968.

Chase, H. P., and O'Brien, D.: Effect of excess phenylalanine and of other amino acids on brain development in the infant rat. Pediat. Res. *4*:96–102, 1970.

Christensen, H. N., Feldman, B. H., and Hastings, A. B.: Concentrative and reversible character of intestinal amino acid transport. Amer. J. Physiol. *205*:255–260, 1963.

Cleland, W. W.: The kinetics of enzyme-catalyzed reactions with two or more substrates or products. I. Nomenclature and rate equations. Biochim. Biophys. Acta *67*:104–137, 1963.

Clow, C., Reade, T., and Scriver, C. R.: Management of hereditary metabolic disease. The role of Allied Health Personnel. New Eng. J. Med. *284*:1292–1298, 1971.

Cohn, G. H., Ouellette, E. M., Moser, H. W., and Efron, M. L.: Atypical phenylketonuria in a seven-year-old profoundly retarded girl. Development of phenylalanine tolerance in spite of apparently continued failure to convert phenylalanine to tyrosine. (Abstract.) Neurology *18*:310–311, 1968.

Coleman, D. L.: Phenylalanine hydroxylase activity in dilute and non-dilute strains of mice. Arch. Biochem. Biophys. *91*:300–306, 1960.

Colombo, J. P.: Plasma glutamine in a phenylketonuric family with normal and mentally defective members. Arch. Dis. Child. *46*:720–721, 1971.

Copenhaver, J. H., Carver, M. J., and Schaine, R. J.: Effects of folic and folinic acids on the metabolism of phenylalanine in phenylketonuria. Metabolism *14*:1233–1236, 1965.

Crome, L., and Pare, C. M. B.: Phenylketonuria: a review and a report of the pathological findings in four cases. J. Ment. Sci. *106*:862–883, 1960.

Crome, L., Tymms, V., and Woolf, L. I.: A chemical investigation of the defects of myelination in phenylketonuria. J. Neurol. Neurosurg. Psychiat. *25*:143–148, 1962.

Cunningham, G. C., Day, R. W., Berman, J. L., and Hsia, D. Y. Y.: Phenylalanine tolerance tests in families with phenylketonuria and hyperphenylalaninemia. Amer. J. Dis. Child. *117*:626–635, 1969.

Denniston, J. C.: Children of mothers with phenylketonuria. J. Pediat. *63*:461–462, 1963.

Dent, C. E.: Discussion of paper by Armstrong, M. D. *In* Report of 23rd Ross Conference, Etiological Factors in Mental Retardation. Ross Laboratories, Columbus, Ohio, pp. 22–23, 1956.

Dobson, J., Koch, R., Williamson, M., Spector, R., Frankenburg, W., O'Flynn, M., Warner, R., and Hudson, F.: Cognitive development and dietary therapy in phenylketonuric children. New Eng. J. Med. *278*:1142–1144, 1968.

Dodge, P. R., Mancall, E. L., Crawford, J. D., Knapp, J., and Paine, R. S.: Hypoglycemia complicating treatment of phenylketonuria with a phenylalanine-deficient diet. New Eng. J. Med. *260*:1104–1111, 1959.

Drummond, K. N., Michael, A. F., and Good, R. A.: Tryptophan metabolism in a patient with phenylketonuria and scleroderma; a proposed explanation of the indole defect in phenylketonuria. Canad. Med. Ass. J. *94*:834–838, 1966.

Efron, M. L., Kang, E. S., Visakorpi, J., and Fellers, X. F.: Effect of elevated plasma phenylalanine levels on other amino acids in phenylketonuric and normal subjects. J. Pediat. *74*:399–405, 1969.

Embden, G., and Baldes, K.: Über den Abbau des Phenylalanins im tierischen Organismus. Biochem. Z. *55*:301–322, 1913.

Fellman, J. H., and Devlin, M. K.: Concentration and hydroxylation of free phenylalanine in adrenal glands. Biochim. Biophys. Acta *28*:328–332, 1958.

Fisch, R. O., Torres, F., Gravem, H. J., Greenwood, C. S., and Anderson, J. A.: Twelve years' clinical experience with phenylketonuria. A statistical evaluation of symptoms, growth, mental development, electroencephalographic records, serum phenylalanine levels and results of dietary management. Neurology *19*:659–666, 1969.

Fisch, R. O., Doeden, D., Lansky, L. L., and Anderson, J. A.: Maternal phenylketonuria. Detrimental effects on embryogenesis and fetal development. Amer. J. Dis. Child. *118*:847–859, 1969.

Fisch, R. O., Jenness, R., Doeden, D., and Anderson, J. A.: The effect of excess L-phenylalanine on mothers and on their breast fed infants. J. Pediat. *71*:176–180, 1967.

Følling, A.: Über Ausscheidung von Phenylbrenztraubensaure in den Harn als Stoffwechselanomalie in Verbindung mit Imbezillitat. Z. Physiol. Chem. *227*:169–176, 1934.

Fox, J. G., Hall, D. L., Haworth, J. C., Maniar, A., and Sekla, L.: Newborn screening for hereditary metabolic disorders in Manitoba 1965–1970. Canad. Med. Ass. J. *104*:1085–1088, 1971.

Frankenburg, W. K., Duncan, B. R., Coffelt, R. W., Koch, R., Coldwell, J. G., and Son, C. D.: Maternal phenylketonuria: Implications for growth and development. J. Pediat. *73*:560–570, 1968.

Friedman, P. A., Fisher, D. B., Kang, E. S., and Kaufman, S.: Detection of hepatic phenylalanine 4-hydroxylase in classical phenylketonuria. Proc. Nat. Acad. Sci. U.S.A. *70*:552–556, 1973.

Friedman, P. A., and Kaufman, S.: A study of the development of phenylalanine hydroxylase in fetuses of several mammalian species. Arch. Biochem. Biophys. *146*:325–326, 1971.

Fuller, R. N., and Shuman, J. B.: Phenylketonuria and intelligence: Trimodal response to dietary treatment. Nature (London) *221*:639–642, 1969.

Fuller, R., and Shuman, J.: Treated phenylketonuria: Intelligence and blood phenylalanine levels. Amer. J. Ment. Defic. *75*:539–545, 1971.

Gallagher, B. B.: The effect of phenylpyruvate on oxidative phosphorylation in brain mitochondria. J. Neurochem. *16*:1071–1076, 1969.

Grant, E. H.: The structure of water neighboring proteins, peptides and amino acids as deduced from dielectric measurements. Ann. N.Y. Acad. Sci. *125*:418–427, 1965.

Grau, C. R., and Steele, R.: Phenylalanine and tyrosine utilization in normal and phenylalanine-deficient young mice. J. Nutr. *53*:59–71, 1954.

Grumer, H. D., Hetland, L. B., and Costantinic, M. L.: L-Benzylalanine as a model amino acid for the study of accumulation diseases. Clin. Chem. *17*:115–118, 1971.

Guroff, G.: Irreversible *in vivo* inhibition of rat liver phenylalanine hydroxylase by *p*-chlorophenylalanine. Arch. Biochem. Biophys. *134*:610–611, 1969.

Guroff, G., and Udenfriend, S.: Studies on aromatic amino acid uptake by rat brain *in vivo*. Uptake of phenylalanine and of tryptophan; inhibition and stereoselectivity in the uptake of tyrosine by brain and muscle. J. Biol. Chem. *237*:803–806, 1962.

Hackney, I. M., Hanley, W. B., Davidson, W., and Linsao, L.: Phenylketonuria: mental development, behavior, and termination of low phenylalanine diet. J. Pediat. *72*:646–655, 1968.

Hambraeus, L., Holmgren, G., and Samuelson, G.: Dietary treatment of adult patients with phenylketonuria. Nutr. Metabol. *13*:298–317, 1971.

Hambraeus, L., and Wranne, L.: The plasma phenylalanine level in newborn infants of normal and low birth weights fed on human milk. Biol. Neonat. *13*:315–324, 1968.

Hanley, W. B., Linsao, L., Davidson, W., and Moes, C. A. F.: Malnutrition with early treatment of phenylketonuria. Pediat. Res. *4*:318–327, 1970.

Hanley, W. B., Linsao, L. S., and Netley, C.: The efficacy of dietary therapy for phenylketonuria. Canad. Med. Ass. J. *104*:1089–1092, 1971.

Heffernan, A. G. A.: Glucose tolerance and insulin response in phenylketonuria. New Eng. J. Med. *285*:57, 1971.

Hill, J. B.: A climatological factor influencing the determination of phenylalanine in blood of newborn infants in North Carolina. Biochem. Med. *2*:261–272, 1969.

Holton, J. B., and West, P. M.: An assessment of an automated fluorimetric blood phenylalanine technique for phenylketonuric screening and for accurate estimations. J. Clin. Path. *23*:440–444, 1970.

Horner, F. A., Streamer, C. W., Alejandrino, L. L., Reed, L. H., and Ibbott, F.: Termination of dietary treatment of phenylketonuria. New Eng. J. Med. *266*:79–81, 1962.

Howell, R. R., and Stevenson, R. E.: The offspring of phenylketonuric women. Soc. Biol. *18*:519–529, 1971.

Hsia, D. Y. Y.: Phenylketonuria, 1967. Devel. Med. Child. Neurol. *9*:531–540, 1967.

Hsia, D. Y. Y.: Phenylketonuria and its variants. Progr. Med. Genet. *VII*:29–68, 1970.

Hsia, D. Y. Y.: Phenylketonuria: Clinical, genetic and biochemical aspects. *In* Primrose, D. A. A., ed., Proceedings of the 2nd Congress of the International Association for the Scientific Study of Mental Deficiency, Warsaw, 1970. Polish Med. Pub., Warsaw, pp. 105–113, 1971.

Hsia, D. Y. Y., Berman, J. L., and Slatis, H. M.: Screening newborns for phenylketonuria. J.A.M.A. *188*:203–206, 1964.

Hsia, D. Y. Y., and Dobson, J.: Altered sex ratio in phenylketonuric infants ascertained by screening newborns. Lancet (i), 905–907, 1970.

Hudson, F. P., Morduant, V. L., and Leaky, I.: Evaluation of treatment begun in first three months of life in 184 cases of phenylketonuria. Arch. Dis. Child. *45*:5–12, 1970.

Hunt, M. M., Sutherland, B. S., and Berry, H. K.: Nutritional management in phenylketonuria. Amer. J. Dis. Child. *122*:1–6, 1971.

Huntley, C. C., and Stevenson, R. E.: Maternal phenylketonuria. Course of two pregnancies. Obstet. Gynec. *34*:694–700, 1969.

Jackson, S. H., Hanley, W. B., Gero, T., and Gosse, G. D.: Detection of phenylketonuric heterozygotes. Clin. Chem. *17*:538–543, 1971.

Jakubovic, A.: Phenylalanine-hydroxylating system in the human fetus at different developmental ages. Biochim. Biophys. Acta *237*:469–475, 1971.

Jervis, G. A.: Phenylpyruvic oligophrenia: deficiency of phenylalanine oxidizing system. Proc. Soc. Exp. Biol. Med. *82*:514–515, 1953.

Jervis, G. A.: Phenylpyruvic oligophrenia (phenylketonuria). Res. Publ. Ass. Res. Nerv. Ment. Dis. *33*:259–282, 1954.

Jones, T. C., Levy, H. L., MacCready, R. A., Shih, V. E., and Garcia, F. G.: Phenylalanine tolerance tests in simian primates. Proc. Soc. Exp. Biol. Med. *136*:1087–1090, 1971.

Justice, P., O'Flynn, M. E., and Gerald, P. S.: Clinical and biochemical observations of patients with atypical phenylketonuria. Pediatrics *45*:83–92, 1970.

Kang, E. S., Kennedy, J. L., Jr., Gates, L., Burwash, I., and McKinnon, A.: Clinical observations in phenylketonuria. Pediatrics *35*:932–943, 1965.

Kang, E., and Paine, R. S.: Elevation of plasma phenylalanine during pregnancies of women heterozygous for phenylketonuria. J. Pediat. *63*:283, 1963.

Kang, E. S., Sollee, N. D., and Gerald, P. S.: Results of treatment and termination of the diet in phenylketonuria. Pediatrics *46*:881–890, 1970.

Kaufman, S.: Enzymatic conversion of phenylalanine to tyrosine. J. Biol. Chem. *226*:511–524, 1957.

Kaufman, S.: A new cofactor required for the enzymatic conversion of phenylalanine to tyrosine. J. Biol. Chem. *230*:931–939, 1958a.

Kaufman, S.: Phenylalanine hydroxylation cofactor in phenylketonuria. Science *128*:1506–1508, 1958b.

Kaufman, S.: The structure of the phenylalanine-hydroxylation cofactor. Proc. Nat. Acad. Sci. U.S.A. *50*:1085–1093, 1963.

Kaufman, S.: Phenylalanine hydroxylase of human liver: Assay and some properties. Arch. Biochem. Biophys. *134*:249–252, 1969.

Kaufman, S.: The phenylalanine hydroxylating system from mammalian liver. Advances Enzym. *35*:245–319, 1971.

Kennedy, J. L., Wertelecki, W., Gates, L., Sperry, B. P., and Cass, V. M.: The early treatment of phenylketonuria. *In* Hsia, D. Y. Y., ed., Symposium on Treatment of Amino Acid Disorders. Amer. J. Dis. Child *113*:16–21, 1967.

Kerr, G. R., Chamove, A. S., Harlow, H. F., and Waisman, H. A.: "Fetal PKU": The effect of maternal hyperphenylalaninemia during pregnancy in the rhesus monkey *(Macaca mulatta)*. Pediatrics *42*:27–36, 1968.

Kerr, G. R., and Waisman, H. A.: Phenylalanine: Transplacental concentrations in rhesus monkeys. Science *151*:824–825, 1966.

Kerr, G. R., and Waisman, H. A.: Dietary induction of hyperphenylalaninemia in the rat. J. Nutr. *92*:10–18, 1967.

Klein, M., Clow, C., and Scriver, C. R.: Genetic heterogeneity for phenylalanine metabolism in man, II. (Abstract.) Clin. Res. *17*:650, 1969.

Kleinman, D. S.: Phenylketonuria: a review of some deficits in our information. Pediatrics *33*: 123–134, 1964.

Knox, W. E.: An evaluation of the treatment of phenylketonuria with diets low in phenylalanine. Pediatrics *26*:1–11, 1960.

Knox, W. E.: Retrospective study of phenylketonuria. Morbidity and mortality among phenylketonurics. Phenylketonuria Newsletter #1, Jan. 1970.

Knox, W. E.: Retrospective study of phenylketonuria: Relation of phenylpyruvate excretion to plasma phenylalanine. Phenylketonuria Newsletter #2, Feb. 1970.

Knox, W. E.: Phenylketonuria. *In* Stanbury, J. B., Wyngaarden, J. B., and Fredrickson, D. S., eds., The Metabolic Basis of Inherited Disease. McGraw-Hill, New York, pp. 266–295, 1972.

Koch, R., Shaw, K. N., Acosta, P. B., Fishler, K., Schaeffler, G., Wenz, E., and Wohlers, A.: An approach to management of phenylketonuria. J. Pediat. *76*:815–828, 1970.

Koe, B. K., and Weissman, A. J.: *p*-Chlorophenylalanine: a specific depletor of brain serotonin. J. Pharmacol. Exp. Ther. *154*:499–516, 1966.

Kretchmer, N., Levine, S. Z., McNamara, H., and Barnett, H. L.: Certain aspects of tyrosine metabolism in the young. I. The development of the tyrosine oxidizing system in human liver. J. Clin. Invest. *35*:236–244, 1956.

LaDu, B. N.: Genetic variation in metabolic disorders. *In* Nyhan, W. L., ed., Amino Acid Metabolism and Genetic Variation. McGraw-Hill, New York, pp. 121–130, 1967.

LaDu, B. N., Howell, R. R., Michael, P. J., and Sober, E. K.: A quantitative micromethod for the determination of phenylalanine and tyrosine in blood and its application in the diagnosis of phenylketonuria in infants. Pediatrics *31*:39–46, 1963.

LaDu, B. N., and Zannoni, V. G.: Inhibition of phenylalanine hydroxylase in liver. *In* Anderson, J. S., and Swaiman, K. F., eds., Proceedings of a Conference on Phenylketonuria and Allied Metabolic Diseases. U.S. Department of Health, Education and Welfare, U.S. Govt. Printing Office, Washington, D.C., 1967-0-282-371, pp. 193–204, 1967.

Leung, P. M-B., Rogers, Q. R., and Harper, A. E.: Effect of amino acid imbalance on dietary choice in the rat. J. Nutr. *95*:483–492, 1968.

Levy H. L.: Genetic screening. *In* Harris, H., and Hirschhorn, K., eds., Advances in Human Genetics. Plenum Press, New York, 1972.

Levy, H. L., Baullinger, P. C., and Madigan, P. M.: A rapid procedure for the determination of phenylalanine and tyrosine from blood filter paper specimens. Clin. Chim. Acta *31*:447–452, 1971.

Levy, H. L., Karolkewicz, V., Houghton, S. A., and MacCready, R. A.: Screening the "normal" population in Massachusetts for phenylketonuria. New Eng. J. Med. *282*:1455–1458, 1970.

Levy, H. L., Shih, V. E., Karolkewicz, V., Frerich, W. A., Carr, J. R., Cass, V., Kennedy, J. L., Jr., and MacCready, R. A.: Persistent mild hyperphenylalaninemia in the untreated state. A prospective study. New Eng. J. Med. *285*:424–429, 1971.

Lin, E. C. C., Hagihira, H., and Wilson, T. H.: Specificity of the transport system for neutral amino acids in the hamster intestine. Amer. J. Physiol. *202*:919–925, 1962.

Lin, E. C. C., and Knox, W. E.: Effect of vitamin B$_6$ deficiency on the basal and adapted levels of rat liver tyrosine and tyrptophan transaminases. J. Biol. Chem. *233*:1183–1185, 1958.

Lin, E. C. C., Rivlin, R. S., and Knox, W. E.: Effect of body weight and sex on activity of enzymes involved in amino acid metabolism. Amer. J. Physiol. *196*:303–306, 1959.

Lindroos, O. F. C., and Oja, S. S.: Hyperphenylalaninaemia and the exchange of tyrosine in adult rat brain. Exp. Brain Res. *14*:48–60, 1971.

Lines, D. R., and Waisman, H. A.: Renal amino acid reabsorption in hyperphenylalaninemic monkeys infused with β-2-thienylalanine. Proc. Soc. Exp. Biol. Med. *134*:1061–1064, 1970.

Lines, D. R., and Waisman, H. A.: Urinary amino acid excretion in phenylketonuric, hyperphenylalaninemic and normal patients. J. Pediat. *78*:474–480, 1971a.

Lines, D. R., and Waisman, H. A.: Placental transport of phenylalanine in the rat: maternal and fetal metabolism. Proc. Soc. Exp. Biol. Med. *136*:790–793, 1971b.

Linneweh, F., and Ehrlich, M.: Die renalen und prarenalen Storungen des Aminosauren-stoffwechsels bei phenylalaninarmer Ernahrung. Klin. Wschr. *38*:904–910, 1960.

Linneweh, F., and Ehrlich, M.: Zur Pathogenese des Schwachsinns bei Phenylketonurie. Klin. Wschr. *40*:225–226, 1962.

Linneweh, F., Ehrlich, M., Graul, E. H., and Hundeshagen, H.: Über den Aminosauren-transport bei phenylketonurischer Oligophrenie. Klin. Wschr. *41*:253–255, 1963.

Lipton, M. A., Gordon, R., Guroff, G., and Udenfriend, L. S.: *p*-Chlorophenylalanine-induced chemical manifestations of phenylketonuria in rats. Science *156*:248–250, 1967.

Longenecker, J. B., Reed, P. B., Lo, G. S., Chang, D. Y., Nasby, M. W., White, M. N., and Ide, S.: Temporary induction of phenylketonuria-like characteristics in infant rats. Nutr. Rep. Internat. *1*:105–112, 1970.

Loo, Y. H., and Ritman, P.: New metabolites of phenylalanine. Nature (London) *203*:1237–1239, 1964.

Lowden, J. A., and LaRamée, M. A.: Hyperphenylalaninemia: the effect on cerebral amino acid levels during development. Canad. J. Biochem. *47*:883–888, 1969.

Lush, I. E.: The biochemical genetics of vertebrates except man. *In* Neuberger, A., and Tatum, E. L., eds., Frontiers of Biology, Vol. 3. North-Holland Publ. Co., Amsterdam, 1967.

Mabry, C. C., Denniston, J. C., and Coldwell, J. G.: Mental retardation in children of phenylketonuric mothers. New Eng. J. Med. *275*:1331–1336, 1966.

Mabry, C. C., Denniston, J. C., Nelson, T. L., and Choon, D. S.: Maternal phenylketonuria: A cause of mental retardation in children without the metabolic defect. New Eng. J. Med. *269*:1404–1408, 1963.

McBean, M. S., and Stephenson, J. B. P.: Treatment of classical phenylketonuria. Arch. Dis. Child. *43*:1–7, 1968.

McCarthy, M. A., Orr, M. L., and Watt, B. K.: Phenylalanine and tyrosine in vegetables and fruit. J. Amer. Diet. Ass. *52*:130–134, 1968.

McKean, C. M.: Growth of phenylketonuric children on chemically defined diets. Lancet (i), 148–149, 1970.

McKean, C. M.: Effects of totally synthetic low phenylalanine diet on adolescent phenylketonuric patients. Arch. Dis. Child. *46*:608–615, 1971.

McKean, C. M., Boggs, D. E., and Peterson, N. A.: The influence of high phenylalanine and tyrosine on the concentrations of essential amino acids in brain. J. Neurochem. *15*:235–241, 1968.

McKean, C. M., and Peterson, N. A.: Glutamic acid in the phenylketonuric central nervous system. New Eng. J. Med. *283*:1364–1367, 1970.

McKean, C. M., Schanberg, S. M., and Giarman, N. J.: Aminoacidemias: effects on maze performance and cerebral serotonin. Science *157*:213–215, 1967.

Medical Research Council, Treatment of Phenylketonuria. Brit. Med. J. *2*:1691–1697, 1963.

Medical Research Council Working Party on Phenylketonuria. Present status of different mass screening procedures for phenylketonuria. Brit. Med. J. *4*:7–13, 1968.

Meister, A.: Phenylpyruvic oligophrenia. Pediatrics *21*:1021–1031, 1958.

Menkes, J. H.: The pathogenesis of mental retardation in phenylketonuria and other inborn errors of amino acid metabolism. Pediatrics *39*:297–308, 1967.

Menkes, J. H.: Cerebral proteolipids in phenylketonuria. Neurology *18*:1003–1008, 1968.

Menkes, J. H., and Aeberhard, E.: Maternal phenylketonuria. The composition of cerebral lipids in an affected offspring. J. Pediat. *74*:924–931, 1969.

Menkes, J. H., and Avery, M. E.: The metabolism of phenylalanine and tyrosine in the premature infant. Bull. Johns Hopkins Hosp. *113*:301–319, 1963.

Milne, M. D., Scribner, B. H., and Crawford, M. A.: Nonionic diffusion and the excretion of weak acids and bases. Amer. J. Med. *24*:709–729, 1958.

Mitoma, C.: Studies on partially purified phenylalanine hydroxylase. Arch. Biochem. Biophys. *60*:476–484, 1956.

Mitoma, C., Auld, R. M., and Udenfriend, S.: On the nature of enzymic defect in phenylpyruvic oligophrenia. Proc. Soc. Exp. Biol. Med. *94*:634–635, 1957.

Moss, A. R., and Schoenheimer, R.: Conversion of phenylalanine to tyrosine in normal rats. J. Biol. Chem. *135*:415–429, 1940.

Murthy, L. I., and Berry, H. K.: Characteristics of phenylalanine hydroxylase (PAHase) activity in liver and kidney. (Abstract 1841.) Fed. Proc. *30*:460, 1971.

Neal, J. L.: Thermal expansibilities of leucine, phenylalanine, alanine and proline in water. (Abstract.) Proc. Canad. Fed. Biol. Soc. *14*:59, 1971.

Neubauer, O.: Über den Abbau der Aminosauern im gesunden und kranken Organismus. Deutsch. Arch. Klin. Med. *95*:211–256, 1909.

Oates, J. A., Nirenberg, P. Z., Jepson, J. B., Sjoerdsma, A., and Udenfriend, S.: Conversion of phenylalanine to phenylethylamine in patients with phenylketonuria. Proc. Soc. Exp. Biol. Med. *112*:1078–1081, 1963.

O'Brien, D., and Ibbot, F. A.: Effect of prolonged phenylalanine loading on the free amino acid and lipid content of the infant monkey brain. Devel. Med. Child. Neurol. *8*:724–728, 1966.

O'Flynn, M. E., Tillman, P., and Hsia, D. Y. Y.: Hyperphenylalaninemia without phenylketonuria. *In* Hsia, D. Y. Y., ed., Symposium on Treatment of Amino Acid Disorders. Amer. J. Dis. Child. *113*:22–27, 1967.

O'Grady, D. J., Berry, H. K., and Sutherland, B. S.: Cognitive development in early treated phenylketonuria. Amer. J. Dis. Child *121*:20–23, 1971.

Paine, R. S.: The variability in manifestations of untreated patients with phenylketonuria (phenylpyruvicaciduria). Pediatrics *20*:290–301, 1957.

Pare, C. M., Sandler, M., and Stacey, R. S.: 5-Hydroxytryptamine deficiency in phenylketonuria. Lancet (i), 551–553, 1957.

Pare, C. M. B., Sandler, M., and Stacey, R. S.: Decreased 5-hydroxytryptophan decarboxylase activity in phenylketonuria. Lancet (ii), 1099–1101, 1958.

Pare, C. M. B., Sandler, M., and Stacey, R. S.: The relationship between decreased 5-hydroxyindole metabolism and mental defect in phenylketonuria. Arch. Dis. Child. *34*:422–425, 1959.

Partington, M. W.: Observations on phenylketonuria in Ontario. Canad. Med. Ass. J. *84*:985–991, 1961.

Partington, M. W.: Case finding in phenylketonuria. III. One-way chromatography of the amino acids in blood. Canad. Med. Ass. J. *99*:638–644, 1968.

Penrose, L., and Quastel, J. H.: Metabolic studies in phenylketonuria. Biochem. J. *31*:266–271, 1937.

Perry, T. L.: The incidence of mental illness in the relatives of individuals suffering from phenylketonuria or mongolism. J. Psychiat. Res *4*:51–57, 1966.

Perry, T. L., Hansen, S., Tischler, B., and Bunting, R.: Determination of heterozygosity for phenylketonuria on the amino acid analyzer. Clin. Chim. Acta *18*:51–56, 1967.

Perry, T. L., Hansen, S., Tischler, B., Bunting, R., and Diamond, S.: Glutamine depletion in phenylketonuria. A possible cause of the mental defect. New Eng. J. Med. *282*:761–766, 1970.

Perry, T. L., Ling, G. M., Hansen, S., and MacDougall, L.: Unimpaired learning ability of rats made artificially phenylketonuric during fetal and neonatal life. Proc. Soc. Exp. Biol. Med. *119*:282–287, 1965.

Perry, T. L., Tischler, B., Hansen, S., and MacDougall, L.: A simple test for heterozygosity for phenylketonuria. Clin. Chim. Acta *15*:47–55, 1967.

Pitt, D.: Phenylalanine maintenance in phenylketonuria. Austral. Paed. J. *3*:161–163, 1967.

Pitt, D.: The natural history of untreated phenylketonuria. Med. J. Aust. (i), 378–383, 1971.

Polidora, V. J., Cunningham, R. F., and Waisman, H. A.: Phenylketonuria in rats: reversibility of behavioral deficit. Science *151*:219–220, 1966.

Poser, C. M., and Van Bogaert, L.: Neuropathologic observations in phenylketonuria. Brain *82*:1–9, 1959.

Rampini, S., Anders, P. W., Curtius, H. C., and Marthaler, T.: Detection of heterozygotes for phenylketonuria by column chromatography and discriminatory analysis. Pediat. Res. *3*:287–297, 1969.

Richards, B. W.: Maternal phenylketonuria. Lancet (i), 829, 1964.

Rosenberg, L. E., and Scriver, C. R.: Amino acid metabolism. *In* Bondy, P. K., ed., Duncan's Diseases of Metabolism, 6th edition. W. B. Saunders Company, Philadelphia, pp. 366–515, 1969.

Rosenblatt, D., and Scriver, C. R.: Heterogeneity in genetic control of phenylalanine metabolism in man. Nature *218*:677–678, 1968.

Rouse, B. M.: Phenylalanine deficiency syndrome. J. Pediat. *69*:246–249, 1966.

Saugstad, L. F.: Birthweights in children with phenylketonuria and in thier siblings. Lancet (i), 809–813, 1972.

Scriver, C. R.: Membrane transport functions and their relation to phenylketonuria. *In* Anderson, J. A., and Swaiman, K. F., eds., Proceedings of a Conference on Phenylketonuria and Allied Metabolic Diseases. U.S. Department of Health, Education and Welfare, U.S. Govt. Printing Office, Washington, D.C., 1967-0-282-371, pp. 181–192, 1967.

Scriver, C. R.: Diagnosis and treatment: interpreting the positive screening test in the newborn infant. Pediatrics *39*:764–768, 1967.

Scriver, C. R.: The use of human genetic variation to study membrane transport of amino acids in kidney. Amer. J. Dis. Child. *117*:4–12, 1969.

Scriver, C. R.: Phenylketonuria: the glutamine hypothesis. New Eng. J. Med. *282*:808–809, 1970.

Scriver, C. R., Davies, E., and Lamm, P.: Accelerated selective short column chromatography of neutral and acidic amino acids on a Beckman-Spinco Analyzer, modified for simultaneous analysis of two samples. Clin. Biochem. *1*:179–191, 1968.

Scriver, C. R., Katz, L., and Clow, C.: Phenylketonuria and diet. Canad. Med. Ass. J. *98*:125, 1968.

Shah, S. N., Peterson, N. A., and McKean, C. M.: Cerebral lipid metabolism in experimental hyper-phenylalaninemia: incorporation of ^{14}C-labelled glucose into total lipids. J. Neurochem. *17*:279–284, 1970.

Shah, S. N., Peterson, N. A., and McKean, C. M.: Impaired myelin formation in experimental hyper-phenylalaninemia. J. Neurochem. *19*:479–485, 1972.

Shih, V., Efron, M. L., and Mechanic, G. L.: Rapid short column chromatography of amino acids: a method for blood and urine specimens in the diagnosis and treatment of metabolic diseases. Anal. Biochem. *20*:299–311, 1967.

Solomons, G., Keleske, L., and Opitz, E.: Evaluation of the effects of terminating the diet in phenyl-ketonuria. J. Pediat. *69*:596–602, 1966.

Stevenson, R. E., and Huntley, C. C.: Congenital malformations in offspring of phenylketonuric mothers. Pediatrics *40*:33–45, 1967.

Swaiman, K. F., and Lemieux, B.: The effect of phenylalanine and its metabolites on glucose utiliza-tion in developing brain. J. Neurochem. *16*:385–388, 1969.

Tada, K., Yoshida, T., Mochizulli, K., Konno, T., Nakagawa, H., Yokoyama, Y., Takada, G., and Arakawa, T.: Two siblings of hyperphenylalaninemia: suggestion to a genetic variant of phenyl-ketonuria. Tohoku J. Exp. Med. *100*:249–253, 1969.

Tourian, A.: Activation of phenylalanine hydroxylase by phenylalanine. Biochim. Biophys. Acta *242*:345–354, 1971.

Tourian, A., Goddard, J., and Puck, T. T.: Phenylalanine hydroxylase activity in mammalian cells. J. Cell. Physiol. *73*:159–170, 1969.

Udenfriend, S.: The primary enzymatic defect in phenylketonuria and how it may influence the central nervous system. *In* Anderson, J. A., and Swaiman, K. F., eds., Proceedings of a Con-ference on Phenylketonuria and Allied Metabolic Diseases, U.S. Department of Health, Edu-cation and Welfare, U.S. Govt. Printing Office, Washington, D.C., 1967-0-282-371, pp. 1–8, 1967.

Udenfriend, S., and Cooper, J. R.: The enzymatic conversion of phenylalanine to tyrosine. J. Biol. Chem. *194*:503–511, 1952.

Umbarger, B., Berry, H. K., and Sutherland, B. S.: Advances in the management of patients with phenylketonuria. J.A.M.A. *193*:784–790, 1965.

Vanderman, P. R.: Termination of dietary treatment for phenylketonuria. Amer. J. Dis. Child. *106*:492–495, 1963.

Vassella, F., Colombo, J. P., Humbel, R., and Rossi, E.: L-Tryptophan Stoffwechsel bei der Phenyl-ketonurie. Helvet. Paediat. Acta *23*:22–36, 1968.

Vink, C. L. J., and Kroes, A. A.: The renal clearance of phenylpyruvate. Clin. Chim. Acta *6*:813–818, 1961.

Waisman, H. A.: Induced phenylketonuria in experimental animals—opportunities and limita-tions. *In* Anderson, J. A. and Swaiman, K. F., eds., Phenylketonuria and Allied Metabolic Diseases, U.S. Department of Health, Education and Welfare, U.S. Govt. Printing Office, Washington, D.C., 1967-0-282-371, pp. 21–31, 1967.

Wallace, H. W., Moldave, K., and Meister, A.: Studies on conversion of phenylalanine to tyrosine in phenylpyruvic oligophrenia. Proc. Soc. Exp. Biol. Med. *94*:632–633, 1957.

Watson, C. W., Nigam, M. P., and Paine, R. S.: Electroencephalographic abnormalities in phenyl-pyruvic oligophrenia. Neurology *18*:203–207, 1968.

Weber, G.: Inhibition of human brain pyruvate kinase and hexokinase by phenylalanine and phenyl-pyruvate: Possible relevance to phenylketonuric brain damage. Proc. Nat. Acad. Sci. *63*:1365–1369, 1969.

Weber, W. W., and Zannoni, V. G.: Reduction of phenylpyruvic acids to phenyllactic acids in mam-malian tissues. J. Biol. Chem. *241*:1345–1349, 1966.

Weil-Malherbe, H.: The concentration of adrenaline in human plasma and its relation to mental activity. J. Ment. Sci. *101*:733–755, 1955.

Williamson, M., Koch, R., and Henderson, R.: Phenylketonuria in school age retarded children. Amer. J. Ment. Defic. *72*:740–747, 1968.

Wong, P. W. K., Berman, J. L., Partington, M. W., Vickery, S. K., O'Flynn, M. E., and Hsia, D. Y. Y.: Glutamine in PKU. New Eng. J. Med. *285*:580, 1971.

Woolf, L. I.: Phenylketonuria and phenylalaninemia. *In* J. Wortis, ed., Mental Retardation: An Annual Review, Vol. II. Grune & Stratton, New York, pp. 29–45, 1970.

Woolf, L. I., Cranston, W. I., and Goodwin, B. L.: Genetics of phenylketonuria. Heterozygosity for phenylketonuria. Nature (London) *213*:882–883, 1967.

Woolf, L. I., Goodwin, B. L., Cranston, W. I., Wade, D. N., Woolf, F., Hudson, F. P., and McBean, M. S.: A third allele at the phenylalanine-hydroxylase locus in mild phenylketonuria (hyperphenylalaninemia). Lancet (i), 114–117, 1968.

Woolf, L. I., Griffiths, R., Moncrieff, A., Coates, S., and Dillistone, F.: Dietary treatment of phenylketonuria. Arch. Dis. Child. *33*:31–45, 1958.

Woolf, L. I., Jakubovic, A., Woolf, F., and Bary, P.: Metabolism of phenylalanine in mice homozygous for the gene "dilute lethal." Biochem. J. *119*:895–903, 1970.

Woolley, D. W.: Serotonin deficiencies in relation to mental defect of phenylketonuria and galactosemia. *In* Proceedings of a Conference on Nutrition and the Inherited Diseases of Man as Related to Public Health, Minneapolis, pp. 155–165, 1966.

Woolley, D. W., and Van der Hoeven, T.: Serotinin deficiency in infancy as one cause of a mental defect in phenylketonuria. Science *144*:883–884, 1964a.

Woolley, D. W., and Van der Hoeven, T.: Prevention of a mental defect in phenylketonuria with serotonin congeners such as melatonin and 5-hydroxytryptophan. Science *144*:1593–1594, 1964b.

World Health Organization: Screening for inborn errors of metabolism. Technical Report Series, #401, Geneva, 1968.

Yarbro, M. T., and Anderson, J. A.: L-Tryptophan metabolism in phenylketonuria. J. Pediat. *68*: 895–904, 1966.

Yu, J. S., Stuckey, S. J., and O'Halloran, M. T.: The dangers of dietary therapy in phenylketonuria. Med. J. Aust. *2*:404–406, 1970.

Zannoni, V. G., and Moraru, E.: "Phenylketonuria" and phenylalanine metabolism in dilute-lethal mice. *In* Sols, A., and Grisolia, S., eds., FEBS Symposium, Vol. 19, Metabolic Regulation and Enzyme Action. Academic Press, New York, p. 347, 1970.

Zannoni, V. G., Rivkin, I., and LaDu, B. N.: Phenylalanine hydroxylase activity in mammalian liver. Fed. Proc. *26*:840, 1967.

Zannoni, V. G., Weber, W. W., VanValen, P., Rubin, A., Bernstein, R., and LaDu, B. N.: Phenylalanine metabolism "phenylketonuria" in dilute lethal mice. Genetics *54*:1391–1399, 1966.

Chapter Sixteen

TYROSINE

The free tyrosine of body fluids is derived primarily from the conversion of dietary or endogenous phenylalanine as well as from peptide-bound tyrosine in proteins. A small amount of tyrosine may also be derived from nitrogen fixation by intestinal bacteria in the presence of the equivalent keto acid, p-hydroxyphenylpyruvic acid (p-HPPA). Tyrosine, like its precursor phenylalanine, is oxidized by tissues to fumarate and acetoacetate.

The normal catabolic pathway is impaired in several conditions of clinical interest (Table 16–1).

Table 16–1 Disorders of Tyrosine Oxidation

Clinical Trait	Enzyme Deficiency	Characteristic Features
Hypertyrosinemia (Oregon type)	Hepatic cytosol tyrosine aminotransferase	One patient known; 2 others possible. Mental retardation?
"Tyrosinosis" (Medes' type)	Unknown. *p*-HPPA oxidase proposed initially; transaminase more likely	One patient (probably benign)
Neonatal tyrosinemia	*p*-HPPA oxidase (ascorbic acid and low-protein responsive)	Usually benign. Lethargy in some premature infants, and IQ deficit perhaps
Hereditary tyrosinemia	*p*-HPPA oxidase (secondary to unidentified event?)	*Acute form* — liver failure. *Chronic form* — nodular cirrhosis, porphyria-like state, Fanconi syndrome, hepatoma
Alcaptonuria	Homogentisic acid oxidase	Alcaptonuria (homogentisic aciduria) from birth. Ochronosis, arthropathy and spondylitis in later life

In the *"Oregon type" of tyrosinemia*, a disorder of transamination has been described in which the soluble (cytosol) form of tyrosine aminotransferase is deficient. *Medes'* (1932) classical description of "tyrosinosis" may also be relevant to this first step in tyrosine metabolism.

p-Hydroxyphenylpyruvic acid oxidase (*p*-HPPA), which catalyzes the second step in tyrosine oxidation, is affected in two diseases: *transient neonatal tyrosinemia*, which is of interest because it elucidates several important facets of postnatal enzyme development; and *hereditary tyrosinemia*, a complex disease accompanied by grave illness, in which the oxidase step is impaired either primarily or secondarily.

Alcaptonuria is one of the classical inborn errors of metabolism mentioned by Garrod in his Croonian lectures of 1908. It is a disorder affecting the conversion of homogentisic acid to 4-maleylacetoacetic acid at the third step of tyrosine oxidation to fumarate and acetate.

There are other diseases in which alternate routes of tyrosine metabolism are abnormal. *Albinism* is a disturbance of pigment metabolism; it, too, was mentioned in the Croonian lectures by Garrod. The many disturbances of tyrosine incorporation into thyroid hormone lie beyond the scope of this discussion but may be read about elsewhere (Stanbury, 1972). Several "miscellaneous" disorders of tyrosine metabolism continue to attract attention; some of these are mentioned briefly in this section.

METABOLISM OF TYROSINE

The enzymes which catalyze the conversion of tyrosine to fumarate and acetoacetate have been isolated and purified. Consequently, much is known about the normal oxidation of this amino acid (Fig. 16–1).

Tyrosine is converted to the corresponding keto acid, *p*-HPPA, by transamination; the cosubstrate for the aminotransferase is α-ketoglutarate or pyruvate,

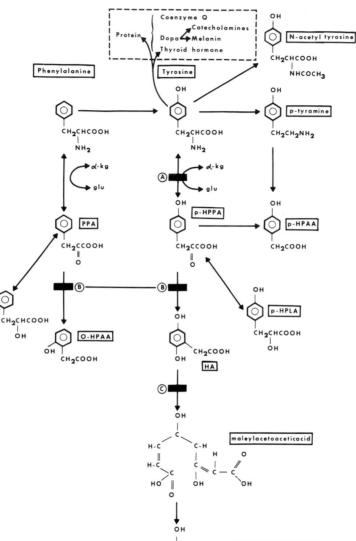

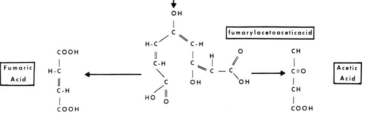

Figure 16–1 Metabolism of tyrosine with an indication of the homologous aspects of phenyl-alanine metabolism. Catabolism is indicated by downward flow; biosynthesis involving tyrosine conversion or incorporation is indicated by upward flow to the box at the top. The inborn errors of tyrosine metabolism are indicated by solid bars: Ⓐ, cytosol tyrosine aminotransferase deficiency (in the Oregon type of hypertyrosinemia). Ⓑ, *p*-HPPA oxidase deficiency (in neonatal tyrosinemia and apparently in hereditary tyrosinemia; In the latter disease, the enzyme deficiency may reflect secondary inhibition of activity). Note that *p*-HPPA oxidase catalyzes the conversion of two different substrates, *p*-HPPA and PPA. Ⓒ, homogentisic acid oxidase deficiency (in alcaptonuria).

PPA = Phenylpyruvic acid; *o*-HPAA = ortho-hydroxyphenylacetic acid; *p*-HPPA = para-hydroxyphenylpyruvic acid; *p*-HPLA = para-hydroxyphenyllactic acid; *p*-HPAA = para-hydroxyphenylacetic acid; HA = homogentisic acid.

and pyridoxal phosphate coenzyme is required for optimal activity. The enzyme is not specific for L-tyrosine, and it is also active toward 3,4-dihydroxyphenyl-alanine and other tyrosine analogues, phenylalanine and tryptophan (Jacoby and LaDu, 1964). These other substances can inhibit tyrosine transamination competitively. The transamination reaction is normally rate-limiting for tyrosine oxidation (Lin and Knox, 1958), and although it is reversible, the equilibrium favors keto acid formation in vivo. Most of the p-HPPA in the body is formed from tyrosine by the forward reaction, but accumulation of the keto acid for any reason will lead to synthesis of tyrosine by reverse transamination.

Tyrosine aminotransferase exists in at least two forms (Canellakis and Cohen, 1956; Litwak et al., 1963; Rowsell et al., 1963; Holt and Oliver, 1969; Fellman et al., 1969; Miller and Litwak, 1969), both of which are present in liver, kidney, brain, heart and muscle. A soluble form of the enzyme is found in cytosol, while another type is present in mitochondria. Several different agents which are known to induce total tyrosine aminotranferase activity seem to affect the two forms differently and independently (Litwak et al., 1963; Holt and Oliver, 1969). The substrate itself, corticosteroids, insulin, glucagon, adrenalin, 3′,5′-cyclic AMP and pyridoxine are all able to induce the enzyme. Tyrosine aminotransferase activity is depressed in liver of the fetal rodent (Kretchmer et al., 1956b; Wicks, 1968) and of the human fetus (Kretchmer et al., 1956a), but activity can be augmented under appropriate conditions even in the fetus.

Deamination of tyrosine (Meister, 1965) can also form p-HPPA, and this alternative source of p-HPPA becomes important for the interpretation of certain diseases of tyrosine metabolism.

Most of the p-HPPA formed in vivo is oxidized to homogentisic acid by the enzyme p-hydroxyphenylpyruvic acid oxidase, which is present in liver and, to a lesser extent, in kidney. LaDu (1967) mentions that this enzyme also exists in different molecular forms and may have subunits. p-HPPA oxidase has been purified and has been shown to have activity when either phenylpyruvate or p-hydroxyphenylpyruvate is the substrate (Taniguchi and Armstrong, 1963; Taniguchi et al., 1964). The relative rates of activity toward the two substrates remain constant during purification of the enzyme (Taniguchi et al., 1964), suggesting that a single enzyme serves both substrates.

The conversion of p-HPPA to homogentisic acid is a complex reaction consuming two atoms of oxygen and yielding one molecule of CO_2 (Lindblad et al., 1970). During hydroxylation of the aromatic ring, there is migration and oxidative decarboxylation of the side chain (pyruvic acid) to form an acetate side chain. How this sequence of reactions is ordered, and on what site(s) of the enzyme protein(s) it takes place, is still unknown. p-HPPA oxidase requires ascorbic acid or other reducing agents (Zannoni and LaDu, 1960; Goswami and Knox, 1961; Knox et al., 1963; Knox et al., 1964) to prevent inhibition of the reaction by its substrate (p-HPPA). The participation of ascorbic acid is rather nonspecific and not analogous to a genuine coenzyme function (Knox, 1958).

Homogentisic acid is oxidized by cleavage of the ring to yield 4-maleylaceto-acetate (Knox and Edwards, 1955). Fumarylacetoacetate is then formed by isomerization of the maleyl analogue (Edwards and Knox, 1956), following which hydrolysis yields fumarate and acetoacetate.

Tyrosine participates in a number of side reactions; these are not discussed in detail here except where relevant to interpretation to the disease processes discussed. They are indicated in Figure 16–1. The biosynthesis of coenzyme Q (ubiquinone) has been discussed by Olson (1966). Thyroid hormone and catecholamine biosyntheses have been the subject of many reviews.

DISTRIBUTION OF TYROSINE IN BODY FLUIDS

Tyrosine is found in plasma, urine, cerebrospinal fluid, saliva, feces and other body fluids. It is also present in the tissues as free and peptide-bound tyrosine. The amino acid is filtered by the renal glomerulus and reabsorbed in the proximal tubule, and the subsequent urinary loss is normally less than 2 per cent of the filtered load.

The keto acid analogue (p-HPPA) can be secreted by the renal tubule into urine in a manner analogous to the renal excretion of other aromatic acids (Vink and Kroes, 1961; Milne et al., 1960). When tyrosine accumulates in plasma it enters kidney cells, where deamination (or transamination) will yield p-HPPA. The keto acid can then be secreted rapidly into urine without formation of the lactic acid analogue in the liver. The urinary excretion pattern of tyrosine metabolites will differ when p-HPPA accumulates initially. Under these circumstances, tyrosine synthesis can take place by reverse transamination of the keto acid. There will also be formation of p-HPLA from p-HPPA by specific enzymatic reduction in the liver (Zannoni and Weber, 1966; Weber and Zannoni, 1966). The kidney will then excrete the lactic acid derivative, as well as p-HPPA and tyrosine, into urine. These relationships are pertinent to the interpretation of the metabolic phenotypes in some of the hereditary disorders of tyrosine metabolism.

DISORDERS OF TYROSINE OXIDATION

Cytosol Tyrosine Aminotransferase Deficiency

Hypertyrosinemia, Oregon Type

Only one patient has been reported with this condition, but it is likely that other patients have been observed. The disorder is of considerable interest for what it teaches us about tyrosine metabolism.

The patient was first reported in an abstract by Campbell et al. (1967) because of an extraordinary degree of hypertyrosinemia (1.9 to 3.0 mM; normal <0.07 mM). Several congenital anomalies and severe mental retardation were also present, and although these findings may have been only coincidental, their presence did bring about the subsequent investigations at various times during the first five years of the patient's life. A re-evaluation of the clinical phenotype suggests that the patient has keratosis palmoplantaris with corneal dystrophy (Richner-Hanhart syndrome), a rare autosomal recessive trait associated with mental retardation. Another proband, a 14-year-old boy with the same syndrome and with hypertyrosinemia, has recently been described (Goldsmith et al., 1972); in the latter patient, dietary control of the tyrosinemia ameliorated the keratosis and corneal dystrophy. Tyrosine excretion is increased in this condition, but renal handling of tyrosine is normal, and, of the amino acids in plasma, only tyrosine is elevated. Consequently, the excessive tyrosinuria is of "prerenal" origin. About 75 per cent of the *unoxidized* tyrosine is excreted as the N-acetyl derivative; this substance is formed when plasma tyrosine exceeds 0.25 mM.

Plasma tyrosine accumulated excessively when the Oregon patient was given a load of phenylalanine or phenylpyruvic acid. A number of unusual tyrosine metabolites were formed and appeared in excessive amounts in the urine and plasma. Even when a low-tyrosine and plant-free diet was given, p-HPPA, *p*-HPLA, *p*-HPAA and *p*-tyramine were formed, and, of these metabolites, *p*-HPLA predominated. Neomycin sterilization of the intestinal lumen caused little change in the metabolite pattern, and *p*-HPAA and *p*-HPLA continued to be excreted in about equal amounts; both were present in amounts twofold greater than the amount of *p*-HPPA. *p*-Tyramine was also excreted in abnormal amounts which were not modified by neomycin treatment.

Drastic restriction of tyrosine intake reduced the excretion of aromatic metabolites to the normal range, but any increase in phenylalanine or tyrosine intake caused their output to increase in proportion to the intake of the amino acids.

Large doses of cortisone, pyridoxine and ascorbic acid did not correct the abnormality of tyrosine metabolism in vivo. Fellman et al. (1969) demonstrated a specific deficiency of the soluble (cytosol) hepatic tyrosine aminotransferase in liver biopsy material, whereas activity of the mitochondrial enzyme was normal (Fig. 16–2).

A seeming paradox thus presented itself to the investigators. Stated simply, Why should *p*-HPPA and related tyrosine derivatives be present in excess when they are the *product* of a deficient enzyme and when hepatic *p*-HPPA oxidase activity (the next enzyme in the sequence) was proven to be normal in the patient's liver in vitro? The findings are contrary to any classical "Garrodian" interpretation.

A likely interpretation of the paradox is summarized in Figure 16–3. Tyrosine accumulates because the amount of mitochondrial aminotransferase is small and rate-limiting. *p*-HPPA will be formed in mitochondria by transamination of tyrosine transported in from cytoplasm. However, once formed, the keto acid cannot be oxidized further because normal mitochondria lack *p*-HPPA oxidase (Fellman et al., 1969). *p*-HPPA will therefore accumulate in mitochondria but can be reaminated to tyrosine or be transported back to cytoplasm, where the increased amount of substrate may inhibit *p*-HPPA oxidase (LaDu and Zannoni, 1955; LaDu, 1967). Under such conditions, *p*-HPPA can

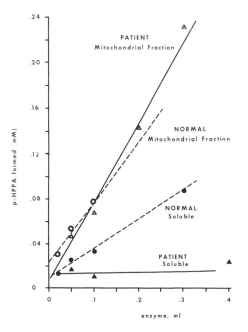

Figure 16–2 Tyrosine-α-keto-glutarate aminotransferase activity in liver fractions obtained from a patient with abnormal aminotransferase activity (△, ▲) and from normal control subjects (○, ●). The patient is deficient only in the soluble (cytosol) fraction of hepatic aminotransferase. The enzyme was assayed by measuring *p*-hydroxyphenylpyruvate (*p*-HPPA) synthesis after 30 minutes incubation. (From Fellman et al.: Biochemistry 8:621, 1969. Copyright 1969 American Chemical Society. By permission of the authors.)

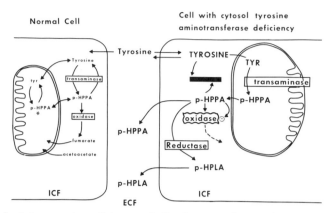

Figure 16–3 Interpretation of the metabolic phenotype in a patient with cytosol tyrosine-α-ketoglutarate aminotransferase deficiency (Fellman et al., 1969; Kennaway and Buist, 1971). The normal pathway of tyrosine metabolism in the cytoplasm and mitochondrion is indicated on the left. The patient (right-hand model) has deficient cytosol transaminase activity, as indicated by the solid bar; the corresponding mitochondrial isoenzyme remains active. Tyrosine will accumulate in cytoplasm but can be converted to *p*-HPPA in mitochondria. Oxidation of *p*-HPPA does not normally occur in mitochondria; therefore *p*-HPPA will move back into cytoplasm, where it may inhibit *p*-HPPA oxidase. The keto acid will leave the cell and appear in plasma. Aromatic reductase in liver will also convert the keto acid to the lactic acid derivative (*p*-HPLA), which can also leave the cell. An additional reaction to dispose of tyrosine is available in kidney. Tyrosine may be converted directly to *p*-HPPA by deamination; the keto acid can then be excreted into urine directly. The three mechanisms can account for the formation of *p*-HPPA and *p*-HPLA and their urinary excretion in cytosol aminotransferase deficiency.

accumulate in the cytoplasm in vivo. This form of substrate inhibition will not be apparent in vitro because, under the usual conditions of the assay for *p*-HPPA oxidase activity (LaDu, 1967), substrate inhibition is prevented by the addition of a large excess of reducing agent.

Kennaway and Buist (1971) and Goldsmith et al. (1972) state that ascorbic acid did not reduce the hypertyrosinemia in their patients. Unfortunately, no detailed comment was made about *p*-HPPA excretion; this point should be restudied carefully.

Fellman, Buist and colleagues (1972) have offered a different but analogous interpretation. They propose that tyrosine which accumulates in blood because of a *hepatic* deficiency of cytosol transaminase could be converted to the corresponding keto acid by other tissues which possess ample mitochondrial transaminase but normally lack *p*-HPPA oxidase. The combined quantities of mitochondrial transaminase in liver and skeletal and cardiac muscle are enough to produce keto acid, whose subsequent oxidation is blocked in those tissues and is then handled in the manner described in the preceding discussion. The authors incidentally pointed out that analogous reasoning may also be used to explain keto acid formation and excretion in phenylketonuria.

When *p*-HPPA accumulates in vivo, there is an opportunity for the aromatic α-keto acid reductase in liver to form *p*-HPLA from *p*-HPAA. Both substances can then be excreted from the blood into urine. At the same time, some of the excess tyrosine might be converted to *p*-HPPA by deamination in kidney (Meister, 1965) and secreted directly into urine, thus by-passing the deficient cytoplasmic transamination by a second route in that tissue.

Kennaway and Buist (1971) noted that phenylpyruvic, phenyllactic and *o*-hydroxyphenylacetic acids were excreted by the patient. This finding also suggests that *p*-HPPA oxidase activity is deficient in vivo, since phenylpyruvate and *p*-HPPA are presumably oxidized by the same enzyme (Taniguchi et al., 1964).

Cytosol aminotransferase deficiency is of interest for some of its negative findings. Neither hepatic failure nor nephropathy are apparent, despite the striking and chronic accumulation of tyrosine metabolites in body fluids. Similar biochemical findings are associated with life-threatening hepatic failure and nephropathy in hereditary tyrosinemia, a disease in which p-HPPA oxidase activity is also deficient (see subsequent text).

Other Possible Examples of Transaminase Deficiency

Two unusual patients with severe persistent hypertyrosinemia, with exaggerated p-HPPA and p-HPLA excretion and without hepatorenal abnormalities have been described by Wadman and associates (1968) and by Holston et al. (1971). Both patients were mentally retarded. The similarities of the biochemical findings in the new patients and in the Oregon patient are noteworthy. Neither of the new patients had enzyme studies performed.

Comment

The importance of tissue enzyme studies, the need for cell fractionation and kinetic studies and the careful interpretation required of data obtained from in vivo and in vitro studies is apparent from the work on the patient with cytosol tyrosine aminotransferase deficiency. The latter study is likely to catalyze similar investigation of other inborn errors of metabolism and a yield of analogous results will bear witness to the many mechanisms by which the genetic control of cellular metabolism is diversified in human tissues.

Tyrosinosis (Medes' Type)

A "new error of tyrosine metabolism" called "tyrosinosis" was first described in 1932 by Grace Medes. Her paper remains a classic model for any student of clinical investigation. The patient was a 49-year-old male with myasthenia gravis who excreted an unusual reducing substance identified as p-HPPA (Medes et al., 1927). Medes attributed the excretion of p-HPPA and 3,4-dihydroxyphenylalanine (dopa), with little p-HPLA excess, to a block in p-HPPA oxidase. However, after review of the original data, LaDu (1972) has suggested that the findings are also compatible with a deficiency of tyrosine aminotransferase activity. Technological limitations at the time prevented Medes from demonstrating hypertyrosinemia, which should have been present if her patient had transaminase deficiency.

Certain findings in Medes' study of "tyrosinosis" suggest that the postulated transaminase deficiency differs from that reported by Fellman et al. (1969) and by Kennaway and Buist (1971). In tyrosinosis (Medes, 1932), the block in tyrosine metabolism is relatively greater at high levels of tyrosine intake than at low levels. Furthermore, almost no p-HPLA was formed at any time, suggesting that most of the urinary p-HPPA was formed in kidney (presumably by deamination), with immediate excretion into urine. These findings could indicate a tissue-specific enzyme deficiency—in this case perhaps a deficiency of renal tyrosine aminotransferase.

Neonatal Tyrosinemia

The commonest disorder of amino acid metabolism in man is transient neonatal tyrosinemia. The condition, first described by Levine, Marples and

Gordon in 1939, elicited the term *tyrosyluria* to indicate the excessive urinary excretion of tyrosine, *p*-HPPA, *p*-HPLA and *p*-HPAA which characterized the condition. It is now known that N-acetyl tyrosine is also excreted by the new-born infant with tyrosinemia (Dubovsky and Dubovska, 1965) and that the *p*-tyramine which is also found in urine is of endogenous origin (Bremer et al., 1969). Levine, in his 1946 Harvey Lecture, described the role of relative vita-min C deficiency in the etiology of the condition. When simple methods became available to estimate tyrosine in plasma, the condition came to be recognized most readily by its tyrosinemia (Hsia et al., 1962; LaDu et al., 1963; Menkes and Avery, 1963; Mathews and Partington, 1964; Light et al., 1966; Bremer et al., 1966; Avery et al., 1967; Wong et al., 1967; Levy et al., 1969; Rizzardini and Abeliuk, 1971). It then became obvious that the neonatal tyrosyluria was al-ways associated with tyrosinemia and that a transient adaptive impairment in the oxidation of tyrosine was usually responsible for the finding.

Kretchmer (1959) and colleagues (1956a, 1956b) showed that neonatal tyrosinemia reflected a partial impairment of *p*-hydroxyphenylpyruvic acid oxidase activity. The amount of this enzyme in the liver of the premature infant is not sufficient to oxidize the *p*-HPPA formed from the relatively large amount of tyrosine normally ingested in the diet of the neonate. Kennaway and Buist (1971) have suggested that an altered pattern of intracellular transamina-tion activity may also contribute to the hypertyrosinemia of the newborn infant.

Neonatal tyrosinemia occurs more frequently in premature infants than in full-term subjects, and under appropriate conditions it may occur in 30 per cent of prematures and in up to 10 per cent of full-term infants (Mathews and Partington, 1964; Avery et al., 1967; Levy et al., 1969). Gestational immaturity is a more likely predisposition to hypertyrosinemia than is a low birth-weight itself (Rizzardini and Abeliuk, 1971; Menkes et al., 1972), and males are more often affected than females (Wong et al., 1967). The hypertyrosinemia peaks at the end of the first week of life and will persist for several weeks after birth in 0.5 per cent of surviving infants. However, it is only a transient phenomenon in the majority of infants.

Investigation of ascorbic acid-depleted guinea pigs and rats (Zannoni and LaDu, 1960; Goswami and Knox, 1961; Knox and Goswami, 1963; Knox et al., 1964) revealed the probable enzymatic basis of the neonatal form of tyrosinemia* in man. In the immature subject, *p*-hydroxyphenylpyruvic acid oxidase is sus-ceptible to inhibition by its substrate, which can be formed from the large quantity of tyrosine in the diet of the newborn. Inhibition of the enzyme is also encouraged by a relative deficiency of ascorbic acid in newborn tissues and by the reduced amount of the apoenzyme in the cell. From the known relationships between total and basal amounts of *p*-HPPA oxidase in the maturing liver (Fig. 16–4), one can predict that very immature infants with little hepatic enzyme will have more severe tyrosinemia, particularly if the protein intake is high, and that ascorbic acid will be of little benefit. Older infants with more basal enzyme activity can tolerate a higher protein intake without developing tyro-sinemia. The predicted physiological relationships between age and degree of tyrosinemia have been clearly documented in the human infant (Mathews and Partington, 1964; Avery et al., 1967; Wong et al., 1967; Komrower and Robins, 1969; Levy et al., 1969; Rizzardini and Abeliuk, 1971).

Since the tyrosine concentration in plasma can exceed 2 mM (normal value

---

*The tyrosyluria of nutritional scurvy in infancy includes the excretion of *p*-HPPA and *p*-HPLA, and impairment of *p*-HPPA oxidase is implied (Huisman and Jonxis, 1957).

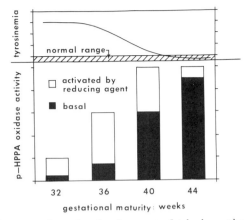

Figure 16–4 A scheme to show the development of *p*-hydroxyphenylpyruvic acid oxidase activity in human liver during perinatal development. The total amount of apoenzyme is small initially. Premature birth and exposure to tyrosine in the diet will cause *p*-HPPA (tyrosine) to accumulate under these conditions. With maturation, more apoenzyme is synthesized in liver cells. However, the enzyme can be inhibited if the tyrosine intake is large. Basal activity (black bar) can be augmented (open bar) with a reducing agent such as ascorbic acid or by reduction of substrate accumulation through a reduction of protein intake. With further maturation there will be sufficient enzyme to prevent inhibition of *p*-HPPA oxidase by *p*-HPPA, and under the usual dietary conditions, hypertyrosinemia will not occur. Tyrosinemia reflects reverse transamination from *p*-HPPA; tyrosine aminotransferase activity is adequate in newborn liver. (Adapted from Goswami and Knox: Biochim. Biophys. Acta *50*:35–40, 1961; Avery et al.: Pediatrics *39*:378–384, 1967.)

<0.07 mM) in infants with neonatal tyrosinemia, it is important to know whether this common condition is harmful. Most observers believe that neonatal tyrosinemia is probably harmless (Menkes et al., 1966; Partington and Mathews, 1966; Avery et al., 1967; Partington et al., 1968). However, some premature infants manifest lethargy (Scriver et al., 1965; Avery et al., 1967) and obtunded motor activity (Partington et al., 1971), during the period of hypertyrosinemia. Moreover, Menkes and colleagues (1972) have reported that neonatal tyrosinemia exceeding levels in plasma of about 1 mM in premature infants with birth weights over 2000 g may be associated with impaired mental development which is detectable only in later childhood. These facts should be weighed in the balance with two other reports (Menkes and Jervis, 1961; Auerbach et al., 1963) of infants with impaired mental development in whom severe persisting tyrosinemia was found which, upon treatment with ascorbic acid and a reduction of protein intake, was followed by immediate biochemical and clinical improvement. Observations of this nature encourage a note of caution before the claim is made that neonatal tyrosinemia is wholly benign for *all* infants.

It is very important to distinguish neonatal tyrosinemia from other forms of tyrosinemia. This can be done relatively well by two simple procedures (Avery et al., 1967). A modest reduction of protein intake to about 2 to 3 g/kg/day will assuage the tyrosinemia in most infants. A similar and immediate effect can be achieved with ascorbic acid (50 to 100 mg/day) if the basal amount of enzyme (Fig. 16–4) is adequate (Light et al., 1966; Avery et al., 1967).

The prevalence of tyrosinemia under the particular adaptive conditions of the neonate encourages a redefinition of the recommended daily allowance of ascorbic acid in this age group. If maintenance of normal tyrosine metabolism is a criterion for the adequacy of vitamin C intake, the recommended daily allowance for the adult (30 mg/day) is not sufficient for the infant. If the re-

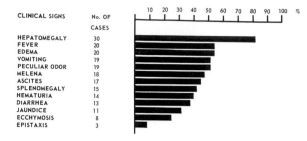

Figure 16–5 Relative frequency of clinical symptoms in the "acute" or "infantile" form of hereditary tyrosinemia occurring in a French-Canadian geographic subisolate. Infantile and "late-onset" ("chronic") forms of hereditary tyrosinemia are known to occur in the same sibship and in the same subisolate, indicating that they are probably manifestations of the same genetic trait. The "chronic" phenotype is sometimes known as Baber's syndrome (1956) and involves nodular hepatic cirrhosis and a Fanconi-like nephropathy. (Graph adapted from Larochelle et al., 1967, describing 37 patients with the condition.)

quirement is expressed as a coefficient of body weight, that for the adult is about 0.5 mg/kg per day, whereas it is about 25 times greater for the newborn infant. In other words, the neonate is transiently "vitamin C-dependent" relative to his adult counterpart.

Hereditary Tyrosinemia*

This inherited disease, which is now known to be pan-ethnic, received its first integrated biochemical and clinical description from Sakai and colleagues in Japan (1957a, 1957b, 1959). The disease has subsequently been the subject of three extensive reviews (Gjessing, 1966; Hsia, 1967; Partington, Scriver, and Sass-Kortsak, 1967), and the most recent review (LaDu and Gjessing, 1972) refers to over 100 patients.

Clinical Aspects

The clinical features of the disorder appear to segregate into two forms, both of which can appear within the same family. The typical "acute" form has been well described by Larochelle and colleagues (1967) (Fig. 16–5). Symptoms appear in the first six months after birth, and death occurs rapidly in about 90 per cent of the untreated patients as the result of liver failure. A characteristic cabbage-like odor (Cone, 1968) is often observed, which many believe is caused by a derivative of methionine. There is hyperplasia of islets of Langerhans and hypoglycemia in these patients.

Some probands, for reasons which are still unclear, escape the acute phase of the disease and present in later childhood with an equally typical "chronic" form; this type has been given several definitive descriptions by investigators

---

*This term is preferred by the authors, rather than "tyrosinosis," which is commonly assigned to the condition by others. "Tyrosinosis" has a classical connotation stemming from Medes' use of the term (Medes, 1932). In view of the fact that the disease she described may have been a benign disorder of tyrosine transaminase activity, the same term should not be used to describe another condition which is of grave clinical significance and in which a different enzyme in the oxidative pathway of tyrosine is involved.

in Scandinavia (Fritzell et al., 1964; Gentz et al., 1965; Halvorsen et al., 1966; Gentz et al., 1967), in France (Lelong et al., 1963), in Canada (Scriver and Davies, 1967) and in the United States (Kogut et al., 1967). Severe nodular hepatic cirrhosis, a nephropathy causing the Fanconi syndrome, susceptibility to hypoglycemia (Silverberg, 1967), an associated hyperplasia of the islets of Langerhans and failure to thrive are all found in the chronic phenotype. Many patients first come to medical attention because of hypophosphatemic rickets secondary to the nephropathy. Patients with the "chronic" phenotype also develop hepatic carcinoma with relatively high frequency.

Biochemical Aspects

The principal biochemical features of the condition include massive tyrosyluria with p-HPPA and p-HPLA predominating over other metabolites of tyrosine (Sakai and Kitagawa, 1957b; Halvorsen et al., 1966; Gentz et al., 1967; Scriver et al., 1967; Gentz et al., 1969). Hypertyrosinemia with tyrosinuria occurs even in the fasting state, and there is an inability to metabolize L-tyrosine and p-HPPA normally via the main oxidative pathway (Scriver and Davies, 1967). p-HPPA is present in excess in plasma, and homogentisic acid is not formed when p-HPPA is infused (Gentz et al., 1969). The impairment of tyrosine metabolism cannot be corrected in vivo with ascorbic acid, steroids or folic acid (Scriver et al., 1967; Scriver and Davies, 1967).

Several important biochemical abnormalities in the trait have been identified.

Hypermethioninemia occurs, particularly in the "acute" phenotype. This finding may only reflect acute liver failure (Gjessing and Halvorsen, 1965; Scriver et al., 1966; Scriver, 1968), but many investigators (Perry et al., 1965; Gaull et al., 1968, 1970) believe the hypermethioninemia represents a more basic disturbance of amino acid metabolism in hereditary hypertyrosinemia. Gaull and colleagues (1970) have demonstrated significant deficiencies of enzyme activity at critical steps in methionine disposal in the liver of patients believed to have "tyrosinosis."

Excessive formation and excretion of δ-aminolevulinic acid and symptoms resembling acute porphyria occur in patients with the severe chronic liver failure of hereditary tyrosinemia, perhaps because the normal feedback control of porphyrin synthesis is lost in hepatocytes in this disease (Gentz et al., 1967, 1969a, 1969b; Kang and Gerald, 1970; Gaull et al., 1970). Catecholamines are also produced and excreted in excess (Gentz et al., 1967, 1969a, 1969c) and may cause hypertension.

Studies in French-Canadian patients indicate that disordered tyrosine metabolism *precedes* the onset of liver failure and the other abnormalities associated with the trait. The activity of several enzymes involved in aromatic amino acid metabolism has been assayed in liver obtained at autopsy (Sakai and Kitagawa, 1957b) and in fresh biopsy samples (Gentz et al., 1965; Taniguchi and Gjessing, 1965; LaDu, 1967). A severe deficiency of p-HPPA oxidase activity was identified, with residual activity being less than 5 per cent of normal in many of the liver samples. These findings encourage one to believe that hereditary tyrosinemia may be a primary disorder of p-HPPA oxidase activity (Scriver, 1967). However, the situation is likely to be less simple, and it has also been appropriate to ask whether the apparent enzyme deficiency is secondary to an unidentified cause of p-HPPA oxidase inhibition (Scriver, 1967; LaDu, 1967; Gaull et al., 1970; LaDu and Gjessing, 1972). It should be noted that no one has yet been able to activate p-HPPA oxidase in liver biopsy samples obtained from these patients under the usual conditions of assay in vitro. More-over, treatment with a low-tyrosine diet prevents clinical tyrosinemia and reverses most of the abnormal biochemical findings. Nonetheless, the impairment of tyrosine metabolism in vivo persists and can be divulged with ease (Gentz et al., 1967; Scriver, Larochelle and Silverberg, 1967). It is often asked why patients with neonatal tyrosinemia or other causes of severe tyrosinemia do not have hepatonephropathy; there is no simple answer to this pertinent question. p-HPPA oxidase deficiency, liver disease and renal tubular failure in hereditary tyrosinemia may all be secondary to an unknown event. On the other hand, it may be said that the degree of p-HPPA oxidase deficiency is more severe in hereditary tyrosinemia and that this circumstance somehow influences the clinical course. The problem is more than academic because even though a tyrosine-restricted diet can benefit the patient, it may not be possible to prevent the liver damage by this means (Hsia, 1967).

Comment. It should be noted, before leaving this discussion at a necessarily unsatisfactory stage of resolution, that most assays of p-HPPA oxidase in liver of patients with hereditary tyrosinemia have been done on cirrhotic liver obtained at operation or post-mortem. There are no reports on enzyme activity in the liver of probands *before* hepatic damage occurs, nor have assays been performed on kidney in which there is a small but measurable p-HPPA oxidase activity. Observations of this type might discern whether low p-HPPA oxidase activity is merely a function of the abnormal liver tissue which must be used for the assay or whether it is a function of inhibitory events secondary to the liver failure itself. Such studies could answer some of the important questions raised by Gaull and colleagues (1970). The possibility that hereditary tyrosinemia as we know it is, in fact, hereditary fructosemia due to an abnormality of hepatic fructose-1-phosphate aldolase activity has become of increasing concern to students of the disease (see following discussion). The striking fructose intolerance in some patients and the amelioration of symptoms with a fructose-free diet encourage further examination of this hypothesis in future patients with "hereditary tyrosinemia."

Diagnosis. The observed deficiency of p-HPPA oxidase activity is irreversible; this finding differentiates hereditary tyrosinemia from neonatal tyrosinemia. This evidence can usually be obtained by metabolic studies in vivo as described by Scriver and Davies (1967) and Gentz and colleagues (1969) or by means of liver biopsy and in vitro assay of the enzyme (LaDu, 1967). Tyrosinemia can be detected initially by simple screening methods (Crawhall et al., 1971), and the tyrosine metabolites will yield positive tests with the Benedict's, ferric chloride and 1-nitrosonaphthol reagents (Perry et al., 1966).

The differential diagnosis of hereditary tyrosinemia is not always simple. Hereditary fructosemia due to hepatic fructose-1-phosphate aldolase deficiency produces many of the biochemical and clinical manifestations of hereditary tyrosinemia (Lindemann et al., 1970; Gentz et al., 1970). A specific search for fructose in urine and plasma should be made, and a fructose tolerance test under carefully controlled conditions may be indicated to facilitate diagnosis. Galactosemia may also cause nephropathy with the Fanconi syndrome and hepatic damage.

The "physiological" tyrosinemia associated with high protein feeding of the newborn should be considered, and in some infants this feeding regimen may also cause transient hypermethioninemia (Komrower and Robins, 1969; Levy et al., 1968). The methioninemia also causes problems in diagnosis and interpretation. Gaull et al. (1968, 1970) consider the finding of primary significance. On the other hand, Scriver and colleagues (1966, 1968) consider the finding representative of nonspecific liver failure as recognized many years ago (Kinsell et al., 1948, 1949, 1950).

Animal Models of Hereditary Tyrosinemia

The unresolved debate over pathogenesis of the trait and interpretation of the hypertyrosinemia and hypermethioninemia has called forth some interesting studies in animals. In this work, rats or guinea pigs have been exposed to toxic diets containing an excess of L-methionine or L-tyrosine or both in the knowledge that these two amino acids are toxic when ingested at high levels (Harper, 1964).

It should be stressed that an animal model of this type is not analogous to the human disease. In the model, input to and outflow from the catabolic pathway under investigation are both greatly augmented; in the disease, input is unimpeded but outflow is reduced. Nonetheless, some observations of interest have been obtained by Perry et al. (1967), who induced the biochemical findings of tyrosinemia in an animal model. Chronic dietary loading with methionine but not with tyrosine caused biochemical imbalance and hepatic and renal damage somewhat similar to that in the naturally occurring human disease. Hardwick and colleagues (1970) confirmed that chronic methionine loading (10 mM/kg per day) in guinea pigs caused a tyrosinemia-like state; and they went on to show that hepatic ATP decreased and that S-adenosylmethionine and S-adenosylhomocysteine accumulated under these conditions. Intraperitoneal adenine injection offset some of the toxic effects of methionine feeding. This finding is interesting because it is known that fructose toxicity in animals depletes liver nucleotides (Maenpaa et al., 1968; Goldblatt et al., 1970; Woods et al., 1970). The clinical similarities between hereditary fructose intolerance and hereditary tyrosinemia suggest that some mechanism of ATP depletion may be active in the latter disease.

Genetics

Hereditary tyrosinemia is autosomal recessive in a French-Canadian sub-isolate in Chicoutimi, where the frequency of homozygotes is high and the estimated carrier rate is between 1 in 20 and 1 in 30 persons (Laberge and Dallaire, 1967). Laberge (1969) traced French-Canadian pedigrees to identify a "founder effect" probably originating from a single couple, Louis Gagné and his wife, who settled in New France in the mid-1600's.

It is not known whether the trait is caused by the same mutant allele in all pedigrees. It seems likely that the "acute" and "chronic" forms of hereditary tyrosinemia are only different clinical manifestations of the same mutant allele (Partington, Scriver, and Sass-Kortsak, 1967; Bodegard et al., 1969). However, the current disagreements between scientists over the apparent pathogenesis of hereditary tyrosinemia may indicate that the effects of different mutant alleles are being observed and interpreted by the investigators whose patients reside in different ethnic groups and geographic regions.

Treatment

It is known that tyrosine and methionine are toxic to mammals when ingested in large amounts (Harper, 1964). Therefore, it seems prudent to prevent the accumulation of these two amino acids in hereditary tyrosinemia despite the reservations concerning the pathogenesis of their accumulation. It is now clearly apparent that restriction of dietary tyrosine and phenylalanine in a manner analogous to the treatment of phenylketonuria is of decided benefit to most patients with the acute and chronic forms of the disease (Halvorsen and Gjessing, 1964; Gjessing, 1966; Partington, Scriver, and Sass-Kortsak, 1967; Hsia, 1967; Aronssen et al., 1968; Tada et al., 1968; Fiarney et al., 1968). Dietary control in the acute form of the disease is associated with dramatic clinical improvement, while long-term treatment in the chronic phenotype can reverse the nephropathy (Fig. 16–6). Relaxation of dietary control is usually followed by immediate reappearance of clinical and biochemical signs of hereditary tyrosinemia. In cases where this has not occurred and in which long-term dietary treatment was not necessary (Harries et al., 1969; Gaull et al., 1970), the diagnosis of "classical" hereditary tyrosinemia is possibly in doubt.

Methionine restriction in the diet is advisable in the acute stage of the disease if hypermethioninemia is present. Prevention of hypoglycemia, with correction of electrolyte imbalance, is also very important. The use of ascorbic acid and other agents to activate p-HPPA oxidase has not been successful in hereditary tyrosinemia.

Whether long-term therapy prevents progression of the liver disease is unknown. Most workers feel that after the liver damage is established the diet does not improve it, and death has been reported from liver failure in the face of treatment (Bodegard et al., 1969). (It is unclear, however, whether hereditary fructosemia was ruled out in this latter patient and others like him.) On the other hand, there are only a few patients who have received dietary treatment from birth. In one such patient, with a confirmed diagnosis, growth and development have been good, and there is no clinical or biochemical evidence of hepatic damage at 8 months of age (Laberge, 1972).

Dietary formulations and instruction for the use of a semisynthetic diet have been described (Hill et al., 1970), and the tyrosine content of many foods is known (McCarthy et al., 1968).

Alcaptonuria

Alcaptonuria, or homogentisic aciduria, is the predecessor to ochronosis, the deposition of oxidized homogentisic acid pigment in connective tissue, and to spondylitis and arthropathy, the degenerative conditions which follow deposition of this pigment.

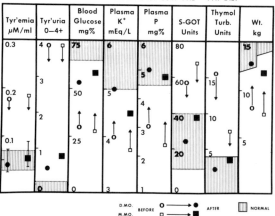

RESPONSE TO 7 MONTHS OF LOW PHE - TYR DIET

Figure 16–6 The effect of a low-phenylalanine–low-tyrosine diet on two patients with hereditary tyrosinemia. Pretreatment values are indicated by open symbols; post-treatment values are indicated by closed symbols. The range of normal values is indicated by the hatched portions of the bar graphs. Dietary treatment for seven months ablated tyrosinemia and tyrosyluria and corrected the hypoglycemia and abnormal liver function. The tubular nephropathy also improved. Significant weight gain also occurred with tyrosine restriction.

Alcaptonuria was one of the four inborn errors of metabolism described by Garrod in the Croonian lectures of 1908. It is also the first disease of man for which Mendelian recessive inheritance was proposed (Garrod, 1902). The disease has a long history, probably because the darkening of urine which occurs when it is exposed to air (Cone, 1968) has attracted the attention of patients for centuries. Boedeker (1859, 1861) was the first person to study and report on the reducing property of alcaptonuric urine and to distinguish it from the reducing property of glucose. The darkening of urine upon standing was attributed to increasing alkalinity and uptake of oxygen; Boedeker called the substance responsible for this finding *Alkapton*, a hybrid of the Arabic word for "alkali" and the Greek word for "to suck up (oxygen) greedily in alkali." Thereafter, the condition was known as alcaptonuria. The trait is encountered throughout the human species, and because of widespread interest, it continues to be the subject of informative reviews (Knox, 1958; O'Brien et al., 1963; LaDu, 1972).

The Metabolic Defect

Alcaptonuria occurs when homogentisic acid is not oxidized to maleylacetoacetic acid (Fig. 16–1). It is now recognized that homogentisic acid is a normal intermediate formed during the enzymatic conversion of tyrosine to fumaric and acetoacetic acid in the liver. The characteristics of homogentisic acid oxidase have been well described (Knox and Edwards, 1955; O'Brien et al., 1963), and it is estimated that the normal adult liver can oxidize 1600 g homogentisic acid per day (LaDu, 1972). The normal destination of the carbon atoms of homogentisic acid is shown in Fig. 16–1.

The view that homogentisic acid is a normal metabolite in the main pathway of tyrosine oxidation was not always accepted (Dakin, 1911), even after Garrod perceived that homogentisic acid probably accumulated because of the absence of a normal hepatic enzyme. Proposals for an enzyme deficiency in blood (Gross, 1914) — an erroneous observation on several counts — an intestinal origin for the homogentisic acid (Wolkow and Baumann, 1891) and an abnormal pathway of tyrosine metabolism (Dakin, 1911) caused an ebb and flow of confusion as to the true nature of alcaptonuria, and it was not until 1958 that LaDu and colleagues finally confirmed Garrod's own proposal about the nature of the defect by demonstrating that the liver of the alcaptonuric patient was specifically deficient in homogentisic acid oxidase activity. The presence of an inhibitor to account for the deficient enzyme activity was ruled out. Zannoni, Seegmiller, and LaDu (1962) later showed that the homogentisic acid oxidase was also deficient in kidney of the alcaptonuric patient.

The effects of the enzyme deficiency are evident soon after birth (Garrod, 1901), and the postnatal urine of the affected infant usually contains large amounts of homogentisic acid, of which the amount excreted is proportional to the dietary intake of phenylalanine and tyrosine. Alcaptonuria is the only manifestation of the trait in childhood, and it is symptomless. Ochronosis does not occur in tissues until there is long exposure to homogentisic acid. Patients may not even know for many years that they carry the trait, since with modern sanitation they may never encounter the darkening of their urine after it has remained exposed to air for a period of time.

Homogentisic acid is normally present in only trace amounts in human urine or plasma (Lustberg et al., 1971). However, even in the alcaptonuric patient there is very little homogentisic acid in plasma. The explanation for the appearance of homogentisic aciduria without significant homogentisic acidemia was found by Neuberger et al. (1947) to reflect the mechanism of its renal excretion. Homogentisic acid is secreted into the tubular lumen, and consequently its renal clearance rate exceeds the glomerular filtration rate. Actually, it was this physiological feature of homogentisic acid metabolism which led investigators away from the concept of an endogenous metabolic defect of tyrosine oxidation and led them to propose an abnormality in the renal excretion of homogentisic acid as the basis for alcaptonuria (Neuberger et al., 1947).

Diagnosis

The patient whose urine darkens to blackness on standing in air or with the addition of alkali may have alcaptonuria. Other compounds, such as bile, porphyrin, myoglobin and hemoglobin, which may also darken the urine, are readily distinguished from homogentisic acid. However the spontaneous appearance of dark urine does not always occur in alcaptonuria, particularly if the urine remains acid or if it contains large amounts of a reducing agent.

Homogentisic acid in urine can be identified by a number of simple procedures:

(i) A dark color will follow the addition of sufficient alkali to raise the pH above neutrality. Alkaline urine left to oxidize in air will darken downward from the exposed surface.

(ii) Homogentisic acid will react with Benedict's reagent and will itself darken under the alkaline conditions of the reaction; the normal orange color of the positive reducing test will thus be changed to a brown color.

(iii) The ferric chloride reagent can yield a purple-black reaction with homogentisic acid.

(iv) Urine (0.5 ml) added to 5 ml of saturated $AgNO_3$ in water (redissolved with NH_3) produces an immediate black color. Ascorbic acid gives a false-positive result with this reagent.

These screening tests can be confirmed by thin-layer chromatography (Sankoff and Sourkes, 1963), by a specific enzymatic method (Seegmiller et al., 1961) and by spectrophotometry (Lustberg et al., 1971).

Genetics

Subsequently published pedigrees confirmed Garrod's original contention (1902; 1908b) that alcaptonuria is a simple recessive trait. Studies of certain pedigrees apparently showing dominant inheritance (viz. Hogben et al., 1932; Khachadurian and Abu Feisal, 1958; Milch, 1961) contained many consanguineous matings, and careful review shows that the alcaptonuric allele(s) behave(s) as a simple autosomal recessive in these pedigrees.

The mutant allele (or alleles, if the trait is genetically heterogeneous) is found widely throughout the world, but the precise frequency of the trait is not known. One patient per quarter-million persons is probably a reasonable estimate (note that the frequency is similar to that of maple syrup urine disease), but since most estimates depend on ascertainment of ochronosis, the true frequency of alcaptonuria may be higher than apparent.

Treatment

There is no effective treatment once ochronosis is established in alcaptonuria. However, it is conceivable that the crippling spondylitis and arthropathy which result from ochronosis could be prevented if homogentisic acid accumulation and polymerization could be curbed by restriction of phenylalanine and tyrosine intake beginning early in life. Ingestion of 200 to 500 mg/day of phenylalanine and a similar amount of tyrosine will support normal growth during childhood in patients with phenylketonuria or hereditary tyrosinemia, and a similar mode of treatment could perhaps be of assistance in alcaptonuria. No one, to our knowledge, has tried this approach to therapy. If attempts are made to identify the patient with alcaptonuria early in life and if palatable diets low in phenylalanine and tyrosine become available for lifelong use, a controlled experiment in treatment could probably be initiated with reasonable justification. It has also been suggested that large doses of ascorbic acid may prevent deposition of the polymerized ochronotic pigment and may therefore prevent subsequent symptoms (Sealock et al., 1940).

DISORDERS OF TYROSINE METABOLISM NOT AFFECTING THE MAIN OXIDATION PATHWAY

Albinism

Albinism is an inherited disorder of melanin synthesis. A number of mutant alleles distributed throughout the biological realm cause the phenotype. In man, albinism visibly affects the melanocyte system of skin or eyes or both.

Garrod postulated that albinism was an inborn error of metabolism in his first Croonian lecture of 1908. Recent work has shown that the melanocyte and its melanin-producing organelles (the melanosomes) are normal in the affected tissue, but the important chemical product (melanin) is not synthesized adequately by the organelles. Therefore albinism is indeed an inborn error of metabolism. In one form of albinism (tyrosinase-negative), a key enzyme required for melanin synthesis is missing. In another form of albinism (tyrosinase-positive), the defect appears to involve tyrosine utilization by the melanosome; once tyrosine enters the organelle, melanin synthesis can occur in this trait.

Albinism is a fascinating topic which, like alcaptonuria, has a long history because the obvious features of the condition attracted attention readily. There are several excellent reviews on albinism—for example, Knox, 1958; Witkop, 1971; Fitzpatrick and Quevedo, 1972—and on the biology of melanin pigmentation (see Fitzpatrick et al., 1961, 1971). Upon reading these discussions, it becomes apparent that albinism is a set of experiments of nature which alter specialization in structure and function at the subcellular level for the purpose of ordering a biosynthetic sequence.

Melanin Metabolism

The melanocyte is the site of the defect in albinism. Melanocytes are dendritic and nondendritic in form, and they are specialized for the synthesis of melanin. They occur in skin, dermis, dermal-epidermal junction, hair bulb, mucous membranes, mesentery, nervous system (pia-arachnoid), internal ear and eye (uveal tract and retinal pigment epithelium). Melanocytes are unicellular secretory glands which elaborate melanosomes; the latter are the end product of an intracellular organization for the biosynthesis of melanin. Seiji and coworkers (1963) studied melanosome development (Fig. 16–7) and observed that the process begins with synthesis of tyrosinase on melanocyte ribosomes, whence it is transferred via the endoplasmic reticulum to the Golgi area;

KERATINOCYTE

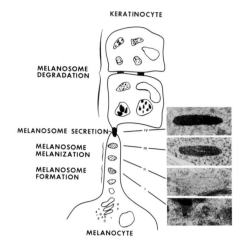

MELANOSOME DEGRADATION

MELANOSOME SECRETION

MELANOSOME MELANIZATION

MELANOSOME FORMATION

MELANOCYTE

Figure 16–7 Development of melanosomes in melanocytes. The melanocyte is a specialized cell whose dendrites serve approximately 36 keratinocytes. Mature melanosomes (Type IV) are transferred from the apex of a dendrite to the keratinocytes. Electron photomicrographs of developing melanosomes are shown. The density of melanin increases as melanosomes mature. The biogenesis of melanosomes and melanin is discussed in the text. (Figure adapted from Seiji et al., 1963; Witkop et al., 1971/72; and Fitzpatrick et al.: *In* Fitzpatrick et al., eds., Dermatology in General Practice. McGraw-Hill, New York, pp. 117–146, 1971.)

assembly into units surrounded by a membrane completes stage I of melanin synthesis. The specialized organelle then develops into a premelanosome (stage II) containing membranous filaments with distinct periodicity (100 Å). Melanin can be synthesized at stage III when tyrosine is brought into contact with tyrosinase and the melanosome. Hydroxylation of tyrosine to form 3,4-dihydroxyphenylalanine (dopa) is followed by oxidation to dopa-quinone (Fig. 16–8). At this point, the internal structure of the melanosome becomes obscured by electron-dense melanin. Stage IV is a more densely packed form of the stage III melanosomes.

Keratinocytes in skin phagocytose melanosomes from neighboring melano-

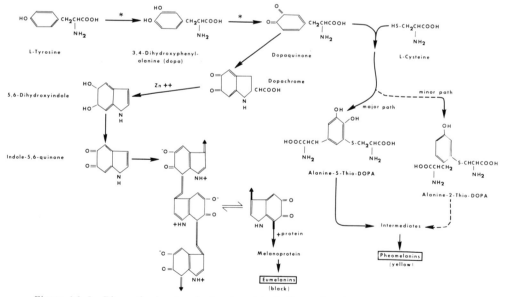

Figure 16–8 Biosynthesis of melanin. Asterisks indicate the place of action of tyrosinase in melanin synthesis. The later steps of biosynthesis probably occur nonenzymatically in the presence of zinc. The synthesis of black eumelanin is the normal major pathway of melanin synthesis. An alternate pathway apparently synthesizes the yellow pheomelanins (Prota, 1968). Pheomelanin synthesis appears to involve two routes as indicated.

cytes which secrete the melanin-containing organelles via their dendrites. About three dozen keratinocytes are supplied by a single melanocyte, and this group of cells composes the epidermal melanin unit.

Melanin is a sunscreen. Its formation in the melanocyte is enhanced upon exposure to ionizing and ultraviolet radiation. Melanin may protect cells from such radiation by its function as a conductor and a repository of electrons produced by photoenergy (Daniels, 1959), and the capture of free radicals may be the focus of melanin's function.

Melanin Biosynthesis in Albinism

In one form of oculocutaneous albinism the melanocyte is present, but melanin synthesis fails to differentiate beyond the premelanosome stage (Seiji et al., 1963). The presence of melanocytes in albinotic tissues is revealed also by the presence of benign melanocytic nevi (Ito et al., 1956) and malignant melanomas (Kennedy and Zelickson, 1963) in the very tissues which exhibit the albino trait.

Melanocyte tyrosinase activity is deficient in one form of oculocutaneous albinism (Witkop, 1971). Tyrosinase catalyzes the first step in the conversion of tyrosine to the melanin polymer (Fig. 16–8). The copper-containing enzyme participates in ortho-hydroxylation of tyrosine to form 3,4-dihydroxyphenylalanine (dopa), which is then oxidized further by the same enzyme to form dopa-quinone (Cromartie and Harley-Mason, 1957). Subsequent oxidation of dopa-quinone and cyclization occurs nonenzymatically in the presence of zinc, which is found in high concentration in melanosomes (Seiji et al., 1963). The monomer is polymerized in the melanosome until a polymer of large molecular weight is formed which is absorbed to the melanosome protein by quinone-amino or quinone-sulfhydryl linkages. The final product is a black pigment (eumelanin).

Some dopa-quinone is diverted from the main polymerization sequence when thioether linkages are formed with free cysteine or protein bound cysteine (Prota, 1969). The resulting pheomelanins are yellow-red (Fig. 16–8).

Tyrosinase can be inhibited in its *soluble* form by certain unidentified biological substances whose molecular weight is below 5000 (Chian and Wilgram, 1967). These substances will not inhibit tyrosinase when it is aggregated with the

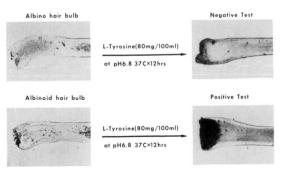

Figure 16–9   The tyrosine incubation hair bulb test has been used to identify two types of albinism. As indicated, upon incubation of hair bulbs, there may be no eumelanin formation. This finding indicates absent, inactive or inaccessible tyrosinase activity. This phenotype is found in classical albinism. On the other hand, after incubation, there may be some enhancement of melanin formation (a positive test). This response indicates that tyrosinase activity is present and accessible in melanosomes; it is the response in "albinoidism" and other mutant forms of albinism. (Figure adapted from Witkop, 1971.)

melanosome, and they are inactivated by ultraviolet light. It is conceivable that a structural gene mutation which altered the site controlling tyrosinase binding to melanosomes could expose the enzyme to inhibitors and that this might produce a form of albinism.

Tyrosinase also initiates the biosynthesis of catecholamines in the adrenal medulla and chromaffin system. However, there is no deficiency of catecholamine formation in the albino because the enzyme in the adrenal medulla and in the chromaffin system is a specific hydroxylase with a function analogous to the hydroxylation of phenylalanine (Nagatsu et al., 1964). The albinism traits reveal that chromaffin tyrosinase is controlled by a gene which is different from that in melanosomes.

Mechanisms of Albinism

Of the many classifications of albinism, those proposed by Fitzpatrick and Quevedo (1972) and by Witkop (1971) and colleagues (1971/72), are most cognizant of the recent advances in melanin biology. The merit of these excellent discussions lies in their attempt to classify hypopigmentation on a biological basis.

There are many levels at which melanin biosynthesis can go wrong (Fitzpatrick and Quevedo, 1972):

(i) Melanocyte deficiency secondary to a failure of melanoblasts to colonize an area of skin.

(ii) Failure of the melanocyte to form melanosomes.

(iii) Failure of melanosomes to form melanin due to tyrosinase deficiency.

(iv) Failure of melanosomes to form melanin due to substrate deficiency.

(v) Failure of melanosomes to store melanin or to transport it to keratinocytes.

(vi) Excessive destruction of functional melanosomes.

The forms of hypopigmentation and albinism tabulated in Table 16–2 have been sufficiently well studied to allow accurate classification of some traits in functional terms.

Two distinct forms of oculocutaneous albinism are now recognized, one of which is "tyrosinase-negative"* and the other, "tyrosinase-positive." Witkop (1971) and colleagues (1970) showed that melanin formation occurs in the hair bulb of some albino subjects after incubation for 10 hours in a concentrated solution of L-tyrosine or L-dopa (Fig. 16–9). Production of melanin under these conditions implies that some tyrosinase activity persists in the melanosomes. Either an impairment of substrate transport is overcome or unfavorable kinetics of tyrosinase activity at the normal concentration of substrate is offset by the higher concentration used in the incubation test. Other interpretations may, of course, be equally relevant and will be discerned in time.

The discovery of tyrosinase-positive and tyrosinase-negative phenotypes introduced the appropriate evidence for genetic heterogeneity in oculocutaneous albinism, and provided an explanation for the birth of normally pigmented children to albino parents, in two famous pedigrees (Trevor-Roper, 1952, 1963; Witkop et al., 1970, 1971/72). In the English family (Trevor-Roper, 1963; Fitzpatrick and Quevedo, 1972), the father was hair-test positive; his hair

---

*The term is less precise than Witkop's own usage. He described the phenotype as "hair-bulb, tyrosine-test positive" or "negative." The more cumbersome term recognized that "negative" tests do not exclude the presence of inaccessible but intact tyrosinase activity in melanosomes.

Table 16–2 Functional Classification of Albinism and Hypomelanoses of Man

Terminology	Inheritance	Features
Albinism		
Tyrosinase-negative*		
Oculocutaneous albinism	AR	Diffuse hypopigmentation of hair, skin and fundus oculi; translucent irides; nystagmus
Albinism-hemorrhagic diathesis (Hermansky-Pudlak syndrome)	AR (probably)	Oculocutaneous hypopigmentation with bleeding tendency and platelet defect
Tyrosinase-positive		
Oculocutaneous albinism	AR	Manifestations of albinism less severe than in tyrosinase-negative type
Tyrosinase negative/positive (variable)		
Yellow-type albino (ym— yellow-mutant)	AR (probably)	Early in life, severe signs of albinism, but improvement with age, when pheomelanin synthesis may occur
Ocular albinism	X-linked	Eye signs similar to oculocutaneous albinism; skin, normal
Hypopigmentation Syndromes		
Piebaldism	AD	Patchy cutaneous depigmentation of limbs and central thorax. White forelock. Eyes normal. Many syndromes, including Waardenburg's. (Melanocyte deficiency?)
Chediak-Higashi Syndrome (tyrosine-positive)	AR	Diffuse hypopigmentation of skin and eyes. Increased susceptibility to infection. Peroxidase-positive leukocytic inclusions—leukomelanopathy. (Melanosome membrane defect?)

*Indicates failure to obtain melanin after incubation of hair bulb for 12 hours at 37°C in L-tyrosine solution (80 mg/100 ml, 0.1M phosphate buffer, pH 6.8). L-dopa can replace L-tyrosine as substrate.

had a yellow tinge when compared with that of his wife, who was hair-test negative. The American family was Negro; the father had a negative hair-bulb test, while his wife, who had "albinoidism" with light golden and red-tinted hair and light pigmentation in nevi and irides, was tyrosinase-positive on the hair bulb test. It is presumed that the two forms of oculocutaneous albinism are nonallelic. The tyrosinase-positive phenotype has been studied further; salivary fluid tyrosine is 3.7 ± 0.3 mg per 100 ml (half normal) in the tyrosinase-positive trait, and serum copper levels are normal in the mutant trait (Witkop et al., 1971/72).

After removal of the outer keratinized layer, tyrosinase-positive albino skin becomes pigmented upon exposure to ultraviolet radiation if a tyrosine-containing solution is applied to the skin. No pigmentation develops in the absence of exogenous tyrosine. Limited pigmentation occurs if the tyrosine solution is used in the absence of UV light. These observations parallel the in vitro incubation studies with hair bulbs, and they suggest that pigmentation of hair, skin and eyes might be achieved in the patient if the tyrosine content of tissue and body fluids were raised sufficiently. A preliminary attempt to induce pigmentation in tyrosinase-positive oculocutaneous albinism by tyrosine supplementation of the diet has not yet been successful (Witkop et al., 1971/72).

Types of Albinism

The clinical manifestations of aberrant tyrosine-dependent pigment metabolism have attracted attention for centuries. Some of the many forms of albinism are classified in Table 16–2 and are discussed in the following sections.

Autosomal Recessive Albinism

OCULOCUTANEOUS ALBINISM.   This is the "classical" disease recognized in men of all races and in many species of animals throughout recorded history. It occurs in two nonallelic forms known as tyrosinase-negative albinism and tyrosinase-positive albinism; the former has the more severe phenotypic manifestations.

In the *tyrosinase-negative type* the fundus oculi is underpigmented, and the irides are transparent gray or gray-blue; the pupil is red only in infancy, and in later life it is black. Photophobia and nystagmus cripple the subject; habitual squinting imprints its effects on the facies. Visual acuity is usually reduced from normal, and central scotomata cause nystagmus. Color vision and night vision are normal.

The skin is underpigmented, milk-white in Caucasians and resembling lightly-tanned "white" skin in the Negro. Erythema, instead of tanning, occurs upon exposure to ultraviolet radiation. The hair is underpigmented, and in Caucasians it tends also to be finer than usual. Albino skin can develop nevi (Ito et al., 1956) and malignant melanomas (Kennedy and Zelickson, 1963); normal freckles (ephelides) occur on exposed skin (Barnicot, 1952).

The evidence for simple autosomal recessive causation of the trait is found in Hogben's analysis (1931) of more than 600 pedigrees. In Northern Ireland, where the frequency of first-cousin matings is 4.49 per cent, the frequency for tyrosinase-negative oculocutaneous albinism is about 1 in 15,000 (Witkop, 1971), and for both types of oculocutaneous albinism in this population the overall frequency is about 1 in 10,000 (Froggatt, 1960). The frequency among Caucasians and Negroes elsewhere in the world for the tyrosinase-negative trait is about 1 in 35,000 persons (Witkop, 1971).

The *tyrosinase-positive type*, or albinoidism, as it has been called, is characterized by light yellow or red-tinged pigmentation of oculocutaneous structures. Albinism is detected at birth, but skin and hair may darken with age.

It has long been suspected that this type of albinism is not allelic with the more severe type (Barnicot, 1957), and the hair bulb, tyrosine-incubation test has borne out this idea. Matings between parents with the two types of albinism produce normally pigmented offspring (Trevor-Roper, 1963; Witkop et al., 1970). Albinoidism behaves as an autosomal recessive trait.

CHEDIAK-HIGASHI SYNDROME.   This is characterized by tyrosinase-positive hypopigmentation of skin, hair and eyes (Stegmaier and Schmender, 1965), photophobia, nystagmus and inclusion bodies in the myeloblasts and promyelocytes of bone marrow. There are also neutropenia and reduced resistance to infection; malignant lymphoma develops with high frequency, and death is common in the first decade of life. The peroxidase-positive leukocytic inclusions are probably large lysosomal bodies, and the hypopigmentation is associated with giant melanosomes in melanocytes (Windhorst et al., 1966). The disease occurs in man, mink and cattle (Leader et al., 1966) and has been termed a "hereditary leukomelanopathy." Its cause is obscure, but the ability to form and deposit melanin, coupled with the morphologic abnormality of the melanosome, and evidence for degeneration in the melanocytes with deficient transfer of pigment to keratinocytes, suggests that there is a membranous defect in the specific intracellular organelle which may be shared with lysosomes in leukocytes.

Hermansky-Pudlak syndrome (albinism with hemorrhagic diathesis). This syndrome, first described by Hermansky and Pudlak (1959) and reviewed by Witkop and colleagues (1971/72) comprises oculocutaneous albinism, bleeding tendency and accumulation of ceroid-like pigment in reticuloendothelial cells. Platelets lack the dense bodies normally visible by electron microscopy and are deficient in serotonin and adenosine diphosphate release (Logan et al., 1971). A deficiency of melanocytes has been postulated but awaits confirmation (Witkop et al., 1971/72). Logan et al. (1971) have proposed two closely linked mutant genes to account for the syndrome.

Yellow mutant albinism. An interesting form of autosomal recessive albinism has been found in several pedigrees, both in genetic isolates and elsewhere (Witkop, 1971/72). The hair bulb test for tyrosine-induced melanin formation is equivocal, being negative in some hair bulbs and positive in others. The clinical phenotype resembles tyrosinase-positive oculocutaneous albinism, but characteristically the findings are more severe at birth and lessen with age. Pigment formation and tanning under UV light are evident. The hair bulb test gives a novel result when cysteine is added to the incubation medium in the presence of L-tyrosine and L-dopa. Under these conditions the formation of *yellow* pigment intensifies, but no black pigment is formed (Witkop, 1971). Stage III premelanosomes and a rare melanized stage IV melanosome are found before incubation; the pattern does not "mature" after incubation as it does in tyrosine-positive albino hair bulbs. These findings suggest a defect in polymerization to form eumelanin and a tendency to form pheomelanin instead (see Figure 16–9); the role of Zn^{++} in this trait has not been examined.

X-linked Albinism: Ocular Albinism

In males with ocular albinism, the fundus is depigmented, choroid vessels are visible, the iris is translucent and nystagmus is present. Females exhibit a mosaic of depigmentation in the fundus, and partial pigmentation occurs in the iris (Falls, 1951). Lyons (1962) used this observation to develop a concept of random inactivation of the X chromosome in the female. There are no cutaneous manifestations in patients of either sex with X-linked albinism.

Apparently, more than one mutant allele can cause ocular albinism. A pedigree living on the Aland islands in the Sea of Bothnia, reported by Fersius and Erikson (1964), contained an X-linked trait in which the females did not have the characteristic patchy depigmentation of the fundus.

Autosomal Dominant Traits

Cutaneous albinism. Albinism can be limited to skin and hair with no effect on the eyes. A piebald effect may be seen, and white forelock is frequent in this form of albinism (Froggatt, 1959). The appearance of partial or complete pigmentation during and after adolescence is not uncommon, but the mechanism for initiation of melanogenic activity is unexplained. Excessive removal of melanin has not been ruled out, and the role of zinc in this disease has not been investigated. Breathnach (1963) proposed that Langerhans cells in the dermal-epidermal junction may differentiate into melanocytes to account for repigmentation. Deficient melanocyte formation and development may be the initial source of piebald albinism (Breathnach et al., 1965).

DiGeorge and coauthors (1960) drew attention to the patchy depigmentation of skin in dominantly inherited Waardenburg's syndrome. The pigmentary disorder is also expressed in the heterochromia of the irides (a common finding in the "piebald" Dalmatian coach hound). Deafness is often part of piebaldism and other forms of albinism (Witkop et al., 1971/72). DiGeorge et al. (1960) have discoursed in an entertaining fashion on deafness in albino animals in general and on the tendency for deaf, white cats with blue eyes to be run over by automobiles.

TYROSINE METABOLISM IN LIVER DISEASE
AND OTHER ILLNESSES

Liver disease impairs the oxidation of tyrosine and of other amino acids (Miller, 1962). Therefore, a distinction may be required between the tyrosyluria of primary liver disease and that which occurs in hereditary tyrosinemia which is associated with liver disease. Frerichs reported in 1854 that tyrosine and leucine crystals were present in the urine of patients with acute yellow atrophy of the liver. Many years later, Dent and Walshe (1954) confirmed the profound disturbance of amino acid metabolism which occurs in this circumstance. Modest hyperaminoacidemia—especially hypertyrosinemia—occurs in adult patients with hepatitis and cirrhosis (Knauff et al., 1964; Levine and Conn, 1967); and the more severe the liver disease, the greater the hypertyrosinemia and hyperaminoacidemia. Tyrosyluria also occurs in acquired liver disease (Robinson, 1962) but not with the intensity found in hereditary and neonatal tyrosinemia; the peak of tyrosinemia in patients with liver disease is greater and more delayed after tyrosine loading than in normal subjects (Levine and Conn, 1967), and the return to preload levels is slower.

Scurvy is associated with an extensive disturbance of amino acid reabsorption by the renal tubule (Jonxis and Huisman, 1954; Huisman, 1954; Huisman and Jonxis, 1957). Tyrosyluria occurs in the human infant with scurvy, but it may not always be observed in older scorbutic patients (Robinson and Warburton, 1966), perhaps because tyrosine intake per kg body weight is less in the adult. Tyrosine clearance from plasma is impaired in scurvy (Rivlin et al., 1965); this, in combination with the other findings, also suggests that scurvy imposes an inhibition on tyrosine oxidation at the p-HPPA oxidase step.

Hyperthyroidism at any age, and in either sex, is accompanied by hypertyrosinemia and impaired tyrosine oxidation; *hypothyroidism* produces the opposite effect (Rivlin et al., 1965). The finding reflects an imbalance between delivery of tyrosine from muscle and catabolism in liver (see p. 86).

Patients with *cystic fibrosis* and other *disorders of intestinal absorption* excrete excessive amounts of p-HPAA and p-hydroxypropionic and p-hydroxyacrylic acids in their urine, whereas p-HPPA and p-HPLA excretion are likely to be normal (Gibbons et al., 1967; Van der Heiden et al., 1971a, 1971b). The plasma tyrosine levels are normal (Zach et al., 1968). The feces contain excessive amounts of the aromatic acids, tyramine and amino acids, including tyrosine. The findings are of interest because they demonstrate in a simple, clear fashion how artifacts can influence the interpretation of disordered amino acid metabolism. In this case, malabsorption of tyrosine is followed by bacterial decarboxylation and conversion to tyramine. p-HPAA and other derivatives are also formed in the gut, whence these compounds are absorbed and excreted in urine. The composition of the tyrosyluria (p-HPAA predominance) gives the clue as to its origin.

The symptoms of *Parkinsonism* can often be alleviated by large doses of the L-isomer of 3,4-dihydroxyphenylalanine (L-dopa). In the untreated patient the amount of dopamine in the brain is decreased. Martin (1971) has suggested that an inherited deficiency of tyrosine hydroxylase in brain would account for many findings in this disease. The hypothesis requires testing.

REFERENCES

Aronsson, S., Engleson, G., Jagenburg, R., and Palmgren, B.: Long term dietary treatment of tyrosinosis. J. Pediat. 72:620–627, 1968.

Avery, M. E., Clow, C. L., Menkes, J. H., Ramos, A., Scriver, C. R., Stern, L., and Wasserman, B. P.:

Transient tyrosinemia of the newborn: Dietary and clinical aspects. Pediatrics *39*:378–384, 1967.

Auerbach, V. H., DiGeorge, A. M., Brigham, M. P., and Dobbs, J. M.: Delayed maturation of tyrosine metabolism in a full-term sibling of a child with phenylketonuria. J. Pediat. *62*:938–940, 1963.

Baber, M. D.: A case of congenital cirrhosis of the liver with renal tubular defects akin to the Fanconi syndrome. Arch. Dis. Child. *31*:335–339, 1956.

Barnicot, N. A.: Albinism in South-Western Nigeria. Ann. Eugen. *17*:38–73, 1952.

Barnicot, N. A.: Human pigmentation. Man *57*:114–120, 1957.

Bloxam, H. R., Day, M. G., Gibbs, N. K., and Woolf, L. I.: An inborn defect in the metabolism of tyrosine in infants on a normal diet. Biochem. J. *77*:320–325, 1960.

Bodegard, G., Gentz, J., Lindblad, B., Lindstedt, S., and Zetterstrom, R.: Hereditary tyrosinemia. III. On the differential diagnosis and the lack of effect of early dietary treatment. Acta Paediat. Scand. *58*:37–48, 1969.

Boedeker, C.: Ueber das Alcapton; ein neuer Beitrag zur Frage: welche Stoffe des Harns konnen Kupferreduction newirken? Ztschr. Rat. Med. 7:130–145, 1859.

Boedeker, C.: Das Alkapton; ein Beitrag zur Frage: welche Stoffe des Harns konnen aus einer alkalischen Kupferoxydlosung Kupferoxydul reduciren? Ann. Chem. Pharm. *117*:98–106, 1861.

Breathnach, A. S.: A new concept of the relation between the Langerhans cell and the melanocyte. J. Invest. Derm. *40*:279–281, 1963.

Breathnach, A. S., Fitzpatrick, T. B., and Wyllie, L. M.: Electron microscopy of melanocytes in human piebaldism. J. Invest. Derm. *45*:28–37, 1965.

Bremer, H. J., Tosberg, P., and Hönscher, U.: Untersuchungen über die Tyrosin-Stoffwechselstörung. Frühgeborenor. Ann. Paediat. (Basel) *206*:12–27, 1966.

Bremer, H. J., Jaenicke, U., and Leupold, D.: Urinary *p*-tyramine excretion in hypertyrosinemia. Clin. Chim. Acta *23*:244–246, 1969.

Campbell, R. A., Buist, N. R. M., Jacinto, E. Y., Koler, R. D., Hecht, F., and Jones, R. T.: Supertyrosinemia (tyrosine transaminase deficiency), congenital anomalies and mental retardation. (Abstract.) Proceedings of the Society for Pediatric Research, 37th Annual Meeting, Atlantic City, N.J., p. 80, 1967.

Canellakis, Z. N., and Cohen, P. P.: Kinetic and substrate specificity study of tyrosine-α-ketoglutaric acid transaminase. J. Biol. Chem. *222*:63–71, 1956.

Chian, L. T. Y., and Wilgram, G. F.: Tyrosinase inhibition: Its role in suntanning and in albinism. Science *155*:198–200, 1967.

Cone, T. E., Jr.: Diagnosis and treatment: Some syndromes, diseases and conditions associated with abnormal coloration of the urine or diaper. Pediatrics *41*:645–658, 1968.

Cone, T. E., Jr.: Diagnosis and treatment: Some diseases, syndromes and conditions associated with an unusual odor. Pediatrics *41*:993–995, 1968.

Crawhall, J. C., Mamer, O., Tjoa, S., and Claveau, J. C.: Urinary phenolic acids in tyrosinemia. Identification and quantitation by gas chromatography-mass spectrometry. Clin. Chim. Acta *34*:47–54, 1971.

Cromartie, R. I. T., and Harley-Mason, J.: Melanin and its precursors. 8. The oxidation of methylated 5:6-dihydroxyindoles. Biochem. J. *66*:713–720, 1957.

Dakin, H. D.: The chemical nature of alkaptonuria. J. Biol. Chem. *9*:151–160, 1911.

Daniels, F., Jr.: Physiological effects of sunlight. J. Invest. Derm. *32*:147–155, 1959.

Dent, C. E., and Walshe, J. M.: Amino-acid metabolism. Brit. Med. Bull. *10*:249–250, 1954.

DiGeorge, A. M., Olmsted, R. W., and Harley, R. D.: Waardenburg's syndrome. A syndrome of heterochromia of the irides, lateral displacement of the medial canthi and lacrimal puncta, congenital deafness and other characteristic associated defects. J. Pediat. *57*:649–669, 1960.

Dubovsky, J., and Dubovska, E.: The excretion of N-acetyl tyrosine in tyrosyluria. Clin. Chim. Acta *12*:118–119, 1965.

Edwards, S. W., and Knox, W. E.: Homogentisate metabolism: The isomerization of maleylacetoacetate by an enzyme which requires glutathione. J. Biol. Chem. *220*:79–91, 1956.

Fairney, A., Francis, D., Ersser, R. S., Seakins, J. W. T., and Cottom, D.: Diagnosis and treatment of tyrosinosis. Arch. Dis. Child. *43*:540–547, 1968.

Falls, H. F.: Sex-linked ocular albinism displaying typical fundus changes in the female heterozygote. Amer. J. Ophthal. *34*:41–50, 1951.

Fellman, J. H., Buist, N. R. M., Kennaway, N. G., and Swanson, R. E.: The source of aromatic ketoacids in tyrosinaemia and phenylketonuria. Clin. Chim. Acta *39*:243–246, 1972.

Fellman, J. H., Vanbellinghen, P. J., Jones, R. T., and Koler, R. D.: Soluble and mitochondrial forms of tyrosine aminotransferase. Relationship to human tyrosinemia. Biochemistry *8*:615–622, 1969.

Fitzpatrick, T. B., Quevedo, W. C., Jr., Szabo, G., and Seiji, M.: The melanocyte system. Biology of the melanin pigmentary system. *In* Fitzpatrick, T. B., Arndt, K. A., Clark, W. H., Eisen, A. Z.,

Van Scott, E. J., and Vaughan, J. H., eds., Dermatology in General Practice. McGraw-Hill, New York, pp. 117–146, 1971.

Fitzpatrick, T. B., and Quevedo, W. C., Jr.: Albinism. *In* Stanbury, J. B., Wyngaarden, J. B., and Fredrickson, D. S., eds., The Metabolic Basis of Inherited Disease, 3rd edition. McGraw-Hill, New York, pp. 326–337, 1972.

Fitzpatrick, T. B., Seiji, M., and McGuigan, A. D.: Melanin pigmentation. New Eng. J. Med. *265*: 328–332, 374–378, 430–434, 1961.

Forsius, H., and Eriksson, A. W.: Ein neues Augensyndrome mit x-chromosomal transmission. Eine Sippe mit Fundusalbinismus. Foveahypoplasia, Nystagmus, Myopie, Astigmatismus und Dyschromatopsie. Klin. Mbl. Augenheilk. *144*:447–457, 1964.

Frerichs, F. T.: Offenes Schreiben und den. Herm. Hofrath Dr. oppolzor in Wien. Wien Med. Wschr. *4*:465–470, 1854.

Fritzell, S., Jagenburg, O. R., and Schnurer, L. B.: Familial cirrhosis of the liver, renal tubular defects with rickets and impaired tyrosine metabolism. Acta Paediat. Scand. *53*:18–32, 1964.

Froggatt, P.: An outline with bibliography of human piebaldism and white forelock. Irish J. Med. Sci. No. 398:86–94, 1959.

Froggatt, P.: Albinism in Northern Ireland. Ann. Hum. Genet. *24*:213–238, 1960.

Garrod, A. E.: About alkaptonuria. Lancet (ii), 1484–1486, 1901.

Garrod, A. E.: The incidence of alkaptonuria. A study in chemical individuality. Lancet (ii), 1616–1620, 1902.

Garrod, A. E.: The Croonian lectures. II. Albinsim. Lancet (ii), 1–7, 1908a.

Garrod, A. E.: The Croonian lectures. III. Alkaptonuria. Lancet (ii), 73–79, 1908b.

Gaull, G. E., Rassin, D. K., Solomon, G. E., Harris, R. C., and Sturman, J. A.: Biochemical observations on so-called hereditary tyrosinemia. Pediat. Res. *4*:337–344, 1970.

Gaull, G. E., Rassin, D. K., and Sturman, J. A.: Significance of hypermethioninemia in acute tyrosinosis. Lancet (i), 1318–1319, 1968.

Gentz, J., Heinrich, J., Lindblad, B., Lindstedt, S., and Zetterstrom, R.: Enzymatic studies in a case of hereditary tyrosinemia with hepatoma. Acta Paediat. Scand. *58*:393–396, 1969a.

Gentz, J., Jagenburg, R., and Zetterstrom, R.: Tyrosinemia, an inborn error of tyrosine metabolism with cirrhosis of the liver and multiple renal tubular defects (deToni-Debré-Fanconi syndrome). J. Pediat. *66*:670–696, 1965.

Gentz, J., Johansson, S., Lindblad, B., Lindstedt, S., and Zetterstrom, R.: Excretion of δ-aminolevulinic acid in hereditary tyrosinemia. Clin. Chim. Acta *23*:257–263, 1969b.

Gentz, J., Lindblad, B., Lindstedt, S., Levy, L., Shasteen, W., and Zetterstrom, R.: Dietary treatment in tyrosinemia. Amer. J. Dis. Child *113*:31–37, 1967.

Gentz, J., Lindblad, B., Lindstedt, S., and Zetterstrom, R.: Studies on the metabolism of the phenolic acids in hereditary tyrosinemia by a gas-liquid chromatographic method. J. Lab. Clin. Med. *74*:185–202, 1969c.

Gibbons, I. S. E., Seakins, J. W. T., and Ersser, R. S.: Tyrosine metabolism and faecal amino acids in cystic fibrosis of the pancreas. Lancet (i), 877–878, 1967.

Gjessing, L. R., ed.: Symposium on Tyrosinosis. (Norwegian Monographs on Medical Science.) Universitetsforlaget, Oslo, 1966.

Gjessing, L. R., and Halvorsen, S.: Hypermethioninemia in acute tyrosinosis. Lancet (ii), 1132, 1965.

Goldblatt, P. J., Witschi, H., Friedman, M. A., Sullivan, R. J., and Schull, K. H.: Some structural and functional consequences of hepatic adenosine triphosphate deficiency induced by intraperitoneal D-fructose administration. Lab. Invest. *23*:378–385, 1970.

Goldsmith, L., Kang, E., Bienfang, D., and Baden, H.: Tyrosinemia with phenolicaciduria in the Richner-Hanhart syndrome. (Abstract.) Amer. J. Hum. Genet. *24*:25a, 1972.

Goswami, M. N. D., and Knox, W. E.: Developmental changes of *p*-hydroxy-phenylpyruvate oxidase activity in mammalian liver. Biochem. Biophys. Acta *50*:35–40, 1961.

Gross, O.: Über den Einfluss des Blutserums des Normalen und des Alkaptonurikers auf Homogentisinsäure. Biochem. Ztschr. *61*:165–170, 1914.

Halvorsen, S., and Gjessing, L. R.: Studies on tyrosinosis. 1. Effect of low-tyrosine and low-phenylalanine diet. Brit. Med. J. *2*:1171–1173, 1964.

Halvorsen, S., Pande, H., Loken, A. C., and Gjessing, L. R.: Tyrosinosis: A study of six cases. Arch. Dis. Child *41*:238–249, 1966.

Hardwick, D. F., Applegarth, D. A., Cockcroft, D. M., Ross, P. M., and Calder, R. J.: Pathogenesis of methionine-induced toxicity. Metabolism *19*:381–391, 1970.

Harper, A. E.: Amino acid toxicities and imbalances. *In* Munro, H. N., and Allison, J. B., eds., Mammalian Protein Metabolism, Vol. II. Academic Press, New York, pp. 87–134, 1964.

Harries, J. T., Seaking, J. W. T., Ersser, R. S., and Lloyd, J. K.: Recovery after dietary treatment of an infant with features of tyrosinosis. Arch. Dis. Child *44*:258–267, 1969.

Hermansky, F., and Pudlak, P.: Albinism associated with hemorrhagic diathesis and unusual pigmented reticular cells in bone marrow. Report of two cases with histochemical studies. Blood *14*:162–170, 1959.

Hill, A., Nordin, P. M., and Zaleski, W. A.: Dietary treatment of tyrosinosis. J. Amer. Diet. Ass. 56:308–312, 1970.

Hogben, L. T.: The genetic analysis of familial traits. J. Genet. 25:97–112, 1931.

Hogben, L. T., Worrall, R. L., and Zieve, I.: The genetic basis of alkaptonuria. Proc. Roy. Soc. Edinburgh 52:264–295, 1932.

Holston, J. L., Levy, H. L., Tomlin, G. A., Atkins, R. J., Patton, T. H., and Hosty, T. S.: Tyrosinosis: A patient without liver or renal disease. Pediatrics 48:393–400, 1971.

Holt, P. G., and Oliver, I. T.: Multiple forms of tyrosine aminotransferase in rat liver and their hormonal induction in the neonate. Federation of European Biochemical Societies Letters 5:89–91, 1969.

Hsia, D. Y. Y., ed.: Symposium on treatment of amino acid disorders. Amer. J. Dis. Child. 113: 1–174, 1967.

Hsia, D. Y. Y., Litwack, M., O'Flynn, M., and Jakovic, S.: Serum phenylalanine and tyrosine levels in the newborn infant. New Eng. J. Med. 267:1067–1070, 1962.

Huisman, T. H. J.: The concentration of different amino acids in the blood plasma in children suffering from rickets and scurvy. Pediatrics 14:245–253, 1954.

Huisman, T. H. J., and Jonxis, J. H. P.: Some investigations on the metabolism of phenylalanine and tyrosine in children with vitamin C deficiency. Arch. Dis. Child. 32:77–81, 1957.

Ito, M., Noguchi, I., and Komatsu, A.: Lentigo achromiant in albinos. Ann. Derm. Syph. (Paris) 83:631–635, 1956.

Jacoby, G. A., and LaDu, B. D.: Studies on the specificity of tyrosine-α-ketoglutarate transaminase. J. Biol. Chem. 239:419–424, 1964.

Jonxis, J. H. P., and Huisman, T. H. J.: Aminoaciduria and ascorbic acid deficiency. Pediatrics 14:238–244, 1954.

Kang, E. S., and Gerald, P. S.: Hereditary tyrosinemia and abnormal pyrrole metabolism. J. Pediat. 77:397–406, 1970.

Kennaway, N. G., and Buist, N. R. M.: Metabolic studies in a patient with hepatic cytosol tyrosine aminotransferase deficiency. Pediat. Res. 5:287–297, 1971.

Kennedy, B. J., and Zelickson, A. S.: Melanoma in an albino. J.A.M.A. 186:839–841, 1963.

Khachadurian, A., and Abu Feisal, K.: Alkaptonuria. Report of a family with seven cases appearing in four successive generations, with metabolic studies in one patient. J. Chronic Dis. 7:455–465, 1958.

Kinsell, L. W., Harper, H. A., Barton, H. C., Hutchin, M. E., and Hess, J. R.: Studies in methionine and sulfur metabolism I. J. Clin. Invest. 27:677, 1948.

Kinsell, L. W., Harper, H. A., Giesse, G. K., Margen, S., McCallie, D. P., and Hess, J. R.: Studies in methionine and sulfur metabolism II. J. Clin. Invest. 28:1439, 1949.

Kinsell, L. W., Margen, S., Tarver, H., Franz, J. McB., Flannagan, E. K., Hutchin, M. E., Michaels, G. D., and McCallie, D. P.: Studies in methionine metabolism III. J. Clin. Invest. 29:238, 1950.

Knauff, H. G., Seybold, D., and Miller, B.: Die freien Plasmaaminosäuren bie Lebercirrhose und Hepatitis. Klin. Wschr. 42:326–332, 1964.

Knox, W. E.: Coenzyme functions of ascorbic acid. Symposium on vitamin metabolism. In Proceeding of the Fourth International Congress of Biochemistry, Vol. XI, Vienna, 1958. Pergamon Press, London, 1958a.

Knox, W. E.: Sir Archibald Garrod's "Inborn errors of metabolism." III. Albinism. Amer. J. Hum. Genet. 10:249–267, 1958b.

Knox, W. E.: Sir Archibald Garrod's "Inborn errors of metabolism." II. Alkaptonuria. Amer. J. Hum. Genet. 10:95–124, 1958c.

Knox, W. E., and Edwards, S. W.: Homogentisate oxidase of liver. J. Biol. Chem. 216:479–487, 1955.

Knox, W. E., Goswami, M. N. D., and Lynch, R. D.: The induction of tyrosyluria in young rats. Ann. N. Y. Acad. Sci. 111:212–219, 1963.

Knox, W. E., Linder, M. C., Lynch, R. D., and Moore, C. L.: The enzymatic basis of tyrosyluria in rats fed tyrosine. J. Biol. Chem. 239:3821–3825, 1964.

Kogut, M. D., Shaw, K. N., and Donnell, G. N.: Tyrosinosis. Amer. J. Dis. Child. 113:47–53, 1967.

Komrower, G. M., and Robins, A. J.: Plasma amino acid disturbance in infancy I. Arch. Dis. Child. 44:418–421, 1969.

Kretchmer, N.: Enzymatic patterns during development. Pediatrics 23:606–617, 1959.

Kretchmer, N., Levine, S. Z., McNamara, H., and Barnett, H. L.: Certain aspects of tyrosine metabolism in the young. I. The development of the tyrosine oxidizing system in human liver. J. Clin. Invest. 35:236–244, 1956a.

Kretchmer, N., and McNamara, H.: Certain aspects of tyrosine metabolism in the young. II. The tyrosine oxidizing system of fetal rat liver. J. Clin. Invest. 35:1089–1093, 1956b.

Laberge, C.: Hereditary tyrosinemia in a French Canadian isolate. Amer. J. Hum. Genet. 21:36–45, 1969.

Laberge, C.: Personal communication, 1972.

Laberge, C., and Dallaire, L.: Genetic aspects of tyrosinemia in the Chicoutimi region. *In* Partington, M., Scriver, C. R., and Sass-Kortsak, A., eds., Conference on Hereditary Tyrosinemia. Canad. Med. Ass. J. *97*:1099–1100, 1967.

LaDu, B. N.: The enzymatic deficiency in tyrosinemia. *In* Hsia, D. Y. Y., ed., Symposium on Treatment of Amino Acid Disorders. Amer. J. Dis. Child. *113*:54–57, 1967.

LaDu, B. N.: Alcaptonuria. *In* Stanbury, J. B., Wyngaarden, J. B., and Fredrickson, D. S., eds., The Metabolic Basis of Inherited Disease, 3rd edition. McGraw-Hill, New York, pp. 308–325, 1972.

LaDu, B. N., and Gjesssing, L. R.: Tyrosinosis and tyrosinemia. *In* Stanbury, J. B., Wyngaarden, J. B., and Fredrickson, D. S., eds., The Metabolic Basis of Inherited Disease, 3rd edition. McGraw-Hill, New York, pp. 296–307, 1972.

LaDu, B. N., Howell, R. R., Michael, P. J., and Sober, E. K.: A quantitative micromethod for the determination of phenylalanine and tyrosine in blood and its application in the diagnosis of phenylketonuria in infants. Pediatrics *31*:39–46, 1963.

LaDu, B. N., and Zannoni, V. G.: The tyrosine oxidation system of liver. II. Oxidation of *p*-hydroxyphenylpyruvic acid to homogentisic acid. J. Biol. Chem. *217*:777–787, 1955.

LaDu, B. N., Zannoni, V. G., Laster, L., and Seegmiller, J. E.: The nature of the defect in tyrosine metabolism in alcaptonuria. J. Biol. Chem. *230*:251–260, 1958.

Larochelle, J., Mortezai, A., Belanger, M., Tremblay, M., Claveau, J. C., and Aubin, G.: Experience with 37 infants with tyrosinemia. *In* Partington, M., Scriver, C. R., and Sass-Kortsak, A., eds., Conference on Hereditary Tyrosinemia. Canad. Med. Ass. J. *97*:1051–1056, 1967.

Leader, R. W., Padgett, G. A., and Gorham, J. R.: Hereditary leukomelanopathy (Chediak-Higashi syndrome of man, mink, and cattle). *In* Gajdusek, D. C., Gibbs, C. J., Jr., and Alpers, M., eds., Slow, Latent and Temperate Virus Infections. pp. 393–399, 1966.

Lelong, M., Alagille, D., Gentil, Cl., Colin, J., LeTan, V., and Gabilar, J.-C.: Cirrhose congénitale et familiale avec diabète phospho-gluco-amine, rachitisme vitamine-résistante et tyrosinurie massive. Etude métabolique et anatomique. Rev. Franc. Etud. Clin. Biol. *8*:37–50, 1963.

Levine, R. J., and Conn, H. O.: Tyrosine metabolism in patients with liver disease. J. Clin. Invest. *46*:2012–2020, 1967.

Levine, S. Z.: Tyrosine and phenylalanine metabolism in infants and the role of vitamin C. Harvey Lect. Series 42:303, 1946–47.

Levine, S. Z., Marples, E., and Gordon, H. H.: Defect in metabolism of aromatic amino acids in premature infants: Role of vitamin C. Science *90*:620–621, 1939.

Levy, H. L., Madigan, P. M., MacCready, R. A., and Crawford, J. D.: Hypermethioninemia and evaluation of other free amino acids in infants on high protein intakes. Proceedings of the American Pediatrics Society, 78th Annual Meeting, Atlantic City, p. 19, 1968.

Levy, H. L., Shih, V. E., Madigan, P. M., and MacCready, R. A.: Transient tyrosinemia in full-term infants. J.A.M.A. *209*:249–250, 1969.

Light, I. J., Berry, H. K., and Sutherland, J. M.: Aminoacidemia of prematurity. Its response to ascorbic acid. Amer. J. Dis. Child. *112*:229–236, 1966.

Lin, E. C. C., and Knox, W. E.: Effect of vitamin B_6 deficiency on the basal and adapted levels of rat liver tyrosine and tryptophan transaminases. J. Biol. Chem. *233*:1183–1185, 1958.

Lindblad, B., Lindstedt, G., and Lindstedt, S.: The mechanism of enzymic formation of homogentisate from *p*-hydroxy-phenylpyruvate. J. Amer. Chem. Soc. *92*:25,7446–7449, 1970.

Lindemann, R., Gjessing, L. R., Morton, B., Loken, A. C., and Halvorsen, S.: Amino acid metabolism in hereditary fructosemia. Acta Paediat. Scand. *59*:141–147, 1970.

Litwak, G., Sears, M. L., and Diamondstone, T. I.: Intracellular distribution of tyrosine-α-ketoglutarate transaminase and 4-C^{14}-hydroxycortisone activities during induction. J. Biol. Chem. *238*:302–305, 1963.

Logan, L. J., Rapaport, S. I., and Maher, T.: Albinism and abnormal platelet function. New Eng. J. Med. *284*:1340–1345, 1971.

Lustberg, T. J., Schulman, J. D., and Seegmiller, J. E.: The preparation and identification of various adducts of oxidized homogentisic acid and the development of a new sensitive colorimetric assay for homogentisic acid. Clin. Chim. Acta *35*:325–333, 1971.

Lyon, M. F.: Sex chromatin and gene action in the mammalian X-chromosome. Amer. J. Hum. Genet. *14*:135–148, 1962.

Maenpaa, P. H., Raivio, K. O., and Kekkomaki, M. P.: Liver adenine nucleotides: Fructose-induced depletion and its effect on protein synthesis. Science *161*:1253–1254, 1968.

Martin, W. E.: Tyrosine hydroxylase deficiency: A unifying concept of Parkinsonism. Lancet (i), 1050–1051, 1971.

Mathews, J., and Partington, M. W.: The plasma tyrosine levels of premature babies. Arch. Dis. Child. *39*:371–378, 1964.

McCarthy, M. A., Orr, M. L., and Watt, B. K.: Phenylalanine and tyrosine in vegetables and fruit. J. Amer. Diet. Ass. *52*:130–134, 1968.

Medes, G.: A new error of tyrosine metabolism: tyrosinosis. The intermediary metabolism of tyrosine and phenylalanine. Biochem. J. 26:917–940, 1932.

Medes, G., Berglund, H., and Lohmann, A.: An unknown reducing urinary substance in myasthenia gravis. Proc. Soc. Exp. Biol. Med. 25:210–211, 1927.

Meister, A.: Intermediary metabolism of amino acids: Phenylalanine and tyrosine. In Biochemistry of the Amino Acids. Academic Press, New York, Chap. VI, pp. 885–928, 1965.

Menkes, J. H., and Avery, M. E.: The metabolism of phenylalanine and tyrosine in the premature infant. Bull. Johns Hopkins Hosp. 113:301–319, 1963.

Menkes, J. H., Chernik, V., and Ringel, B.: Effect of elevated blood tyrosine on subsequent intellectual development of premature infants. J. Pediat. 69:583–588, 1966.

Menkes, J. H., and Jervis, G. A.: Developmental retardation associated with an abnormality in tyrosine metabolism. Pediatrics 28:399–409, 1961.

Menkes, J. H., Welcher, D. W., Levi, H. S., Dallas, J., and Gretsky, N. E.: Relationship of elevated blood tyrosine to the ultimate intellectual performance of premature infants. Pediatrics 49:218–224, 1972.

Milch, R. A.: Studies of alcaptonuria: A genetic study of 58 cases occurring in eight generations of seven interrelated Dominican kindreds. Arthritis Rheum. 4:131–136, 1961.

Miller, J. E., and Litwack, G.: Subcellular distribution of tyrosine aminotransferase in rat brain. Arch. Biochem. Biophys. 134:149–159, 1969.

Miller, L. L.: The role of the liver and the non-hepatic tissues in the regulation of free amino acid levels in the blood. In Holden, J. T., ed., Amino Acid Pools. Elsevier, New York, pp. 708–721, 1962.

Milne, M. D., Crawford, M. A., Girac, C. B., and Loughridge, L.: The excretion of indolylacetic acid and related indolic acids in man and the rat. Clin. Sci. 19:165–179, 1960.

Nagatsu, T., Levitt, M., and Udenfriend, S.: Conversion of L-tyrosine to 3,4-dihydroxyphenylalanine by cell-free preparations of brain and sympathetically innervated tissues. Biochem. Biophys. Res. Commun. 14:543–549, 1964.

Neuberge, A., Rimington, C., and Wilson, J. M. G.: Studies on alcaptonuria. 2. Investigations on a case of human alcaptonuria. Biochem. J. 41:438–449, 1947.

O'Brien, W. M., LaDu, B. N., and Bunim, J. J.: Biochemical, pathologic and clinical aspects of alcaptonuria, ochronosis and ochronotic arthropathy. Amer. J. Med. 34:813–838, 1963.

Olson, R. E.: Biosynthesis of ubiquinones in animals. Vitamins Hormones (N.Y.) 24:551–574, 1966.

Partington, M. W., Campbell, D., Kuyck, J., and Mehlomakulu, M.: Motor activity in early life. III. Premature babies with neonatal tyrosinemia; a pilot study. Biol. Neonat. 18:121–128, 1971.

Partington, M. W., Delahaye, D. J., Masotti, R. E., Read, J. H., and Roberts, B.: Neonatal tyrosinaemia. A follow-up study. Arch. Dis. Child. 43:195–199, 1968.

Partington, M. W., and Mathews, J.: The relation of plasma tyrosine level to weight gain of premature infants. J. Pediat. 68:749–753, 1966.

Partington, M. W., Scriver, C. R., and Sass-Kortsak, A., eds., Conference on Hereditary Tyrosinemia. Canad. Med. Ass. J. 97:1045–1101, 1967.

Perry, T. L., Hansen, S., and MacDougall, L.: Urinary screening tests in the prevention of mental deficiency. Canad. Med. Ass. J. 95:89–95, 1966.

Perry, T. L., Hardwick, D. F., Dixon, G. H., Dolman, C. L., and Hansen, S.: Hypermethioninemia: A new metabolic disease producing cirrhosis, islet cell hyperplasia and renal tubular degeneration. Pediatrics 36:236–250, 1965.

Perry, T. L., Hardwick, D. F., Hansen, S., Pohlmann, L., and Warrington, P. D.: Methionine induction of experimental tyrosinemia. J. Ment. Defic. Res. 4:246–253, 1967.

Prota, G.: Structure and biogenesis of pheomelanin. Corsi Seminars Chem. 11:136–139, 1968.

Rivlin, R. S., Melman, K. L., and Sjoerdsma, A.: An oral tyrosine tolerance test in thyrotoxicosis and myxedema. New Eng. J. Med. 272:1143–1148, 1965.

Rowsell, E. U., Turner, K. V., and Carrie, J. A.: Subcellular distribution of α-ketoglutarate and pyruvate transaminase in rat liver. Biochem. J. 89:65, 1963.

Rizzardini, M., and Abelink, P.: Tyrosinemia and tyrosinuria in low-birth-weight infants. A new criterion to assess maturity at birth. Amer. J. Dis. Child. 121:182–185, 1971.

Robinson, R.: Urinary phenolic acids in infectious hepatitis. Nature (London) 194:879, 1962.

Robinson, R., and Warburton, F. G.: Tyrosine metabolism in human scurvy. Nature (London) 212:1605, 1966.

Sakai, K., and Kitagawa, T.: An atypical case of tyrosinosis (1-para-hydroxyphenyllactic aciduria). I. Clinical and laboratory findings. Jikeikai Med. J. 4:1–10, 1957a.

Sakai, K., and Kitagawa, T.: An atypical case of tyrosinosis (1-para-hydroxyphenyllactic aciduria). II. A research on the metabolic block. Jikeikai Med. J. 4:11–15, 1957b.

Sakai, K., Kitagawa, T., and Yoshioka, K.: An atypical case of tyrosinosis (1-para-hydroxyphenyllactic aciduria). III. The outcome of the patient; pathological and biochemical observation of the organ tissues. Jikeikai Med. J. 6:15–23, 1959.

Sankoff, I., and Sourkes, T. L.: Determination of thin-layer chromatography of urinary homovanillic acid in normal and disease states. Canad. J. Biochem. Physiol. *41*:1381–1388, 1963.

Scriver, C. R.: The phenotypic manifestations of hereditary tyrosinemia and tyrosyluria: A hypothesis. *In* Partington, M., Scriver, C. R., and Sass-Kortsak, A., eds., Conference on Hereditary Tyrosinemia. Canad. Med. Ass. J. *97*:1073–1075, 1967.

Scriver, C. R.: Hypermethioninemia in acute tyrosinosis. Lancet (i), 1319, 1968.

Scriver, C. R., Clow, C., Davies, E., Ramos, A., and Stern, L.: A commentary on multiple screening for aminoacidopathies in the newborn infant. Canad. Med. Ass. J. *92*:1331–1333, 1965.

Scriver, C. R., Clow, C., and Silverberg, M.: Hypermethioninemia in acute tyrosinosis. Lancet (i), 153, 1966.

Scriver, C. R., and Davies, E.: Investigation in vivo of the biochemical defect in hereditary tyrosinemia and tyrosyluria. *In* Partington, M., Scriver, C. R., and Sass-Kortsak, A., eds., Conference on Hereditary Tyrosinemia. Canad. Med. Ass. J. *97*:1076–1078, 1967.

Scriver, C. R., Larochelle, J., and Silverberg, M.: Hereditary tyrosinemia and tyrosyluria in a French Canadian geographic isolate. Amer. J. Dis. Child. *113*:41–46, 1967.

Sealock, R. R., Galdston, M., and Steel, J. M.: Administration of ascorbic acid to an alkaptonuric patient. Proc. Soc. Exp. Biol. Med. *44*:580–583, 1940.

Seegmiller, J. E., Zannoni, V. G., Laster, L., and LaDu, B. N.: An enzymatic spectrophotometric method for the determination of homogentisic acid in plasma and urine. J. Biol. Chem. *236*:774–777, 1961.

Seiji, M., Fitzpatrick, T. B., Simpson, R. T., and Birbeck, M. S. C.: Chemical composition and terminology of specialized organelles (melanosomes and melanin granules) in mammalian melanocytes. Nature (London) *197*:1082–1084, 1963.

Silverberg, M.: *In* Partington, M., Scriver, C. R., and Sass-Kortsak, A., eds., Conference on Hereditary Tyrosinemia. Canad. Med. Ass. J. *97*:1086–1088, 1967.

Stanbury, J. B.: Familial goitre. *In* Stanbury, J. B., Wyngaarden, J. B., and Fredrickson, D. S., eds., The Metabolic Basis of Inherited Disease, 3rd edition. McGraw-Hill, New York, pp. 223–265, 1972.

Stegmaier, O. C., and Schneider, L. A.: Chediak-Higashi syndrome, dermatologic manifestations. Arch. Derm. (Chicago) *91*:1–8, 1965.

Tada, K., Wada, Y., Yazaki, N., Yokayama, Y., Nakagawa, H., Yoshida, T., Sato, T., and Arakawa, T.: Dietary treatment of infantile tyrosinemia. Tohoku J. Exp. Med. *95*:337–344, 1968.

Taniguchi, K. and Armstrong, M. D.: The enzymatic formation of *o*-hydroxyphenylacetic acid. J. Biol. Chem. *238*:4091–4097, 1963.

Taniguchi, K., and Gjessing, L. R.: Studies on tyrosinosis. 2. Activity of transaminase, para-hydroxyphenylpyruvate oxidase and homogentisic acid oxidase. Brit. Med. J. (i), 968–969, 1965.

Taniguchi, K., Kappe, T., and Armstrong, M. D.: Further studies on phenylpyruvate oxidase. Occurrence of side-chain rearrangement and comparison with *p*-hydroxyphenylpyruvate oxidase. J. Biol. Chem. *239*:3389–3394, 1964.

Trevor-Roper, P. D.: Marriage of two complete albinos with normally pigmented offspring. Brit. J. Ophthal. *36*:107–108, 1952.

Trevor-Roper, P. D.: Albinism. Proc. Roy Soc. Med. (Sect. Ophthalm.) *56*:21–24, 1963.

Van der Heiden, C., Wadman, S. K., Ketting, D., and deBree, P. K.: Urinary and faecal excretion of metabolites of tyrosine and phenylalanine in a patient with cystic fibrosis and severely impaired amino acid absorption. Clin. Chim. Acta *31*:133–141, 1971a.

Van der Heiden, C., Wauters, E. A. K., Ketting, D., Dwan, M., and Wadman, S. K.: Gas chromatographic analysis of urinary tyrosine and phenylalanine metabolites in patients with gastrointestinal disorders. Clin. Chim. Acta *34*:289–296, 1971b.

Vink, C. L. J., and Kroes, A. A.: The renal clearance of phenylpyruvate. Clin. Chim. Acta *6*:813–818, 1971.

Wadman, S. K., Van Sprang, F. J., Maas, J. W., and Ketting, D.: An exceptional case of tyrosinosis. J. Ment. Defic. Res. *12*:269–281, 1968.

Wadman, S. K., Van der Heiden, C., Ketting, D., and Van Sprang, F. J.: Abnormal tyrosine and phenylalanine metabolism in patients with tyrosyluria and phenylketonuria; gas-liquid chromatographic analysis of urinary metabolites. Clin. Chim. Acta *34*:277–287, 1971.

Weber, W. W., and Zannoni, V. G.: Reduction of phenylpyruvic acids to phenyllactic acids in mammalian tissues. J. Biol. Chem. *241*:1345–1349, 1966.

Wicks, W. D.: Induction of tyrosine-α-ketoglutarate transaminase in fetal rat liver. J. Biol. Chem. *243*:900–908, 1968.

Windhorst, D. B., Zelickson, A. S., and Good, R. A.: Chediak-Higashi syndrome. Hereditary gigantism of cytoplasmic organelles. Science *151*:81–83, 1966.

Witkop, C. J., Jr.: Albinism. *In* Harris, H., and Hirschhorn, K., eds., Advances in Human Genetics, Vol. 2. Plenum Publishing Co., New York, 1971, pp. 61–142.

Witkop, C. J., Jr., Nance, W., Ravols, R., and White, J.: Autosomal recessive oculocutaneous albinism in man: evidence for genetic heterogeneity. Amer. J. Hum. Genet. *22*:55–74, 1970.

Witkop, C. J., Jr., White, J. G., Nance, W. E., Jackson, C. E., and Desnick, S.: Classification of albinism in man. Birth Defects: Original Article Series VII, No. 8, Part XII, Skin, Hair and Nails, pp. 13–25, 1971/72.

Wolkow, M., and Baumann, E.: Über das Wesen der Alkaptonurie. Ztschr. Physiol. Chem. *15*: 228–285, 1891.

Wong, P. W. K., Lambert, A. M., and Komrower, G. M.: Tyrosinemia and tyrosyluria in infancy. Develop. Med. Child. Neurol. *9*:551–562, 1967.

Woods, H. F., Eggleston, L. U., and Krebs, H. A.: The cause of hepatic accumulation of fructose-1-phosphate on fructose loading. Biochem. J. *119*:501–570, 1970.

Zack, P., Ross, R. T., Applegarth, D. A., and Israels, S.: Tyrosine in fibrocystic disease. J. Pediat. *72*:692–693, 1968.

Zannoni, V. G., and LaDu, B. N.: Tyrosyluria resulting from inhibition of *p*-hydroxyphenylpyruvic acid oxidase in vitamin C-deficient guinea pigs. J. Biol. Chem. *235*:2667–2671, 1960.

Zannoni, V. G., Seegmiller, J. E., and LaDu, B. N.: Nature of the defect in alcaptonuria. Nature (London) *193*:952–953, 1962.

Zannoni, V. G., and Weber, W. W.: Isolation and properties of aromatic α-keto acid reductase. J. Biol. Chem. *241*:1340–1344, 1966.

Chapter Seventeen

HISTIDINE

Histidinemia is an autosomal recessive trait characterized by an increase in the concentration of histidine in blood and urine and by deficient "histidase" (L-histidine ammonia-lyase, E.C. 4.3.1.3) activity in tissues. The formation of urocanic acid is impaired, and this can be detected most easily in sweat. Imidazole pyruvic acid is often, but not always, present in excessive amounts in urine and may be detected by a positive (green) ferric chloride reaction. About two thirds of the histidinemic patients suffer modest mental retardation and disordered speech development. The trait is probably genetically heterogeneous, because although all patients are apparently deficient in liver histidase, some have normal enzyme activity in the stratum corneum. The accumulation of histidine and its derivatives can be stemmed by the use of a low-histidine diet, but the effect of this on the evolution of clinical manifestations has not yet been sufficiently evaluated.

METABOLISM OF HISTIDINE

Nutritional Requirements

Histidine is an essential nutrient for most mammals. Unexpectedly, Rose et al. (1951) observed no obligatory requirement for dietary histidine by the adult human male in short-term studies. On the other hand, Snyderman and colleagues (1963) found a requirement in the growing human infant for dietary L-histidine in amounts of about 16 to 35 mg/kg/day.

In the absence of sufficient dietary histidine, physical growth is retarded, the plasma concentrations of other essential amino acids rise, and a dermatitis akin to infantile eczema may appear (Snyderman et al., 1963). The significance of an obligatory need for dietary histidine during infancy, and yet independence of this requirement in the adult human, is unclear. To explain this finding,

370

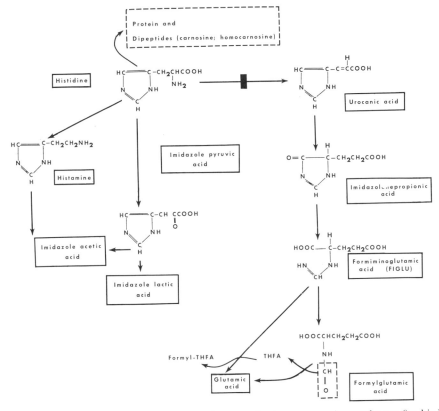

Figure 17-1 The main degradative pathway and minor conversion pathways for histidine. The oxidation pathway yields a formyl group and glutamic acid; the block in histidinemia is in this pathway at the urocanase step.

whether biosynthesis by intestinal microorganisms (as discussed by Meister, 1965) or endogenous biosynthesis of histidine ever occurs in man must still be determined.

Degradative Pathways

Histidine is converted by five different pathways into a number of derivatives (Fig. 17-1):

(i) The major degradative pathway of histidine metabolism yields glutamate and the carbon chain can enter the tricarboxylic acid cycle via α-ketoglutarate. This pathway is initiated by nonoxidative deamination to form urocanic acid,* which is then converted to formiminoglutamic acid (FIGlu). The α-amino group of the side chain and the nitrogen in the third position of the ring are introduced into ammonia metabolism by this pathway; the second carbon atom of the ring is used in one-carbon transfer reactions via FIGlu, which is an important

---

*Urocanic acid was identified in canine urine in 1874 by Jaffe, 22 years before histidine was isolated from a biological source.

donor of formyl groups to tetrahydrofolic acid for purine and pyrimidine biosynthesis.

(ii) Imidazolepyruvic acid (IPA) is formed by transamination or deamination of histidine. This substance reacts with ferric chloride to give a green color in solution. Development of the transaminase may be delayed after birth. For this reason, the ferric chloride reaction should not be relied upon to detect hyperhistidinemic traits in the neonatal period (Levy et al., 1971). IPA can also be metabolized to lactate, acetate and acetate riboside derivatives.

(iii) Decarboxylation of histidine forms histamine, and imidazoleacetic acid, after oxidative deamination.

(iv) Histidine may be incorporated with activated β-alanine to form carnosine in muscle; and with γ-aminobutyric acid to form homocarnosine in brain. Anserine, which is β-alanyl-1-methylhistidine, is not found in human tissues. (See Chapter 18.) There is no convincing evidence that free L-histidine can be converted directly to 1-methylhistidine in man.

(v) Histidine is activated and incorporated into protein.

Distribution

Free histidine is present in extracellular fluids in appreciable amounts. Its endogenous renal clearance rate is normally one of the highest for the plasma amino acids. O'Brien and Butterfield (1963) have questioned whether this phenomenon is a determinant of the nutritional requirement for histidine in infancy.

Several histidine metabolites are present normally in tissues. For example, imidazolepyruvic acid appears in urine, perhaps by tubular excretion, in very small amounts (0 to 11 mg/day) (Auerbach et al., 1962). The compound tends to be unstable unless protected during analysis. Urocanic acid is found in sweat, but it is not excreted as a true constituent of the fluid formed by the sweat glands; it is apparently eluted from stratum corneum across the sweat-epidermis interface (Brusilow and Ikai, 1968). Urocanic acid may have a role in epidermis as a physiological sunscreen (Zenisek et al., 1955; Hais and Zenisek, 1959).

HISTIDINEMIA

Clinical Features of Histidinemia

Ghadimi and Partington (1967), Ghadimi and Zischka (1967), Wadman and associates (1967) and LaDu (1971) all have reviewed the clinical features and various aspects of histidinemia in the numerous patients brought to medical attention since the first recognition of the trait (Ghadimi et al., 1961, 1962). Most patients are Caucasian, but the trait has been identified in the Negro (Kappelman et al., 1971). The predominant clinical features are the following:

(i) Moderate mental retardation occurs in about two thirds of patients. The IQ values which have been reported fall between 47 and the normal range (LaDu, 1971).

(ii) A defect in speech development occurs in about three quarters of the patients; it is probably attributable to a short auditory memory span (Ghadimi et al., 1961; LaDu, 1972). There is no abnormality of hearing. The speech or articulation defect does not necessarily coincide with overt evidence of mental retardation, nor even with the presence of histidinemia, in some sibships (Waisman, 1967). Moreover, many children with speech defects have now been screened without detection of histidinemia.

(iii) There is no history in histidinemic patients of intolerance to ultraviolet light or urticaria.

(iv) As in other aminoacidopathies, it is difficult to know whether the clinical features of this particular trait are closely related to the histidinemia or whether they are coincidental features. At present, it is probably justified to suspect that histidinemia is a condition which, when accompanied by a histidine concentration in plasma exceeding 0.5 mM, may have impaired development of the nervous system. Consequently, careful supervision and prophylactic treatment of the patient is probably justified as early as possible in life.

Biochemical Features of the Trait

Hyperhistidinemia is the hallmark of the condition. The degree of histidinemia is dependent to some extent upon the amount of protein in the diet (Ghadimi and Partington, 1967). The histidine concentration will also be raised in spinal fluid when its concentration in plasma is about 1 mM.

A number of chemical findings are directly related to the histidinemia. When histidine transamination is adequate, excretion of imidazolepyruvic acid in urine is augmented and yields a green ferric chloride reaction (Levy et al., 1971). However, this test will be positive only when the plasma concentration of histidine exceeds about 0.5 mM (Rosenblatt et al., 1970). The excretion of urocanic acid, imidazolepropionic acid and FIGlu is suppressed in histidinemic patients, even after administration of L-histidine in large amounts (Auerbach et al., 1963, 1967; LaDu, 1967; Rosenblatt et al., 1970) and even when the plasma histidine concentration has been raised to very high levels for 24 hours or more. FIGlu is formed by histidinemic patients only when urocanic acid is given (Auerbach et al., 1962; LaDu et al., 1963).

Ghadimi and colleagues (1967) commented on the relative deficiency of glutamic acid and glutamine in the plasma of histidinemic patients, while others have found hyperalaninemia in some patients (Ghadimi and Zischka, 1967; Auerbach et al., 1967; Rosenblatt et al., 1970). The clinical significance of these observations has not been determined.

The concentration of serotonin in blood is reduced in untreated patients (Auerbach et al., 1962; Corner et al., 1968). The serotonin content of blood rises when the plasma histidine concentration is lowered.

Urocanic acid is absent from the sweat and epidermal cells of most histidinemic patients, and this finding has been used by Levy et al. (1969) and Rosenblatt and coworkers (1970) to develop a simple indirect method to detect histidase deficiency in the stratum corneum of patients with the trait. In one sibship reported by Woody et al. (1965), there were three histidinemic probands who had urocanic acid in sweat, and their stratum corneum also contained adequate histidase activity; it is believed that these probands have a different form of histidinemia.

The Enzymatic Defect

LaDu and colleagues (1963) and Zannoni and LaDu (1963) confirmed the proposal of Auerbach et al. (1962) that L-histidine ammonia-lyase (E.C. 4.3.1.3; trivial term, histidase) is deficient in the histidinemic patient. LaDu and his colleagues found evidence for deficiency of this enzyme by examination of the stratum corneum of their patients, and Auerbach (1967) has examined liver activity and found it to be deficient in the enzyme in two probands with the trait. Kihara et al. (1968) have improved the assay of histidase in stratum corneum and shown that there is twofold greater activity in the skin of the hand than of the foot.

Not all histidinemic patients exhibit the "classical" phenotype. In the consanguineous pedigree reported by Woody et al. (1965), there were three affected sibs with modest histidinemia, and yet histidase activity was intact in stratum corneum. This suggests that the human histidinemic trait may comprise more than one mutant genotype.

Diagnosis

The histidinemic trait is recognized by the excessive accumulation of histidine in plasma. Because the simple screening methods, which employ partition chromatography and ninhydrin staining in sequence with a more specific stain for histidine, are not sensitive enough to detect histidine below about 0.5 mM (Scriver et al., 1964), it may not be possible to detect all histidinemic patients by simple plasma screening. Levy et al. (1971) recommend primary staining of the plasma amino acid chromatogram with diazotized sulfanilic acid to improve the screening test.

Histidine is rapidly cleared from plasma into urine; thus, the recognition of abnormal histidinuria, particularly in the postprandial state, is a reliable way to detect the disease in the newborn (Levy et al., 1971a). The histidinuria can be identified by chromatographic methods or by a color test (Gerber and Gerber, 1969).

A positive (green) ferric chloride reaction for imidazolepyruvicaciduria may identify the trait. However, this test is unreliable in the neonatal period (Levy et al., 1971a). Furthermore, a positive ferric chloride test must be confirmed by other procedures, since it may also indicate the excretion of phenylketones and other substances. In fact, patients with histidinemia have actually been misdiagnosed as having phenylketonuria on the basis of this test (Wadman et al., 1967). Green ferric chloride reactions are also found in association with 1-methylhistidinuria. The various histidine metabolites in urine can be analyzed by column chromatographic methods for purposes of confirmatory study of patients (Wadman et al., 1971).

Hyperhistidinuria by itself cannot be taken as an indication of histidinemia, particularly in adult female patients, since the renal clearance of histidine may be altered by the menstrual cycle and by pregnancy (Armstrong and Yates, 1964). Histidine, in free and peptide forms, is also excreted in excess under certain dietary conditions (see Chapter 18), as well as in conditions which do not involve hyperhistidinemia.

A secure diagnosis of histidinemia requires direct or indirect evidence of impaired histidase activity. However, normal activity in stratum corneum does *not* rule out the diagnosis of histidinemia because of genetic heterogeneity in the trait.

Genetics

The trait (of any genotype) appears at birth with a frequency of about six cases per 100,000 births (Levy, 1971b); this figure is derived from mass screening surveys of the newborn. Most cases exhibit an autosomal recessive inheritance pattern, and these are of at least two phenotypes (with or without normal histidase activity in stratum corneum). A third type of histidinemia, with apparent dominant inheritance, has been observed in a pedigree with consanguinity (Bruckman et al., 1970). These patients had little or no histidase activity in skin, but they formed small amounts of FIGlu in contrast to the patients with the autosomal recessive trait.

Segregation of heterozygotes for the trait cannot be performed reliably by the fasting histidine concentration of plasma or by simple histidine loading and a measure of the plasma histidine response. Even skin histidase activity does not discriminate heterozygotes efficiently (Bruckman et al., 1970), probably because this parameter does not necessarily reflect hepatic histidase activity. At present, the most useful test to identify the heterozygote in the autosomal recessive form of the disease has been to measure urine FIGlu during the first four hours after an L-histidine load; heterozygotes show deficient FIGlu excretion (LaDu et al., 1963; Rosenblatt et al., 1970). Simultaneous comparison of the plasma histidine response and FIGlu excretion after L-histidine loading can improve classification of heterozygotes.

Treatment

There has been only limited experience with the treatment of histidinemia. Some authors have noted a reverse correlation between the degree of histidinemia and the degree of mental retardation (Ghadimi and Partington, 1967; Ghadimi and Zischka, 1967). It is not yet known whether the mental retardation has anything to do with blood serotonin depletion in the trait. If this is the case, then prevention of hyperhistidinemia may be warranted. A few investigators have attempted dietary restriction of histidine intake. LaDu and colleagues (1963) were unable to reduce the plasma histidine concentration of their two older patients, an experience also reported by Cain and Holton (1968) for their patient. Treatment of older patients may fail because of insufficient selective reduction of histidine intake, or over-restriction of protein intake, which causes catabolism of tissue protein and release of incorporated histidine; the inessential nature of histidine beyond infancy may also compromise the effect of histidine restriction. However, it does seem possible that careful, selective histidine restriction, even in the older patient, can reduce histidine levels in plasma (Gatfield et al., 1969).

There have been reports of successful biochemical control by selective restriction of histidine intake in young patients. A low-histidine diet (25 mg/kg/day), beginning at 7 months (Van Sprang and Wadman, 1967) or 12 months (Croner et al., 1968) maintained biochemical control in two infants for more than a year and supported adequate physical growth. Auerbach and colleagues (1967) temporarily exposed one of their patients to a complete absence of dietary histidine for one month; serine intake was also restricted to determine whether the patient would develop megaloblastic anemia. On this regime, the biochemical signs of histidinemia were ablated, hyperalaninemia was suppressed and megaloblastosis of bone marrow failed to appear, even though the average percentage of five-lobed polymorphic leukocytes increased temporarily. On the other hand, there is a danger that somatic growth can be impaired if patients maintain a histidine-restricted diet for several months (Corner et al., 1968; Van Spring and Wadman, 1967). Whether this is a function of the histidine restriction or of the general nature of artificial diets is not clear. None of the treated patients have developed the dermatitis of histidine deficiency as described by Snyderman et al. (1963).

No claims can be made yet for clinical improvement of histidinemic patients treated by diet alone. The use of serotonin congeners has not been investigated. If clinical well-being can ever be achieved, it is likely that a therapeutic diet should be started as soon after birth as possible. Only by early detection and investigation can the natural history of this aminoacidopathy be properly evaluated and the true relation between apparent clinical and biochemical features established.

MATERNAL HISTIDINEMIA

It is not known yet whether maternal histidinemia requires treatment. One woman with modest histidinemia (0.5 to 0.75 mM plasma histidine) is known to have given birth to a child who at 4½ years of age is healthy and not retarded (Neville et al., 1971). Since the fetal:maternal gradient for histidine is about 2.3 (Butterfield and O'Brien, 1963), it is possible for the fetus to be exposed to considerable intrauterine hyperhistidinemia. This fact should be kept in mind when counseling female patients with histidinemia.

REFERENCES

Armstrong, M. D., and Yates, K. N.: Amino acid excretion during pregnancy. Amer. J. Obstet. Gynec. 88:381–390, 1964.

Auerbach, V. H., DiGeorge, A. M., Baldridge, R. C., Tourtelotte, C. D., and Brigham, M. P.: Histidinemia: A deficiency in histidase resulting in the urinary excretion of histidine and of imidazolepyruvic acid. J. Pediat. 60:487–497, 1962.

Auerbach, V. H., DiGeorge, A. M., and Carpenter, G. G. (with technical assistance of Black, M., and Rensch, D.): Histidinemia. In Nyhan, W. L., ed., Amino Acid Metabolism and Genetic Variation. McGraw-Hill, New York, pp. 145–160, 1967.

Bruckman, C., Berry, H. K., and Dasenbrock, R. J.: Histidinemia in two successive generations. Amer. J. Dis. Child. 119:221–227, 1970.

Brusilow, S. W., and Ikai, K.: Urocanic acid in sweat, an artifact of elution from epidermis. Science 160:1257–1258, 1968.

Butterfield, L. J., and O'Brien, D.: The effect of maternal toxaemia and diabetes on transplacental gradients of free amino acids. Arch. Dis. Child. 38:326–327, 1963.

Cain, A. R. R., and Holton, J. B.: Histidinaemia: A child and his family. Arch. Dis. Child. 43:62–68, 1968.

Corner, B. D., Holton, J. B., Norman, R. M., and Williams, P. M.: A case of histidinemia controlled with a low histidine diet. Pediatrics 41:1074–1081, 1968.

Gatfield, P. D., Knights, R. M., Devereux, M., and Pozsonyi, J. P.: Histidinemia: Report of four new cases in one family and the effect of low-histidine diets. Canad. Med. Ass. J. 101:465–469, 1969.

Gerber, M. G., and Gerber, D. A.: A simple screening test for histidinuria. Pediatrics 43:40–43, 1969.

Ghadimi, H., and Partington, M. W.: Salient features of histidinemia. In Hsia, D. Y. Y., ed., Symposium on Treatment of Amino Acid Disorders. Amer. J. Dis. Child. 113:83–87, 1967.

Ghadimi, H., Partington, M. W., and Hunter, A.: Inborn error of histidine metabolism. Pediatrics 29:714–728, 1962.

Ghadimi, H., Partington, M. W., and Hunter, A.: A familial disturbance of histidine metabolism. New Eng. J. Med. 265:221–224, 1961.

Ghadimi, H., and Zischka, R.: Histidinemia. In Nyhan, W. L., ed., Amino Acid Metabolism and Genetic Variation. McGraw-Hill, New York, pp. 133–143, 1967.

Hais, I. H., and Zenisek, A.: Urocanic acid: A physiological sunscreen. Amer. Perfumer Aromatics 73:26–28, 1959.

Jaffe, M.: Ueber einen neuen Bestandtheil des Hundeharns. Dtsch. Chem. Ges. Berlin, 7:1669–1673, 1874.

Kappelman, M., Thomas, G. H., and Howell, R. R.: Histidinemia in a Negro child. Amer. J. Dis. Child. 122:212–214, 1971.

Kihara, H., Boggs, D. E., Lassila, E. L., and Wright, S. W.: Histidinemia: Studies on histidase activity in stratum corneum. Biochem. Med. 2:243–250, 1968.

LaDu, B. N.: Histidinemia. In Hsia, D. Y. Y., ed., Symposium on Treatment of Amino Acid Disorders. Amer. J. Dis. Child. 113:88–92, 1967.

LaDu, B. N.: Histidinemia. In Stanbury, J. B., Wyngaarden, J. B., and Fredrickson, D. S., eds., The Metabolic Basis of Inherited Disease, 3rd edition. McGraw-Hill, New York, pp. 338–350, 1972.

LaDu, B. N., Howell, R. R., Jacoby, G. A., Seegmiller, J. E., Sober, E. K., Zannoni, V. G., Canby, J. P., and Ziegler, L. K.: Clinical and biochemical studies on two cases of histidinemia. Pediatrics 32:216–227, 1963.

Levy, H. L., Baden, H. P., and Shih, V. E.: A simple indirect method of detecting the enzyme defect in histidinemia. J. Pediat. 75:1056–1058, 1969.

Levy, H. L., Madigan, P. M., and Peneva, P.: Evidence for delayed histidine transamination in neonates with histidinemia. Pediatrics 47:128–132, 1971.

Levy, H. L., Shih, V. E., and MacCready, R. A.: Inborn errors of metabolism and transport: Prenatal and neonatal diagnosis. Proceedings of the Eighth International Congress on Pediatrics V-1:1–16, 1971.

Meister, A.: Histidine. In Meister, A., ed., Biochemistry of the Amino Acids, 2nd edition. Academic Press, New York, pp. 818–841, 1965.

Neville, B. G. R., Harris, R. F., Stern, D. J., and Stern, J.: Maternal histidinaemia. Arch. Dis. Child. 46:119–121, 1971.

O'Brien, D., and Butterfield, L. J.: Further studies on renal tubular conservation of free amino acids in early infancy. Arch. Dis. Child. 38:437–442, 1963.

Rose, W. C., Haines, W. J., Warner, D. T., and Johnson, J. E.: The amino acid requirements of man. II. The role of threonine and histidine. J. Biol. Chem. 188:49–58, 1951.

Rosenblatt, D., Mohyuddin, F., and Scriver, C. R.: Histidinemia discovered by urine screening after renal transplantation. Pediatrics 46:47–53, 1970.

Snyderman, S. E., Boyer, A., Roitman, E., Holt, L. E., Jr., and Prose, P. H.: The histidine requirement of the infant. Pediatrics 31:786–801, 1963.

Van Sprang, F. J., and Wadman, S. K.: Treatment of a patient with histidinemia. Acta Paediat. Scand. 56:493–497, 1967.

Wadman, S. K., De Bree, P. K., Van Der Heiden, C., and Van Sprang, F. J.: Automatic column chromatographic analysis of urinary and serum imidazoles in patients with histidinaemia and normals. Clin. Chim. Acta 31:215–224, 1971.

Wadman, S. K., Van Sprang, F. J., Van Skelenburg, G. J., and DeBree, P. K.: Three new cases of histidinemia. Acta Paediat. Scand. 56:485–492, 1967.

Waisman, H. A.: Variations in clinical and laboratory findings in histidinemia. In Hsia, D. Y. Y., ed., Symposium on Treatment of Amino Acid Disorders. Amer. J. Dis. Child. 113:93–94, 1967.

Woody, N. C., Snyder, C. H., and Harris, J. A.: Histidinemia. Amer. J. Dis. Child. 110:606–613, 1965.

Zannoni, V. G., and LaDu, B. N.: Determination of histidine α-deaminase in human stratum corneum and its absence in histidinaemia. Biochem. J. 88:160–162, 1963.

Zenisek, A., Ural, J. A., and Hais, I. M.: Sunscreening effect of urocanic acid. Biochim. Biophys. Acta 18:589–591, 1955.

Chapter Eighteen

FREE AND PEPTIDE-BOUND BETA-AMINO ACIDS

HYPER-β-ALANINEMIA

Hyper-β-alaninemia has been described in one male infant (Scriver et al., 1966). Associated clinical symptoms include somnolence and seizures not controlled by anticonvulsant medication. Large amounts of β-aminoisobutyric acid and taurine, in addition to β-alanine, are excreted in the urine in direct proportion to the degree of hyper-β-alaninemia. Gamma-aminobutyric acid (GABA), a compound that is synthesized in brain and kidney but not normally excreted in human urine, was excreted in large amounts by the patient without relation to the degree of β-alaninuria. The brain and other tissues of the hyper-β-alaninemic patient contain excessive amounts of free β-alanine and carnosine (β-alanyl-histidine).

The relative importance of this extremely rare condition is related to the new information about a tubular transport system with preference for β-alanine compounds; with a sizeable metabolic pool of free β-alanine in man; the dependence of the peptide-bound β-alanine pool on the availability of free β-alanine; and the likelihood that carnosine and β-alanine in excess impair brain function. This information was derived from observation of the single patient.

β-Alanine Metabolism

Free β-alanine (H_2N—CH_2—CH_2—$COOH$) accounts for an insignificant fraction of the free amino acids in extracellular fluids. Liver and kidney contain small amounts of free β-alanine (Scriver et al., 1966; Roberts and Simonsen, 1962). Because the substance has no asymmetric carbon and, moreover, has its amino group in the beta position, this amino acid is poorly transported across plasma membranes (Christensen, 1960) and is therefore rapidly cleared by kidney.

Synthesis

The principal endogenous source of free β-alanine in mammalian tissues is the degradation of uracil and β-alanine-containing dipeptides (Fig. 18–1). Microorganisms form β-alanine by α-decarboxylation of aspartic acid. This reaction does not occur in mammalian tissues (Meister, 1965), although the large bowel contents of man can serve as an exogenous source of β-alanine derived from bacterial metabolism.

Catabolism

Free β-alanine can be removed by two reactions in mammalian tissues. It may be degraded first to malonic semialdehyde by the action of β-alanine: α-ketoglutarate aminotransferase (E.C. 2.6.1.18), an enzyme which has been well characterized in *Pseudomonas* (Hayaishi et al., 1961); impairment of this enzyme, by mutation, completely blocks oxidative catabolism of β-alanine in *Pseudomonas* (Hechtman and Scriver, 1970). Much less is known about the characteristics of this initial step of β-alanine oxidation in human or other mammalian tissues, but it is believed to be analogous to the situation in bacteria. It has been suggested by Roberts and Bregoff (1953) that β-alanine, GABA and β-aminoisobutyric acid (βAIB) utilize the same aminotransferase. Malonic semialdehyde is presumably decarboxylated to form acetate in human tissues, as it does in microorganisms (Hayaishi et al., 1961) but the reaction has not been well characterized in man.

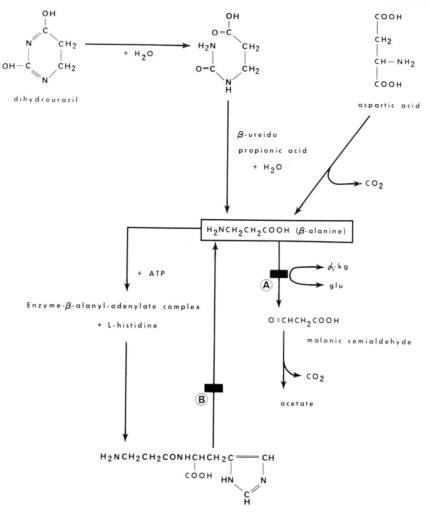

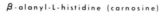

Figure 18–1   Metabolic relationships of β-alanine in free and peptide-linked forms. Ⓐ is proposed block in hyper-β-alaninemia; Ⓑ is site of block in carnosinemia.

Incorporation

The majority of β-alanine in the human body is found in the dipeptide carnosine (Fig. 18–2). In skeletal muscle, the concentration of this bound form may be 500 times greater than that of free β-alanine. Incorporation of β-alanine into carnosine (Fig. 18–1) is an important reaction which has been studied intensively in the skeletal muscles of mammals and birds (Crush, 1970). Carnosine is not present in cardiac muscle (Schmidt and Cubiles, 1955; Reddy and Hegstedt, 1962). It is synthesized by carnosine synthetase, an enzyme which requires ATP during the formation of an enzyme–β-alanyl-adenylate complex (Kalyankar and Meister, 1959; Stenesh and Winnick, 1960; McManus and Benson, 1967); L-histidine is united with the β-alanine complex, and the dipeptide β-alanyl-L-histidine is then released from the enzyme.

Skeletal muscle of birds and certain species of mammals, notably the rabbit, rat and whale (DuVigneaud and Behrens, 1939; Davey, 1960), can also form anserine (β-alanyl-1-methyl-L-histidine) (Fig. 18–2). Human skeletal muscle is characterized by the absence of anserine (Perry et al., 1967; Davies and Scriver, 1967). The methyl group of anserine is donated to the peptide after formation of carnosine; the enzyme S-adenosylmethionine:carnosine N-methyl transferase is required for this reaction (McManus and Benson, 1967; McManus, 1962). Vitamin E deficiency causes impaired synthesis of anserine (McManus, 1960) and a concomitant loss of dipeptides from muscle.

The physiological function of β-alanyl-imidazole dipeptides in tissues is not yet completely understood. Davey (1960) has suggested that they may serve as buffers in stabilizing the pH of anaerobically contracting muscle. Avena and Bowen (1969) have shown that carnosine and anserine, in concentrations comparable to those found in skeletal muscle, serve as potent in vitro activators of myosin ATPase. It is noteworthy that anserine is most prominent in muscles and species where rapid contractile activity is a function of successful adaptation and survival (e.g., limb muscle of rabbit and pectoral muscle of bird) (Fig. 18–3). Apparently anserine has some particular function, apart from that of carnosine, which is worth the additional genetic and enzymatic apparatus required for its synthesis.

β-Alanine is a constituent of the pantothenate moiety of coenzyme-A (Fig. 18–2). Incorporation into pantothenic acid does not occur in mammalian tissues; pantothenate is thus an essential nutrient in human nutrition.

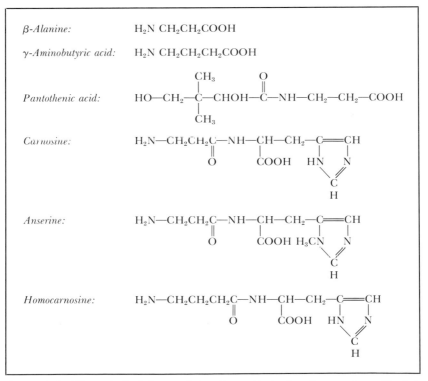

Figure 18–2 The principal forms of β-amino acids in free form and peptide linkage encountered in human metabolism. Carnosine is β-alanyl-histidine; anserine is β-alanyl-1-methyl-histidine; homocarnosine is γ-aminobutyryl-histidine. Carnosine (and homocarnosine) occur in human tissues, but anserine does not; the latter can appear in urine after dietary intake.

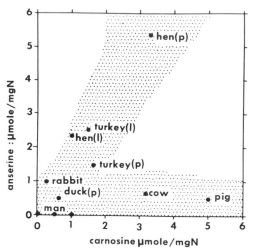

Figure 18–3 Carnosine and anserine content of muscle in various species. In all cases, skeletal muscle was analyzed. *P* = pectoral muscle; *l* = leg muscle; limb muscles examined where not specified. (By permission, from Scriver and Perry: *In* Stanbury, J. B., Wyngaarden, J. B., and Fredrickson, D. S., eds., The Metabolic Basis of Inherited Disease, 3rd edition. McGraw-Hill, New York, 1972.)

Biochemical Abnormalities in Hyper-β-Alaninemia

The important features of the disorder are persistent hyper-β-alaninemia (20 to 50 μM; normal <14 μM), and elevated β-alanine concentration in CSF; elevated renal clearance and urinary excretion of β-alanine, β-amino-isobutyric acid (βAIB) and taurine; normal plasma concentrations of βAIB and taurine; excretion of γ-aminobutyric acid (GABA) in urine, and detectable amounts in CSF and plasma; and excessive accumulation of GABA in brain, and of β-alanine and carnosine in brain and muscle.

These findings indicate a defect in the catabolism of β-alanine. An absence of malonic semialdehyde in the urine of the patient suggests that the amino-transferase is the site of the block in catabolism of β-alanine. This enzyme requires pyridoxal phosphate as a coenzyme, and it is of interest that a transient biochemical improvement was recorded when a pyridoxine was given to the patient. This suggests that the enzyme defect was partial and that activity could be enhanced in the presence of excess coenzyme.

Expansion of the tissue carnosine pool was thought to reflect a diversion of free β-alanine into its bound form, since free and bound concentrations in muscle were each about sevenfold greater than normal.

Accumulation of free GABA in brain and extracellular fluids, including urine, is an exceptional finding. Impaired catabolism of GABA and displacement from binding sites by the excess of β-alanine may occur in the hyper-β-alaninemic patient, particularly if β-alanine and GABA use a common amino-transferase (Roberts and Bregoff, 1953; Baxter and Roberts, 1961).

β-Aminoaciduria in hyper-β-alaninemia is directly proportional to the concentration of β-alanine in plasma. A prerenal or saturation mechanism accounts for the β-alaninuria (Scriver et al., 1966) while the excretion of βAIB and taurine reflects inhibition of their tubular reabsorption in the presence of β-alanine. These observations imply that a membrane system shared by β-amino acids is present in mammalian kidney. The impression is supported by more extensive investigation of tubular reabsorption of β-amino acids in vivo in mouse (Gilbert et al., 1960) and rat (Goldman and Scriver, 1967).

Genetics

Hyper-β-alaninemia has been identified only once in those large surveys where partition chromatography and other methods were used which could easily identify β-alaninuria. Therefore, the trait is probably very rare, and if inherited, it is probably autosomal recessive.

The parents of the original proband are not related. There is one living healthy sib, but another sib died at birth with "breathing difficulties" and there was also one stillbirth at term and one miscarriage in the first trimester. A previous marriage of the mother produced two healthy half-sibs.

Clinical Findings

The white male patient was two months old when admitted to hospital because of somnolence and lethargy since birth. In retrospect, fetal movement was thought to be diminished. Grand mal seizures appeared at six weeks and continued until death at 22 weeks of age. The striking lethargy interfered with feeding, and somatic growth was slow. The important clinical features were limited to the nervous system. They included poor Moro and suck reflexes, active deep tendon reflexes, hypotonia between the recurrent and frequent grand mal seizures and very sluggish response to pain and other stimuli. Many observers commented on the peaceful, sleepy appearance of the infant between convulsions. A variety of anticonvulsant medications were unsuccessful in controlling the seizures, but pyridoxine (10 mg/day) did ameliorate the biochemical features of the disease. The clinical symptoms presumably reflected the effect of β-alanine and related compounds on nervous tissue (Krnjević, 1965).

Treatment

If there is deficient β-alanine transaminase activity in this disease, subsequent patients should be given large doses of vitamin B_6. It is possible that the correlation between biochemical improvement and pyridoxine therapy in the original patient (Scriver et al., 1966) was an important clue to the nature of this disease. The absence of clinical improvement during the biochemical amelioration probably indicates that brain damage was irreparable in the patient. However, the possibility that hyper-β-alaninemia belongs in a group of diseases classified as "vitamin-responsive inborn errors of metabolism" should be considered, since it may lead to an important therapeutic option for future patients.

ACQUIRED ABNORMALITIES OF β-ALANINE METABOLISM

β-alanine excretion in urine is increased under some acquired circumstances. For example, Gras and colleagues (1968) reported β-alaninuria following transplantation of the kidney in man; the finding was most prominent during rejection crises. Plasma β-alanine was apparently not increased, and the authors suspected that the urinary β-alanine originated in the renal parenchyma from uracil turnover. Since β-alaninuria is not a feature of renal disease in our own experience, the finding may reflect some feature of the immunological reaction to transplantation. The study reported by Gras et al. did not describe plasma levels, nor did it indicate whether the clearance of β-alanine exceeded its rate of filtration at the glomerulus, as one would expect if the amino acid were being added to the urine directly from the kidney. To our knowledge no studies of the β-alanine content in human kidney after transplantation have been reported.

Takao et al. (1968) reported β-alaninuria in patients with tuberculosis of various organs. Plasma β-alanine was clearly increased in these patients, and the authors concluded that endogenous β-alanine catabolism was impaired, since the content of β-alanine in the tuberculous tissue was not elevated. The authors also excluded the possibility that isoniazid (an inhibitor of β-alanine transaminase and a commonly used antitubercle drug) caused the defect in β-alanine metabolism. The significance of the finding awaits interpretation.

β-AMINOISOBUTYRICACIDURIA

Excessive urinary excretion of β-aminoisobutyric acid (βAIB) in man is most often a benign polymorphism. It also occurs in a transient, acquired form during tissue catabolism.

Metabolism of β-Aminoisobutyric Acid

The stepwise degradation of thymine (Fig. 18–4) leads to the formation of βAIB (Meister, 1965), this pathway being analogous to the degradation of uracil to form β-alanine (Fig. 18–1). The pyrimidine pathway is apparently the most important endogenous source of βAIB (Fink et al., 1951, 1952). An alternate source of βAIB, found in valine metabolism through transamination of methylmalonate semialdehyde (Fink et al., 1952; Kupiecki and Coon, 1957), is not quantitatively important in man. A single aminotransferase is believed to serve the transamination of βAIB and β-alanine (Kupiecki and Coon, 1957); however, the activity of βAIB-α-ketoglutarate transaminase toward the natural D-(−)-βAIB isomer is negligible in human tissues, suggesting that this enzyme does not catabolize βAIB conversion (Kakimoto et al., 1968).

Distribution

βAIB was identified first in human urine (Fink et al., 1951; Crumpler et al., 1951). Although this amino acid is present in tissues in small amounts, its concentration in normal plasma is scarcely measurable by the usual chromatographic methods.

The capacity to metabolize βAIB is apparently limited in man (Armstrong et al., 1963); this finding has been confirmed by Kakimoto et al. (1968). The form derived from thymine is the natural D-(−) isomer, which is excreted very rapidly through the kidney by a mechanism which probably involves glomerular filtration and net tubular "secretion." Its very high endogenous clearance rate caused Dent (1957) to identify βAIB as a "no-threshold" substance in his discussion of the mechanisms of aminoaciduria. The unnatural isomer L-(+)-βAIB is metabolized more rapidly by other, as yet unidentified, enzymes; it passes through the kidney by glomerular filtration and net reabsorption (Armstrong et al., 1963).

Clinical Abnormalities of βAIB Excretion

Hereditary Variation

The "high-excretor" state (Sutton, 1960)* constitutes one of the more common forms of hereditary variation in amino acid metabolism in the human

---

*A precise quantitative definition of the high-excretor trait is not readily available, but Harris (1953) suggests that a βAIB spot on a partition chromatogram of greater intensity than α-alanine is a suitable index. Others use an excretion rate in excess of about 25 mg (0.25 millimole)/g creatinine as a criterion for abnormal βAIB excretion.

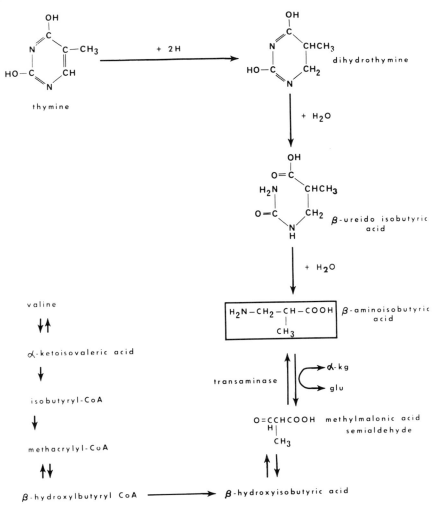

Figure 18–4   Metabolic relationships of β-aminoisobutyric acid.

species. Although only about 5 to 10 per cent of Caucasians are high βAIB excretors (Crumpler et al., 1951; Harris, 1953), high excretors occur in frequencies up to 95 per cent among the Mongoloid race in Southeast Asia (McEvoy-Bowe and Lugg, 1961).

The basis for the high excretion phenotype was thought to be a disturbance in the enzymatic conversion of βAIB derived from thymine. Armstrong and colleagues (1963) showed that high excretors are unable to metabolize D-(–)-βAIB as efficiently as control subjects. They also found that valine does not contribute to the formation of βAIB in high excretors or in normal subjects. Although it seemed likely that a deficiency of βAIB transaminase would explain the high-excretor state, Kakimoto and colleagues (1968) disposed of this popular interpretation by demonstrating normal βAIB transaminase activity in the tissues of high excretors. The basis for the trait remains unknown at the present time.

The inheritance pattern of the βAIB excretor phenotype is also somewhat obscure, and it is not known whether the same mutant allele accounts for the trait in all species or in all individuals in a given race. A pattern of "incomplete" autosomal recessive inheritance (with partial expression of the trait in carriers) is apparent in some Caucasian pedigrees (Fig. 18–5), but there are other situations where this simple interpretation is not appropriate. However, in populations with a high frequency of excretors, it is believed that simple autosomal recessive inheritance with expression of the trait in heterozygotes can be demonstrated with confidence (Gartler et al., 1957). The genetic advantage or disadvantage conferred by the trait is not known.

Acquired Variation

Limitations on the capacity for βAIB metabolism in normal subjects may predispose to the appearance of the high-excretor "status" under certain conditions. A number of workers have observed transient high excretion of βAIB in infants and children (Berry, 1960) and in adults (Levey et al., 1963) after typical catabolic stimuli. For example, malignancies, infection, burns, surgical intervention and fasting are each capable of producing the finding in subjects who do not otherwise manifest it. Tissue degradation and release of thymine, or diversion of thymine prior to incorporation, probably provides the excess of βAIB. This form of the elevated βAIB excretion is important in pedigree studies, where it must be differentiated from the hereditary form.

CARNOSINEMIA

The rare disorder carnosinemia is characterized by an elevated concentration of carnosine in body fluids. A deficiency of the serum enzyme carnosinase has been identified in probands with this trait. Excessive carnosine accumulation in brain may be associated with neurological dysfunction.

Metabolism of β-Alanine Dipeptides and Related Compounds

β-Alanine in tissues occurs predominantly in dipeptide linkage (Crush, 1970) (Fig. 18–2). In human tissues, the dipeptide is carnosine (β-alanyl-histidine); in other species, anserine (β-alanyl-1-methylhistidine) is prominent,

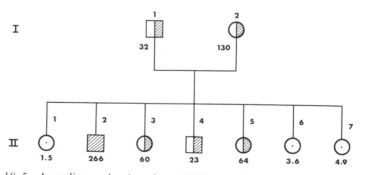

Figure 18–5 A pedigree showing three βAIB excretion phenotypes. Numbers beneath symbols are βAIB excretion in urine expressed as mg/g creatinine; the normal value is <25 mg/g creatinine. Each subject except II-4 expressed the phenotype consistently on repeated examination; the exception was of both normal and high-excretor status on various occasions. The excretion patterns suggest that II-2 is a homozygous βAIB excretor, while others (I-1, I-2, II-3, II-4, II-5) are heterozygous for the trait.

particularly in the muscle of fowl. Dipeptides incorporating other forms of histidine have also been identified in vertebrate tissues.

Intestinal absorption of carnosine is slower than the equivalent uptake of free β-alanine or free L-histidine (Asatoor et al., 1970), and separate types of intestinal transport sites serve absorption of free and bound β-amino acids (Navab and Asatoor, 1970). Absorption of the intact dipeptide is not the source of tissue carnosine.

Carnosine is synthesized in muscle and brain from β-alanine and histidine by the tissue enzyme carnosine synthetase (Fig. 18–1). The same enzyme can synthesize anserine, in vitro, from β-alanine and 1-methylhistidine. Anserine can also be formed by transmethylation of carnosine in the presence of the enzyme carnosine N-methyltransferase. In human tissues there is very little free 1-methylhistidine, and the transferase enzyme has yet to be demonstrated; these observations explain the absence of tissue anserine in this species.

The enzyme system which synthesizes carnosine can also employ γ-amino-butyric acid (GABA) in the place of β-alanine to form homocarnosine (γ-amino-butyryl-histidine) (Fig. 18–2). Homocarnosine is found in brain, CSF and urine (Pisano et al., 1961), but in the latter instance, its occurrence probably reflects the synthesis of GABA in kidney (Scriver et al., 1969; Whelan et al., 1969). Kanazawa and Sano (1967) have investigated the regional distribution of homo-carnosine in human brain; its concentration varies from 15 to 60 μmoles/g wet weight in different areas of brain. Homocarnosine may be synthesized in brain by the same enzyme that forms carnosine in skeletal muscle, although the presence of carnosine synthetase in brain has not yet been demonstrated. Homocarnosine is not hydrolyzed by the carnosinase which has been isolated from swine kidney. The physiologic role of homocarnosine in human brain remains unknown.

The turnover rate of these dipeptides in tissues reflects their net rates of synthesis and degradation. Vitamin E deficiency will, for instance, diminish synthesis and allow increased dipeptide loss from tissue pools. There is an increase in tissue carnosine in hyper-β-alaninemia (Scriver et al., 1966), but in this condition there is no apparent defect in carnosine degradation; carnosine synthesis must, therefore, exceed degradation when free β-alanine is present in excess. The increased tissue carnosine in carnosinemia is apparently related to carnosinase deficiency. Carnosinase would thus appear to be the rate-limiting enzyme in the turnover of the dipeptides. Carnosinase is present in mammalian liver, spleen and kidney. It is a metalloprotein, containing zinc; it hydrolyzes carnosine and anserine and probably also homocarnosine.

Distribution of Dipeptides

Exogenous or dietary carnosine and anserine play little role in the tissue metabolism of these dipeptides. The compounds are normally split either in the intestine or in blood (Perry et al., 1967); the fraction escaping hydrolysis is excreted into urine with a high clearance rate in the kidney. Thus, urinary carnosine and anserine reflect dietary intake, primarily and particularly meat or fowl in the diet (Block et al., 1965; Perry et al., 1967; Davies and Scriver, 1967). If anserine is a component of the diet, urinary excretion of free 1-methyl-histidine will also occur (Davies and Scriver, 1967; Butts and Fleshler, 1965), since the latter compound is poorly metabolized in man, and it is excreted with high renal clearance in the urine (Cusworth and Dent, 1960; Scriver and Davies, 1965). L-Methylhistidinuria can cause a green ferric chloride reaction (Davies and Scriver, 1967).

The distribution of the β-alanine dipeptides in man can be summarized as follows:

Carnosine is present in muscle and brain; while normally detectable in plasma, it is present in small quantities in urine and in very small amounts in CSF. Excretion is normally increased after ingestion of meat and fowl, and abnormally, in carnosinemia.

Homocarnosine is present in CSF and in brain (about 50 μmoles/100 g white matter). It is also detectable in small quantities in urine (2 to 10 μmoles/day), the amount not being influenced by diet. It is excreted abnormally in urine in carnosinemia.

Anserine is not present in human tissues but is found in brain and muscle of other mammalian species. When present in human urine, and particularly when 1-methylhistidine is also present, it reflects the dietary intake of this dipeptide.

Clinical and Biochemical Features of Carnosinemia

Two unrelated male probands were described by Perry and colleagues (1967), and one male child has been reported from Holland (van Heeswijk et al., 1969). Perry's first patient had a condition which can be called "carnosinemia," while the second patient had intermittent carnosinemia and fewer clinical abnormalities. The third (Dutch) patient did not have "carnosinemia" but did have seizures and striking carnosinuria; a symptomatic carnosinuria was also detected in the newborn sib of the latter patient, but the significance of this is unknown since dietary controls were unspecified and serum carnosinase activity is normally low in the human infant.

The fasting plasma concentration of carnosine was constantly elevated (more than 1 μM) in only one of the patients reported by Perry. The fasting plasma dipeptide concentration was not elevated in Perry's second patient, and it was never elevated in the Dutch patient. The level of dipeptide in urine was always abnormal, even on a meat-free diet, in all three patients, and the concentrations of homocarnosine and carnosine were elevated in cerebrospinal fluid.

No anserine was excreted except when it was administered in the diet. Anserine appeared unchanged in urine after a dietary load, in contrast to the response of normal subjects, who excrete large amounts of 1-methylhistidine under these conditions.

The three patients had a neurological disorder in association with the "carnosinemic" trait. They were all mentally retarded, and each had a seizure disorder. However, it is not possible to say yet whether the metabolic abnormality is primarily responsible for the CNS findings. Follow-up reports on the carnosinuric infant sib of the Dutch proband will be important to determine more about the constancy of clinical symptoms in this phenotype.

The Probable Enzymatic Defect

Perry and colleagues (1967, 1968) presented evidence for a deficiency of carnosinase in the blood of their patients. Serum from normal adult subjects hydrolyzes 19.5 ± 8.3 μmoles of carnosine/ml/16 hr (mean and SD); the values are lower for children matched for age with the patients (5.5 ± 2.6 μmoles/ml/ 16 hr; range 1.7 to 11.8). Serum carnosinase activity in the patients varied between 0 and 0.8 units. The Dutch proband and one of his sibs had no carnosinase activity in serum despite the absence of "carnosinemia" (van Heeswijk et al., 1970). Postmortem tissues of Perry's second patient contained some carnosinase-like activity. The significance of the tissue activity in relation to the deficiency of serum carnosinase activity is not clear.

Genetics

The parents of Perry's first patient were first cousins, and an older female sib had died at three months of age with symptoms suggestive of the trait. Neither parent had abnormal serum carnosinase activity. Parental consanguinity was also present in the Dutch pedigree, but these parents had partial deficiency of serum carnosinase activity with modest dipeptiduria. Simple autosomal recessive inheritance of the trait is suggested by these findings, but whether the Dutch and Canadian traits result from the same mutant allele is unknown and is perhaps unlikely on the basis of the present evidence.

Numerous urine screening programs throughout the world have not detected other patients with hereditary carnosinuria. However, the trait can be easily ignored because of its known dietary origin.

Treatment

No therapy is known. Dietary restriction is not possible in hereditary carnosinemia, since the major source of serum carnosine is endogenous. The possibility that the enzyme could respond to administration of zinc cofactor should be considered in future patients.

IMIDAZOLEAMINOACIDURIA AND PEPTIDURIA

Bessman and Baldwin (1962) described a dominantly inherited trait present in three families of a single kinship and in two other unrelated families. The trait was characterized by excessive urinary excretion of carnosine, anserine and 1-methylhistidine. The index disease which brought the patients to medical attention was a recessively inherited form of juvenile cerebromacular degeneration, which did not occur in all patients with the imidazoleaminoaciduria. Levenson and colleagues (1964) also reported histidine peptiduria in four of 15 children with the same type of cerebromacular degeneration. Neither group of authors mentions dietary control during the study of their patients, and therefore it is possible, although unlikely, that a dietary artifact accounted for the observation. Tocci and Bessman (1967) reported the results of further investigation of the original patients. Their results are at variance with current knowledge of human metabolism of carnosine and anserine, making it impossible at present to interpret their data or to understand the relevance of histidine peptiduria to cerebromacular degeneration.

TAURINE METABOLISM

Taurine, a ubiquitous metabolite, has not yet been identified with a primary aberration of its own metabolism in man. However, it is involved secondarily in a number of metabolic disorders, and it is of quantitative importance in several tissues. An extensive review of taurine metabolism is available (Jacobson and Smith, 1968).

Taurine is a β-amino compound in which the carboxyl group in the corresponding amino acid series is replaced by SO_3^- thus:

$$^+H_3NCH_2CH_2SO_3$$

Taurine is an intermediate of cysteine oxidation, and it participates in some interconversions of metabolic interest.

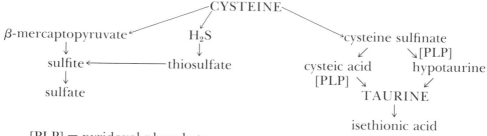

[PLP] = pyridoxal phosphate

The principal pathway of cysteine oxidation is via sulfite to sulfate, and this is well illustrated by the careful studies in the patient with sulfite oxidase deficiency (see p. 226). Any inorganic sulfate derived directly from taurine in mammals is almost certainly formed by intestinal bacterial conversion and not from tissue conversion of taurine.

Three metabolites of taurine have now been identified in man which indicate that taurine is not merely an end product of cysteine metabolism, as it once was thought to be.

ISETHIONIC ACID.   This deaminated analogue of taurine has been isolated from human urine. Its normal urinary excretion is about 5 to 25 mg/24 hours in the adult (or about 10 per cent of taurine excretion), and the main site of biosynthesis is believed to be striated muscle. Its physiological role is unknown, but isethionic acid may influence the distribution of ions across membranes of excitable tissues.

TAUROCYAMINE (GUANIDOTAURINE).   This compound has no known role in mammalian physiology or biochemistry. It is excreted in human urine in trace amounts.

TAUROCHOLIC ACID.   Taurine is conjugated with bile acids to form taurocholate, but these biliary excretion products are of less significance than the corresponding glycine conjugates in man.

Taurine itself is found in blood plasma, urine, bile, breast milk, saliva, cerebrospinal fluid and sweat of man, and in platelets, leukocytes, muscle, brain, skin and liver; 75 per cent of the total body taurine is in striated muscle. The tissue concentration of taurine is higher in the fetus than in the adult, and blood and urine levels are higher after birth than in later life. Taurine is actively transported across the placenta to the fetus, and transport across plasma membranes is served by the β-amino-preferring system (see earlier section on β-alanine metabolism).

The role of taurine in human tissues has not been extensively studied. Transmission of nerve impulses is known to be inhibited by taurine, and the chemical analogies between taurine and GABA invite further investigation of a neurohumoral type of function. Taurine, and its derivative isethionic acid, may regulate excitability of cardiac muscle, in particular by modifying potassium efflux from the cell. The preponderance of taurine in platelets and leukocytes suggests that it may function in platelet contractibility and in leukocyte mobility and phagocytosis.

Taurine levels in blood are influenced by *age* (higher in the immediate postnatal period), by *venipuncture* (transient fall after the procedure) and by artifacts of sample collection (higher in serum than in plasma and when leakage occurs from leukocytes and platelets during improper processing of blood samples). The normal concentration in plasma is 25 to 150 μM; higher values occur for the reasons given and particularly in the blood dyscrasias which augment the platelet and leukocyte fraction of formed elements in blood.

The urinary excretion of taurine is high relative to other amino acids. This finding reflects its inefficient tubular reabsorption, which is to be expected of a β-amino substance; tubular reabsorption of taurine is less than 95 per cent of the normal filtered load and less than that when its plasma concentration increases. The excretion rate of taurine is considered to be abnormal when it exceeds 2500 μmoles/day in the adult and when it is more than 1200 μmoles/day in children under 12 years.

Catabolic stimuli which produce negative nitrogen balance increase taurine excretion; hypertaurinuria occurs postoperatively and after trauma, burns and so forth. High protein intake, acute liver failure and leukemia also cause hypertaurinuria. All of these conditions produce "prerenal hypertaurinuria." Disorders of renal tubular function may also cause increased taurinuria. Diseases which involve muscle atrophy cause hypotaurinuria. Vitamin B_6 deficiency impairs the synthesis of taurine from cysteine, and taurine excretion diminishes under these conditions (see sites of action of pyridoxal phosphate coenzyme (PLP) in the foregoing diagram of taurine metabolism). Taurine excretion is usually normal in the inborn errors of sulfur amino acid catabolism.

DISORDERS OF PHOSPHOETHANOLAMINE METABOLISM

Phosphoethanolamine (or O-phosphorylethanolamine) is analogous to a β-amino acid in that an acidic group exists and the amino group is attached to the β-carbon:

$$^+NH_3CH_2CH_2OPO_3^-$$

The acidic group in this compound can yield inorganic phosphate (P_i) upon enzymatic hydrolysis.

Metabolism of Phosphoethanolamine

Metabolism in Animal Liver

Mammalian liver (rat and rabbit) metabolizes phosphoethanolamine by the reaction

$$^+NH_3CH_2CH_2OPO_3^= \rightarrow NH_4 + CH_3CHO + P_i$$

according to the work of Fleshood and Pitot (1970). The reaction is catalyzed by the enzyme O-phosphorylethanolamine phospho-lyase, of approximate molecular weight 168,000; the pH optimum is 7.8, and the enzyme is unstable at temperatures above 55°. The apparent K_m for the substrate is 6.1×10^{-4}M; the reaction requires pyridoxal phosphate as coenzyme, the apparent K_m for which is 2.7×10^{-7}M. The enzyme is highly specific, rejecting many compounds structurally similar to substrate; P_i is, however, a competitive inhibitor at high physiological concentrations (K_m, P_i, 1.3×10^{-3}M).

Whether this enzyme occurs in plasma and accounts for any of the "alkaline phosphatase activity" there is unknown at present but should be investigated.

Metabolism in Man

Phosphoethanolamine occurs in tissues and is excreted in small amounts in normal urine (Harris and Robson, 1959; Cusworth and Dent, 1960; Goyer, 1963; Rasmussen, 1968). It was first isolated from human urine by two independent groups of investigators (Fraser et al., 1955; McCance et al., 1955) during the investigation of patients affected with the disease now known as hypophosphatasia (Rathbun, 1948; Fraser, 1957; Rasmussen, 1968). Phosphoethanolamine is not a derivative of phosphatidyl ethanolamine, as might be expected, and its metabolic origin in mammalian tissues is still unclear. Phosphoethanolamine has also been found in brain (Tallan, 1962) and in saliva (Rose and Kerr, 1958; Westall, 1962).

The subject of phosphoethanolamine metabolism and its relation to hypophosphatasia has been exhaustively reviewed by Rasmussen (1968). Phosphoethanolamine is a β-amino compound, and it is therefore rapidly cleared from plasma by the kidney; it appears in the urine when its plasma concentration is scarcely detectable, and on this basis, Dent (1957) placed phosphoethanolamine in the "no-threshold" category in his classification of aminoaciduria. The normal excretion rate is 62 ± 20 μmoles/m^2 per 24 hours in the first four years of life; the excretion rate falls in later childhood to the adult range (24 to 44 μmoles/m^2 per 24 hours) (Rasmussen, 1968). The methods presently available for chromatographic analysis of phosphoethanolamine show that, in most conditions associated with increased phosphoethanolaminuria, there is an increase of phosphoethanolamine in plasma as well. The common feature in each of these conditions is some disturbance of circulating alkaline phosphatase activity. In conditions where bone-derived alkaline phosphatase activity is increased, phosphoethanolaminuria may actually be diminished (Rasmussen, 1968).

Hypophosphatasia

Subjects who are homozygous for this trait excrete large amounts of phosphoethanolamine in urine and have clearly elevated plasma levels of the compound (Rasmussen, 1968). However, the metabolic relationship between phosphoethanolamine and alkaline phosphatase activity has not been particularly clarified by any studies of this trait so far. Heterozygotes for the trait can be identified with about 60 per cent efficiency on the basis of their phosphoethanolamine excretion in urine (Harris and Robson, 1959; Goyer, 1963). Slight deviation of plasma phosphoethanolamine in heterozygotes has been clearly shown in most heterozygotes (Rasmussen, 1968). Several alleles are believed to control the phenotypic expression of hypophosphatasia and hyperphosphoethanolaminuria, but to conclude, as did Rasmussen (1968), that phosphoethanolamine transport is impaired in the trait is erroneous, since the normal phenomenon of saturable transport is sufficient to explain the phosphoethanolaminuria.

The reader should consult Bartter (1972), Rasmussen (1968) and Fraser (1957) for detailed reviews of the disease. The bone disease is said by some to benefit from a high-phosphate diet (Bongiovanni et al., 1968), but others disagree (Teree and Klein, 1968). The latter opinion is more likely correct, since the disease is known to undergo spontaneous remission in the period of infancy, and the efficiency of therapy is difficult to evaluate under such conditions.

Pseudohypophosphatasia

A female infant has been described (Scriver and Cameron, 1969) whose clinical phenotype closely mimics classical hypophosphatasia, with the important exception that the plasma alkaline phosphatase activity is normal. The parents of the proband both have abnormal phosphoethanolaminuria. A study of the patient's "alkaline phosphatase activity" in plasma showed it to be composed of the isozymes from bone (heat-labile) and intestine (L-phenylalanine-inhibitable) in the normal proportion. The pH optimum for activity of the total enzyme was normal. However, at phosphoethanolamine concentrations between 1.6 and 8 mM, the enzyme in the patient's plasma cleaved phosphoethanolamine less efficiently than normal, whereas the activity toward other substrates was normal.

The possibility that pseudohypophosphatasia is a specific disorder of the pyridoxal-requiring enzyme O-phosphorylethanolamine phospho-lyase merits specific investigation—first as to the presence or absence of the enzyme in normal plasma, and then as to its status in the hereditary disease. The effect of vitamin B_6 on the trait should also be evaluated.*

Miscellaneous

Phosphoethanolamine is excreted in elevated amounts in a variety of conditions, including liver disease, scurvy and hypothyroidism (Fraser, 1957).

ETHANOLAMINE METABOLISM

Ethanolamine ($NH_2CH_2CH_2OH$) is a derivative of serine and glycolate, and it is a normal constituent of body fluids. Its excretion is augmented synchronously with βAIB in the newborn (Scriver, 1962), and it is excreted in some types of liver disease (Dent and Walshe, 1953).

γ-AMINOBUTYRIC ACID (GABA)

The role of γ-aminobutyric acid in cellular metabolism is still not completely understood, despite over 20 years of intensive study. GABA is present in significant amounts in two tissues: brain and kidney cortex. In both organs, it participates in the formation of succinate from glutamate by an alternate pathway which bypasses the usual direct transformation of glutamate to α-ketoglutarate and thence to succinate. In gray matter, GABA may serve a neuro-inhibitory function. Glutamate conversion to GABA may be impaired in hereditary pyridoxine dependency.

Metabolism of GABA

GABA is synthesized from L-glutamic acid by a decarboxylation reaction catalyzed by the vitamin B_6-dependent enzyme L-glutamate 1-decarboxy-lyase (E.C. 4.1.1.15). An α-ketoglutarate-requiring transaminase converts GABA to succinic semialdehyde, and the latter then appears as succinate. This "GABA shunt" (depicted in Figure 18–6) has been identified in brain (see compendium edited by Roberts, 1960) and in kidney (Scriver and Whelan, 1969; Whelan et al., 1969).

Two types of glutamate decarboxylase (trivial name of L-glutamate 1-decarboxy-lyase) have been found in brain: one in glial cells and the other in

---

*We are grateful to Dr. Paul Benke for bringing this suggestion to our attention.

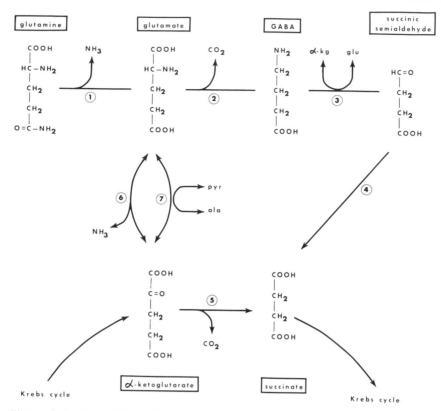

Figure 18–6 The GABA pathway in mammalian brain and kidney cortex, indicating the relationships of GABA to glutamate, α-ketoglutarate and succinate metabolism.

neurons (Haber et al., 1970a, 1970b). The type of decarboxylase found in kidney cortex resembles the glial form (Whelan et al., 1969). These new and important observations suggest that GABA function differs at the various cellular sites at which biosynthesis occurs.

The amount of glutamate converted to succinate by the GABA shunt is not more than one third of that converted via α-ketoglutarate, according to our own estimates (Lancaster et al., 1973). The GABA shunt can serve the oxidation of glutamate in brain and kidney cortex, where the concentration of the latter is high (about 5 mM, or 50 to 100 times greater than the equivalent concentration in extracellular fluid). The GABA shunt in kidney may particularly facilitate glutamate oxidation to succinate in acidosis, since glutamate will be formed from glutamine during ammoniagenesis. Under these circumstances, glutamate oxidation would be achieved without stoichiometric consumption of pyruvate, as is the case when glutamate is transaminated to α-ketoglutarate, and this may be of significance in supporting the increased renal gluconeogenesis which occurs in acidosis.

The GABA pathway may serve a supportive role in oxidative metabolism in brain (McKhann and Tower, 1959; McKhann et al., 1960), but it also yields high concentrations of intracellular GABA. This neurohumoral substance has inhibitory activity at synaptic membranes (Roberts et al., 1964; Elliott, 1965; Steiner, 1969).

Distribution

GABA occurs almost exclusively as an intracellular metabolite in man, and its appearance in any more than trace amounts in extracellular fluids is abnormal. GABA is present in concentrations exceeding $10^{-3}M/g$ wet weight in human kidney (Scriver and Whelan, 1969); by comparison, its concentration is insignificant (10^{-10} to $10^{-8}M/g$ wet weight) in other tissues. It is not known whether intracellular GABA exists in the free state in brain, but most evidence suggests that it is bound to synaptic sites there (Elliott, 1964); the amino acid appears to be free in kidney (Lancaster et al., 1973). GABA penetrates the plasma membrane by mediated diffusion, but only slowly, and its renal clearance is very rapid.

Disturbances of GABA Metabolism

Pharmacological and Nutritional States

Drugs which inhibit glutamate decarboxylase or GABA transaminase (e.g., carbonyl trapping agents) can modify the cellular concentration of GABA; vitamin B_6 deficiency is rare in man, but the presumed impairment of GABA formation in this nutritional state may account for the convulsive disorder which often accompanies the deficiency state in man (Scriver, 1967).

Hyper-β-Alaninemia

GABA excretion in urine and its concentration in brain are both abnormally elevated in this disease (see discussion in section on β-alanine metabolism). The striking somnolence in clinical hyper-β-alaninemia may reflect the neuroinhibitory effects of GABA.

Vitamin-B_6 Dependency

This autosomal recessive trait (Scriver and Whelan, 1969) has a high mortality (80 per cent in the first year of life), is recognizable at or soon after birth and is dramatically responsive to pharmacologic doses of pyridoxine (10 to 50 mg/day). Early diagnosis and treatment with the vitamin is apparently compatible with normal mental and neurological development in the patient.

It has been suggested that a specific disturbance of pyridoxal-5-phosphate binding by glutamate decarboxylase apoprotein may exist in this condition (Scriver, 1960; Scriver and Whelan, 1969). The finding by Yoshida et al. (1971) of deficient conversion of glutamate to GABA in kidney, and correction of the conversion defect by addition of pyridoxal phosphate to kidney homogenate in a patient affected with pyridoxine dependency, is compatible with this hypothesis. Immediate correction by pyridoxal phosphate in vitro of impaired activity of the specific decarboxylase in the brain of such patients should also be evident, if the defective binding hypothesis is to be proven ultimately. The biological significance of the vitamin B_6 dependency trait for the student of pyridoxal phosphate-dependent enzymes has been discussed at length by Mudd (1970) (see Chapter 22).

REFERENCES

Hyper-β-Alaninemia

Avena, R. M., and Bowen, W. J.: Effects of carnosine and anserine on muscle adenosine triphosphatase. J. Biol. Chem. *244*:1600–1604, 1969.

Baxter, C. F., and Roberts, E.: Elevation of γ-aminobutyric acid in brain: Selective inhibition of γ-aminobutyric-α-ketoglutaric acid transaminase. J. Biol. Chem. *236*:3287–3294, 1961.

Christensen, H. N.: Reactive sites and biological transport. Advances Protein Chem. *15*:239–314, 1960.

Crush, K. C.: Carnosine and related substances in animal tissues. Comp. Biochem. Physiol. *34*: 3–30, 1970.

Davey, C. L.: Significance of carnosine and anserine in striated skeletal muscle. Arch. Biochem. *89*:303–308, 1960.

Davies, E., and Scriver, C. R.: 1-Methylhistidinuria in man: A festive index. Proceedings of the Society for Pediatric Research, Atlantic City, N.J., p. 134, 1967.

DuVigneaud, V., and Behrens, O.: Carnosine and anserine. Ergebn. Physiol. *41*:917–973, 1939.

Gilbert, J. B., Ku, Y., Rogers, L. L., and Williams, R. L.: The increase in urinary taurine after intraperitoneal administration of amino acids to the mouse. J. Biol. Chem. *235*:1055–1060, 1960.

Goldman, H., and Scriver, C. R.: A transport system in mammalian kidney with preference for β-amino compounds. Pediat. Res. *1*:212–213, 1967.

Hayaishi, O., Nishizuka, Y., Tatibana, M., Takeshita, M., and Kuno, S.: Enzymatic studies on the metabolism of β-alanine. J. Biol. Chem. *236*:781–790, 1961.

Hechtman, P., and Scriver, C. R.: Neutral amino acid transport in *Pseudomonas fluorescens*. J. Bact. *104*:857–863, 1970.

Hechtman, P., and Scriver, C. R.: The isolation and properties of β-alanine permeaseless mutant of *Pseudomonas fluorescens*. Biochim. Biophys. Acta *219*:428–436, 1970.

Kalyankar, G. D., and Meister, A.: Enzymatic synthesis of carnosine and related β-alanyl and γ-aminobutyryl peptides. J. Biol. Chem. *234*:3210–3218, 1959.

Krnjevic, K.: Action of drugs on single neurones in the cerebral cortex. Brit. Med. Bull. *21*:10–14, 1965.

McManus, I. R.: Metabolism of anserine and carnosine in normal and vitamin E-deficient rabbits. J. Biol. Chem. *235*:1398–1403, 1960.

McManus, I. R.: Enzymatic synthesis of anserine in skeletal muscle by N-methylation of carnosine. J. Biol. Chem. *237*:1207–1211, 1962.

McManus, I. R., and Benson, M. S.: Studies on the formation of carnosine and anserine in pectoral muscle of the developing chick. Arch. Biochem. *119*:444–453, 1967.

Meister, A.: β-Alanine and β-aminoisobutyric acid. *In* Biochemistry of the Amino Acids, Vol. II, 2nd edition. Academic Press, New York, pp. 601–606, 1965.

Reddy, W. J., and Hegsted, D. M.: Measurement and distribution of carnosine in rat. J. Biol. Chem. *237*:705–706, 1962.

Roberts, E., and Bregoff, H. M.: Transamination of γ-aminobutyric acid and β-alanine in brain and liver. J. Biol. Chem. *201*:393–398, 1953.

Roberts, E., and Simonsen, D. G.: Free amino acids in animal tissues. *In* Amino Acid Pools: Distribution, Formation and Function of Free Amino Acids, J. T. Holden, ed., Elsevier, New York, pp. 285–349, 1962.

Schmidt, G., and Cubiles, R.: Comparative studies on occurrence of carnosine-anserine fraction in skeletal muscle and heart. Arch. Biochem. *58*:227–231, 1955.

Scriver, C. R., Pueschel, S., and Davies, E.: Hyper-β-alaninemia associated with β-aminoaciduria and γ-aminobutyricaciduria, somnolence and seizures. New Eng. J. Med. *274*:636–643, 1966.

Stenesh, J. J., and Winnick, T.: Carnosine-anserine synthetase of muscle. 4: partial purification of the enzyme and further studies of β-alanyl peptide synthesis. Biochem. J. *77*:575–581, 1960.

Acquired Abnormalities of β-Alanine Metabolism

Gras, J., Tuset, N., Caralps, A., Gil-Vernet, J. M., Magrina, N., Brulles, A., and Conde, M.: β-alaninuria following human renal allotransplantation. Clin. Chim. Acta *20*:295–298, 1968.

Takao, T., Yasumitsu, T., Uozumi, T., Kakimoto, Y., and Kanazawa, A.: β-alaninuria in patients with tuberculosis. Nature (London) *217*:365–366, 1968.

β-Aminoisobutyricaciduria

Armstrong, M. D., Yates, K., Kakimoto, Y., Taniguchi, K., and Kappe, T.: Excretion of β-amino isobutyric acid by man. J. Biol. Chem. *238*:1447–1455, 1963.

Berry, H. K.: Individual metabolic patterns. II. Excretion of β-aminoisobutyric acid. Metabolism *9*:373–376, 1960.

Crumpler, H. R., Dent, C. E., Harris, H., and Westall, R. G.: β-Aminoisobutyric acid (α-methyl-β-alanine): A new amino acid, obtained from human urine. Nature (London) *167*:307–308, 1951.

Dent, C. E.: Clinical applications of amino acid chromatography. Scand. J. Clin. Lab. Invest. (Suppl. 31) *10*:122–127, 1957.

Fink, K., Henderson, R. B., and Fink, R. M.: β-Aminoisobutyric acid, a possible factor in pyrimidine metabolism. Proc. Soc. Exp. Biol. Med. *78*:135–141, 1951.

Fink, K., Henderson, R. B., and Fink, R. M.: β-Aminoisobutyric acid in rat urine following the administration of pyrimidines. J. Biol. Chem. *197*:441–452, 1952.

Gartler, S. M., Firschein, I. L., and Kraus, B. S.: An investigation into the genetics and racial variation of βAIB excretion. Amer. J. Hum. Genet. *9*:200–207, 1957.

Harris, H.: Family studies on the urinary excretion of β-aminoisobutyric acid. Ann. Eugen. *18*: 43–49, 1953.

Kakimoto, Y., Kanazawa, A., Taniguchi, K., and Saro, I.: β-aminoisobutyrate-α-ketoglutarate transaminase in relation to β-aminoisobutyric aciduria. Biochim. Biophys. Acta *156*:374–380, 1968.

Kupiecki, F. P., and Coon, M. J.: The enzymatic synthesis of β-aminoisobutyrate, a product of valine metabolism, and of β-alanine, a product of β-hydroxypropionate metabolism. J. Biol. Chem. *229*:743–754, 1957.

Levey, S., Woods, T., and Abbott, W. E.: Urinary excretion of β-aminoisobutyric acid following surgical procedures. Metabolism *12*:148–156, 1963.

McEvoy-Bowe, E., and Lugg, T. W. H.: A direct quantitative paper chromatography of amino acids and its application to the urinary excretions of some human ethnic groups. Biochem. J. *80*: 616–623, 1961.

Meister, A.: β-Alanine and β-aminoisobutyric acid. *In* Meister, A., ed., Biochemistry of the Amino Acids, Vol. II, 2nd edition. Academic Press, New York, pp. 601–606, 1965.

Sutton, H. E.: β-Aminoisobutyricaciduria. *In* Stanbury, J. B., Wyngaarden, J. B., and Fredrickson, D. S., eds., The Metabolic Basis of Inherited Disease. McGraw-Hill, New York, pp. 792–806, 1960.

Carnosinemia

Asatoor, A. M., Bandoh, J. K., Lant, A. F., Milne, M. D., and Navab, F.: Intestinal absorption of carnosine and its constituent amino acids in man. Gut *11*:250–254, 1970.

Block, W. D., Hubbard, R. W., and Steele, B. F.: Excretion of histidine and histidine derivatives by human subjects ingesting protein from different sources. J. Nutr. *85*:419–425, 1965.

Butts, J. H., and Fleshler, B.: Anserine, a source of 1-methylhistidine in urine of man. Proc. Soc. Exp. Biol. Med. *118*:722–725, 1965.

Crush, K. C.: Carnosine and related substances in animal tissues. Comp. Biochem. Physiol. *34*:3–30, 1970.

Cusworth, D. C., and Dent, C. E.: Renal clearances of amino acids in normal adults and in patients with aminoaciduria. Biochem. J. *74*:550–561, 1960.

Davies, E., and Scriver, C. R.: 1-Methylhistidinuria in man: a festive index. Proceedings of the Society for Pediatric Research, Atlantic City, N.J., p. 134, 1967.

Kanazawa, A., and Sano, I.: Method of determination of homocarnosine and its distribution in mammalian tissues. J. Neurochem. *14*:211–214, 1967.

Navab, F., and Asatoor, A. M.: Studies on intestinal absorption of amino acids and a dipeptide in a case of Hartnup disease. Gut *11*:373–379, 1970.

Perry, T. L., Hansen, S., and Love, D. L.: Serum-carnosinase deficiency in carnosinaemia. Lancet, (i), 1229–1230, 1968.

Perry, T. L., Hansen, S., Tischler, B., Bunting, R., and Berry, K.: Carnosinemia: a new metabolic disorder associated with neurologic disease and mental defect. New Eng. J. Med. *277*:1219–1227, 1967.

Pisano, J. J., Wilson, J. D., Cohen, L., Abraham, D., and Udenfriend, S.: Isolation of γ-aminobutyrylhistidine (homocarnosine) from brain. J. Biol. Chem. *236*:499–502, 1961.

Scriver, C. R., and Davies, E.: Endogenous renal clearance rates of free amino acids in pre-pubertal children. Pediatrics *32*:592–598, 1965.

Scriver, C. R., Pueschel, S., and Davies, E.: Hyper-β-alaninemia associated with β-aminoaciduria and γ-aminobutyricaciduria, somnolence and seizures. New Eng. J. Med. *274*:636–643, 1966.

Scriver, C. R., and Whelan, D. T.: Glutamic acid decarboxylase (GAD) in mammalian tissue outside the central nervous system and its possible relevance to hereditary vitamin B₆ dependency with seizures. Ann. N.Y. Acad. Sci. *166*:83–96, 1969.

Van Heeswijk, P. J., Trybels, J. M. F., Schretlen, E. D. A. M., van Munster, P. J. J., and Monnens, L. A. H.: A patient with a deficiency of serum carnosinase activity. Acta Paediat. Scand. *58*: 584–592, 1969.

Whelan, D. T., Scriver, C. R., and Mohyuddin, F.: Glutamic acid decarboxylase and γ-aminobutyric acid in mammalian kidney. Nature (London) *224*:916–917, 1969.

Imidazoleaminoaciduria and Peptiduria

Bessman, S. P., and Baldwin, R.: Imidazole aminoaciduria in cerebromacular degeneration. Science *135*:789–791, 1962.

Levenson, J., Lindahl-Kiessling, K., and Rayner, S.: Carnosine excretion in juvenile amaurotic idiocy. Lancet (ii), 756–757, 1964.

Tocci, P. M., and Bessman, S. P.: Histidine peptiduria. *In* Nyhan, W. L., ed., Amino Acid Metabolism and Genetic Variation. McGraw-Hill, New York, pp. 161–166, 1967.

Taurine Metabolism

Jacobson, J. G., and Smith, H., Jr.: Biochemistry and physiology of taurine and taurine derivatives. Physiol. Reviews *48*:424–511, 1968.

Disorders of Phosphoethanolamine Metabolism

Bartter, F. C.: Hypophosphatasia. *In* Stanbury, J. B., Wyngaarden, J. B., and Fredrickson, D. S., eds., The Metabolic Basis of Hereditary Disease, 3rd edition. McGraw-Hill, New York, 1972.

Bongiovanni, A. M., Album, M. M., Root, A. W., Hope, J. W., Marino, J., and Spencer, D. M.: Studies in hypophosphatasia and response to high phosphate intake. Amer. J. Med. Sci. *255*: 163–170, 1968.

Cusworth, D. C., and Dent, C. E.: Renal clearance of amino acids in normal adults and in patients with aminoaciduria. Biochem. J. *74*:550–561, 1960.

Dent, C. E.: Clinical applications of amino acid chromatography. Scand. J. Clin. Lab. Invest. *10*: 122–127, 1957.

Fleshood, H. L., and Pitot, H. C.: The metabolism of O-phosphorylethanolamine in animal tissues. I. O-phosphorylethanolamine phospho-lyase: partial purification and characterization. J. Biol. Chem. *245*:4414–4420, 1970.

Fraser, D.: Hypophosphatasia. Amer. J. Med. *22*:730–746, 1957.

Fraser, D., Yendt, E. R., and Christie, F. H. E.: Metabolic abnormalities in hypophosphatasia. Lancet (i), 286, 1955.

Goyer, R. A.: Ethanolamine phosphate excretion in a family with hypophosphatasia. Arch. Dis. Child. *38*:205–207, 1963.

Harris, H., and Robson, E. B.: A genetical study of ethanolamine phosphate excretion in hypophosphatasia. Ann. Hum. Genet. *23*:421–441, 1959.

McCance, R. A., Morrison, A. B., and Dent, C. E.: The excretion of phosphoethanolamine and hypophosphatasia. Lancet (i), 131, 1955.

Rasmussen, K.: Phosphorylethanolamine and hypophosphatasia. Danish Med. Bull. *15*:1–112, 1968.

Rathbun, J. C.: Hypophosphatasia, a new developmental anomaly. J. Dis. Child. *75*:822–831, 1948.

Rose, G. A., and Kerr, A. C.: The amino acids and phosphoethanolamine in salivary gland secretions of normal men and of patients with abnormal calcium, phosphorus and amino acid metabolism. Quart. J. Exp. Physiol. *43*:160–168, 1958.

Scriver, C. R., and Cameron, D.: Pseudohypophosphatasia. New Eng. J. Med. *281*:604–606, 1969.

Tallan, H. H.: A survey of the amino acids and related compounds in nervous tissue. *In* Holden, J. T., ed., Amino Acid Pools: Distribution, Formation and Function of Free Amino Acids. Elsevier, New York, pp. 471–485, 1962.

Teree, T. M., and Klein, L.: Hypophosphatasia. Clinical and metabolic studies. J. Pediat. *72*:41–50, 1968.

Westall, R. G.: The free amino acids of body fluids and some hereditary disorders of amino acid metabolism. *In* Holden, J. T., ed., Amino Acid Pools: Distribution, Formation and Function of Free Amino Acids. Elsevier, New York, pp. 195–219, 1962.

Ethanolaminuria

Dent, C. E., and Walshe, J. M.: Primary carcinoma of the liver: Description of a case of ethanolaminuria, a new and obscure metabolic defect. Brit. J. Cancer *7*:166–180, 1953.

Scriver, C. R.: Hereditary amino aciduria. *In* Bearn, A., and Steinberg, A. G., Progress in Medical Genetics, Vol. 2. Grune & Stratton, New York, pp. 83–186, 1962.

γ-Aminobutyric Acid

Elliott, K. A. C.: γ-Aminobutyric acid and other inhibitory substances. Brit. Med. Bull. *21*:70–75, 1965.

Haber, B., Kuriyama, K., and Roberts, E.: L-Glutamic acid decarboxylase: A new type in glial cells and human brain gliomas. Science *168*:598–599, 1970a.

Haber, B., Kuriyama, K., and Roberts, E.: An anion stimulated L-glutamic acid decarboxylase in non-neural tissues. Occurrence and subcellular localization in mouse kidney and developing child brain. Biochem. Pharmacol. *19*:1119–1136, 1970b.

Lancaster, G. A., Mohyuddin, F., Scriver, C. R., and Whelan, D. T.: Unpublished observations, 1973.

McKhann, G. M., and Tower, D. B.: γ-Aminobutyric acid: A substrate for oxidative metabolism of cerebral cortex. Amer. J. Physiol. *196*:36–38, 1959.

McKhann, G. M., Albers, R. W., Sokoloff, L., Mickelsen, O., and Tower, D. B.: The quantitative significance of the γ-aminobutyric acid pathway in cerebral oxidative metabolism. *In* Roberts, E., ed., Inhibition in the Nervous System and γ-Aminobutyric Acid. Pergamon Press, New York, pp. 169–181, 1960.

Mudd, S. H.: Pyridoxine-responsive genetic disease. Fed. Proc. *30*:970–976, 1971.

Okamura, M., Otsuki, S., and Kameyama, A.: Studies on free amino acids in human brain. J. Biochem. (Tokyo) *47*:315–320, 1960.

Roberts, E., ed.: Inhibition in the Nervous System and γ-Aminobutyric Acid. Pergamon Press, New York, p. 591, 1960.

Roberts, E., Wein, J., and Simonson, D. G.: γ-Aminobutyric acid (γABA), vitamin B₆ and neuronal function: A speculative synthesis. Vitamins Hormones *22*:503–539, 1964.

Scriver, C. R.: Vitamin B₆ dependency and infantile convulsions. Pediatrics *26*:62–71, 1960.

Scriver, C. R.: Vitamin B₆ deficiency and dependency in man. Amer. J. Dis. Child. *113*:109–114, 1967.

Scriver, C. R., and Whelan, D. T.: Glutamic acid decarboxylase (GAD) in mammalian tissue outside the central nervous system and the possible relevance to hereditary vitamin B₆ dependency with seizures. Ann. N.Y. Acad. Sci. *166*:83–96, 1969.

Steiner, F. A.: L-Glutamic acid, GABA and pyridoxal-5'-phosphate at single unit level in brain. Ann. N.Y. Acad. Sci. *166*:199–209, 1969.

Whelan, D. T., Scriver, C. R., and Mohyuddin, F.: Glutamic acid decarboxylase and γ-aminobutyric acid in mammalian kidney. Nature (London) *224*:916–917, 1969.

Yoshida, T., Tada, K., and Arakawa, T.: Vitamin B₆-dependency of glutamic acid decarboxylase in the kidney from a patient with vitamin-B₆ dependent convulsion. Tohoku J. Exp. Med. *104*:195–198, 1971.

Chapter Nineteen

GLYCINE

Glycine is structurally the simplest of all the naturally occurring amino acids. It is another natural amino acid without an asymmetric carbon atom and, hence, without D- and L-stereoisomers. Glycine is abundantly present in nearly all animal proteins. It constitutes 25 or more per cent of the amino acid residues of collagen, gelatin and elastin but is found in much smaller amounts in proteins such as casein or lactalbumin. Three to five grams of glycine are ingested per day by an American adult on an average protein diet; but glycine is also readily synthesized within the body and is, therefore, not a dietary essential amino acid. It is classified as a glycogenic amino acid since it is readily converted to glucose by way of pyruvate.

Abnormalities in glycine metabolism exist in many human diseases. We have already discussed conditions in which defects in renal tubular transport of this amino acid result in excessive excretion of glycine in the urine (Chapters 6 and 8), and further mention of hyperglycinuria will be found in Chapter 20. In addition, there is a growing list of inherited diseases in which glycine and its metabolic products accumulate in the blood or spill over into the urine. Some of these disease states almost certainly reflect primary enzymatic defects in the

400

complex pathways of glycine metabolism (Fig. 19–1), but others are caused by distant metabolic aberrations which affect glycine metabolism secondarily.

METABOLISM OF GLYCINE

Glycine Utilization and Turnover

As noted in Figure 19–1, glycine has more metabolic fates than any other amino acid. It is incorporated intact into proteins, purines and glutathione. It is a key substrate in the formation of creatine, via guanidoacetate, and of porphyrins, via δ-aminolevulinic acid. About 1 g of glycine is utilized per day in several conjugation reactions: with benzoate to form hippurate; with choline to form the bile acid glycocholate; and with salicylates, steroids and bromsulphalein.

The metabolic pool of glycine is large and nonhomogeneous and turns over rapidly. Watts and Crawhall (1959) administered glycine-1-^{13}C to humans and estimated the glycine pool to be about 80 mg per kg body weight. Gutman and his colleagues (1958) obtained almost identical estimates in their study of the incorporation of glycine-1-^{14}C into urinary uric acid. After oral or parenteral administration of isotopically labeled glycine, there was greater labeling of urinary hippurate (Elder and Wyngaarden, 1960). These results indicate that the miscible glycine pool is not homogeneous but rather is composed of several intracellular and extracellular compartments in poor equilibrium with one another. The rate of glycine turnover in man has been estimated to be about 1 g per kg body weight per day, implying that the glycine pool turns over completely about 10 to 12 times in a 24-hour period.

Glycine Formation

Serine is the principal source of nondietary glycine. Shemin (1946) first demonstrated that ingested, labeled serine was rapidly converted to glycine. Subsequent studies showed that glycine can also be converted to serine (Winnick et al., 1948; Siekevitz and Greenberg, 1949; Kisliuk and Sakami, 1955). The

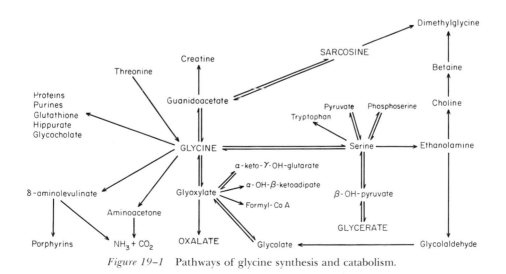

Figure 19–1 Pathways of glycine synthesis and catabolism.

details of this glycine-serine interconversion system have been studied in bacteria, avian liver and rat liver (Nyhan, 1972), but we shall detail only the mammalian system (Kawasaki et al., 1966; Sato et al., 1969a, 1969b; Motokawa and Kikuchi, 1969). The enzyme system involved in this catalysis is called serine hydroxymethyl transferase or serine aldolase. In rat liver mitochondria, glycine is synthesized by a unique CO_2-fixation reaction in which serine, bicarbonate and ammonia combine to yield two molecules of glycine. The β-carbon of serine and bicarbonate carbon are incorporated stoichiometrically into the α-carbon and carboxyl carbon of glycine, respectively. Methylenetetrahydrofolate may replace serine in the synthesis of glycine, supporting the following reaction schema:

$$\text{serine} + \text{tetrahydrofolate} \leftrightarrow \text{glycine} + \text{methylenetetrahydrofolate} \quad \textbf{(1)}$$
$$\text{methylenetetrahydrofolate} + CO_2 + NH_3 \leftrightarrow \text{glycine} + \text{tetrahydrofolate} \quad \textbf{(2)}$$

Additional studies have revealed that this reaction sequence requires at least two protein species, uses pyridoxal phosphate as a cofactor and catalyzes the decarboxylation as well as the synthesis of glycine. The reaction appears to operate predominantly in the direction of glycine synthesis (Arnstein and Neuberger, 1953) and is of little quantitative significance in the catabolism of glycine, except when glycine loads are administered.

Appreciable amounts of glycine are also formed from the irreversible degradation of threonine. In rats 20 to 30 per cent of dietary threonine is converted to glycine via this reaction (Meltzer and Sprinson, 1952), which is catalyzed by a widely distributed enzyme called glycinogenase or hydroxamino acid aldolase (Karasek and Greenberg, 1957). Acetaldehyde is the other product of this cleavage reaction. Sequential oxidative methylation of dimethyl glycine and sarcosine (N-methyl glycine) may also lead to glycine formation, but the quantitative importance of this pathway appears to be small (Hoskins and Mackenzie, 1961).

Finally, glycine is synthesized by the transamination of glyoxylate. The latter compound will be discussed in greater detail subsequently. Its conversion to glycine is catalyzed by several transaminases in vitro, but two specific transaminases that function with glutamic acid or alanine as the amino donors appear to be most important (Nakada, 1964). This reaction is reversible, but its thermodynamics markedly favor glycine synthesis.

Glycine Catabolism

The carbon skeleton of glycine may be oxidized completely to carbon dioxide by three routes: conversion to pyruvate via serine; condensation with succinyl Co A to yield α-amino-β-ketoadipic acid; and condensation with acetyl Co A to form α-amino-β-ketobutyric acid. The pathway to pyruvate is of quantitatively little import except after glycine loads (Arnstein and Neuberger, 1953). The condensation reactions are of considerable interest. Decarboxylation of α-amino-β-ketoadipic acid yields δ-aminolevulinic acid (ALA), the first specific precursor of the porphyrin ring, and carbon dioxide, the latter being derived from the carboxyl carbon of glycine (Kikuchi et al., 1958). The α-carbon of glycine, which becomes the C-5 of ALA, has two fates. ALA may be oxidized back to succinate (Nemeth et al., 1957) and enter the tricarboxylic acid cycle, the α-carbon of glycine ultimately appearing as carbon dioxide. Alternately, the ALA may be utilized in porphyrin biosynthesis, a pathway of greater quantitative significance. In a similiar way, glycine condenses with acetyl CoA to form α-amino-β-ketobutyric acid, which decarboxylates to aminoacetone (Elliott, 1960). The latter compound is ultimately dissimilated to ammonia and carbon dioxide via the aminoacetone cycle, described in animal liver by Urata and Granick (1963). The quantitative significance of this pathway in mammalian systems has not been established, but its distinction from the ALA pathway is secure. ALA synthetase is found in the soluble portion of the cell, whereas aminoacetone synthetase has been found only in the mitochondria (Urata and Granick, 1963). Both enzymes require pyridoxal phosphate.

Glycine may also be catabolized to glyoxylate. Glycine oxidase, now considered to be identical with D-amino acid oxidase (Neims and Hellerman, 1962), catalyzes the oxidative deamination of glycine to glyoxylate and ammonia. This enzyme is present in animal liver and kidney, but its contribution to glycine turnover is minimal. It has been estimated that only 0.2 to 0.4 per cent of net glycine turnover can be accounted for by the sum of the oxidative deamination and transamination reactions which convert glycine to glyoxylate (Elder and Wyngaarden, 1960).

Oxalate and Glyoxylate

The metabolism of glyoxylate assumes special significance in human biochemistry because of its relationship to hyperoxaluria, an inherited disorder of oxalate biosynthesis (Fig. 19–1). Three immediate precursors of glyoxylate have been identified in man: glycine; glycolic acid; and α-keto-γ-hydroxyglutarate (Goldstone and Adams, 1962; Maitra and Dekker, 1963). Although only a small proportion of glycine is metabolized via glyoxylate, this pathway is quantitatively important in oxalate and glyoxylate biosynthesis. As shown in Figure 19–1, glycine is converted to glyoxylate in two ways: first, by direct deamination; and second, via interconversion of glycine to serine followed by the formation of ethanolamine, glycolaldehyde glycolate and finally glyoxylate (Williams and Smith, 1972). The oxidation of glycolate to glyoxylate is catalyzed by the flavoprotein, glycolic acid oxidase, found in liver, kidney and other tissues (Kun et al., 1954). Lactic dehydrogenase also catalyzes the reversible interconversion of glycolate and glyoxylate (Nakada and Weinhouse, 1953). Glyoxylate is also synthesized from hydroxyproline via catabolic reactions in which α-keto-γ-hydroxyglutarate acts as the immediate precursor of glyoxylate. This sequence is reversible since labeled glyoxylate has been shown to label hydroxyproline.

In addition to these reversible processes, glyoxylate is irreversibly catabolized in three ways: It is decarboxylated to formyl CoA (Nakada and Sund, 1958). It undergoes a complex synergistic decarboxylation with α-OH-β-ketoadipate, a reaction demonstrated initially by Crawhall and Watts (1962a) and catalyzed by an enzyme called α-ketoglutarate:glyoxylate carboligase (Koch and Stokstad, 1966). Finally, glyoxylate may be oxidized to oxalic acid.

Oxalic acid, a dicarboxylic acid which readily forms a calcium salt of very low solubility in neutral or alkaline pH, is a nonessential end product of metabolism in mammalian tissues. Isotopically labeled oxalate is excreted unchanged in urine and feces and does not label expired carbon dioxide (Williams and Smith, 1972). It is absorbed poorly from the intestine (Archer et al., 1958) and cleared rapidly by the kidney. A small amount of oxalate may be synthesized in man from the catabolism of ingested ascorbic acid (Hellman and Burns, 1958). With this minor exception, all oxalate is synthesized from glyoxylate. Three, and possibly four, enzymes catalyze this reaction. Glycolic acid oxidase will convert glyoxylate to oxalate as well as glycolate to glyoxylate (Richardson and Tolbert, 1961). Xanthine oxidase, another flavoprotein, also catalyzes the conversion of glyoxylate to oxalate (Booth, 1938), as does lactic dehydrogenase (Williams and Smith, 1972). There may also be a mutase enzyme in kidney, liver and muscle (Nyhan et al., 1967), which converts two glyoxylate residues into oxalate and glycolate, respectively. The rate of oxalate synthesis depends on the size of the glyoxylate pool. Nakada and Weinhouse (1953) found that when the glyoxylate concentration in an in vitro pigeon liver homogenate system was 0.001 M or less, glyoxylate was largely oxidized to carbon dioxide, but when the glyoxylate concentration was increased to 0.01 M, oxalate synthesis equaled carbon dioxide evolution.

THE HYPERGLYCINEMIAS

In 1961 Childs and Nyhan and their coworkers described a male infant with profound metabolic ketoacidosis, protein intolerance and remarkably elevated plasma and urinary glycine concentrations. Hyperglycinemia has since been observed in children with a great diversity of clinical and biochemical abnormalities. In some, the hyperglycinemia is irregular and represents a secondary manifestation of some underlying biochemical lesion; in others, the hyperglycinemia reflects a primary dysfunction of one of the many anabolic or catabolic pathways of glycine utilization.

Classification of the Hyperglycinemias

The hyperglycinemia syndromes may be conveniently subdivided into two groups. Children with ketosis and hyperglycinemia have been designated as having the "ketotic hyperglycinemia" syndrome (Nyhan et al., 1967). It is now known that such children have primary disturbances in isoleucine, propionate or methylmalonate metabolism (see Chapter 14). The mechanism of the hyperglycinemia in these children is not known, but probably it reflects inhibition of glycine-serine interconversion by the organic acid intermediates which accumulate in these disorders (Hillman et al., 1972).

Hyperglycinemia without ketosis was first reported by Gerritsen and coworkers (1965), who noted a five-year-old boy with severe mental retardation, spastic paraplegia and seizures who had markedly elevated plasma glycine concentrations and distinctly reduced urinary oxalate. Additional patients with "nonketotic hyperglycinemia" have been described subsequently (Nyhan et al., 1967; Prader, 1967), but hypo-oxaluria has not been a constant feature. Since these patients very likely suffer from a primary disturbance in glycine catabolism, they will be discussed here.

Nonketotic Hyperglycinemia

Biochemical Abnormalities

The index case reported by Gerritsen and coworkers (1965) had plasma glycine concentrations which were 3 to 5 times normal (plasma values from 0.85 to 1.25 mM). Plasma glycine concentrations greater than 1.5 μM were noted in patients described subsequently by Ziter (1968), Baumgartner

(1969) and their colleagues. Urinary excretion of glycine is also increased 10- to 20-fold, as is the glycine concentration in the cerebrospinal fluid (Gerritsen et al., 1965; Ziter et al., 1968). All other amino acids have been found in normal amounts in these patients. Hypo-oxaluria was found in the index patient (Gerritsen et al., 1965), but subsequent investigations indicate that this is not a constant feature of the disease. Oxalate excretion was not decreased in the patients reported by Baumgartner (1969), Rampini (1967) and their associates. Furthermore, the index patient had normal urinary oxalate values when he was restudied (Gerritsen et al., 1969).

The mechanism of the hyperglycinemia in these patients has been investigated in vivo and in vitro. Affected patients are unable to clear glycine normally from the plasma after oral or parenteral loads (Gerritsen et al., 1965; Baumgartner et al., 1969). After such glycine loading, the normal increase in plasma serine concentrations was not observed, but serine loading was followed by the expected increase in plasma serine and plasma glycine values, indicating that serine metabolism was normal and that glycine utilization was impaired. The metabolism of radioisotopically labeled glycine has been evaluated in patients with nonketotic hyperglycinemia. Ando (1968), Baumgartner (1969) and their associates administered glycine-1-^{14}C and glycine-2-^{14}C to three patients and to controls. They found that the rate of formation of $^{14}CO_2$ from glycine-1-^{14}C was much slower in the patients than in controls and that this abnormality could not be attributed to differences in the glycine pool size. Whereas $^{14}CO_2$ production in controls was much faster after administration of glycine-1-^{14}C than glycine-2-^{14}C, the patients converted both isotopic forms of glycine to $^{14}CO_2$ with similar time courses. Furthermore, patients with nonketotic hyperglycinemia converted much less of the carbon-2 of glycine to carbon-3 of serine. These observations led to the thesis that the glycine decarboxylating system identified in bacteria, avian liver and mouse liver is also present in man and is defective in ketotic hyperglycinemia (Nyhan, 1972). Support for this thesis has been provided by in vitro investigations. DeGroot et al. (1970) found that the livers of three patients with nonketotic hyperglycinemia converted glycine-2-^{14}C and glycine-1-^{14}C to serine at about equal rates, whereas normal rat liver converted considerably more glycine-2-^{14}C than glycine-1-^{14}C to serine. Tada and his colleagues (1969) found that $^{14}CO_2$ production from glycine-1-^{14}C was much lower in their patient's liver than in controls and that the rate of ^{14}C incorporation into serine from glycine-1-^{14}C and glycine-2-^{14}C was also distinctly reduced. Thus, there is now convincing evidence that the primary lesion in nonketotic hyperglycinemia is a defect in the glycine cleavage reaction which gives rise to CO_2, methylenetetrahydrofolate and ammonia (see Reaction (2), p. 402).

Clinical Findings

Severe mental retardation has been the hallmark of all of the reported patients with nonketotic hyperglycinemia. The first patient reported by Gerritsen et al. (1965) lacked spontaneous movements, was listless even in the neonatal period and was admitted to an institution for retarded children at the age of 9 months. By the age of 5 years, he lay in an opisthotonic position, had seizures and was unable to move or feed himself. This clinical description has subsequently been confirmed by several groups (Ziter et al., 1968; Baumgartner et al., 1969; Tada et al., 1969), all of whom have emphasized that profound developmental retardation and seizures from the time of birth appear to be regular features of affected children.

Diagnosis

Since hyperglycinemia and hyperglycinuria occur in patients with primary disturbances of branched chain amino acid catabolism as well as in children with primary defects in glycine cleavage, one cannot make the diagnosis of nonketotic hyperglycinemia by amino acid analysis alone. This difficulty is accentuated by the hyperglycinuria which is a normal finding in newborns. At present, nonketotic hyperglycinemia should be suspected in an infant with neonatal developmental arrest, hyperglycinemia and the absence of protein-induced ketosis or acidosis. In vivo or in vitro assays of glycine-^{14}C utilization are required to confirm this diagnostic impression.

Treatment

No effective therapy is available at this time. The plasma concentrations of glycine may be lowered by dietary restriction or sodium benzoate administration (Ziter et al., 1968; Baumgartner et al., 1969), but these measures do not appear to alter the course of the disease. A transient decrease in plasma glycine was observed following administration of N^5-formyl-tetrahydrofolate (DeGroot et al., 1970). Treatment with methionine to provide free methyl groups returned plasma glycine values to normal in one patient (DeGroot et al., 1970), but it is too early to determine if such therapy has any lasting biochemical or clinical value.

Genetics

The mode of inheritance of nonketotic hyperglycinemia has not been defined. Autosomal recessive inheritance is suggested by the following features: involvement of approximately equal numbers of males and females; consanguinity among the parents of two affected female sibs (DeGroot et al., 1970); and failure to observe clinical abnormalities in the parents of affected children.

HYPERSARCOSINEMIA

Sarcosine (N-methylglycine) is an intermediate in the metabolism of glycine and serine (Fig. 19–1). It is derived from N-dimethylglycine by an oxidative demethylation reaction catalyzed by a hepatic mitochondrial enzyme (Mackenzie and Frisell, 1958). Sarcosine dehydrogenase, another mitochondrial enzyme which requires flavin adenine dinucleotide as cofactor, catalyzes the oxidative demethylation of sarcosine to glycine (Hoskins and Mackenzie, 1961). This reaction sequence is of significance because it adds methyl groups to the 1-carbon pool. No other specific metabolic role for sarcosine has been defined. In some normal humans it is undetectable in blood plasma, while in others concentrations less than 0.01 mM have been found (Gerritsen and Waisman, 1966).

Sarcosine was not implicated in human disease until 1966, when Gerritsen and Waisman described a one-year-old boy with markedly increased quantities of sarcosine in blood and urine. The patient suffered from profound developmental retardation from birth and died at one year of age. He excreted more than 1 millimole of sarcosine daily in the urine and had plasma concentrations recorded of 0.13 to 0.26 mM. The patient's mildly retarded sister also had distinct hypersarcosinemia and sarcosinuria, but another retarded sister had a normal plasma sarcosine value. Oral loads of sarcosine or dimethylglycine were administered to the patient's parents, sibs and relatives. His mother, brother and two maternal relatives excreted abnormal amounts of sarcosine after such loads, but his father did not. No other abnormalities in plasma or urinary amino acids were noted in the family or the patient. Gerritsen and Waisman proposed that the patient had an inherited defect of sarcosine dehydrogenase, but they were unable to carry out the necessary in vitro studies prior to the patient's death.

Several children with hypersarcosinemia have been described subsequently (Hagge et al., 1967; Scott et al., 1970; Glorieux et al., 1970). No reproducible clinical phenotype has emerged, suggesting that hypersarcosinemia is a benign trait (Hagge et al., 1967; Glorieux et al., 1970). Oral loading studies in parents of affected children have usually shown either elevated plasma or urinary sarcosine values, suggesting that such parents are heterozygous carriers for a mutant gene which, in double dose, results in sustained hypersarcosinemia. Since sarcosine dehydrogenase activity has not been found in peripheral blood leukocytes or cultured skin fibroblasts (Scott et al., 1970; Glorieux et al., 1970), verification of the presumed enzymatic defect still awaits in vitro assays with liver or kidney tissue.

HYPEROXALURIA

Oxalate is the major constituent of 65 to 75 per cent of all kidney stones. Most patients who form calcium oxalate stones have no apparent defect in oxalate metabolism. In this group nephrolithiasis is caused by excessive excretion of calcium or by a presumed physiochemical abnormality of the urine which predisposes to stone formation despite normal concentrations of calcium and oxalate. A small fraction of patients with calcium oxalate stones, however, have *primary hyperoxaluria*. This is a general term for two rare, inherited disorders which are characterized by excretion of large amounts of oxalate, nephrolithiasis, nephrocalcinosis and the early onset of renal failure. In these patients calcium oxalate deposits may be found in the kidney and extrarenal tissues, a condition referred to as *oxalosis*. Family studies indicate that both types of primary hyperoxaluria (I and II) are inherited as autosomal recessive traits. Recent studies have demonstrated that the mutant phenotype in Type I hyperoxaluria (also called glycolic aciduria) is produced by a defect in glyoxylate metabolism, whereas Type II hyperoxaluria (also called L-glyceric aciduria) is caused by a defect in hydroxypyruvate metabolism.

Early Description

In 1950 Davis and coworkers described extensive extrarenal deposits of calcium oxalate in a 12-year-old boy who had died of uremia secondary to calcium oxalate nephrolithiasis and nephrocalcinosis. Newns and Black (1953) recorded excessive oxalate excretion in a patient with recurrent nephrolithiasis in 1953, but no tissue examinations or stone analyses were performed. All the essential criteria for primary hyperoxaluria and oxalosis were present in twin boys described in 1954 by Aponte and Fetter. These children excreted 180 to 200 mg of oxalate in the urine, formed calcium oxalate kidney stones and showed calcium oxalate deposits in the bone marrow at autopsy. Many additional patients with this constellation have been described since, but only recently has the nature of the biochemical lesion been elucidated.

Chemical Abnormalities

The oxalate content of normal urine is less than 50 mg per 25 hours (Williams and Smith, 1972; Smith and Williams, 1967a). Patients with primary hyperoxaluria excrete 150 to 650 mg of oxalate per day. Most patients with hyperoxaluria excrete as much glycolate as oxalate, the former being a precursor of glyoxylate (Fig. 19–2). (The absence of glycolicaciduria in patients with hyperoxaluria was responsible for defining a new genetic variant of this disorder, and we shall return to this matter subsequently.) Since the widespread deposition of oxalate in these patients is obviously not produced by failure to excrete this compound, only three other general pathophysiological mechanisms need be entertained: decreased catabolism, increased absorption or increased biosynthesis. Decreased catabolism can be excluded because oxalate is a metabolic end product in man (Williams and Smith, 1972). Oxalate is poorly absorbed from the intestine, and patients with primary hyperoxaluria do not absorb increased amounts of this organic acid (Archer et al., 1958); therefore, hyperoxaluria must be caused by excessive biosynthesis of oxalic acid.

Only two known pathways for oxalate biosynthesis exist. A small amount of oxalate is synthesized from the catabolism of ascorbic acid (Hellman and Burns, 1958), but the amount formed in this way could not explain the findings in hyperoxaluria. Most oxalate is formed by the irreversible oxidation of glyoxylate. Hence, excessive oxalate synthesis in hyperoxaluria can be explained only by an increased activity of the enzymes which catalyze the oxidation of glyoxylate to oxalate or an increased concentration or pool size of glyoxylate. Crawhall and Watts (1962b) and Frederick et al. (1963) found that oxidation of glyoxylate-^{14}C to oxalate by hepatic mitochondria from patients with hyperoxaluria was normal. This observation indicates that the activity of glycolic acid oxidase, xanthine oxidase and lactic dehydrogenase, all of which may convert glyoxylate to oxalate, is normal in this disorder. By exclusion, the basis for the excessive oxalate synthesis had to be found in the pathways of glyoxylate metabolism.

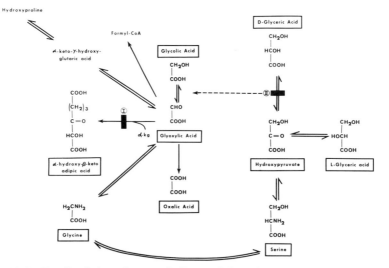

Figure 19–2 Details of glyoxylate metabolism and sites of metabolic defects in hyperoxaluria Types I and II. The solid bar marked I denotes the reaction catalyzed by glyoxylate: α-ketoglutarate carboligase, the enzyme deficient in Type I hyperoxaluria. The bar marked II denotes the reaction catalyzed by D-glyceric acid dehydrogenase, the enzyme deficient in Type II hyperoxaluria. The dotted line represents the postulated identity of D-glycerate dehydrogenase and glyoxylate reductase.

Type I Hyperoxaluria

As noted in Figure 19–2, glyoxylate is formed and dissimilated in several ways. A block in any of these pathways could lead to an accumulation of glyoxylate and, secondarily, to excessive oxalate formation. Since most patients with hyperoxaluria excrete excess glycolate as well as oxalate, a block in the interconversion of glycolate and glyoxylate can be ruled out. Frederick et al. (1963) administered glyoxylate-^{14}C to patients with hyperoxaluria and found that the rate of incorporation of label into carbon dioxide and glycine was decreased. This observation suggested a defect in the transamination of glyoxylate to glycine, but in vitro studies failed to confirm such an abnormality (Smith and Williams, 1967a), and the in vivo observations probably reflected dilution of the labeled glyoxylate in an enlarged glyoxylate pool rather than a defect in glycine synthesis. Glyoxylate may be decarboxylated to formyl CoA, but this conversion is quantitatively so minor that it has not been studied in human tissues (Smith and Williams, 1967a). Similarly, the aldolase reaction whereby glyoxylate condenses with pyruvate to yield α-keto-γ-hydroxyglutarate was found to be of very low activity in human liver and has not been studied in hyperoxaluria (Smith and Williams, 1967a).

Crawhall and Watts (1962a) demonstrated that the synergistic decarboxylation of α-ketoglutarate and glyoxylate in intact mitochondria leads to the formation of α-hydroxyl-β-ketoadipic acid. The activity of the enzyme which catalyzes this carboligase reaction in mitochondria from patients with hyperoxaluria was found to be normal by Crawhall and Watts (1962b) and by Koch et al. (1967). The latter group found, however, that the carboligase activity in the soluble fraction of hepatic, splenic and renal tissue was markedly reduced in five patients with hyperoxaluria (Koch et al., 1967). Furthermore, mixtures of enzyme preparations from controls and patients failed to demonstrate inhibition. These results indicate that patients with hyperoxaluria and glycolic aciduria (Type I) suffer from an inherited defect of the soluble α-ketoglutarate:glyoxylate carboligase which leads to an accumulation of glyoxylate and secondarily, to increased biosynthesis of oxalate and glycolate.

Type II Hyperoxaluria

Williams and Smith (1967, 1968) described four patients in two families who had hyperoxaluria and calcium oxalate nephrolithiasis but who did not excrete excessive amounts of glycolic acid. These patients excreted large amounts of D-glyceric acid in the urine, a compound not detectable in normal urine or in that of patients with the usual type of hyperoxaluria. These findings suggested that a different biochemical defect was responsible for the hyperoxaluria in this group of patients, and additional studies have confirmed this concept.

Patients with D-glycericaciduria and oxaluria failed to incorporate glyoxylate-^{14}C into urinary glycolate, in sharp contrast to the extensive incorporation found in patients with glycolicaciduria and oxaluria. Administration of β-hydroxypyruvate-^{14}C to a patient with glycericaciduria led to significant labeling of urinary glycerate but *not* oxalate or glycolate, indicating the lack of any precursor-product relationship between hydroxypyruvate and glyoxylate (Fig. 19–2). Finally, D-glyceric acid dehydrogenase activity was assayed in leukocytes from four patients with glycericaciduria and hyperoxaluria. No detectable enzymatic activity was found when compared with leukocyte preparations from 12 control subjects (Williams and Smith, 1968). These results demonstrate a defect in the interconversion of D-glycerate and β-hydroxypyruvate and provide a logical basis for the glycericaciduria.

Williams and Smith suggest that D-glyceric acid dehydrogenase and glyoxylate reductase (which converts glyoxylate to glycolate) are the same enzyme and that a block in the pathway from glyoxylate to glycolate produced by the enzymatic defect shown in Figure 19–2 leads to hyperoxaluria and reduced glycolic acid excretion. D-Glyceric acid could also act as an inhibitor of glyoxylate reductase and lead to the same chemical consequences. They suggested that the disorder characterized by excessive excretion of oxalate and D-glycerate be called "hyperoxaluria Type II."

Genetics

Approximately equal numbers of affected males and females have been reported in Type I hyperoxaluria (Hockaday et al., 1964). Hyperoxaluria and oxalosis have been described in siblings several times (Williams and Smith, 1972) and in identical twins (Aponte and Fetter, 1954). Consanguinity has been demonstrated in several families (Hockaday et al., 1964). These findings are all consistent with autosomal recessive inheritance and suggest that affected patients are homozygous for the carboligase defect described previously. Heterozygous carriers do not excrete oxalate or glycolate in increased amounts, but carboligase assays in such individuals have not been reported. Williams and Smith (1968) found that D-glyceric acid dehydrogenase activity in the leukocytes of the mother of three patients with hyperoxaluria Type II was below that observed in controls, but the father's cells were normal. Additional families must be identified and studied before a definitive statement about the mode of inheritance of Type II hyperoxaluria can be made.

A dominant mode of inheritance has apparently been demonstrated in a few families. Shepard and his colleagues (1960) reported hyperoxaluria in two, and possibly three, successive generations in a single family. In addition, hyperoxaluria has been noted in one parent of affected children in at least three families (Williams and Smith, 1972). These observations are hard to reconcile with a recessive trait and suggest that there may be other genetic disturbances which lead to excessive oxalate synthesis.

Clinical Considerations

Nephrolithiasis and oxalosis may become manifest during the first year of life (Williams and Smith, 1972; Hockaday et al., 1964). Most patients experience initial symptoms of renal colic or hematuria between two and ten years of age and succumb because of uremia before age 20. In patients with a delayed onset of symptoms, survival to age 50 or 60 has been reported. The symptoms of renal colic and uremia which these patients develop are identical to those noted in patients with other kinds of calculi and renal disease. X-rays reveal radiopaque calculi and nephrocalcinosis, but these findings are nonspecific.

Pathology

Renal lithiasis, nephrocalcinosis, pyelonephritis, hydronephrosis and scarring have all been reported in the kidneys of patients with hyperoxaluria. Refractile crystals may be seen in the proximal tubule or in small blood vessels, but these abnormalities are not diagnostic. Extrarenal deposits of oxalate have had a predilection for the heart, male urogenital tract and bone (both Haversian systems and marrow). Crystals are frequently found in the walls of arteries and veins and have thus appeared in all tissues. No corneal deposits have been described.

Diagnosis

Since calcium oxalate stones are most common, a diagnosis of hyperoxaluria must depend on quantitative measurements of urinary oxalate. Acquired hyperoxaluria has been reported with rhubarb ingestion (Jeghers and Murphy, 1945), ethylene glycol poisoning (Gessner et al., 1960), pyridoxine deficiency (Faber et al., 1963) and thiamine deficiency (Liang, 1962), but these conditions may be excluded with relative ease. Hyperoxaluria and recurrent calcium oxalate nephrolithiasis have also been reported in several patients with ileal resections (Smith et al., 1972; Admirand et al., 1971; Dowling et al., 1971). The mechanism of hyperoxaluria in this setting remains undefined, but the beneficial effect of taurine and cholestyromine administration suggest an acquired abnormality of bile salt metabolism. These patients do not excrete excesses of glycolic acid or L-glyceric acid and hence can be distinguished readily from patients with either form of primary hyperoxaluria.

Treatment

The treatment of inherited hyperoxaluria has been far from satisfactory (Smith and Williams, 1967b). Urine oxalate concentration can be reduced by increasing urine flow rate or by decreasing oxalate synthesis. Frederick (1963), McLaurin (1961) and their associates found that a high phosphate diet seemed to reduce the frequency of attacks of renal colic without changing urinary oxalate. Administration of calcium carbimide, a potent inhibitor of the enzyme which catalyzes the conversion of glycolaldehyde to glycolate (Fig. 19–1), was reported initially to produce promising reductions in urinary oxalate excretion (Solomons et al., 1967). Other workers (Gibbs and Watts, 1970; Smith et al., 1969; Williams and Smith, 1972) have failed to confirm these findings. Several groups have reported distinct decreases in urinary oxalate after large doses of pyridoxine (Smith and Williams, 1967b; Gibbs and Watts, 1970; Williams and Smith, 1972). This approach must now be evaluated in a larger number of patients. Finally, renal transplantation has been attempted in patients with primary hyperoxaluria, but the results have been disappointing.

REFERENCES

Admirand, W., Earnest, D., and Williams, H. E.: Hyperoxaluria and bowel disease. Trans. Ass. Amer. Physicians 84:307–312, 1971.

Ando, T., Nyhan, W. L., Gerritsen, T., Gong, L., Heiner, D. C., and Bray, P. F.: Metabolism of glycine in the nonketotic form of hyperglycinemia. Pediat. Res. 2:254–263, 1968.

Aponte, B. E., and Fetter, T. R.: Familial idiopathic oxalate nephrocalcinosis. Amer. J. Clin. Path. 24:1363–1373, 1954.

Archer, H. E., Dormer, A. E., Scowen, E. F., and Watts, R. W. E.: The aetiology of primary hyperoxaluria. Brit. Med. J. 1:175–181, 1958.

Arnstein, H. R. V., and Neuberger, A.: The synthesis of glycine and serine by the rat. Biochem. J. 55:271–280, 1953.

Baumgartner, R., Ando, T., and Nyhan, W. L.: Nonketotic hyperglycinemia. J. Pediat. 75:1022–1030, 1969.

Booth, V. H.: The specificity of xanthine oxidase. Biochem. J. 32:494–502, 1938.

Childs, B., Nyhan, W. L., Borden, M., Bard, L., and Cooke, R. E.: Idiopathic hyperglycinemia and hyperglycinuria: A new disorder of amino acid metabolism. I. Pediatrics 27:522–538, 1961.

Crawhall, J. C., and Watts, R. W. E.: The metabolism of glyoxylate by human- and rat-liver mitochondria. Biochem. J. 85:163–171, 1962a.

Crawhall, J. C., and Watts, R. W. E.: The metabolism of (1-^{14}C) glyoxylate by the liver mitochondria of patients with primary hyperoxaluria and nonhyperoxaluric subjects. Clin. Sci. *23*:163–168, 1962b.

Davis, J. S., Klingberg, W. G., and Stowell, R. E.: Nephrolithiasis and nephrocalcinosis with calcium oxalate crystals in kidneys and bones. J. Pediat. *36*:323–334, 1950.

DeGroot, C. J., Troelstra, J. A., and Hommes, F. A.: The enzymatic defect of the nonketotic form of hyperglycinemia. Pediat. Res. *4*:238–243, 1970.

Dowling, R. H., Rose, G. A., and Sutor, D. J.: Hyperoxaluria and renal calculi in ileal disease. Lancet (i), 1103–1106, 1971.

Elder, T. D., and Wyngaarden, J. B.: The biosynthesis and turnover of oxalate in normal and hyperoxaluric subjects. J. Clin. Invest. *39*:1337–1344, 1960.

Elliot, W. H.: Aminoacetone formation by Staphylococcus aureus. Biochem. J. *74*:478–485, 1960.

Faber, S. R., Feitler, W. W., Bleiler, R. E., Ohlson, M. A., and Hodges, R. E.: The effects of an induced pyridoxine and pantothenic acid deficiency in excretions of oxalic and xanthurenic acids in the urine. Amer. J. Clin. Nutr. *12*:406–412, 1963.

Frederick, E. W., Rabkin, M. T., Richie, R. H., Jr., and Smith, L. H., Jr.: Studies on primary hyperoxaluria. I. In vivo demonstration of a defect in glyoxylate metabolism. New Eng. J. Med. *269*:821–829, 1963.

Gerritsen, T., Kaveggia, E., and Waisman, H. A.: A new type of idiopathic hyperglycinemia with hypo-oxaluria. Pediatrics *36*:882–891, 1965.

Gerritsen, T., Nyhan, W. L., Rehberg, M. L., and Ando, T.: Metabolism of glyoxylate in nonketotic hyperglycinemia. Pediat. Res. *3*:269–274, 1969.

Gerritsen, T., and Waisman, H. A.: Hypersarcosinemia. An inborn error of metabolism. New Eng. J. Med. *275*:66–69, 1966.

Gessner, P. K., Parke, D. V., and Williams, R. T.: Studies in detoxication: The metabolism of glycols. Biochem. J. *74*:1–5, 1960.

Gibbs, D., and Watts, R. W. E.: The action of pyridoxine in primary hyperoxaluria. Clin. Sci. *38*: 277–286, 1970.

Glorieux, F. H., Scriver, C. R., Delvin, E., and Mohyuddin, F.: Transport and metabolism of sarcosine in hypersarcosinemic and normal phenotypes. J. Clin. Invest. *50*:2313–2322, 1970.

Goldstone, A., and Adams, E.: Metabolism of α-hydroxyglutamic acid. J. Biol. Chem. *237*:3476–3485, 1962.

Gutman, A. B., T'sai, F. Y., Black, H., Yalow, R. S., and Berson, S. A.: Incorporation of glycine-1-C^{14}, glycine-2-C^{14} and glycine-N^{15} into uric acid in normal and gouty subjects. Amer. J. Med. *25*:917–932, 1958.

Hagge, W., Brodehl, J., and Gellissen, K.: Hypersarcosinemia. Pediat. Res. *1*:409, 1967.

Hellman, L., and Burns, J. J.: Metabolism of 1-ascorbic acid-1-C^{14} in man. J. Biol. Chem. *230*: 923–930, 1958.

Hillman, R. E., Feigin, R. D., Tenebaum, S. M., and Keating, J. P.: Defective isoleucine metabolism as a cause of the "ketotic hyperglycinemia" syndrome. (Abstract.) Pediat. Res. *6*:394, 1972.

Hockaday, T. D. R., Clayton, J. E., Frederick, E. W., and Smith, L. H., Jr.: Primary oxaluria. Medicine *43*:315–345, 1964.

Hoskins, D. D., and Mackenzie, C. G.: Solubilization and electron transfer flavoprotein requirement of mitochondrial sarcosine dehydrogenase and dimethylglycine dehydrogenase. J. Biol. Chem. *236*:177–183, 1961.

Jeghers, H., and Murphy, R.: Practical aspects of oxalate metabolism. New Eng. J. Med. *233*:208–215, 1945.

Karasek, M. A., and Greenberg, D. M.: Studies on the properties of threonine aldolases. J. Biol. Chem. *227*:191–205, 1957.

Kawasaki, H., Sato, T., and Kikuchi, G.: A new reaction for glycine biosynthesis. Biochem. Biophys. Res. Commun. *23*:227–233, 1966.

Kikuchi, G., Kumar, A., Talmage, P., and Shemin, D.: The enzymatic synthesis of α-aminolevulinic acid. J. Biol. Chem. *233*:1214–1219, 1958.

Kisliuk, R. L., and Sakami, W.: A study of the mechanism of serine biosynthesis. J. Biol. Chem. *214*:47–57, 1955.

Koch, J., and Stokstad, E. L. R.: Partial purification of a 2-oxo-glutarate:glyoxylate carboligase from rat liver mitochondria. Biochem. Biophys. Res. Commun. *23*:585–591, 1966.

Koch, J., Stokstad, E. L. R., Williams, H. E., and Smith, L. H.: Deficiency of 2-oxo-glutarate:glyoxylate carboligase activity in primary hyperoxaluria. Proc. Nat. Acad. Sci. U.S.A. *57*:1123–1129, 1967.

Kun, E., Dechary, J. M., and Pitot, H. C.: The oxidation of glycolic acid by a liver enzyme. J. Biol. Chem. *210*:269–280, 1954.

Liang, C. C.: Studies of experimental thiamine deficiency. 2. Tissue breakdown and glyoxylic acid formation. Biochem. J. *83*:101–106, 1962.

Mackenzie, C. G., and Frisell, W. R.: The metabolism of dimethylglycine by liver mitochondria. J. Biol. Chem. *232*:417–427, 1958.

Maitra, U., and Dekker, E. E.: Enzymatic steps in the conversion of α-hydroxyglutamate to glyoxylate and alanine. J. Biol. Chem. *238*:3660–3669, 1963.

McLaurin, A. W., Beisel, W. R., McCormick, G. J., Scalettar, R., and Herman, R. H.: Primary hyperoxaluria. Ann. Intern. Med. *55*:70–80, 1961.

Meltzer, H. L., and Sprinson, D. B.: The synthesis of 4-C^{14},N^{15}-1-threonine and a study of its metabolism. J. Biol. Chem. *197*:461–474, 1952.

Motokawa, Y., and Kikuchi, G.: Glycine metabolism by rat liver mitochondria. II. Methylene tetrahydrofolate as the direct one carbon donor in the reaction of glycine synthesis. J. Biochem. *65*:71–76, 1969.

Nakada, H. I.: Glutamic-glycine transaminase from rat-liver. J. Biol. Chem. *239*:468–471, 1964.

Nakada, H. I., and Sund, L. P.: Glyoxylic acid oxidation by rat liver. J. Biol. Chem. *233*:8–13, 1958.

Nakada, H. I., and Weinhouse, S.: Studies of glycine oxidation in rat tissues. Arch. Biochem. *42*: 257–270, 1953.

Neims, A. H., and Hellerman, L.: Specificity of the D-amino acid oxidase in relation to glycine oxidase activity. J. Biol. Chem. *237*:PC976, 1962.

Nemeth, A. M., Russell, C. S., and Shemin, D.: The succinate-glycine cycle. II. Metabolism of α-aminolevulinic acid. J. Biol. Chem. *229*:415–422, 1957.

Newns, G. H., and Black, J. A.: Case of calcium oxalate nephrocalcinosis. Gt. Ormond Str. J. *5*:40–44, 1953.

Nyhan, W. L.: Nonketotic hyperglycinemia. *In* Stanbury, J. B., Wyngaarden, J. B., and Fredrickson, D. S., eds., The Metabolic Basis of Inherited Disease, 3rd edition. McGraw-Hill, New York, pp. 464–475, 1972.

Nyhan, W. L., Ando, T., and Gerritsen, T.: Hyperglycinemia. *In* Nyhan, W. L., ed., Amino Acid Metabolism and Genetic Variation. McGraw-Hill, New York, pp. 255–265, 1967.

Paik, W. K., and Benoiten, L.: Purification and properties of hog kidney ε-lysine acylase. Canad. J. Biochem. *41*:1643–1654, 1963.

Prader, A.: Discussion of papers on hyperglycinemia. Amer. J. Dis. Child. *113*:137, 1967.

Rampini, S., Vischer, D., Curtius, H. C., Anders, P. W., Tancredi, F., Frisch-Knecht, W., and Prader, A.: Hereditäre Hyperglycinämie. Klinisches Bild und Bestimmung von Glyoxysäure und Oxalsäure im Urin bei je einem Patienten mit der acidotischen und der nicht-acidotischen Form. Helv. Paediat. Acta *22*:135–159, 1967.

Ratner, S., Nocito, V., and Green, D. E.: Glycine oxidase. J. Biol. Chem. *152*:119–133, 1944.

Richardson, K. E., and Tolbert, N. E.: Oxidation of glyoxylic acid to oxalic acid by glycolic acid oxidase. J. Biol. Chem. *236*:1280–1284, 1961.

Ryan, W. L., and Wells, I. C.: Homocitrulline and homoarginine synthesis from lysine. Science *144*:1122–1127, 1964.

Sato, T., Kochi, H., Motokawa, Y., Kawasaki, H., and Kikuchi, G.: Glycine metabolism by rat liver mitochondria. I. Synthesis of two molecules of glycine from one molecule each of serine, bicarbonate and ammonia. J. Biochem. *65*:63–70, 1969a.

Sato, T., Kochi, H., Sato, N., and Kikuchi, G.: Glycine metabolism by rat liver mitochondria. III. The glycine cleavage and the exchange of carboxyl carbon of glycine with bicarbonate. J. Biochem. *65*:77–83, 1969b.

Schoenheimer, R., and Rittenberg, D.: The study of intermediary metabolism of animals with the aid of isotopes. Physiol. Rev. *20*:218–248, 1940.

Scott, C. R., Clark, S. H., Teng, C. C., and Svedberg, K. R.: Clinical and cellular studies of sarcosinemia. J. Pediat. *77*:805–811, 1970.

Shemin, D.: The biological conversion of L-serine to glycine. J. Biol. Chem. *162*:297–307, 1946.

Shepard, T. H., Lee, L. W., and Krebs, E. G.: Primary hyperoxaluria. II. Genetic studies in a family. Pediatrics *25*:869–871, 1960.

Siekevitz, P., and Greenberg, D. M.: The biological formation of serine from glycine. J. Biol. Chem. *180*:845–856, 1949.

Smith, L. H., Jr., Fromm, H., and Hofmann, A. F.: Acquired hyperoxaluria, nephrolithiasis and intestinal disease. New Eng. J. Med. *286*:1371–1375, 1972.

Smith, L. H., Jr., Jones, J. D., and Keating, F. R., Jr.: Primary hyperoxaluria. *In* Hodgkinson, A., and Nordin, B. E. C., eds., Renal Stone Research Symposium. Churchill, London, p. 297, 1969.

Smith, L. H., Jr., and Williams, H. E.: Hyperoxaluria (glycolic aciduria). *In* Nyhan, W. L., ed., Amino Acid Metabolism and Genetic Variation. McGraw-Hill, New York, pp. 239–247, 1967a.

Smith, L. H., Jr., and Williams, H. E.: Treatment of primary hyperoxaluria. Mod. Treatm. *4*:522–530, 1967b.

Solomons, C. C., Goodman, S. I., and Riley, C. M.: Calcium carbimide in the treatment of primary hyperoxaluria. New Eng. J. Med. *276*:207–210, 1967.

Tada, K., Narisawa, K., Yoshida, T., Konno, T., Yokoyama, Y., Nakagawa, H., Tanno, K., Mochizuki, K., Arakawa, T., Yoshida, T., and Kikuchi, G.: Hyperglycinemia: A defect in glycine cleavage reaction. Tohoku J. Exp. Med. *98*:289–296, 1969.

Urata, G., and Granick, S.: Biosynthesis of α-aminoketones and the metabolism of amino-acetone. J. Biol. Chem. *238*:811–820, 1963.

Wada, Y., Tada, K., Takada, G., Omura, K., Yoshida, T., Kuniya, T., Auyama, T., Hakui, T., and Harada, S.: Hyperglycinemia associated with hyperammonemia: In vitro glycine cleavage in liver. Pediat. Res. *6*:622–625, 1972.

Watts, R. W. E., and Crawhall, J. C.: The first glycine metabolic pool in man. Biochem. J. *73*:277–286, 1959.

Whelan, T., and Scriver, C. R.: Cystathioninuria and renal iminoglycinuria in a pedigree. New Eng. J. Med. *278*:924–927, 1968.

Williams, H. E., and Smith, L. H., Jr.: L-Glyceric aciduria. A new genetic variant of primary hyperoxaluria. New Eng. J. Med. *278*:233–239, 1968.

Williams, H. E., and Smith, L. H., Jr.: Hyperoxaluria (L-glyceric aciduria). *In* Nyhan, W. L., ed., Amino Acid Metabolism and Genetic Variation. McGraw-Hill, New York, pp. 249–254, 1967.

Williams, H. E., and Smith, L. H., Jr.: Primary hyperoxaluria. *In* Stanbury, J. B., Wyngaarden, J. B., and Fredrickson, D. S., eds., The Metabolic Basis of Inherited Disease, 3rd edition. McGraw-Hill, New York, pp. 196–219, 1972.

Winnick, T., Moring-Claesson, I., and Greenberg, D. M.: Distribution of radioactive carbon among certain amino acids of liver homogenate protein, following uptake experiments with labeled glycine. J. Biol. Chem. *175*:127–132, 1948.

Zarembski, P. M., Hodgkinson, A., and Cochran, M.: Treatment of primary hyperoxaluria with calcium carbimide. New Eng. J. Med. *277*:1000–1002, 1967.

Ziter, F. A., Bray, P. F., Madsen, J. A., and Nyhan, W. L.: The clinical findings in a patient with non-ketotic hyperglycinemia. Pediat. Res. *2*:250–253, 1968.

Chapter Twenty

IMINO ACIDS

THE HYPERPROLINEMIAS

Hyperprolinemia is the result of an autosomal recessive trait characterized by accumulation of free L-proline in body fluids as well as iminoglycinuria, reflecting both saturation and competition during tubular absorption of proline, hydroxyproline and glycine. The condition has two known causes: deficiency of proline oxidase (Type I) and deficiency of Δ'pyrroline-5-carboxylic acid dehydrogenase (Type II); the latter form is accompanied by excessive urinary excretion of Δ'pyrroline-5-carboxylic acid (PC). Clinical symptoms of hereditary renal disease or epilepsy have been found in some patients with the trait; it is possible that these clinical features are coincidental and not directly related to the hereditary metabolic disorder.

Proline Metabolism

A thorough review of the metabolism and biochemistry of proline is available for the interested reader in the International Review of Connective Tissue Research (Adams, 1970). L-Proline is a nonessential amino acid for which the

415

trivial term imino acid is often used to indicate the configuration of the amino group of pyrrolidine-2-carboxylic acid.

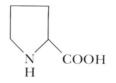

Biosynthesis

Strecker (1957) has shown that proline synthesis in biological systems is achieved by an irreversible pathway (Fig. 20–1). Much of this work was done with bacterial mutants, but earlier studies by Stetten and Schoenheimer (1944) showed that glutamic acid is converted to PC in mammalian tissue; the latter compound is then reduced by a second enzyme (PC reductase) to form L-proline.

Degradation Pathway

L-Proline is catabolized by conversion to PC and then to glutamic acid (Fig. 20–1). The enzymes required for these steps are independent of those employed for proline biosynthesis (Strecker, 1957). Proline oxidase is located on the inner membrane of the mitochondrion, whereas the next enzyme (PC dehydrogenase) in the degradation sequence is found in the cytosol (Brunner and Neupert, 1969).

The degradation of proline introduces its attached nitrogen moiety into the urea cycle through ornithine (Sporn et al., 1959). Entry of the carbon moiety of proline into the tricarboxylic cycle can also occur after transamination of glutamic acid to α-ketoglutaric acid. Proline is also available for conversion to γ-aminobutyric acid via glutamate in brain and kidney. Proline oxidation is known to be active in liver and brain, but the oxidation rate in kidney is probably higher than in any other tissue (Felig et al., 1969; Baerlocher et al., 1971).

Distribution in Body Fluids

The normal concentration of L-proline in plasma is about 0.1 to 0.35 mM; it is scarcely detectable in cerebrospinal fluid. Its renal clearance is normally very low, indicating efficient cellular transport at physiological concentrations (Scriver, 1969). At plasma concentrations above about 0.15 mM, proline reabsorption in the renal tubule is shared with hydroxyproline and glycine (Mohyuddin and Scriver, 1970). Proline has the greatest preference for this transport system, and it will competitively displace the other two solutes if its concentration is raised sufficiently. Scriver and colleagues (1964) demonstrated that tubular absorption of L-proline is saturable, and a maximum rate of reabsorption (T_m) has been demonstrated. These attributes of proline transport in kidney account for some of the characteristic features of the hyperprolinemic traits.

Two forms of hyperprolinemia, which appear to be genetically independent, have been identified; the published pedigrees with Type I hyperprolinemia (oxidase deficiency) and Type II trait (PC-dehydrogenase deficiency) are now quite numerous (Table 20–1).

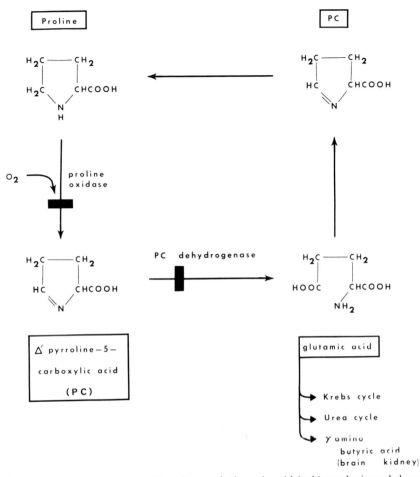

Figure 20–1 Interconversion of proline and glutamic acid in biosynthetic and degradative pathways (adapted from Strecker, 1957). Nonenzymatic interconversion between Δ' pyrroline-5-carboxylic acid and glutamic acid-γ-semialdehyde occurs by the removal or addition of water across the C=N bond, in the step leading to glutamate formation. The outflow of the proline carbon chain and amino group to other metabolic pathways is indicated. The sites of the inherited blocks in Type I hyperprolinemia (oxidase deficiency) and in Type II hyperprolinemia (dehydrogenase deficiency) are indicated.

Type I Hyperprolinemia

The original description of hyperprolinemia by Scriver and colleagues (1961; Schafer et al., 1962) raised the important question of whether the imino-acidopathy causes clinical disease. An association between renal disease and the disturbance of proline oxidation was apparent in some members of the large original pedigree (Fig. 20–2). However, careful perusal of inheritance patterns in this pedigree revealed that hyperprolinemia appears as an autosomal recessive trait, whereas the familial renal disease is dominantly inherited. Consequently, there was no reason to believe that the renal and proline traits were more than coincidentally associated with each other in this family.

This impression gained support when numerous families with various hereditary forms of nephropathy were examined for presence of the imino-acidopathy; no evidence of the latter was found in any of these pedigrees.

Table 20-1 Hyperprolinemia, Types I and II

Pedigree	Reference	Presumed Type[a]	Age of Proband at Diagnosis (yr)	Sex	Plasma Proline mM[b]	In Proband				Consanguinity in Parents	In Relatives (Number Affected)		
						Renal Disease	Deafness	Mental Retardation	Seizures		Proline Defect (alone)	Clinical Disease (alone)	Proline Defect and Clinical Disease
A	Scriver et al., 1961; Schafer et al., 1962	I	5	M	0.67	+	+	+	+	0	0	19	3
B	Kopelman et al., 1964	I(?)	13	M	0.51*	+	?	0	0	?	2	(1)?	1
C	Efron, 1965	I	33	M	1.15–1.8	+	0	+	0	0	0	5	3
D[c]	Berlow and Efron, 1964; Efron, 1966; Selkoe, 1969.	II	19/12	M	3.7	0	0	+	+	0	0	0	0
E	Perry et al., 1968	I	3	M	0.79–1.26	+	0	+	0	+	5	3	5
F	Similä and Visakorpi, 1967; Similä, 1970	II	6/12	M	3.5	0	0	+	+	+	0	?	1
G	Emery et al., 1968	II	18	F	1.75–2.6	0	0	+	+	+	0	0	(1)?
H	Goyer et al., 1968												
I	Piesowicz, 1968;	I(?)	14	F	0.81	+	+	0	0	+	0	10	2
	Harries et al., 1971	I	6/12	M	2.2–2.6	0	0	+	+	0	2	0	0

Table 20-1 Hyperprolinemia, Types I and II (*Continued*)

		Type[a]		Sex	Proline[b]										
J	Fontaine, 1969; Fontaine et al., 1970	I	9/12	F	0.72–1.0	0	0	0	0	0	0	0	0	6	0
K	Woody et al., 1969	I	3/12	M	1.3–1.85*	+	?	+	–	+	?	+	4	Many	3
L	Jeune et al., 1970[d]	II	4/12	M	0.47–1.2	0	?	0	+	+	?	0	0	0	1
M	Goodman, 1970	II	9	F	1.65	0	0	0	0	0	0	0	0	0	0
N	Mollica et al., 1971	I	20/12	F	1.07	0	0	0	0	0	0	0	6	0	0
O	Applegarth et al., 1971	II	13	M	3.1	0	0	0	0[e]	0	0	0	?	0	?

[a]Type I = block at proline oxidase; Type II = block at Δ'pyrroline-5-carboxylic acid (PC dehydrogenase); ? = PC excretion not mentioned—presumed that defect is Type I.

[b]Normal values (range) for all ages, infant to adult, 0.10 to 0.35 mM. Results obtained by quantitative analysis by elution chromatography on ion exchange resin columns, except in pedigrees B and K (where direct chemical methods were used for proline analysis).

[c]An additional patient with Type II hyperprolinemia and convulsions is mentioned by Efron (1967). The details on this patient appear to be equivalent to those presented in detail by Selkoe (1969).

[d]A coexistent transaminase defect in propositus caused hyperleucine-isoleucinemia. The patient thus has a double aminoacidopathy.

[e]One seizure with fever at 2 years of age; EEG mildly abnormal at 13 years, suggesting epileptic disorder without localizing features.

*Direct chemical methods used for proline analysis.

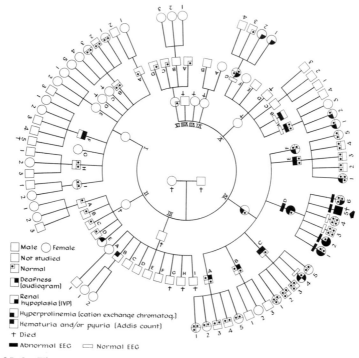

Figure 20-2 The maternal pedigree of original propositus (arrow) with hyperprolinemia (Schafer et al., 1962); the latter appears as a recessive trait. A congenital nephropathy first brought the child to medical attention; this condition is dominantly inherited in a complex manner (Cohen et al., 1961). (Illustration reproduced from Schafer, I. A., et al.: New Eng. J. Med. 267:51–60, 1962, with permission.)

The converse finding—that patients with the iminoacidopathy may have no renal disease—has also been reported in at least two pedigrees (*J* and *N* in Table 20–1).

Under these circumstances, one is reluctant to ascribe nephropathy to the presence of hyperprolinemia. The reverse association may, however, be of some physiological interest. Hyperprolinemia of modest degree (0.5 to 1 mM; normal <0.35 mM) occurs in some patients with advanced renal disease (Scriver, unpublished data) although this is not generally the case in uremia (Condon and Asatoor, 1971). This finding may reflect a considerable decline in the capacity to catabolize proline when renal parenchyma is lost. The point is worth considering in the differential diagnosis of hyperprolinemia and in the interpretation of therapeutic trials for patients with combined hyperprolinemia and renal disease (Goyer et al., 1969).

There is also a possible relationship between hyperprolinemia and central nervous system (CNS) disease (seizures and mental retardation) (Table 20–1). This is discussed further under Type II hyperprolinemia.

The enzyme deficiency in Type I hyperprolinemia was first documented by the late Mary Efron (1965, 1966), who found that proline oxidase activity was greatly diminished in liver obtained from a presumed homozygote at death; conversion of L-proline to PC was impaired under the conditions of the assay. Since proline catabolism is also impaired in vivo in Type I hyperprolinemia, it is assumed that proline oxidase is deficient in tissues other than liver.

Several lines of evidence suggest that the block is incomplete (Efron, 1965, 1966; Harries et al., 1971).

Type II Hyperprolinemia

The original report of this condition by Berlow and Efron in abstract (1964) was followed by later publications which emphasized an association between this trait and CNS disease (Table 20–1). In fact, the probands of four pedigrees came to medical attention because of mental retardation or seizures. Moreover, three of the eight probands with Type I hyperprolinemia have also presented with a history of seizures. Although this does not confirm a cause and effect relationship between hyperprolinemia and CNS disease, the problem clearly requires further study, particularly since proline participates in several metabolic interrelations in brain (Sporn et al., 1959).

The degree of hyperprolinemia is generally greater in Type II hyperprolinemia than in the Type I trait. The reason for this is still unclear; it may well reflect more complete impairment of proline oxidation in the Type II trait. The enzyme deficiency in Type II hyperprolinemia is believed to occur at the second stage of proline oxidation, since Δ'pyrroline-5-carboxylic acid (PC), as well as proline, can be detected in the urine of these patients. PC reacts with o-aminobenzaldehyde, and the test applied to urine can be used to distinguish the two types of hyperprolinemia from each other.

The Mechanism of Hyperaminoaciduria in Hyperprolinemia

The specific hyperaminoaciduria of the hyperprolinemia trait is commonly referred to as an "iminoglycinuria," because it comprises proline, hydroxyproline and glycine. The intensity of iminoglycinuria is directly proportional to the degree of hyperprolinemia (Scriver et al., 1964) if the plasma proline concentration exceeds about 0.8 mM. The hyperprolinuria results from progressive saturation by proline of the transport system shared by the imino acids and glycine. The excretion of proline itself occurs by the "overflow" mechanism. At the same time, glycine and hydroxyproline are competitively displaced from the transport system which they share with proline (Scriver et al., 1964; Mohyuddin and Scriver, 1970). The coexistence of overflow and displacement mechanisms has led to the use of the term "combined hyperaminoacidura" to describe its origin.

The iminoglycinuria produced by hyperprolinemia must be distinguished from that associated with the autosomal recessive trait called *familial renal iminoglycinuria* (Rosenberg et al., 1968; Scriver, 1968). In the latter condition, the renal transport system itself is affected, so that tubular reabsorption of the imino acids and glycine is impaired. The concentration of proline in plasma is normal in this inborn error of membrane transport. Renal iminoglycinuria also occurs in the newborn as a normal postnatal phenomenon, involving a transient deficiency of tubular transport systems (Baerlocher et al., 1970, 1971).

Genetics

The inheritance of both types of hyperprolinemia is likely to be autosomal recessive. Consanguinity of the parents of probands with Type I and Type II hyperprolinemia has been documented frequently (Table 20–1). No pedigree is known to contain Type I and Type II hyperprolinemia together. This observation, and the quite different biochemical phenotypes of the two traits, reveal that the two forms of hyperprolinemia are caused by different mutant alleles. However, the possibility of genetic heterogeneity within either trait has not been ruled out. This consideration is raised because it is now evident that some obligate Type I heterozygotes have modest hyperprolinemia, while other Type I heterozygotes do not (Fig. 20–3). This finding suggests that the Type I trait may be heteroallelic. The obligate heterozygotes for Type II hyperprolinemia do not have hyperprolinemia.

The frequency of hyperprolinemia in the general population is unknown. Large surveys in the newborn period have not yet revealed any patients, although this could be the fault of the screening methods or the failure of the trait to express itself in the newborn.

Treatment

Proline is not an essential amino acid, and nearly all dietary proteins with the exception of lactalbumin (Block and Bolling, 1951) contain proline. Dietary management of hyperprolinemia is therefore likely to be difficult and ineffective. Harries and colleagues (1971) studied the effects of extreme restriction of proline intake (<5 mg/kg/day; normal intake up to 500 mg/kg/day) in a nine-month-old infant with Type I hyperprolinemia; they were able to lower the plasma proline to the normal range. With an intermediate intake of dietary proline (130 mg/kg/day), normal growth occurred and the hyperprolinemia was moderately well controlled. Concomitant improvement in clinical symptoms (seizures and intestinal dysfunction) was recorded during the course of the dietary regimen. This important clinical observation will necessitate fur-

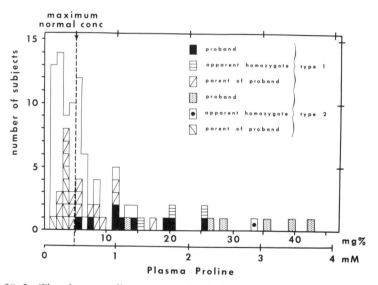

Figure 20–3 The plasma proline concentration in 95 members of hyperprolinemic pedigrees (Types I and II). The maximum normal proline concentration is shown as 5 mg. per cent. This acknowledges the extreme upper limit recorded in the literature; 4 mg per cent is the more usual value. Persons whose probable genotype is unclear are shown by open symbols.

Plasma proline levels are higher in the Type II probands than in the Type I trait. All parents of Type II probands have normal plasma proline; Type II probands probably show the homozygous phenotype.

The situation is less clear with the Type I trait; probands and parents can each show hyperprolinemia. This probably means that the Type I heterozygous phenotype is not always silent.

ther study of the efficacy of dietary management in other patients with hyper-prolinemia, particularly the Type II patient with CNS disease.

Goyer and colleagues (1969) studied the effect of proline restriction on their Type I patient with uremic nephropathy. The diet reduced the plasma proline concentration; however, protein intake was also restricted in this study. In view of the patient's uremic status, it is difficult to know whether the improvement in the hyperprolinemia was merely secondary to improved control of the uremia.

HYDROXYPROLINEMIA

Hydroxyprolinemia is an iminoacidopathy characterized by an increase in the concentration of free hydroxyproline in plasma and urine and by normal urinary excretion of peptide-bound hydroxyproline. The condition has been reported in three unrelated pedigrees (Efron et al., 1962, 1965; Raine, 1970; Pelkonen and Kivirikko, 1970). It is likely that the condition is inherited, but the frequency of the trait is probably very low. The biological importance of the condition lies in its elucidation of hydroxyproline metabolism in man. Hydroxyproline catabolism apparently occurs by a pathway distinct from that serving proline degradation; there is another pathway for endogenous biosynthesis of hydroxyproline, which is independent of that serving hydroxylation of proline in situ in precollagen polypeptides.

Hydroxyproline Metabolism

Adams (1970) has written a superb review of hydroxyproline metabolism which may be consulted for intensive coverage of the subject. Hydroxyproline is classified as an imino acid, a trivial term used to acknowledge the amino group configuration of 4-hydroxypyrrolidine-2-carboxylic acid. Hydroxy-L-proline occurs in mammalian tissue in two forms: as 4-hydroxyproline, representing about 14 per cent of collagen residues (Neumann and Logan, 1950) and 2 per cent in elastin; and as 3-hydroxyproline, comprising about 0.26 per cent of bovine collagen (Ogle et al., 1962). The chemical formulas for these two compounds are as follows:

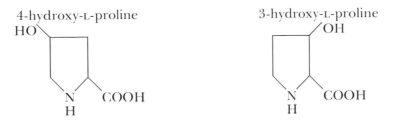

In the equivalent alloepimers of the D- and L-isomers of hydroxyproline, the OH and COOH groups are in the same plane relative to the ring.

The principal source of hydroxyproline in man is collagen, but its role in this protein has not been clearly defined. A small amount of total body hydroxyproline is in the free form in tissue fluids.

Synthesis in Collagen

Most of the hydroxyproline in the body is peptide-bound and is derived directly from proline (Robertson, 1964). Atmospheric oxygen is incorporated during the hydroxylation reaction (Prockop et al., 1963), which may be enzymatic or direct (Bade and Gould, 1968) and during which a hydrogen is also lost (Prockop et al., 1964). The reaction has an absolute requirement for ferrous iron and α-ketoglutarate and a preferential need for ascorbic acid, which can be partially replaced by reduced pteridines (Peterkofsky and Udenfriend, 1965; Hutton et al., 1967).

The hydroxylation reaction has, for many years, been considered to take place on a proline-rich precursor of collagen, either an intermediate attached to polysomes (Urivetsky et al., 1965) or a free precollagen polypeptide (Peterkofsky and Udenfriend, 1963; Prockop and Juva, 1965). The weight of recent evidence (Lazarides et al., 1971) obtained from cultured fibroblast systems suggests that hydroxylation of proline residues in vivo occurs on nascent collagen chains attached to polysomes. Hydroxyproline-containing proteins formed in cultured human fibroblasts are similar to the collagen which can be extracted from normal human skin (Layman et al., 1971). Hydroxylation of collagen appears to be essential for its normal extrusion from the cell following protein synthesis (Ramaley and Rosenbloom, 1971).

Proline hydroxylation in collagen requires a specific enzyme whose specific activity varies with the stage of cell activity and the demand on collagen synthesis (McGee et al., 1971).

Biosynthesis

Formation of a small amount of free hydroxyproline also occurs by a system whose significance is still obscure. Goldstone and Adams (1964) demonstrated free hydroxyproline biosynthesis in the mammal, from glyoxalate and pyruvate (Fig. 20–4). The presence of this pathway in man has also been inferred from studies of normal and hydroxyprolinemic subjects (Efron et al., 1968; Pelkonen and Kivirikko, 1970).

Degradation

Free hydroxyproline can be catabolized by a specific pathway (Fig. 20–5) which has been well defined in mammalian tissues (Goldstone and Adams, 1962, 1964). This pathway has also been detected in human liver and kidney (Efron et al., 1965). About 80 per cent of hydroxyproline oxidation in man occurs by this pathway (Weiss and Klein, 1969; Efron et al., 1968; Pelkonen and Kivirikko, 1970). The remainder escapes into urine, the majority (96 per cent) occurring in the peptide-bound form (Meilman et al., 1963). The excretion rate of bound hydroxyproline serves as a rough index for the turnover of soluble collagen.

Distribution in Body Fluids

Hydroxyproline circulating in plasma is about 70 per cent in protein and 23 per cent in the free form (Kibrick, 1965); the latter is less than 0.01 mM (Øye, 1962). Hydroxyproline peptides account for less than 2 per cent of the total hydroxyproline in plasma, whereas they are the predominant form in urine. The oligopeptides prolylhydroxyproline and glycylprolylhydroxyproline are poorly transported into cells (Christensen and Rafn, 1952) and are poorly hydrolyzed by renal peptidases (Weiss and Klein, 1969). These peptides may also be secreted by the renal tubule (Benoit and Watten, 1968).

Renal clearance of free hydroxyproline is normally very low, but the re-

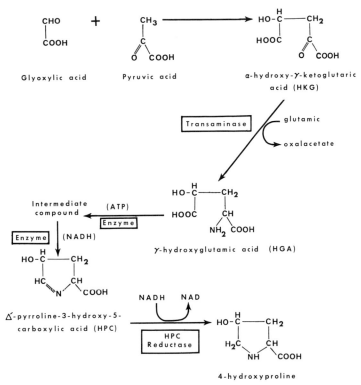

Figure 20–4 Biosynthetic pathway of 4-hydroxyproline.

absorption process is saturable, thus explaining its appearance in urine in hyper-hydroxyprolinemic states (Scriver and Goldman, 1966). Renal uptake occurs on more than one saturable system (Scriver, 1968; Mohyuddin and Scriver, 1970). At high concentrations, hydroxyproline reabsorption is shared with proline and glycine, while at endogenous concentrations it is transported on a system with preference for proline. Finerman and Rosenberg (1966) showed that its transport into bone is also shared with other amino acids. One concludes that hydroxyproline moves across the cell membrane as a parasitic passenger on transport systems primarily serving other amino acids.

Clinical Features of Hydroxyprolinemia

The first patient to be reported with this disease (Efron et al., 1962, 1965) was born prematurely to a low-IQ mother. This female child was herself discovered during screening of an institution for the mentally retarded; retardation had been identified in the patient's early infancy. Physical stature was at the 10th percentile for height and weight, but motor and mental development were severely retarded. The history was negative for fractures, skin defects, abnormal wound healing and hernias. Thus, no phenotype relevant to deviant collagen metabolism was found. The mental retardation was thought to be a coincidental problem unrelated to the hydroxyprolinemia. The dietary history was adequate, and no disturbance of vitamin C metabolism was identified.

A second patient has been identified by Raine and colleagues (1970). She is the second of three sibs born to nonconsanguineous parents. The hydroxyprolinemia (0.5 mM; normal <0.01 mM) was discovered at about six years of age

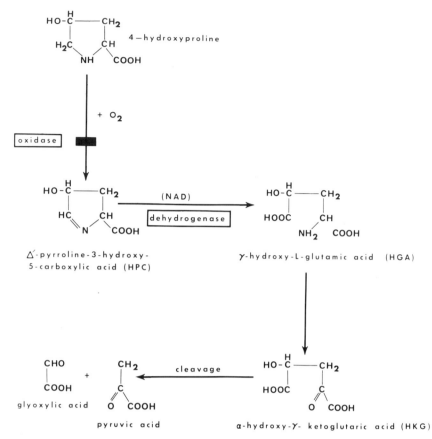

Figure 20–5   Degradative pathway of 4-hydroxyproline in mammalian tissue. The block in *hydroxyprolinemia* is indicated at the oxidase step.

during a work-up for mental retardation evident since six months of age. Although physical growth was normal, there were severe disturbance of mental development, an abnormal electroencephalogram and episodic psychotic-like behavior.

A third proband, also a female, has been described from Finland by Pelkonen and Kivirikko (1970). She was 31 years old when discovered. A family study revealed a brother who was also affected. There were five healthy offspring of the proband. Neither subject with hydroxyprolinemia was mentally retarded, and their life situations clearly indicated an adequately healthy status.

The findings in these three pedigrees indicate either that the "hydroxy-prolinemic" trait is a "non-disease" only incidentally associated with brain damage or that it is genetically heterogeneous with accompanying phenotypic heterogeneity. Both interpretations are equally acceptable at the present state of our understanding of this condition.

The Biochemical Disorder

The plasma concentration of free hydroxyproline is usually about 30 to 50 times greater than normal in hydroxyprolinemia. Urinary excretion of the free imino acid is greatly increased, but excretion of bound hydroxyproline is completely normal (Efron et al., 1965; Pelkonen and Kivirikko, 1970). However, the degree of hydroxyprolinemia is usually not sufficiently elevated to initiate competition on renal tubular transport systems so that prolinuria and hyperglycinuria also occur (Scriver and Goldman, 1966).

The cause of the hydroxyprolinemia can be traced to a defect in the first or "oxidase" step (Fig. 20-5) in free hydroxyproline catabolism (Efron et al., 1965). Hydroxy-L-proline loading will cause a marked and further increase in plasma free hydroxyproline of these patients. Contrary to the excretory response of normal subjects, metabolites distal to the block (Fig. 20-5) are not excreted by hydroxyprolinemic patients, even in the presence of the augmented amounts of substrate.

The source of the excess hydroxyproline lies in the normal turnover of collagen and in the small endogenous biosynthesis of the free substance. There is no abnormal breakdown of collagen, since the excretion pattern and the amount of hydroxyproline peptides in urine are normal (Efron et al., 1968; Pelkonen and Kivirikko, 1970). The normal turnover of collagen, equivalent to about 2 g/day, is sufficient to produce the degree of hydroxyprolinemia found in these patients.

Genetics

It is presumed that the hydroxyprolinemic trait(s) is inherited as a rare autosomal recessive. This assumption is based on the suspected close consanguinity of the parents in the first pedigree and the involvement of sibs in the third. None of the offspring of the hydroxyprolinemic female proband in the third pedigree were apparently hydroxyprolinemic or abnormal in any way.

Treatment

Efron and colleagues attempted biochemical control of their patient (Efron, 1967; Efron et al., 1968). Rigid elimination of hydroxyproline-containing protein, such as gelatin, from the diet had no effect on the degree of hydroxyprolinemia. Restriction of L-ascorbic acid intake for five months did not reduce collagen turnover and did not alter the hydroxyprolinemia. Raine (1970) achieved a modest, transient lowering of plasma hydroxyproline (from 0.5 mM to 0.2 mM) by glycine feeding; however, the latter caused an increase in plasma glycine to distinctly abnormal levels. Production of a second hyperaminoacidemia to ameliorate the first does not seem warranted if hydroxyprolinemia is indeed a benign trait.

IMINOPEPTIDURIA

Normal adults excrete between 10 and 30 mmoles of peptide-bound amino acids in the urine per day. About 750 μmoles of this, or less, is bound proline (Stein, 1953); a similar amount of bound hydroxyproline is also excreted, but age-dependent variation in the excretion rate is an important feature of iminopeptiduria. The imino acids are usually carboxyterminal in their peptide linkage.

Considerable efforts have been made to define the significance of iminopeptiduria in man. A normal, age-dependent pattern has been established, deviation from which may be used to indicate aberrations of growth and development or the presence of disease.

Hydroxyproline Peptides

A reliable method is available for the measurement of peptide-bound or total (bound plus free) hydroxyproline in urine (Prockop and Udenfriend, 1960). Many modifications have subsequently been published to improve the availability of this analysis. The excretion of bound hydroxyproline, which constitutes about 96 per cent of the total hydroxyproline in urine, is not influenced by the usual dietary components, other than gelatin, or by urine flow rate; and there is no circadian variation in excretion rate (Prockop and Sjoerdsma, 1961). Bound hydroxyproline is excreted in urine following degradation of soluble and insoluble collagen (Prockop, 1964). Large changes in collagen turnover are required to modify the excretion pattern, and, as expected, growth itself dramatically influences peptide excretion (Fig. 20–6) (Smiley and Ziff, 1964; Jones et al., 1964; Younazai et al., 1967, 1968). Hydroxyproline excretion correlates well with the velocity curve for linear growth in infancy and, later, with the growth spurt of adolescence and early adulthood.

The component peptides of bound hydroxyproline excretion have been extensively characterized, and appropriate references may be consulted for details (Smiley and Ziff, 1964; Meilman et al., 1963). Benoit and Watten (1965) suggested that peptides are excreted both by glomerular filtration and by tubular secretion. Distortion in the excretion pattern has been claimed in so many conditions that it is probably of little value to review the subject here. It is now apparent that hydroxyproline peptide excretion is not a "wonder" test for growth failure, malnutrition, metastatic disease or inborn errors of connective tissue metabolism. Any condition which is likely to alter collagen turnover (in particular, disorders of parathyroid function and of other endocrine glands) and disturbances of nutrition and nitrogen balance will modify iminopeptide excretion. A clinical interpretation of the findings in the patient will be dependent on a knowledge of the normal age-dependent excretion rates. They are quite unlikely to have any primary diagnostic significance in themselves, except possibly in the following rather specific cases.

Specific Iminopeptidurias

(i) Pelc and Vis (1960) and Paine and Efron (1963) described a peptide composed of proline and hydroxyproline in equal amounts which is excreted

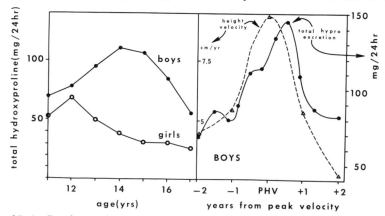

Figure 20–6 Graphs to show total hydroxyproline excretion in relation to growth during adolescence. Left-hand figure from Zorab et al., 1970; right-hand figure from Zorab, 1969. In the latter, hydroxyproline excretion in boys is related to the velocity of linear growth (cm/yr). Hydroxyproline excretion is roughly parallel to the linear growth rate, suggesting that collagen turnover is an important determinant of age-dependent total hydroxyproline excretion.

in urine by some patients with ataxia telangiectasia or clinical variants of that syndrome.

(ii) Seakins (1963) described glycylprolinuria and prolylhydroxyprolinuria in a patient with generalized overgrowth of bone and hyperphosphatasia.

(iii) Scriver (1964) described glycylprolinuria in patients with several forms of severe rickets, each probably encompassing severe hyperparathyroidism. The dipeptiduria correlated with the severity of the osteopathy. Glycylproline is inefficiently reabsorbed by the renal tubule, apparently by a system independent of those serving transport of free glycine and free proline (Scriver, 1964).

(iv) Goodman and colleagues (1968) described an adult male patient with a lathyritic-like condition and striking iminopeptiduria. In addition to a fourfold increase in bound hydroxyproline excretion, six different C-terminal proline dipeptides (asparagyl-glutamyl-, glycyl-, valyl-, leucyl-, and isoleucyl-) were present in abnormal amounts. The renal clearance of glycylproline indicated that more than half of the total excretion probably took place by net tubular "secretion." Tissue collagen was normal in its amino acid composition, and abnormal turnover was postulated.

Further study of the patient by Buist and colleagues (1972) revealed that about 3 g of dipeptide proline and 250 mg of dipeptide hydroxyproline were excreted in 24 hours. All combinations of dipeptide proline with the exception of met-pro and cys-pro were found; gly-pro was 18 per cent of the total proline dipeptide excretion. A generalized defect in imino-carboxyterminal dipeptide catabolism was apparent, perhaps secondary to a defect in tissue prolidase activity. The degradation of 2 to 5 g/day of collagen and 75 to 100 g/day of endogenous protein catabolism was compromised in the patient.

The systemic diseases associated with perturbed hydroxyproline peptiduria are many. Uremia illustrates some of the complexities which determine the qualitative and quantitative aspects of total hydroxyprolinuria. Bone collagen undergoes changes in uremia that are not shared by skin collagen (Hahn and Avioli, 1970). Studies in the rat show that soluble collagen of bone increases, whereas the insoluble collagen fraction is decreased. These changes are believed to originate in abnormalities of parathyroid hormone secretion and of vitamin D metabolism which occur in uremia and which affect bone physiology. Jaworski (1973) found an increase in the nondialyzable fraction of total hydroxyproline in the urine of human subjects in advanced uremia. This fraction is normally about 10 per cent of total urinary hydroxyproline, and it is believed to reflect soluble collagen synthesis in bone. Increased excretion of this fraction was interpreted by Jaworski as evidence for impaired maturation of bone collagen in uremia. The urinary findings in man could be considered analogous to the changes in bone collagen in the experimental animal; they also indicate how difficult it can be to interpret urinary bound hydroxyproline measurements and their relationship to collagen synthesis or degradation or both.

REFERENCES

Hyperprolinemia

Adams, E.: Metabolism of proline and hydroxyproline. Int. Rev. Connect. Tissue Res. 5:2–92, 1970.
Applegarth, D. A., Ingram, P., Hingston, J., Sturrock, S., and Hardwick, D. F.: Hyperprolinemia Type II. Proceedings of the Eighth International Congress of Pediatricians 5:249–251, 1971.
Baerlocher, K., Scriver, C. R., and Mohyuddin, F.: Ontogeny of iminoglycine transport in mammalian kidney. Proc. Nat. Acad. Sci. U.S.A. 65:1009–1016, 1970.

Baerlocher, K. E., Scriver, C. R., and Mohyuddin, F.: The ontogeny of amino acid transport in rat kidney. I. Effect on distribution ratios and intracellular metabolism of L-proline and glycine. Biochim. Biophys. Acta *249*:353–363, 1971a.

Baerlocher, K. E., Scriver, C. R., and Mohyuddin, F.: The ontogeny of amino acid transport in rat kidney. II. Kinetics of uptake and effect of anoxia. Biochim. Biophys. Acta *249*:364–372, 1971b.

Berlow, S., and Efron, M. E.: A new cause of hyperprolinemia associated with the excretion of Δ'-pyrroline-5-carboxylic acid. (Abstract.) Proceedings of the Society for Pediatric Research, 34th Annual meeting, Seattle, Wash. p. 43, 1964.

Block, R. M., and Bolling, D.: The Amino Acid Composition of Proteins and Foods. Charles C Thomas, Springfield, Ill., 1951.

Brunner, G., and Neupert, W.: Localization of proline oxidase and Δ-pyrroline-5-carboxylic acid dehydrogenase in rat liver. FEBS Letters *3*:283–286, 1969.

Cohen, M. M., Cassady, G., and Hanna, B. L.: A genetic study of hereditary renal dysfunction with associated nerve deafness. Amer. J. Hum. Genet. *13*:379–389, 1961.

Condon, J. R., and Asatoor, A. M.: Amino acid metabolism in urinemic patients. Clin. Chim. Acta *32*:333–337, 1971.

Efron, M. L.: Familial hyperprolinemia. Report of a second case, associated with congenital renal malformations, hereditary hematuria and mild mental retardation, with demonstration of an enzyme defect. New Eng. J. Med. *272*:1243–1254, 1965.

Efron, M. L.: Disorders of proline and hydroxyproline metabolism. *In* Stanbury, J. B., Wyngaarden, J. B., and Fredrickson, D. S., eds., The Metabolic Basis of Inherited Disease. McGraw-Hill, New York, pp. 376–392, 1966.

Emery, F. A., Goldie, L., and Stern, J.: Hyperprolinemia Type 2. J. Ment. Defic. Res. *12*:187–195, 1968.

Felig, P., Owen, O. E., Wahren, J., and Cahill, G. F., Jr.: Amino acid metabolism during prolonged starvation. J. Clin. Invest. *48*:584–594, 1969.

Fontaine, G.: Personal communication, 1969.

Fontaine, G., Farniaux, J. P., and Dautrevaux, M.: L'Hyperprolinémie de Type I. Étude d'une observation familiale. Helvet. Paediat. Acta *25*:165–175, 1970.

Goodman, S. I.: Personal communication, 1970.

Goyer, R. A., Mitchell, B. J., and Leonard, D. L.: Dietary reduction of hyperprolinemia. J. Lab. Clin. Med. *73*:819–824, 1969.

Goyer, R. A., Reynolds, J., Burke, J., and Burkholder, P.: Hereditary renal disease with neurosensory hearing loss, prolinuria and icthyosis. Amer. J. Med. Sci. *256*:166–179, 1968.

Harries, J. T., Piesowicz, A. T., Seakins, J. W. T., Francis, D. E. M., and Wolff, O. W.: Low proline diet in Type I hyperprolinemia. Arch. Dis. Child. *46*:72–81, 1971.

Jeune, M., Collambel, C., Michel, M., David, H., Guibaud, P., Guerrier, G., and Albert, J.: Hyperleucine-isoleucinémie par défaut partiel de transamination associée à une hyperprolinémie de Type 2. Observation familiale d'une double amino-acidopathie. Ann. Pediat. *46*:85–99, 1970.

Kopelman, H., Asatoor, A. M., and Milne, M. D.: Hyperprolinemia and hereditary nephritis. Lancet (ii), 1075–1079, 1964.

Mohyuddin, F., and Scriver, C. R.: Amino acid transport in mammalian kidney: Multiple systems for imino acids and glycine in rat kidney. Amer. J. Physiol. *219*:1–8, 1970.

Mollica, F., Pavone, L., and Antener, I.: Pure familial hyperprolinemia: Isolated inborn error of amino acid metabolism without other anomalies in a Sicilian family. Pediatrics *48*:225–231, 1971.

Perry, T. L., Hardwick, D. F., Lowry, R. B., and Haisen, S.: Hyperprolinemia in two successive generations of a North American Indian family. Ann. Hum. Genet. *31*:401–407, 1968.

Piesowicz, A. T.: Hyperprolinemia. Arch. Dis. Child. *43*:748, 1968.

Rosenberg, L. E., Durant, J. L., and Elsas, L. J.: Familial iminoglycinuria. An inborn error of renal tubular transport. New Eng. J. Med. *278*:1407–1413, 1968.

Schafer, I. A., Scriver, C. R., and Efron, M. L.: Familial hyperprolinemia, cerebral dysfunction and renal anomalies occurring in a family with hereditary nephritis and deafness. New Eng. J. Med. *267*:51–60, 1962.

Scriver, C. R.: Renal tubular transport of proline, hydroxyproline and glycine. III. Genetic basis for more than one mode of transport in human kidney. J. Clin. Invest. *47*:823–835, 1968.

Scriver, C. R.: The use of human genetic variation to study membrane transport of amino acids in kidney. Amer. J. Dis. Child. *117*:4–12, 1969.

Scriver, C. R., Efron, M. L., and Schafer, I. A.: Renal tubular transport of proline, hydroxyproline and glycine in health and in familial hyperprolinemia. J. Clin. Invest. *43*:374–385, 1964.

Scriver, C. R., Schafer, I. A., and Efron, M. L.: New renal tubular amino acid transport system and a new hereditary disorder of amino acid metabolism. Nature (London) *192*:672–673, 1961.

Selkoe, D. J.: Familial hyperprolinemia and mental retardation. A second metabolic type. Neurology *19*:494–501, 1969.

Similä, S.: Hyperprolinemia Type II. Ann. Clin. Res. *2*:143–150, 1970.

Similä, S., and Visakorpi, J. K.: Hyperprolinemia without renal disease. (Abstract.) Acta Paed. Scand. (Suppl.) *177*:122–123, 1967.

Sporn, M. B., Dingman, W., Defalco, A., and Davies, R. K.: The synthesis of urea in the living rat brain. J. Neurochem. *5*:62–67, 1959.

Stetten, M. R., and Schoenheimer, R.: The metabolism of L-proline studied with the aid of deuterium and isotopic nitrogen. J. Biol. Chem. *153*:113, 1944.

Strecker, H. J.: The interconversion of glutamic acid and proline. I. The formation of Δ'-pyrroline-5-carboxylic acid from glutamic acid in *Escherichia coli*. J. Biol. Chem. *225*:825–834, 1957.

Woody, N. C., Snyder, C. H., and Harris, J. A.: Hyperprolinemia: Clinical and biochemical family study. Pediatrics *44*:554–563, 1969.

Hydroxyprolinemia

Adams, E.: Metabolism of proline and hydroxyproline. Int. Rev. Connect. Tissue Res. *5*:2–92, 1970.

Bade, M., and Gould, B. S.: Proline hydroxylation by oxygen. Biochim. Biophys. Acta *156*:425–428, 1968.

Benoit, F. L., and Watten, R. H.: Renal tubular transport of hydroxyproline peptides: Evidence for reabsorption and secretion. Metabolism *17*:20–33, 1968.

Christensen, H. N., and Rafn, M. L.: Uptake of peptides by a free-cell neoplasm. Cancer Res. *12*: 495–497, 1952.

Efron, M. L.: Disorders of proline and hydroxyproline metabolism. *In* Stanbury, J. B., Wyngaarden, J. B., and Fredrickson, D. S., eds., The Metabolic Basis of Inherited Disease. McGraw-Hill, New York, pp. 376–392, 1966.

Efron, M. L.: Treatment of hydroxyprolinemia and hyperprolinemia. Amer. J. Dis. Child. *113*: 166–169, 1967.

Efron, M. L., Bixby, E. M., and Pryles, C. V.: Hydroxyprolinemia. II: A rare metabolic disease due to a deficiency of the enzyme "hydroxyproline oxidase." New Eng. J. Med. *272*:1299–1309, 1965.

Efron, M. L., Bixby, E. M., Palattao, L. G., and Pryles, C. V.: Hydroxyprolinemia associated with mental deficiency. New Eng. J. Med. *267*:1193–1194, 1962.

Efron, M. L., Bixby, E. M., Hockaday, T. D. R., Smith, L. M., Jr., and Meshorer, E.: Hydroxyprolinemia. III: The origin of free hydroxyproline in hydroxyprolinemia collagen turnover. Evidence for a biosynthetic pathway in man. Biochim. Biophys. Acta *165*:238–250, 1968.

Finerman, G. A. M., and Rosenberg, L. E.: Amino acid transport in bone: Evidence for separate transport systems for neutral amino and imino acids. J. Biol. Chem. *241*:1487–1493, 1966.

Goldstone, A., and Adams, E.: Metabolism of gamma hydroxyglutamic acid. J. Biol. Chem. *237*: 3476–3485, 1962.

Goldstone, A., and Adams, E.: Further metabolic reactions of hydroxyglutamate: Amidation to hydroxyglutamine; possible reduction to hydroxyproline. Biochem. Biophys. Res. Commun. *16*:71–76, 1964.

Kibrick, A. C., Kitagawa, G., Maskaleris, M. L., Gaines, R., Jr., and Milhorat, A. T.: Hydroxyproline in human blood: Forms in which it is present. Proc. Soc. Exp. Biol. Med. *119*:622–625, 1965.

Layman, D. L., McGoodwin, E. B., and Martin, G. R.: The nature of collagen synthesized by cultured human fibroblasts. Proc. Nat. Acad. Sci. U.S.A. *68*:454–458, 1971.

Lazarides, E. L., Lukens, L. N., and Infante, A. A.: Collagen polysomes: Site of hydroxylation of proline residues. J. Molec. Biol. *58*:831–846, 1971.

McGee, J. O. D., Langness, U., and Udenfriend, S.: Immunological evidence for an inactive precursor of collagen proline hydroxylase in cultured fibroblasts. Proc. Nat. Acad. Sci. U.S.A. *68*:1585–1589, 1971.

Meilman, E., Urivetzky, M. M., and Rapoport, C. M.: Urinary hydroxyproline peptides. J. Clin. Invest. *42*:40–50, 1963.

Mohyuddin, F., and Scriver, C. R.: Amino acid transport in mammalian kidney: Multiple systems for imino acids and glycine in rat kidney. Amer. J. Physiol. *219*:1–8, 1970.

Neumann, R. E., and Logan, M. A.: The determination of hydroxyproline. J. Biol. Chem. *184*: 299–306, 1950.

Ogle, J. D., Arlinghaus, R. B., and Logan, M. A.: 3-Hydroxyproline, a new amino acid of collagen. J. Biol. Chem. *237*:3667–3673, 1962.

Øye, I.: The amount of free hydroxyproline in human blood serum. Scand. J. Clin. Lab. Invest. *14*:259–261, 1962.

Pelkonen, R., and Kivirikko, K. I.: Hydroxyprolinemia. New Eng. J. Med. *283*:451–456, 1970.

Peterkofsky, B., and Udenfriend, S.: Conversion of proline to collagen hydroxyproline in a cell-free system from chick embryo. J. Biol. Chem *238*:3966–3977, 1963.

Peterkosfky, B., and Udenfriend, S.: Enzymatic hydroxylation of proline in microsomal polypeptide leading to formation of collagen. Proc. Nat. Acad. Sci. U.S.A. 53:335–342, 1965.

Prockop, D. J., and Juva, K.: Hydroxylation of proline in particulate fractions from cartilage. Biochem. Biophys. Res. Commun. 18:54–59, 1965.

Prockop, D. J., Ebert, P. S., Shapiro. B. M.: Studies with proline-3, 4-H³ on the hydroxylation of proline during collagen synthesis in chick embryos. Arch. Biochem. 106:112–122, 1964.

Prockop, D., Kaplan, A., and Udenfriend, S.: Oxygen-18 studies on the conversion of proline to collagen hydroxyproline. Arch. Biochem. 101:499–503, 1963.

Raine, D. N.: Defects in renal tubular reabsorption. In Defects in Cellular Organelles and Membranes in Relation to Mental Retardation. Ciba Foundation Study Group, 1971.

Ramaley, P. B., and Rosenbloom, J.: Inhibition of proline and lysine hydroxylation prevents normal extrusion of collagen by 3T6 fibroblasts in culture. FEBS Letters, 15:59–62, 1971.

Robertson, W. van B.: Connective tissue: Intracellular macromolecules. In New York Heart Association Symposium, Boston, Mass., Little, Brown and Company, 1964.

Scriver, C. R.: Renal tubular transport of proline, hydroxyproline, and glycine. III. Genetic basis for more than one mode of transport in human kidney. J. Clin. Invest. 47:823–835, 1968.

Scriver, C. R., and Goldman, H.: Renal tubular transport of proline, hydroxyproline, and glycine. II. Hydroxy-L-proline as substrate and as inhibitor in vivo. J. Clin. Invest. 45:1357–1363, 1966.

Urivetzky, M., Frei, J. M., and Meilman, E.: Cell-free collagen biosynthesis and the hydroxylation of sRNA-proline. Arch. Biochem. 109:480–489, 1965.

Weiss, P. H., and Klein, L.: The quantitative relationship of urinary peptide hydroxyproline excretion to collagen degradation. J. Clin. Invest. 48:1–10, 1969.

Iminopeptiduria

Buist, N. R., Strandholm, J. S., Bellinger, J. F., and Kennaway, N. G.: Further studies on a patient with iminopeptiduria: A probable case of prolidase deficiency. Metabolism, (In press).

Goodman, S. I., Solomons, C. C., Muschenheim, F., McIntyre, C. A., Miles, B., and O'Brien, D.: A syndrome resembling lathyrism associated with iminopeptiduria. Amer. J. Med. 45:152–159, 1968.

Hahn, T. J., and Avioli, L. V.: Effect of chronic uremia on collagen metabolism in skin and bone. Arch. Intern. Med. (Chicago) 126:882–886, 1970.

Jaworski, G.: Personal communication, 1973.

Jones, C. R., Bergman, M. W., Kittner, P. J., and Pigman, W. W.: Urinary hydroxyproline excretion in normal children and adolescents. Proc. Soc. Exp. Biol. Med. 115:85–87, 1964.

Meilman, E., Urivetzky, M. M., and Rapoport, C. M.: Urinary hydroxyproline peptides. J. Clin. Invest. 42:40–50, 1963.

Paine, R. A., and Efron, M. L.: Atypical variants of the atoxia telangiectasia syndrome. Develop. Med. Child Neurol. 5:14–23, 1963.

Pelc, S., and Vis, H.: Ataxie familiale avec télangiectasies oculaires (Syndrome de D. Louis-Bar). Acta Neurol. Belg. 60:905–922, 1960.

Prockop, D. J., and Udenfriend, S.: A specific method for the analysis of hydroxyproline in tissues and urine. Anal. Biochem. 1:228–239, 1960.

Prockop, D. J., and Sjoerdsma, A.: Significance of urinary hydroxyproline in man. J. Clin. Invest. 40:843–849, 1961.

Prockop, D. J.: Isotopic studies on collagen degradation and the urinary excretion of hydroxyproline. J. Clin. Invest. 43:453–460, 1964.

Scriver, C. R.: Glycyl-proline in urine of humans with bone disease. Canad. J. Physiol. Pharmacol. 42:357–364, 1964.

Seakins, J. W. T.: Peptiduria in an unusual bone disorder. Arch. Dis. Child. 38:215–219, 1963.

Smiley, J. D., and Ziff, M.: Urinary hydroxyproline excretion and growth. Physiol. Rev. 44:30–44, 1964.

Stein, W. H.: A chromatographic investigation of the amino acid constituents of normal urine. J. Biol. Chem. 201:45–58, 1953.

Younoszai, M. K., Andersen, D. W., Filer, L. J., Jr., and Fomon, S. J.: Urinary excretion of endogenous hydroxyproline by normal male infants. Pediat. Res. 1:266–270, 1967.

Younoszai, M. K., and Haworth, J. C.: Excretion of hydroxyproline in urine by premature and normal full-term infants and those with intrauterine growth retardation during the first three days of life. Pediat. Res. 2:17–21, 1968.

Zorab, P. A.: Normal creatinine and hydroxyproline excretion in young persons. Lancet (ii), 1164–1165, 1969.

Zorab, P. A., Clark, S., Harrison, A., and Seel, J. R.: Hydroxyproline excretion and height velocity in adolescent boys. Arch. Dis. Child. 45:763–765, 1970.

Chapter Twenty-One

GLUTAMATE, ALPHA-ALANINE, TRYPTOPHAN AND OTHER SUBSTANCES

There are several facets of amino acid metabolism and disorders thereof which do not rightfully belong in the preceding chapters. Discussions of these have therefore been gathered into the present chapter, their links with the appropriate aspects of amino acid metabolism being mentioned where indicated.

GLUTAMATE METABOLISM

L-Glutamate is an important nonessential amino acid whose role in the collection of amino groups and whose participation in gluconeogenesis is described in Chapter 4.

433

The intracellular concentration of glutamate usually greatly exceeds that in the extracellular fluid. In brain, glutamate is one of the most prominent amino acids (10 to 20 μM/g wet weight) (Tallan, 1962); and in kidney there are about 8 μM glutamate/g wet weight (Lancaster et al., 1973). The corresponding concentration in plasma is about 30 to 50 μM/L. Glutamate has important anabolic roles, e.g., γ-aminobutyric acid synthesis in brain and kidney, and it participates in energy metabolism and protein synthesis.

Glutamate is transported from splanchnic to peripheral tissues in the cellular fraction of whole blood, and under the influence of insulin it is rapidly transferred from blood cell to muscle cell during transit through the tissue capillary bed in man (Aoki et al., 1972); the contribution from plasma in this exchange is relatively unimportant. Since the glutamate content in the human blood cell fraction is about three to four times greater than in the plasma component of normal whole blood, it is apparent that the cellular (erythrocyte) fraction is an important vehicle for glutamate transfer into muscle. The similarity between these observations on glutamate transport in blood to regions of protein synthesis in man (Aoki et al., 1972) and those by Elwyn et al. (1972) on whole blood transport of other amino acids away from the liver in the dog (see Chapter 4) suggests that this may be a mechanism for interorgan exchange of amino acids in general.

Measurement of glutamate requires special attention (Pagliara and Goodman, 1968). Careful chromatographic determination or enzymatic assay will allow an accurate estimate of the true glutamate content. Deterioration of the sample is a major pitfall in glutamate analysis, since it will yield increased glutamate as glutamine is degraded on standing at room temperature. The normal content of glutamate in fasting human plasma is 43 ± 14 (SD) μM/L (Pagliara and Goodman, 1968), and that in the blood cell fraction is about 108 ± 3 (SEM) μM/L (Aoki et al., 1972).

Abnormalities of Glutamate Metabolism

Sex-linked Mental Retardation (Kinky Hair Syndrome)

There are at least two reports (Menkes et al., 1962; Yoshida et al., 1964) of a syndrome characterized by failure to thrive after birth, hypothermia and progressive mental retardation with impaired motor development indicative of cerebral and cerebellar degeneration; there is also evidence compatible with sex-linked recessive inheritance of the condition. In one family (Menkes et al., 1962), the pili torti defect of cephalic hair was evident; subsequently the term "kinky hair syndrome" was used to epitomize the condition. Both original reports deserve mention because elevated levels of glutamic acid were found in the plasma (in Menkes' patients) and in the cerebral spinal fluid (in Yoshida's patient). In the former report, the authors were careful to disclaim glutamine degradation as the source of the excess glutamate; this artifact cannot be ruled out in the second report. Both authors drew attention to an earlier report by Paine (1960) of sex-linked mental retardation without pili torti but with elevated α-amino nitrogen content of the cerebrospinal fluid, the source of which was not identified.

Whether there is a specific syndrome of sex-linked retardation with glutamate accumulation remains unproven at the present time. The picture is now more complicated because the kinky hair syndrome has emerged as a probable disorder of copper absorption (Danks et al., 1972a, 1972b). Menkes (1972) has suggested that the associated finding of copper deficiency in body fluids accounts for the abnormalities of hair and connective tissue in the kinky hair syndrome; the deficiency of docosahexanoic acid, the most highly unsaturated fatty acid of gray matter in brain (O'Brien and Sampson, 1966); and the nearly complete absence of copper-containing cytochromes in brain mitochondria (French et al., 1972). Unfortunately, the reports from Danks' group lack data on glutamate levels in plasma and cerebral spinal fluid. Therefore, it is not yet clear whether the abnormalities of glutamate metabolism described in the earlier reports reflect the apparent abnormality of copper metabolism which has been recently discovered or whether the amino acid finding has any etiological significance in the evolution of the clinical phenotype. The matter is of considerable interest because of recent data which imply that glutamate can be toxic under certain conditions.

Glutamate Toxicity In Vivo

Two "toxicity" syndromes are known: one in man; the other in the mouse. In both, glutamate is implicated as the primary toxic agent.

Chinese Restaurant Syndrome. L-Glutamate, as the monosodium salt (monosodium-L-glutamate, or MSG), is widely used as a food additive with flavoring properties. Its use in Chinese cooking and the association of unusual feelings, particularly after eating won ton soup which has been heavily flavored with MSG, is responsible for the piquant name of the syndrome.

When MSG is consumed in sufficient doses (usually more than one gram at once on an empty stomach) it causes a burning sensation over the torso, neck and arms, a sensation of tightness in the malar area sometimes extending to zygomatic and retro-orbital areas and a feeling of chest pressure (Schaumberg et al., 1969). The sensations are dose-related and transient, appearing at about 30 minutes after the ingestion of MSG and lasting for approximately the same length of time. Simultaneous ingestion of food, particularly protein, attenuates the threshold for response. L-Glutamic acid (5 g in 500 ml water at 30°C) will precipitate the symptoms. The ability to experience the Chinese restaurant syndrome is a talent found in all subgroups of the human race; the civil rights movement will find no racial discrimination in this realm. The possibility that heredity influences the threshold at which the symptoms are experienced has been disproved; the modal threshold dose is 4 g (range, 1 to 12 g), and there is no apparent relationship between body weight, sex or age and threshold dose in the adult.

Schaumberg and colleagues (1969) did not report blood glutamate levels in the subjects who were studied for the occurrence of the syndrome after ingestion of MSG. However, McLaughlan and coworkers showed that MSG given by gavage to rats in dosages exceeding 200 mg per kilogram caused at least a fourfold rise in the glutamate level of systemic venous *plasma* within 20 minutes. The *whole blood* glutamate content was not examined in their protocol, but presumably arterial whole blood levels were even higher, for the reasons discussed above. The dose levels on a weight basis which are necessary to cause a change in the blood level in the rat are in excess of those which cause the Chinese restaurant syndrome in man, but interspecies comparisons may not be valid for many reasons.

Glutamate transaminase activity in the intestine may influence the threshold dose required to develop the syndrome. Neame and Wiseman (1957) showed that glutamate is avidly converted to α-ketoglutarate in the dog during transit through the intestinal wall after absorption. Consequently, the blood level of glutamate rises little under these conditions. A threshold level for glutamate intake is required to exceed the capacity of the transamination reaction before the glutamate level in blood will rise after absorption.

Neuronal Necrosis Syndrome. When administered by subcutaneous injection to newborn mice (0.5 to 4 mg/g body weight) MSG will induce acute neuronal necrosis in the hypothalamus, arcuate nucleus and other regions of the developing brain (Olney, 1969; Reynolds et al., 1971). Acute lesions in brain follow injection of large doses (5 to 7 mg/g body weight) into adult mice. Treated newborn mice showed stunted skeletal development as adults, obesity without hyperphagia and female sterility.

Oral dosing of the primate infant with MSG (1, 2 and 4 g/kg) did not cause neuronal necrosis; this finding suggests the possibility of a species difference in the response to MSG (Reynolds et al., 1971). MSG (6 g) given to lactating women does not affect breast milk amino acid composition, indicating protection of the suckling infant should the mother be exposed to MSG (Stegink et al., 1972). Of more pressing interest, it has now been demonstrated that intravenous nourishment of infants with amino acid mixtures containing large amounts of glutamate do not raise plasma glutamate levels, or apparently produce any clinical signs analogous to the mouse toxicity syndrome (Stegink and Baker, 1971).

McLaughlan and colleagues (1970) confirmed that the lowest dosage schedule employed by Olney (0.5 mg MSG/g body weight) raises the plasma glutamate level of the rodent about sixfold above control levels in litter mates. However, this injection regime does *not* change the steady-state level of glutamate in brain. The question remains, How are exposure to MSG and changes in blood glutamate levels in the newborn animal associated with neuronal necrosis? Clearly no one has sufficient information to answer the question; this probably explains why the U.S. Food and Drug Administration adopted a position of caution toward extensive use of MSG in foods and infant formulas.

Hechtman and colleagues (1972) injected large doses of MSG (between 2.2 and 4.4 mg/g body weight) either into pregnant female mice throughout pregnancy or into newborn mice for 10 days after birth. They subsequently studied behavioral components in the treated offspring at 6 to 7 weeks and at 4 months of age. No abnormalities were observed in any of the offspring at 7 weeks. The mice treated postnatally showed performance deficits at 4 months as well as obesity and short stature, whereas the group exposed to MSG prenatally did not. Control litter mates treated with equimolar sodium acetate developed no abnormalities. The data suggest that behavorial deficits are part of the postnatal MSG toxicity syndrome and that the placenta may protect the fetus from toxicity of MSG. Recent studies in the primate (Stegink et al., 1973) show that glutamate does not cross the hemichorial placenta between maternal and fetal circulations.

Comments. Both glutamate toxicity syndromes, as described, leave much to be desired with respect to their interpretation. The implication of glutamate toxicity in the pathogenesis of symptoms or tissue changes is strongly circumstantial, but to our knowledge no mechanism for these sequelae has yet been discovered. Muscle extraction of blood glutamate may explain why symptoms in the Chinese restaurant syndrome involve muscles; but neither the restriction of symptoms to the torso, head and neck nor the concomitant skin sensations are readily accounted for in these terms.

The failure to find a change in mouse brain glutamate content after exposure to glutamate in doses sufficient to produce neuronal necrosis is a paradox. But glutamate flux is not evaluated in steady-state observations, and it is the net flux in the tissue which may be important. Waelsch's group (Van den

Berg et al., 1969) has presented evidence for the presence of two different tri-carboxylic acid cycles in mouse brain and compartmentation of its glutamate metabolism, one component of which is coupled to a Krebs cycle with fast turn-over. Differential and excessive flux of glutamate through these compartments at critical times in the development of mouse brain may yield the syndrome described above.

Lessons learned from the aforementioned syndromes demand caution on the part of clinicians proceeding with intravenous alimentation of infants by means of solutions containing L-glutamate, until we know more about all the consequences of glutamate loading in the human infant. At the same time, caution from overreacting to the supposed damage caused by glutamate is also indicated until we know more (Bessman and Hochstein, 1970).

Glutamate Metabolism Related to Glutathione

Glutathionemia

Glutamate is a component of glutathione, being linked to the amino group of cysteine through its γ-carboxyl group (γ-L-glutamyl-L-cysteinylglycine).

Glutathionemia, with massive glutathionuria but otherwise normal aminoaciduria and a positive cyanide-nitroprusside test in the urine (see Appendix to Chapter 5, Table 5A–1) has been reported in at least two subjects who are mentally retarded (O'Daly, 1968, 1969, 1973; Goodman et al., 1970). Glutathione metabolism and glutathionemia due to serum γ-glutamyl transpeptidase deficiency is described in Chapter 11.

The γ-Glutamyl Cycle

Orlowski and Meister (1970) have found that rat kidney contains a sequence of enzymes for the synthesis and utilization of glutathione. These enzymes apparently function in a cyclic process which the authors have called the *γ-glutamyl cycle* (Fig. 21–1). The high concentration of glutathione and of the enzymes of the cycle in kidney, an organ with an important role to play in transepithelial transport, led Orlowski and Meister to propose that the cycle might serve amino acid transport. Although this hypothesis has not yet been proven it is of interest that γ-glutamyl transpeptidase, the glycoprotein enzyme which transfers free amino acid to gamma glutamylaminoacid via glutathione, is found in highest concentration in rat kidney in the brush border membranes. Glossman and Neville (1972) estimate that 1.5 per cent of the total protein in brush border is γ-glutamyl transferase.

A "new" enzyme had to be postulated to accommodate the γ-glutamyl cycle because L-pyroglutamic acid, an essential product of the cycle, does not accumulate in blood, kidney or urine. This compound is also the N-terminal residue of several proteins. L-Pyroglutamic acid is rapidly oxidized by kidney in vitro (Ramakrishna et al., 1970). Even though the thermodynamics of the equilibrium between glutamate and 5-oxo-L-proline strongly favor the cyclized state, Van der Werf and colleagues (1971) concluded that a catalytic mechanism must exist in kidney for the removal of L-pyroglutamate; accordingly, they sought and identified a reaction which carried out the conversion of 5-oxo-L-proline to L-glutamic acid, consuming ATP in the process and yielding ADP and ortho-phosphate (Equation 1). The enzyme, whose trivial name is *5-oxo-prolinase*, requires Mg^{++} and K^+ (or Mn^{++} and NH_4^+). The equilibrium of the enzyme

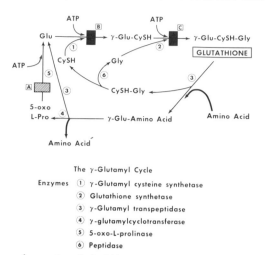

The γ-Glutamyl Cycle

Enzymes
① γ-Glutamyl cysteine synthetase
② Glutathione synthetase
③ γ-Glutamyl transpeptidase
④ γ-glutamylcyclotransferase
⑤ 5-oxo-L-prolinase
⑥ Peptidase

Figure 21–1   The γ-glutamyl cycle in kidney proposed by Orlowski and Meister (1970). The cycle may also exist in other tissues. Enzyme 3, transpeptidase, is tightly bound to cell particles and is probably a glycoprotein. Enzyme 4, also a glycoprotein, is found in the brush border membrane of kidney tubules. Enzyme 5 is located only in the soluble fraction. It has been suggested that the cycle may serve amino acid transport. Enzyme deficiencies have been proposed ▨ or identified ■ at the various steps of glutathione turnover indicated in the cycle; however, a defect in total *cycle* activity is not necessarily implicated in any of these deficiencies.

    Defect A: ? 5-oxo-prolinase deficiency in pyroglutamicaciduria. *Defect B:* erythrocyte γ-glutamyl cysteine synthase deficiency in glutathionepenic hereditary hemolytic anemia. *Defect C:* erythrocyte glutathione synthase deficiency in hereditary hemolytic anemia with almost complete deficiency of erythrocyte glutathione.

catalyzed reaction at pH 7.8 favors glutamate formation, justifying the expenditure of ATP.

$$
\begin{array}{c}
\underset{O}{\overset{\displaystyle H_2C}{\underset{\displaystyle \|}{\underset{\displaystyle C}{|}}}} \underset{NH}{-} \underset{}{\overset{\displaystyle CH_2}{\underset{\displaystyle CHCOOH}{|}}} + ATP + H_2O \xrightarrow[K^+ \ (or \ NH_4^+)]{Mg^{++} \ (or \ Mn^{++})} HOOCCH_2CH_2\underset{NH_2}{\overset{}{\underset{|}{CHCOOH}}}
\end{array}
$$

$$+ \ ADP + P_i \qquad\qquad (1)$$

    5-oxoprolinase has been purified 100-fold (Van der Werf et al., 1971) from rat kidney homogentates, but its location in kidney or in the cell was not reported. The enzyme is found in the kidney of all mammalian species studied so far and also in rat liver, spleen, brain and lung. Focus on the functional significance of 5-oxo-prolinase has been heightened by the recent discovery of a new inborn error of metabolism called *pyroglutamicaciduria* (5-oxo-prolinuria).

Pyroglutamicaciduria

    Jellum and colleagues (1970) discovered large amounts of pyroglutamic acid in the urine and plasma of a 19-year-old retarded male patient. The compound was identified by mass spectrometry after isolation by gas chromatography; it is ninhydrin-negative. Unexplained chronic metabolic acidosis was the index clinical finding which provoked the chemical search. The general clinical phenotype included spastic tetraparesis, a cerebellar disorder with intention tremor and ataxia, and dysarthria. The full-scale IQ level was 57.

The average urinary excretion of 5-oxo-proline was 30.5 g per day when the patient consumed an unrestricted diet; control subjects excrete insignificant amounts of this compound. The concentration of pyroglutamic acid in plasma could only be estimated indirectly from the measurement of "total glutamate" in the extract, but it was clearly increased. The cerebrospinal fluid contained relatively higher amounts, suggesting formation of excess 5-oxo-proline in brain tissue (see discussion of metabolites in CSF, Chapter 3). The proline content of plasma was significantly increased (three times normal), the blood urea level was lower than normal, and aminoaciduria was normal (Eldjarn et al., 1972).

Pyroglutamicaciduria is believed to be caused by a deficiency of 5-oxo-prolinase in kidney, but proof is lacking. Studies have been performed on cultured skin fibroblasts obtained from the patient. Such cells normally contain a pyroglutamic acid "hydrolase" (Strömme and Eldjarn, 1972) whose characteristics closely resemble those of rat kidney 5-oxo-prolinase (Van der Werf et al., 1971). The activity is found exclusively in the soluble fraction of sonicated fibroblasts, and it is not inhibited by L-proline. The K_m for the substrate is about 8 μM, and the V_{max} is about 50 μM. The fibroblast enzyme initiates the conversion of pyroglutamate via glutamate to CO_2, and it is apparently rate-limiting. The conversion rate of substrate to CO_2 is about $1/20$ of that when glutamate is the substrate. However, these interesting observations shed little light on the nature of the defect in pyroglutamicaciduria, because the patient's skin fibroblasts contain normal pyroglutamic "hydrolase" activity. The authors deduced that isozymes may exist, the form in skin fibroblasts being unaffected in the disease, or that the enzyme deficiency in pyroglutamicacidemia does not involve the conversion of 5-oxo-L-proline to glutamate by the step mediated by 5-oxo-prolinase.

The absence of generalized aminoaciduria in the patient with pyroglutamic-aciduria implies that the apparent block in the γ-glutamyl cycle does not impair amino acid transport significantly. However, further speculation is not warranted until the exact enzyme defect, its completeness and its occurrence in kidney have been demonstrated. The likelihood that the γ-glutamyl cycle is a glutathionine-primed mechanism used for detoxification instead should not be ignored.

Glutathione and Hemolytic Anemia

Several forms of hemolytic anemia result from a deficiency of glutathione in the erythrocyte (Oski and Naiman, 1972); two are relevant to the discussion of the γ-glutamyl cycle.

A deficiency of γ-glutamyl-cysteine synthetase in the erythrocyte (Phenotype B, Fig. 21–1) is probably inherited in autosomal recessive fashion and causes reduced glutathione (GSH) to fall to 5 per cent of normal. The amount of activity of the synthetase in other tissues is not well documented. However, leukocytes may be affected and probands may have neurological symptoms (Konrad et al., 1972). Erythrocyte lysates form GSH when incubated with glycine and pre-synthesized γ-glutamyl cysteine, the product of the deficient enzyme.

Erythrocyte glutathione synthetase is normally the rate-limiting enzyme in glutathione synthesis. Its deficiency (Phenotype C, Fig. 21–1) reduces erythrocyte glutathione to about 5 per cent of normal and provokes severe compensated hemolytic anemia.

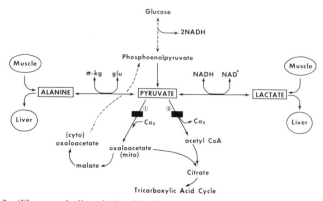

Figure 21–2   The metabolic relationships between α-L-alanine, pyruvate and lactate. Pyruvate is formed by glycolysis and by transamination of alanine or oxidation of lactate. Both of the latter reactions are reversible. Muscle delivers alanine and lactate in the plasma, and liver or kidney can extract these substrates from plasma. A change in pyruvate metabolism which causes it to accumulate will influence lactate and alanine; both will increase concomitantly with pyruvate. The normal molar ratios of alanine:pyruvate:lactate are approximately 3:1:10; the normal pyruvate content of plasma is slightly above 0.1 mM. A state of "excess lactate" occurs when hypoxia generates an excess of NADH. Pyruvate is removed by two routes in mitochondria: pyruvate carboxylase (Enzyme 1) adds CO_2 to pyruvate and generates oxaloacetate which may then leave the mitochondria as malate and enter gluconeogenesis; or pyruvate can lose CO_2 to yield acetyl-CoA by the pyruvate dehydrogenase reaction (Enzyme 2). Blocks in pyruvate metabolism at both enzymes have been described, each causing hyperalaninemia.

α-L-ALANINE METABOLISM

Alpha-L-alanine* is another important nonessential amino acid whose role in fuel metabolism, in gluconeogenesis and in the regulation of glucagon release is described in Chapter 4.

Alanine is among the most abundant of the amino acids in human blood plasma. The normal alanine concentration varies somewhat with age (see Chapter 3, Table 3–1); the range of normal values is from 135 to 650 μM/L, with an overall mean value of 310 ± 73 (SD) μM/L (Perry, 1967). However, these plasma values reflect only one moment in alanine traffic, being sampled at the time of the venipuncture. Plasma alanine is in equilibrium with important tissue pools, and from what we know at the present time it is apparent that deposits by muscle into the plasma alanine "bank," and withdrawal from it by the liver, account for much of the alanine turnover in blood. The central position of alanine in the metabolic interrelationships between amino acids and carbohydrates is indicated in Figure 21–2.

The renal reabsorption of alanine is efficient (see Chapter 3), but any changes which occur in the plasma alanine steady-state will be reflected in the urinary excretion of alanine, since its renal reabsorption at endogenous concentrations is not complete.

The Hyperalaninemias

There are several conditions associated with hyperalaninemia and hyperalaninuria. Their classification is still unclear because, with relatively few ex-

---

*β-Alanine is discussed in Chapter 18.

ceptions, the precise nature of the defect in alanine metabolism is not evident. However, the hyperalaninemias, as a group, tend to have one finding in common: they are often accompanied by lacticacidemia or lacticacidosis. A brief comment on lacticacidosis will help to indicate the relationship between hyperalaninemia and lactic acid metabolism.

Lactate Metabolism

Lactic acid is the end product of anaerobic glucose oxidation via the Embden-Meyerhof pathway (Oliva, 1970). Two moles of lactate are formed from one mole of glucose by the reduction of two moles of pyruvic acid in the presence of lactate dehydrogenase (LDH) and $NADH_2$. The reaction is summarized in Equation 2.

$$CH_3\underset{O}{\overset{\|}{C}}COOH + NADH^+ + H^+ \rightleftharpoons CH_3\underset{OH}{\overset{|}{C}}HCOOH + NAD^+ \qquad (2)$$

The electrons consumed in the reduction reaction are donated by glyceraldehyde-3-phosphate, an earlier intermediate in the pathway of glucose oxidation. The equilibrium of the reaction is toward lactate formation; regeneration of NAD^+ permits glycolysis to continue past the thiose stage under anaerobic conditions.

Tissues dependent on rapid glycolysis for energy metabolism (e.g., white muscle and liver) have isozymes of lactate dehydrogenase in which the M polypeptide subunit predominates; these enzymes are characterized by the configuration M_4 or M_3H, where H represents the other form of subunit in the lactate dehydrogenase tetramer. The M forms of lactate dehydrogenase have a very high affinity for pyruvate as the electron acceptor, and thus they regenerate NAD^+ readily under anaerobic conditions. The H_4 and MH_3 isozymes of LDH have low affinity for pyruvate. They are found in aerobic tissues (e.g., heart and kidney), where NADH can be reoxidized readily during mitochondrial oxidation reactions.

The relationship between lactate and pyruvate can be restated in terms of mass action in terms of Equation 3.

$$\text{Lactate} = \text{Pyruvate} \times K\left[\frac{NADH + H^+}{NAD^+}\right] \qquad (3)$$

According to this statement, the lactate content of body fluids will be dependent on three variables: the pyruvate concentration; the relative amounts of reduced and oxidized NAD; and the type of LDH isozyme present in the tissue. When the $NADH_2:NAD^+$ ratio is constant, any change in lactate must depend on a change in the rate of pyruvate formation and the final concentration of the ketoacid in tissue. Under these conditions the resting lactate:pyruvate ratio (L:P ratio) remains normal (that is, the ratio is less than 10:1).* Any increase

---

*Measurement of lactate and pyruvate requires careful technique. The blood should not be drawn when there is stasis of the blood flow through the tissue, as, for example, after long application of a tourniquet, or during exercise, as may occur when the patient is struggling. Stasis will tend to raise the lactate concentration in the sample. Artifacts which occur during collection of the sample should always be considered when interpreting the laboratory results on lactate and pyruvate values in the pediatric patient.

in lactate unaccompanied by a change in pyruvate is said to indicate "excess lactate" (Huckabee, 1958). Such an abnormality will reflect a change in the $NADH_2:NAD$ ratio.

Because an equilibrium is maintained between alanine and pyruvate, by the transaminase responsible for the conversion of one into the other, when hyperalaninemia occurs in lacticacidosis, it can be assumed that the lactic acidosis is likely to be of the type with a normal L:P ratio; it follows that lactic-acidosis of the type with an elevated L:P ratio may not be accompanied by hyper-alaninemia. An awareness of the distinction between the "excess lactate" type of lacticacidosis and the type where the L:P ratio is normal, should allow the clinician to use the laboratory sign of hyperalaninemia or hyperalaninuria as a guide to the differential diagnosis.

Lacticacidosis with Hyperalaninemia

We have grouped the conditions associated with hyperalaninemia under a heading which emphasizes lacticacidosis because it is the latter abnormality which may first bring the patient to medical attention. However, it should be emphasized that not all patients with hyperalaninemia will present with lacticaci-dosis; the latter may become apparent only under exceptional conditions. Those patients who do not present with acidosis as a major clinical sign may be recog-nized during incidental investigation by virtue of their hyperalaninuria or an elevated level of alanine in plasma.

The literature on the group of diseases associated with incipient or frank lacticacidosis is difficult to classify. Information concerning alanine metabolism is often missing from earlier reports on such patients. For example, the original papers on familial lacticacidosis, by Israels and colleagues (1964) and by Ha-worth et al. (1967), offer no specific data on alanine levels in plasma; that in-formation appears only in a much later report on one of the original patients (Haworth and Ford, 1969), at which time the reader learns that plasma alanine is in fact about four times above the normal range. Hopefully, the alanine data will be provided in all future reports on lacticacidosis.

Excess production of alanine or pyruvate, or diminished utilization of either (see Figure 21–2) will cause both to accumulate. Because of the abundant glutamate-pyruvate aminotransferase in plasma and tissues, alanine is allowed to equilibrate with pyruvate when the latter is formed in excess. Lactate accumulation may follow.

Hyperalaninemia Associated with Pyruvate Dehydrogenase Deficiency. Pyruvate dehydrogenase (EC 1.2.4.1.) is a multienzyme complex analogous to the oxidative decarboxylase for branched-chain ketoacids (see Chapter 14). A block at the dehydrogenase step in glycolysis will lead to pyruvate accumula-tion; hyperalaninemia and lacticacidemia will follow, with lacticacidosis resulting if the accumulation of pyruvate is great enough.

A male patient with deficient pyruvate dehydrogenase activity has been described by Blass and colleagues (1970). The enzyme defect was restricted to the decarboxylase component (2-oxo-acid carboxy-lyase, EC 4.1.1.1.) of the multienzyme complex. The residual activity was somewhat less than 20 per cent of normal in blood leukocytes and in cultured skin fibroblasts. Oxidation of glu-tamate, which requires an analogous dehydrogenase-like enzyme with different substrate specificity in the decarboxylation component, was normal. The metabolism of acetate and palmitate was also normal; both of these substrates enter oxidative metabolism behind the proposed block (see Figure 21–2). Pyruvate decarboxylation activity in one parent of the patient lay in the intermediate zone between the values for the normal controls and the patient, while the other parent had values just below the normal range. Kinetic evaluation of enzyme activity suggested to Blass and colleagues (1970) that more than one form of mutant gene occurred in the family, thus raising the possibility that the propositus was a genetic compound.

The patient presented with a clinical history of intermittent cerebellar ataxia and choreo-athetoid movements brought on by infectious illness or stressful excitement (Blass et al., 1971). The symptoms appeared at 16 months of age; the episodes of neurological symptoms would last from hours to weeks at a time. Involuntary ocular movements were also a prominent part of the choreo-athetoid component (Podos, 1970). Pyruvate and alanine levels in venous blood, urine and cerebrospinal fluid were elevated about four times above normal in the acute attacks; lactate levels were elevated proportionately, and the L:P ratio was normal. Acidosis was not a prominent finding in this patient. Neither the biochemical abnormality or the enzyme deficiency responded to thiamine differently from normal when this coenzyme for the decarboxylase reaction was made available in large supplemental doses either in vivo or in vitro.

The patient of Blass and colleagues is reminiscent of another boy reported earlier by Lonsdale and colleagues (1969). Their patient presented with a similar history of intermittent ataxia and choreoathetosis, ocular incoordination and precipitation of episodes by infection. This patient showed cyclic, parallel changes in alanine and pyruvate accumulation in blood and urine. The levels were higher in the day than at night, and peak accumulation occurred during ataxic episodes. The index laboratory finding which led to the investigation of the patient was striking hyperalaninuria during an episode of ataxia. Lactic acidosis was never recorded in the patient. Thiamine in very large doses (600 mg/day) appeared to ameliorate the clinical and biochemical abnormalities; but there has been no subsequent report to inform whether thiamine actually prevents episodes of ataxia from occurring. Data on pyruvate decarboxylase activity in this patient have not yet been published.

The clinical resemblance between Wernicke's encephalopathy due to thiamine deficiency and the course in the patients with hyperpyruvicacidemia and hyperalaninemia due to pyruvate decarboxylase deficiency (either confirmed or proposed) was noted by Blass and Lonsdale in their reports.

Hyperalaninemia with Pyruvate Carboxylase Deficiency. Pyruvate carboxylase (pyruvate-carbon dioxide ligase [ADP], EC 6.4.1.1) is a biotin-dependent, mitochondrial enzyme which converts pyruvate to oxaloacetate in liver, kidney, adipocytes and brain. Pyruvate carboxylation is believed to be the rate-limiting step in the anaplerotic sequence which commits pyruvate to gluconeogenesis. The enzyme probably has more than one functional component in human liver (Delvin et al., 1972).

Deficiency of the low-K_m component of pyruvate carboxylase (Fig. 21–3) has been described in a female patient with retarded development who presented with postnatal hypoglycemia, hyperpyruvicacidemia and hyperalaninemia, 3 to 10 times above normal (Brunette et al., 1972). The incidental discovery of hyperalaninuria by partition chromatography initiated the studies, which identified the enzymatic basis of the illness in this patient.

Severe intermittent lacticacidosis occurred in the patient described by Brunette and colleagues. The acidosis seemed to correlate with the degree of pyruvate accumulation. The latter became worse when the patient was exposed to conditions which yielded an excess of alanine delivery to liver or an excess of pyruvate formation from glucose. Thus lacticacidosis in this patient was the end result

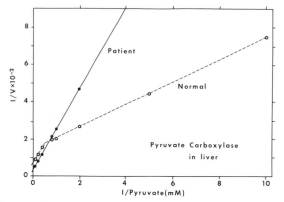

Figure 21–3 Data on the enzyme deficiency in a patient with hyperalaninemia and lactic-acidosis due to pyruvate carboxylase deficiency. A double reciprocal plot showing hepatic pyruvate carboxylase activity in the presence of pyruvate at various concentrations. Pyruvate carboxylase activity in normal liver (O − − −O) has two components, as shown by the deflection in the regression line above 1 mM pyruvate. The patient has only the high-K_m component when her hepatic pyruvate carboxylase activity is measured (●———●). (Activity of the carboxylase measured as amount of labeled oxaloacetate formed from labeled Na_2CO_3.) (From Brunette et al.: Pediatrics *50*:702–711, 1972, with permission).

of pyruvate overproduction under conditions where its removal was constrained. Administration of thiamine (10 to 20 mg/day) had a dramatic clinical effect; lacticacidosis abated immediately, and pyruvate accumulation rapidly subsided. A shunt mechanism with the removal of pyruvate by the dehydrogenase pathway was proposed to explain this interesting response.

Another female patient, with similar biochemical findings, has been reported by Tada and colleagues in Japan (Tada et al., 1969; Yoshida et al., 1969; Yoshida et al., 1970). A retarded sib of the patient died at 5 years of age. The concentrations of alanine and pyruvate in cerebrospinal fluid were higher than in the blood, suggesting that the metabolic defect was expressed in brain as well as in other tissues. Hepatic pyruvate carboxylase was measured and found to be about 15 per cent of normal at an unspecified concentration of pyruvate. The partial deficiency of the enzyme may be analogous to that found in the Canadian patient.

On the basis of the current evidence, it appears that hyperpyruvicacidemia with intermittent lacticacidosis and mental retardation can be a sequela of *partial* pyruvate carboxylase deficiency (modified K_m variety). This "syndrome" should probably be distinguished from another in which almost complete deficiency of hepatic carboxylase activity can be associated with abnormal pyruvate metabolism and a fatal neurological disease called Leigh's necrotizing encephalomyelopathy (Hommes et al., 1968) (see next section).

Other Conditions Potentially Associated With Hyperalaninemia. Subacute necrotizing encephalomyelopathy (Leigh's encephalomyelopathy) is a fatal syndrome with hypotonia, oculomotor palsies and progressive motor deterioration associated with intermittent hypoglycemia and accumulation of pyruvate and lactate in blood (Dunn and Dolman, 1969; Grover et al., 1972). Intermittent lacticacidosis can also occur. Hommes and colleagues (1968) found that pyruvate carboxylase activity in liver biopsy material from one patient was less than 1 per cent of normal at one year of age. However, the kinetics of the assay were not described.

Hommes et al. (1968) and Clayton's group (1967) both showed amelioration of the lacticacidemia and of clinical findings in Leigh's disease upon treatment with lipoic acid. Lipoate is a cofactor for pyruvate dehydrogenase. It is interesting that two different substances, thiamine and lipoic acid, both of which are cofactors for pyruvate dehydrogenase, improve the biochemical and clinical course of patients with pyruvate carboxylase deficiency. A shunt mechanism via pyruvate dehydrogenase for pyruvate disposal seems pertinent.

The similarity of the biochemical findings in the Dutch patient (Hommes et al., 1968) and in the French-Canadian and Japanese patients (Brunette et al., 1972; Tada et al., 1969; Yoshida et al., 1969) encourages one to believe in similar phenotypic mechanisms for these patients. Pyruvate carboxylase occurs in brain (Grover et al., 1972) and an almost complete deficiency of this critical determinant of oxaloacetate availability and gluconeogenesis in brain tissue may explain the severe neurological abnormalities of Leigh's syndrome, while less complete impairment of the enzyme may be compatible with a more benign clinical course, as seen in the Canadian and Japanese patients. However, Grover and coworkers (1972) have shown that hepatic pyruvate carboxylase activity can be normal early in the course of the disease and depressed in liver and brain only at the final stage. This finding makes a primary deficiency of the enzyme unlikely in Leigh's disease, and a search for an inhibitor is indicated.

Necrotizing encephalomyelopathy is also associated with a distrubance in the formation of thiamine triphosphate (TTP) by the enzyme thiamine pyrophosphate-adenosine triphosphate phosphoryl transferase. About 10 per cent of total thiamine in the body occurs as TTP, and it has been suggested that this is the neurophysiologically active form of thiamine. The presence of an inhibitor of TTP formation has been identified in Leigh's encephalomyelopathy (Pincus et al., 1969; Cooper et al., 1969, 1970). The relationship of this finding to the apparent defect in hepatic pyruvate carboxylase activity is unclear at present, but the two findings have been documented simultaneously in the same patient (Tang et al., 1972).

The prominence of ataxia as a clinical sign in patients with hyperpyruvicacidemia has been noted and discussed by Dunn and Dolman (1969) and Blass et al. (1971).

ASPARTYLGLYCOSAMINURIA

A novel ninhydrin-positive, orange-yellow substance was first discovered in the urine of a mentally retarded 30-year-old woman with coarse facial features and signs suggestive of a connective tissue disorder. A sibling, also retarded, excreted the same compound in his urine. Appropriate studies revealed the substance to be 2-acetamido-1-(β^1-L-aspartamido)-1,2-dideoxy-β-D-glucose (AADG) (Jenner and Pollitt, 1967). The trait associated with abnormal urinary excretion of this substance has come to be known by the trivial name aspartylglycosaminuria (Pollitt et al., 1968; Pollitt and Jenner, 1971).

Adult patients excrete about 300 mg per day of AADG, traces of which are also found in plasma and cerebrospinal fluid; AADG is normally absent from all three body fluids. The degradation of AADG is attributed to a specific enzyme, 2-acetamido-1-(β^1-L-aspartamido)-1,2-dideoxyglucose amidohydrolase (or N-aspartyl β-glucosylamine aminidase, EC 3.5.1. __). The enzyme occurs in plasma, and its origin is apparently associated with the lysosomal fraction of tissues including brain, liver and kidney and of semen; the distribution is appropriate for an enzyme whose substrate is a constituent of glycoprotein catabolism. There is a possibility that AADG amidohydrolase occurs as several isozymes.

Serum AADG amidohydrolase activity is severely deficient in probands (Pollitt and Jenner, 1971), and the activity in brain and liver is a fifth of normal (Palo et al., 1971). The presumed heterozygote has normal serum activity (Pollitt and Jenner, 1971).

Over 30 patients are known (Palo et al., 1971); most have been reported from Finland. Adult patients have glial cells and neurons with large lysosomes containing electron-dense membranous material. Hepatocytes also display large lysosomes with inclusions. The activity of several intralysosomal enzymes is concomitantly increased.

This disease occupies a position between the lysosomal storage diseases and the hereditary aminoacidurias. At present, it is not known how early in life the specific peptiduria occurs or whether prenatal and early postnatal diagnosis is possible.

DISORDERS OF TRYPTOPHAN METABOLISM

We have already discussed tryptophan metabolism in some detail with regard to two conditions in which its renal and intestinal transport are impaired (see sections on Hartnup disease and tryptophan malabsorption in Chapter 9). In addition to these disorders of tryptophan transport, there are other disorders of intracellular tryptophan catabolism which deserve mention: tryptophanuria, hydroxykynureninuria and xanthurenic aciduria. These disorders affect the major pathway of tryptophan catabolism by which tryptophan is converted to nicotinic acid and ultimately to nicotinamide adenine dinucleotide (Fig. 21–4).

Tryptophanuria

In 1963 Tada and coworkers reported a nine-year-old dwarfed girl with severe developmental retardation, a skin rash characterized by photosensitivity and hyperpigmentation, cerebellar ataxia and tryptophanuria. Although her pellagra-like clinical findings and tryptophanuria were suggestive of Hartnup disease, other biochemical parameters were very different: her fasting plasma tryptophan concentration was increased, not reduced, as in some patients with Hartnup disease; she responded to an oral tryptophan load with an exaggerated and prolonged rise in plasma tryptophan, not the blunted response seen in Hartnup disease; she had no generalized increase in urinary excretion of neutral aliphatic and aromatic amino acids so characteristic of Hartnup disease; and the urinary excretion of indican and indoleacetic acid was not increased as it is in Hartnup disease. These findings suggested a block in tryptophan catabolism, which was localized further by loading studies with tryptophan and its metabolites. Following an oral tryptophan load, urinary kynurenine and N-methylnicotinamide rose less in the patient than in controls, whereas she responded to oral nicotinic acid loading with the same increment in urinary N-methylnicotinamide as controls did. These observations led Tada et al. to propose that their patient had an enzymatic block in one of the two reactions by which tryptophan is converted to kynurenine: either the tryptophan pyrrolase-catalyzed conversion of tryptophan to N-formylkynurenine (Knox and Mehler, 1950; Tanaka and Knox, 1959) or the formylase-catalyzed conversion of N-formylkynurenine to kynurenine (Mehler and Knox, 1950). Since the patient was the product of a consanguineous mating, and since both parents excreted more tryptophan after an oral load than controls did, it was further concluded that this disorder is most probably inherited as an autosomal recessive trait. No in vitro studies

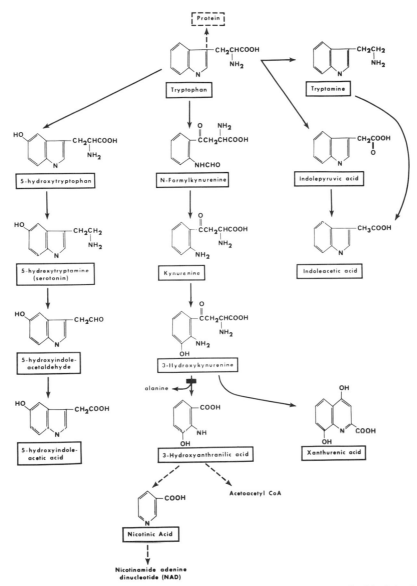

Figure 21–4   Major and minor pathways of tryptophan metabolism. The block in the major pathway between 3-hydroxykynurenine and 3-hydroxyanthranilic acid denotes site of the metabolic lesion in *xanthurenicaciduria* due to hepatic kynureninase deficiency (Tada et al., 1967, 1968) and presumably in the analogous condition, *3-hydroxykynureninuria* (Komrower et al., 1964). The site of the defect in *tryptophanuria* (Tada et al., 1963) is not shown, but it presumably occurs at the first or second step of tryptophan oxidation to kynurenine.

in the patient or her parents have been conducted to confirm these very likely hypotheses.

Xanthurenicaciduria

Kynureninase is the enzyme which catalyzes the conversion of 3-hydroxy-kynurenine to 3-hydroxyanthranilic acid (Fig. 21–4) and kynurenine to anthranilic acid (an analogous reaction not shown in Figure 21–4). This apoenzyme requires pyridoxal phosphate (B_6) as a coenzyme. Its in vivo activity has often been used as an indirect indicator of vitamin B_6 deficiency (Scriver, 1961; Scriver and Hutchison, 1963; Scriver, 1967). Patients depleted of vitamin B_6 respond to an oral load of tryptophan by excreting far more of the substrates (kynurenine and hydroxykynurenine) and their transamination by-products (kynurenic acid and xanthurenic acid) than do normal subjects. Reduction of kynureninase, with xanthurenicaciduria after tryptophan loading, is one of the biochemical reactions to be modulated early by vitamin B_6 deficiency. In this setting, physiologic replacement of vitamin B_6 results in prompt normalization of this aberrant response to tryptophan administration.

Since 1960, 18 patients from seven families in Germany, the United States and Japan have been described with a different kind of xanthurenicaciduria. None of these patients has had microcytic anemia, convulsions, reduced serum pyridoxal phosphate concentrations or decreased urinary 4-pyridoxic acid content, as B_6-deficient patients do. Nonetheless, all of these individuals have responded to oral tryptophan loading with markedly exaggerated urinary excretion of xanthurenic acid as well as kynurenine and 3-hydroxykynurenine. Furthermore, in all patients tested, administration of supraphysiologic amounts of vitamin B_6 (10 to 100 mg/day) has resulted in marked but transient improvement in the observed biochemical abnormalities.

The disorder was first recognized by Knapp (1960), who described 12 affected members of three pedigrees. The probands in all three kindreds were detected in the course of surveying individuals for B_6 deficiency, not because they suffered from any phenotypic abnormality. Importantly, none of these individuals had seizures or mental retardation, though all had typical biochemical findings following an oral tryptophan load. Subsequently, O'Brien and Jensen (1963) described two females with xanthurenicaciduria detected in a survey of mentally retarded patients. In a smiliar way, Tada and his coworkers (1967, 1968) found xanthurenicaciduria in four members of two kindreds referred because of familial mental retardation. These circumstances make it impossible at present to determine whether the abnormalities in tryptophan metabolism are etiologically related to the mental subnormality noted in the last six patients described.

Tada and his associates (1967, 1968) have measured kynureninase activity in liver biopsies from three of their four patients and suitable controls. They found that kynureninase activity was markedly reduced in the absence of pyridoxal phosphate, but rose to nearly normal values when pyridoxal phosphate was added in saturating amounts. Based on this in vitro evidence and the well-documented in vivo responsiveness of these patients to B_6 supplements, these workers concluded that the disorder is due to a mutant kynureninase apoenzyme with much-reduced affinity for its normal coenzyme, pyridoxal phosphate. This concept will be discussed in greater detail in Chapter 22.

The mode of inheritance of this condition is obscure at this time. Fifteen of the 18 reported patients are females, raising the possibility of a sex-limited or sex-linked trait. Knapp (1960) noted biochemical abnormalities in two and even three generations in his kindreds. Tada et al., too, found xanthurenic-aciduria in one of the parents of affected children in both kindreds studied, but they assayed kynureninase only in affected children. Hence, at this time we can say only that the disease is familial and appears to have a most unusual sex ratio.

Hydroxykynureninuria

Komrower and associates (1964, 1967) reported a girl with pyridoxine-resistant xanthurenicaciduria in whom there was an equivalent amount of 3-hydroxykynureninuria (20 to 25 μM/kg per day). This excess of tryptophan derivatives (10 to 20 times normal) was excreted without the necessity of loading the patient with tryptophan, whereas it was necessary to administer a load of L-tryptophan (100 mg/kg) by mouth to produce this degree of xanthurenic acid excretion in pyridoxine-responsive xanthurenicaciduria. L-Tryptophan loading augmented the excretion of this metabolite at least threefold in Komrower's patient, and it was estimated that about 40 per cent of the administered trypto-phan was excreted in the urine in the form of derivatives accumulating proxi-mal to the kynureninase step. Since no metabolites distal to this enzyme were detected, even after loading with L-tryptophan, the authors assumed that a deficiency of kynureninase was present in their patient. A dietary supplement of pyridoxine, up to 100 mg/day given orally or parenterally for long periods of time, did not alter the biochemical trait. The patient exhibited mild mental retardation, transient hepatosplenomegaly and signs interpreted as nicotinic acid deficiency during infancy, when she was fed milk primarily. Her parents were healthy, but the mother excreted xanthurenic acid at three times the normal rate after an oral load of L-tryptophan.

From this evidence it appears that hydroxykynureninuria is indeed a condi-tion associated with deficient kynureninase activity. However, hydroxykynure-ninuria is quite different from pyridoxine-responsive xanthurenicaciduria; and because the former is probably familial also, it may reflect the expression of a different mutant allele at the kynureninase locus.

Tryptophan Metabolism in Other Diseases

There have been many studies of tryptophan metabolism in various disease states. The wealth of by-products excreted in urine after bacterial conversion of malabsorbed tryptophan in the intestinal lumen has intrigued investigators for years. The reports by Scriver (1961) and Kowlessar et al. (1964), among others, describe studies on the urinary excretion of 5-hydroxy-indoleacetic acid, indole-3-acetic acid and indican, as well as of other tryptophan metabolites, by patients with sprue and celiac-like diseases. Sterilization of the intestinal lumen with antibiotics ablates the indoleuria in these conditions in much the same way that it does in the hereditary disorders of tryptophan (Hartnup disease and the blue-diaper syndrome) described in Chapter 9.

REFERENCES

Glutamate Metabolism, α-L-Alanine Metabolism and Aspartylglycosaminuria

Aoki, T. T., Brennan, M. F., Muller, W. A., Moore, F. D., and Cahill, G. F., Jr.: Effect of insulin on muscle glutamate uptake. Whole blood versus plasma glutamate analysis. J. Clin. Invest. *51*:2889–2894, 1972.

Bessman, S. P., and Hochstein, P.: Borscht, beets and glutamate. New Eng. J. Med. *282*:812–813, 1970.

Blass, J. P., Avigan, J., and Uhlendorf, B. W.: A defect in pyruvate decarboxylase in a child with an intermittent movement disorder. J. Clin. Invest. *49*:423–432, 1970.

Blass, J. P., Kark, R. A. P., and Engel, W. K.: Clinical studies of a patient with pyruvate decarboxylase deficiency. Arch. Neurol. (Chicago) *25*:449–460, 1971.

Brunette, M. G., Delvin, E., Hazel, B., and Scriver, C. R.: Thiamine-responsive lactic acidosis in a patient with deficient low-K_m pyruvate carboxylase activity in liver. Pediatrics, *50*:702–711, 1972.

Clayton, B. E., Dobbs, R. H., and Patrick, A. D.: Leigh's subacute necrotizing encephalopathy: Clinical and biochemical study with special reference to therapy with lipoate. Arch. Dis. Child. *42*:467–478, 1967.

Cooper, J. R., Itokawa, Y., and Pincus, J. H.: Thiamine triphosphate deficiency in subacute necrotizing encephalomyelopathy. Science *164*:74–75, 1969.

Cooper, J. R., Pincus, H. J., Itokawa, Y., and Piros, K.: Experience with phosphoryl transferase inhibition in subacute necrotizing encephalomyelopathy. New Eng. J. Med. *283*:793–795, 1970.

Danks, D. M., Campbell, P. E., Stevens, B. J., Mayne, V., and Cartwright, E.: Menkes' kinky hair syndrome. An inherited defect in copper absorption with widespread effects. Pediatrics *50*:188–201, 1972b.

Danks, D. M., Stevens, B. J., Campbell, P. E., Gillespie, J. M., Walher-Smith, J., Blomfield, J., and Turner, B.: Menkes' kinky-hair syndrome. Lancet (i), 1100–1102, 1972a.

Delvin, E., Neal, J. L., and Scriver, C. R.: Pyruvate carboxylase: Two forms in human liver. (Abstract.) Pediat. Res. *6*:392, 1972.

Dunn, H. G., and Dolman, C. L.: Necrotizing encephalomyelopathy. Report of a case with relapsing polyneuropathy and hyperalaninemia and with manifestations resembling Friedrick's ataxia. Neurology (Minneap.) *19*:536–550, 1969.

Eldjarn, L., Jellum, E., and Stokke, O.: Pyroglutamic aciduria. Studies on the enzyme block and on the metabolic origin of pyroglutamic acid. Clin. Chim. Acta *40*:461–476, 1972.

Elwyn, D. H., Launder, W. J., Parikh, H. C., and Wise, E. M., Jr.: Roles of plasma and erythrocytes in interorgan transport of amino acids in dogs. Amer. J. Physiol. *222*:1333–1342, 1972.

French, J. M., Sherard, E. S., Lubell, H., Brotz, M., and Moore, C. L.: Trichopoliodystrophy. 1. Report of a case and biochemical studies. Arch. Neurol. (Chicago) *26*:229–244, 1972.

Glossman, H., and Neville, D. M., Jr.: γ-Glutamyl transferase in kidney brush border membranes. F.E.B.S. Letters *19*:340–344, 1972.

Goodman, S. I., Mace, J. W., and Pollak, S.: Serum gammaglutamyl transpeptidase deficiency. Lancet (i), 234–235, 1971.

Grover, W. D., Auerbach, V. H., and Patel, M. S.: Biochemical studies and therapy in subacute necrotizing encephalomyelopathy (Leigh's syndrome). J. Pediat. *81*:39–44, 1972.

Haworth, J. C., Ford, J. D., and Younozai, M. K.: Familial chronic acidosis due to an error in lactate and pyruvate metabolism. Canad. Med. Ass. J. *97*:773–779, 1967.

Haworth, J. C., and Ford, J. D.: Comment on ketotic hyperglycemia. (Letter to editor.) Lancet (i), 1159, 1969.

Hechtman, L., Morgenstern, G., Fraser, F. C., and Chim, P.: Unpublished observations, 1972.

Hommes, F. A., Polman, H. A., and Reerink, J. D.: Leigh's encephalomyelopathy: An inborn error of gluconeogenesis. Arch. Dis. Child. *43*:423–426, 1968.

Huckabee, W. E.: Relationships of pyruvate and lactate during anaerobic metabolism. I. Effects of infusion of pyruvate or glucose and of hyperventilation. J. Clin. Invest. *37*:244–254, 1958.

Israels, S., Haworth, J. C., Gourley, B., and Ford, J. D.: Curonic acidosis due to an error in lactate and pyruvate metabolism. Pediatrics *34*:346–356, 1964.

Jellum, E., Kluge, T., Borresen, H. C., Stokke, O., and Eldjarn, L.: Pyroglutamic aciduria—a new inborn error of metabolism. Scand. J. Clin. Lab. Invest. *26*:327–335, 1970.

Jenner, F. A., and Pollitt, R. J.: Large quantities of 2-acetamido-1-(β^1-L-aspartamido)-1,2-dideoxyglucose in the urine of mentally retarded siblings. Biochem. J. *103*:488, 1967.

Konrad, P. N., Richards, F., II., Valentine, W. N., and Paglia, D. E.: γ-Glutamyl-cysteine synthetase deficiency. A cause of hereditary hemolytic anemia. New Eng. J. Med. *286*:557–561, 1972.

Lancaster, G., Mohyuddin, F., Scriver, C. R., and Whelan, D. T.: A γ-aminobutyrate pathway in mammalian kidney cortex. Biochim. Biophys. Acta *297*:229–240, 1973.

Lonsdale, D., Faulkner, W. R., Price, J. M., and Smeby, R. R.: Intermittent cerebellar ataxia associated with hyperpyruvic acidemia, hyperphenylalaninemia and hyperalaninuria. Pediatrics *43*:1025–1034, 1969.

McLaughlan, J. M., Neel, F. J., Bolting, H. G., and Knipfel, J. E.: Blood and brain levels of glutamic acid in young rats given monosodium glutamate. Nutr. Rep. Int. *1*:131–138, 1970.

Menkes, J. H.: Kinky hair disease. Pediatrics *50*:181–182, 1972.

Menkes, J. H., Alter, M., Steigleder, G. K., Weakley, D. R., and Surg, J. H.: A sex-linked recessive disorder with retardation of growth, peculiar hair and local cerebral and cerebellar degeneration. Pediatrics *29*:764–779, 1962.

O'Brien, J. S., and Sampson, E. L.: Kinky hair disease. II. Biochemical studies. J. Neuropath. Exp. Neurol. 25:523–530, 1966.

O'Daly, S.: An abnormal sulfhydryl compound in urine. Irish J. Med. Sci. Series VII 1:578, 1968.

O'Daly, S.: Personal communication, 1973.

O'Daly, S.: Reflections on metabolic errors and mental defect. J. Roy. Coll. Surg. Ireland 5:57–60, 1969.

Oliva, P. B.: Lactic acidosis. Amer. J. Med. 48:209–225, 1970.

Olney, J. W.: Brain lesions, obesity and other disturbances in mice treated with monosodium glutamate. Science 164:719–721, 1969.

Orlowski, M., and Meister, A.: The γ-glutamyl cycle: A possible transport system for amino acids. Proc. Nat. Acad. Sci. U.S.A. 67:1248–1255, 1970.

Oski, F. A., and Naiman, J. L.: Hematologic Problems in the Newborn, 2nd edition. W. B. Saunders Company, Philadelphia, 1972.

Pagliara, A., and Goodman, A. D.: Pitfalls in the determination of plasma glutamate. New Eng. J. Med. 279:1402, 1968.

Paine, R. S.: Evaluation of familial biochemically determined mental retardation in children with special reference to aminoaciduria. New Eng. J. Med. 262:658–665, 1960.

Palo, J., Riekkinen, P., Arstila, A., and Antio, S.: Biochemical and fine structural studies on brain and liver biopsies in aspartyl glycosaminuria. Neurology (Minneap.) 21:1198–1204, 1971.

Perry, T. L.: Unpublished observations, 1967. Cited in Dunn, A. G., and Dolman, C. L., Necrotizing encephalomyelopathy. Neurology (Minneap.) 19:536–550, 1969.

Pincus, J. H., Itokawa, Y., and Cooper, J. R.: Enzyme-inhibiting factor in subacute necrotizing encephalomyelopathy. Neurology 19:841–845, 1969.

Podos, S. M.: Hyperpyruvicemia with hyper-alpha-alaninemia. Arch. Ophthal. (Chicago) 83:504–505, 1970.

Pollitt, R. J., Jenner, F. A., and Mersky, H.: Aspartyl glycosaminuria. An inborn error of metabolism associated with mental defect. Lancet 2:253, 1968.

Pollitt, R. J., and Jenner, F. A.: Enzymatic cleavage of 2-acetoamido-1-(β¹-L-aspartamido)-1,2-dideoxy-β-D-glucose by human plasma and seminal fluid. Failure to detect the heterozygous state for aspartylglycosaminuria. Clin. Chim. Acta 25:413, 1969.

Pollitt, R. J., and Jenner, F. A.: Aspartylglycosaminuria. A new inborn error possibly due to a lysosomal enzyme defect. In Institute for Research into Mental Retardation, Study Group No. 2, Ciba Foundation, London, 1970, Benson, P. F., ed., Cellular Organelles and Membranes in Mental Retardation. Churchill Livingstone, London, pp. 95–101, 1971.

Ramakrishna, N., Krishnaswamy, P. R., and Rajagopal Rao, D.: Metabolism of pyrrolidone carboxylic acid in the rat. Biochem. J 118:895–897, 1970.

Reynolds, W. A., Lenkey-Johnston, N., Filer, L. J., Jr., and Pitkin, R. M.: Monosodium glutamate: Absence of hypothalamic lesions after ingestion by newborn primates. Science 172:1342–1344, 1971.

Schaumberg, H. H., Byck, R., Gerstl, R., and Mashman, J. H.: Monosodium L-glutamate: Its pharmacology and role in the Chinese Restaurant Syndrome. Science 163:826–828, 1969.

Stegink, L. D., and Baker, G. L.: Infusion of protein hydrolysates in the newborn infant: Plasma amino acid concentrations. J. Pediat. 78:595–602, 1971.

Stegink, L. D., Filer, L. J., Jr., and Baker, G. L.: Monosodium glutamate: Effect on plasma and breast milk amino acid levels in lactating women. Proc. Soc. Exp. Biol. Med. 140:836–841, 1972.

Stegink, L. D., Pitkin, R. M., Reynolds, W. A., and Filer, L. J., Jr.: Placental transfer of monosodium glutamate (MSG) and its metabolites in the primate. (Abstract #3797.) Fed. Proc. 32:893, 1973.

Strömme, J. H., and Eldjarn, L.: The metabolism of L-pyroglutamic acid in fibroblasts from a patient with pyroglutamic aciduria: The demonstration of an L-pyroglutamate hydrolase system. Scand. J. Clin. Lab. Invest. 29:335–342, 1972.

Tada, K., Yoshida, T., Konno, T., Wada, Y., Yokoyama, Y., and Arakawa, T.: Hyperalaninemia with pyruvicemia. Tohoku J. Exp. Med. 97:99–100, 1969.

Tallan, H. H.: A survey of the amino acids and related compounds in nervous tissue. In Holden, J. T., ed., Amino Acid Pools: Distribution, Formation and Function of Free Amino Acids. Elsevier, New York, pp. 471–485, 1962.

Tang, T. T., Good, T. A., Dyken, P. R., Johnsen, S. D., McCreadie, S. R., Sy, S. T., Lardy, H. A., and Rudolf, F. B.: Pathogenesis of Leigh's encephalomyelopathy. J. Pediat. 81:189–190, 1972.

Van den Berg, C. J., Krzalic, L. J., Mela, P., and Waelsch, H.: Compartmentation of glutamate metabolism in brain. Evidence for the existence of two different tricarboxylic acid cycles in brain. Biochem. J. 113:281–290, 1969.

Van der Werf, P., Orlowski, M., and Meister, A.: Enzymatic conversion of 5-oxo-L-proline (L-pyrrolidone carboxylate) to L-glutamate coupled with cleavage of adenosine triphosphate to adenosine diphosphate, a reaction in the γ-glutamyl cycle. Proc. Nat. Acad. Sci. U.S.A. 68:2982–2985, 1971.

Yoshida, T., Tada, K., and Arakawa, T.: Abnormally high levels of lactate and pyruvate in cerebrospinal fluid of hyperalaninemia with hyperpyruvicemia. Tohoku J. Exp. Med. *101*:375–378, 1970.

Yoshida, T., Tada, K., Konno, T., and Arakawa, T.: Hyperalaninemia with pyruvicemia due to pyruvate carboxylase deficiency of the liver. Tohoku J. Exp. Med. *99*:121–128, 1969.

Yoshida, T., Tada, K., Mizuno, T., Wada, Y., Akabane, J., Ogasawara, J., Minagawa, A., Morikawa, T., and Okamura, T.: A sex-linked disorder with mental and physical retardation characterized by cerebrocortical atrophy and increase of glutamic acid in the cerebrospinal fluid. Tohoku J. Exp. Med. *83*:261–269, 1964.

Tryptophan

Knapp, A.: Über eine neue Hereditäre von Vitamin-B₆ abhängige Störung im Tryptophanstoffwechsel. Clin. Chim. Acta 5:6–13, 1960.

Knox, W. E., and Mehler, A. H.: The conversion of tryptophan to kynurenine in liver. I. The coupled tryptophan peroxidase-oxidase system forming formylkynurenine. J. Biol. Chem. *187*:419–430, 1950.

Komrower, G. M., Wilson, V., Clamp, J. R., and Westall, R. G.: Hydroxykynureninuria. Arch. Dis. Child. *39*:250–256, 1964.

Kowlessar, O. D., Haeffner, L. J., and Benson, G. D.: Abnormal metabolism in patients with adult celiac disease, with evidence for deficiency of vitamin-B₆. J. Clin. Invest. *43*:894–903, 1964.

Mehler, A. H., and Knox, W. E.: The conversion of tryptophan to kynurenine in liver. II. The enzymatic hydrolysis of formylkynurenine. J. Biol. Chem. *187*:431–438, 1950.

O'Brien, D., and Jensen, C. B.: Pyridoxine dependency in two mentally retarded subjects. Clin. Sci. *24*:179–186, 1913.

Scriver, C. R.: Abnormalities of tryptophan metabolism in a patient with malabsorption syndrome. J. Lab. Clin. Med. *58*:908–919, 1961.

Scriver, C. R.: Vitamin B₆ deficiency and dependency in man. Amer. J. Dis. Child. *113*:109–114, 1967.

Scriver, C. R., and Hutchison, J. H.: The vitamin B₆ deficiency syndrome in human infancy. Biochemical and clinical observations. Pediatrics *31*:240–250, 1963.

Tada, K., Ito, H., Wada, Y., and Arakawa, T.: Congenital tryptophanuria with dwarfism. Tohoku J. Exp. Med. *80*:118–134, 1963.

Tada, K., Yokoyama, Y., Nakagawa, H., and Arakawa, T.: Vitamin B₆ dependent xanthurenic aciduria. The second report. Tohoku J. Exp. Med. *95*:107–114, 1968.

Tada, K., Yokoyama, Y., Nakagawa, H., Yoshida, T., and Arakawa, T.: Vitamin B₆ dependent xanthurenic aciduria. Tohoku J. Exp. Med. *93*:115–124, 1967.

Tanaka, T., and Knox, W. E.: The nature and mechanism of the tryptophan pyrrolase (peroxidase-oxidase) reaction of pseudomonas and rat liver. J. Biol. Chem. *234*:1162–1170, 1959.

Chapter Twenty-Two

VITAMIN-RESPONSIVE AMINOACIDOPATHIES

We have chosen to conclude this volume with a discussion of a special group of inherited disorders of amino acid metabolism: those which respond biochemically or clinically to specific vitamin supplementation. Since the clinical and chemical manifestations of each of these conditions have already been discussed in detail elsewhere in this book, the reader may ask why we have chosen to devote a separate chapter to them. We have four reasons. First, these disorders exemplify that class of inherited conditions which physicians are most interested in: eminently treatable ones. Second, they illustrate a cardinal principle of human biochemical genetics—namely, that the study of rare abnormalities is often crucial to an understanding of normal processes. Third, these conditions underscore the kinship between basic biochemistry and clinical medicine. Finally, they represent an area of investigation which has occupied, and sometimes preoccupied, both of the writers of this volume for several years.

HISTORICAL PERSPECTIVE

Although the concept of vitamin-responsive, or, as they have often been called, vitamin-dependent inherited aminoacidopathies is less than 20 years old, the historical roots of this discussion date back to the earliest years of this century. At the same time (1902–1908) that Archibald Garrod was introducing the subject of human biochemical genetics by publishing his classic studies of three "inborn errors" of amino acid metabolism (alcaptonuria, cystinuria and albinism), Hopkins was investigating systematically the significance of a group of "accessory food substances" required for normal human nutrition. Soon thereafter, Funk (1912) coined the term *vitamine* to describe the nature of the beri-beri curing substance, which he believed erroneously to be a vital amine.

Progress in the areas of vitamin and amino acid metabolism has accelerated rapidly during the past three decades. More than 100 disorders have been described which are caused by specific inherited defects in the anabolic or catabolic pathways for individual amino acids, and much has been learned about their biochemical, clinical and genetic hallmarks. In like measure, we have come to recognize that vitamins are organic compounds which must be ingested in minute amounts for normal growth, maintenance and reproduction. Just as the numerous amino acids differ markedly in structure and function, so do the vitamins. Some are obtained from animal sources, others from vegetables; some are water-soluble, others fat-soluble; some function as chemical precursors, others as cofactors for one or more enzymatic reactions.

The two fields have been drawn together logically by the expanding knowledge in each. The demonstration that vitamin B_6 (pyridoxine) functions as a coenzyme in the transamination, decarboxylation and deamination of most amino acids led to the discovery that this vitamin could correct abnormalities in several disorders of amino acid metabolism. Similarly, the more recent identification of patients with aminoacidopathies responsive to thiamine, folic acid, biotin or vitamin B_{12} rested on an understanding of the role that each of these vitamins plays in the catalysis and modulation of reactions involving amino acids or their derivatives.

Vitamin Requirements: Deficiency and Dependency

The explosion of interest in vitamins at the turn of this century terminated a long period of informal awareness about these accessory substances (Needham, 1962).

A text entitled *Medical Experiences of a Frontier Official* had appeared in China in the 8th century A.D. wherein conditions resembling deficiency of vitamin A and vitamin D were described. In the 14th century, again from China, the book *Principles of Correct Diet* described a condition resembling beri-beri. Two hundred years later, the French explorer Cartier (1545) described in a report to his king how the drinking of the liquor from boiled spruce needles, prepared for him by the Indians of the St. Lawrence Valley region, cured the scurvy of his crew members. Cartier's preliminary communication about an antiscorbutic agent was later confirmed by many an English sea captain. This anecdotal approach to vitamins and vitamin deficiencies continued until the end of the 19th century, when certain diseases formerly presumed to be infectious were linked unequivocally to a deficiency of specific food factors.

The human requirements for most vitamins concerned with amino acid metabolism have been carefully defined under a variety of physiological conditions (Table 22–1). When the intake or absorption of a vitamin falls below the minimal requirement, a specific deficiency state will occur which can be corrected simply by supplementing the diet with the vitamin up to the required intake. Thus, vitamin-deficient states are usually characterized by an acquired origin, a broad spectrum of biochemical disarray and responsiveness to a normal intake of the vitamin in question.

Table 22–1   The Recommended Dietary Allowances for Several Vitamins
Concerned with Amino Acid Metabolism*

Vitamin	Unit	Infant (<12 mos)	Child 1–8 yr	Youth 9–17 yr	Adult
Thiamine (B$_1$)	mg	0.4	0.8	1.4	1.2
Riboflavin (B$_2$)	mg	0.6	1.3	2.0	1.7
Pyridoxine (B$_6$)	mg	0.4	1	2	2
Cobalamin (B$_{12}$)	μg	2.5	2.5	5	5
Folic acid	mg	0.05	0.05	0.1	0.1
Niacin†	mg	6	14	22	19
Ascorbic acid (C)	mg	30–100**	60	80	70

*The recommended dietary allowances are intended to serve as a guide in planning food
supplies and for the interpretation of food consumption of groups of people (National Academy of
Sciences, 1968; WHO, 1967, 1970). Minimum and maximum allowable intakes are another concept
(Federal Register, 1966.)

**Higher allowance recommended for premature infants or full-term infants with postnatal
tyrosinemia.

†L-Tryptophan, 60 mg, is equivalent to 1 mg niacin.

On the other hand, we now know that some few individuals have a constant,
specific requirement for a particular vitamin that differs from normal in one
of two ways: either the *route* of vitamin administration must be changed from
oral to parenteral; or the *quantity* of the vitamin must be increased to 5 to 500
times that usually recommended. The prevention of disease in such individuals
is, in fact, dependent upon such altered administration. This group of patients
with *vitamin-dependent* or *vitamin-responsive* conditions can be contrasted to those
with vitamin-deficient states in several ways. First, vitamin dependency states
have a genetic etiology, whereas typical vitamin deficiencies are acquired. If
the inherited abnormality impairs intestinal absorption of the vitamin, then its
clinical and biochemical manifestations will be identical to those of an acquired
deficiency, but the mode of vitamin administration needed to correct these
manifestations will differ. Second, most vitamin-dependent disorders reflect
an underlying biochemical abnormality in only a single reaction, while vitamin
deficiency states commonly lead to interference with several reactions. Third,
most vitamin-dependent conditions respond only to a pharmacologic dose of
a specific vitamin, not to a physiologic one. Only one of these characteristics,
however, is common to all vitamin-responsive aminoacidopathies: their inherited
nature.

GENETIC CONTROL OF VITAMIN METABOLISM

The very fact that all of the compounds we call vitamins must be supplied
in the diet is *prima facie* evidence that, in the course of evolution, the human
species has lost the genetic information required to synthesize these compounds. But it does not follow therefrom that man's genes play no part in vitamin metabolism. On the contrary, it is clear that a number of proteins and, therefore, a number of genes regulate all facets of vitamin metabolism once ingestion
has occurred. These proteins are of two general types: those concerned with
vitamin transport, and those required for intracellular vitamin utilization
(Table 22–2). For example, at least nine proteins are needed if ingested vitamin

Table 22–2   Classes of Proteins Participating in Vitamin-Dependent Reactions

Transport Proteins
1. Intestinal receptor
2. Plasma-binding
3. Tissue receptor

Intracellular Proteins
4. Activating enzyme
5. Holoenzyme synthetase
6. Apoenzyme

B_{12} is to function as a coenzyme: gastric intrinsic factor which binds B_{12} in the stomach and carries it to the small bowel; specific receptors in the ileal mucosa which facilitate absorption of B_{12} to and from tissue cells; two plasma-binding proteins; at least three intracellular activating enzymes which convert the vitamin to its active coenzyme forms; and finally, two apoenzymes which require B_{12} coenzymes for catalytic activity. Even this extensive array of proteins specifically concerned with the use of this vitamin may be incomplete. There may also be specific lysosomal or mitochondrial binding proteins for B_{12} (Pletsch and Coffey, 1971, 1972) and perhaps, as has been shown for biotin, holoenzyme synthetases which act to catalyze the binding of coenzyme to apoenzyme (Cazzulo et al., 1970). Although not all of the vitamins require as intricate a set of regulatory reactions as B_{12}, there is a large body of data which shows that thiamine, riboflavin, niacin, pyridoxine, pantothenic acid and folic acid are each modified by one or more enzyme-catalyzed steps prior to carrying out their intracellular function. Thus, there is a large array of vitamin-regulating proteins whose structure and function could be altered by specific mutations in their respective genomes.

THE BIOCHEMICAL ROLE OF VITAMINS

Some enzymes depend for activity only on their structure as proteins, while others require one or more nonprotein *cofactors* for activity. Some cofactors are simple cations; others are more complex, heat-stable organic compounds called *coenzymes*. Each of the vitamins that concerns us in this discussion of vitamin-responsive aminoacidopathies is a precursor of one or more coenzymes (Table 22–3). Once formed intracellularly, the coenzyme associates with its appropriate protein species, called the *apoenzyme*, to form a *holoenzyme*. The holoenzyme then combines with its substrate, and catalyzes the formation of a product. Each coenzyme has a preferred type of reaction in which it participates (Table 22–3). Thiamine pyrophosphate, for example, functions in aldehyde transfer reactions; pyridoxal phosphate, in transaminations or decarboxylations; and folic acid, in 1-carbon fragment transfer systems. Just as the structure of the coenzyme defines the nature of functions in which it can participate, so the structure of the apoenzyme regulates the substrate specificity of the holoenzyme molecule. The molecular events involved in coenzyme-catalyzed reactions are beyond the scope of this discussion, but some general possibilities are shown in Figure 22–1 (Rosenberg, 1970). In some instances, the coenzyme forms part of the active site that reacts with substrate (Example 1, Figure 22–1). Alternatively, binding of coenzyme may change the apoenzyme's conformation and facilitate binding at a site distant from that for coenzyme attachment (Example 2). Furthermore, coenzymes may act to "glue" apoenzyme subunits together, thereby permitting

Table 22–3 The Coenzyme Role of Vitamins Concerned with
Amino Acid Metabolism

Vitamin	Coenzyme Form	Function
Thiamine (B_1)	Thiamine pyrophosphate	Activation of carboxyl derivatives; aldehyde transfer
Riboflavin (B_2)	Flavin mononucleotide and flavin adenine dinucleotide	Hydrogen atom (electron) transfer
Pyridoxine (B_6)	Pyridoxal-5′-phosphate	Amino group transfer; amino acid decarboxylation, etc.
Cobalamin (B_{12})	Methylcobalamin	Methyl group transfer for N^5-methyltetra-hydrofolate-homocysteine methyl-transferase
	5′-deoxyadenosylcobalamin	Hydrogen transfer in isomerization of L-methylmalonyl-CoA to succinyl-CoA
Folic acid	Tetrahydrofolate	1-Carbon fragment activation and transfer
Niacin	Nicotinamide adenine dinucleotide (phosphate)	Hydrogen atom (electron) transfer
Ascorbic acid (C)	L-Ascorbic acid	Reducing agent
Pantothenic acid	Coenzyme A	Acyl transfer
Biotin	Biotin	CO_2 activation and transfer

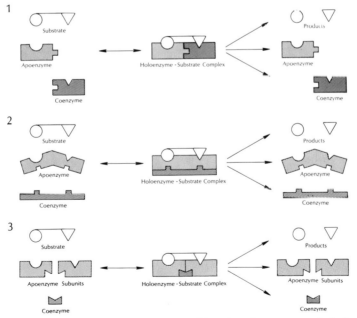

Figure 22–1 Schematic representation of possible roles of a coenzyme in holoenzyme-catalyzed reactions. *1*, coenzyme makes up part of substrate combining site; *2*, coenzyme alters the configuration of its apoenzyme to facilitate substrate binding; *3*, coenzyme unites apoenzyme subunits, thereby enhancing substrate binding.

substrate interaction (Example 3). By these or other mechanisms, coenzymes accelerate or permit catalytic reactions between apoenzyme and substrate.

Coenzyme-dependent apoenzyme proteins bind their specific coenzymes with varying degrees of affinity. In most instances, coenzymes are bound by hydrogen or hydrophobic bonds and may be dissociated from the apoenzyme by dialysis. Some coenzymes, however, are tightly and virtually irreversibly bound to their apoenzyme by covalent linkage. These different mechanisms of apoenzyme-coenzyme binding lead to different kinds of reaction kinetics— some which follow typical Michaelis-Menten formulation, others which do not (Northrop, 1969; Mudd, 1971).

Coenzymes have another important role which is not directly related to their chemical participation in catalysis. The steady-state concentration of certain apoenzymes can be regulated by their coenzymes. Apoenzymes normally undergo a cycle of synthesis and degradation within the cell, and the balance between the two phases of the cycle is an important focal point for regulation of the amount and activity of the enzyme in higher organisms (Wyngaarden, 1970). The rate of inactivation is probably the more important site of enzyme regulation in diploid cells (Barber et al., 1971). Some apoenzymes are induced by exposure to their coenzyme, and the effective concentration of holoenzyme, as well as the absolute concentration of apoenzyme can be increased. Such induction has been well documented for certain amino transferases and for tryptophan pyrrolase (Lin et al., 1958; Greengard, 1963). Binding of coenzyme to apoenzyme may also slow holoenzyme degradation. If the rate of apoenzyme synthesis remains constant, the concentration of holoenzyme will then rise, and enzyme activity (catalytic rate) will increase.

EFFECT OF MUTATION ON VITAMIN FUNCTION: THEORETICAL POSSIBILITIES

From the foregoing discussion, it is clear that a wide variety of different mutations could theoretically interfere with the activity of a vitamin as coenzyme (Fig. 22–2). The mutant allele could impair vitamin transport at one of several points: the intestine; the plasma; the tissue cells; or within intracellular organelles. The mutant allele could block the reaction(s) by which the vitamin is converted intracellularly to coenzyme. The mutant allele could alter the apoenzyme in such a way that its normal interaction with coenzyme would be disturbed. Finally, the mutant allele could lead to the synthesis of an altered apoenzyme whose turnover rate in the presence of normal amounts of coenzyme was distinctly increased. The very fact that any such mutation would demonstrate vitamin responsiveness implies that the effect of the mutation is partial, i.e., in bacterial terms, that the mutant is "leaky." Let us now examine the known vitamin-responsive aminoacidopathies to see how these theoretical considerations relate to observed phenomena.

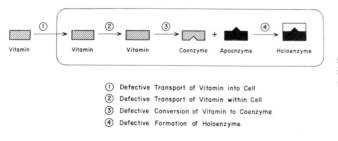

Figure 22–2 Scheme of sites at which mutations could interfere with vitamin-catalyzed reactions.

① Defective Transport of Vitamin into Cell
② Defective Transport of Vitamin within Cell
③ Defective Conversion of Vitamin to Coenzyme
④ Defective Formation of Holoenzyme

Defects of Vitamin Transport and Coenzyme Synthesis

Before any coenzyme can function biochemically, two general processes must be satisfied: its vitamin precursor must be absorbed from the intestinal tract and carried to the tissues; and the inactive vitamin must be converted to its active coenzyme form. There is much more information on the latter process than the former one. Although it is widely held that the water-soluble vitamins are absorbed from the gut by "active" transport, detailed information on this crucial point appears to exist only for vitamin B_{12} and folic acid. It is not surprising, therefore, that well-documented inherited defects of vitamin transport are known only for B_{12} and folate. We shall discuss the absorption and activation of these two vitamins in some detail to illustrate the principles alluded to previously.

Vitamin B_{12} (Cobalamin)

The structure and function of vitamin B_{12} have fascinated biologists of all stripes since Minot and Murphy (1926) demonstrated that crude liver extract was effective in the treatment of pernicious anemia. By 1948 this "antipernicious anemia factor" had been isolated from several animal sources and renamed vitamin B_{12} (Smith and Parker, 1948; Rickes et al., 1948). B_{12} is synthesized almost exclusively by microorganisms in soil, water and the rumen and intestine of animals. Although the exact human requirement has not been defined, less than 1 μg daily is sufficient to prevent signs or symptoms of deficiency.

The chemical structure of B_{12} (cobalamin) is complex (Fig. 22–3). It is composed of a central cobalt (Co) nucleus, a planar corrin ring and a dimethyl-benzimidazole ribose phosphate sidechain (Hodgkin et al., 1955). The molecule is completed by coordinate linkage of one of several different radicals (R) to the cobalt nucleus. Thus, cyanocobalamin, the commercial form of vitamin B_{12}, is formed by attachment of a cyanide radical to the cobalt atom. This compound, however, is an artifact of the chemical procedures used to isolate B_{12} and does not occur naturally in bacteria or animal tissues. Three other cobalamins have been isolated from mammalian tissue. Hydroxocobalamin is the major biological form of the vitamin found in blood plasma. Methylcobalamin (CH_3—B_{12}) and 5'-deoxyadenosylcobalamin (Ad—B_{12}) are the only two coenzyme forms of B_{12}, and each is known in man to cocatalyze only a single reaction: CH_3—B_{12} acts

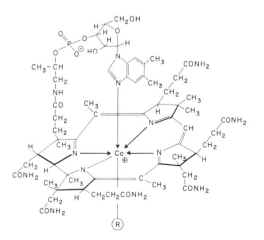

Figure 22–3 Chemical structure of vitamin B_{12} (cobalamin). ⓡ refers to several different radicals which may be coordinately linked to the cobalt atom, such as CN^- (cyanocobalamin), OH^-(hydroxocobalamin), CH_3 (methylcobalamin) or 5'-deoxyadenosyl (5'-deoxyadenosylcobalamin).

with N^5-methyltetrahydrofolate methyltransferase in the methylation of homocysteine to methionine; Ad—B_{12} acts with methylmalonyl-CoA mutase in the isomerization of L-methylmalonyl-CoA to succinyl-CoA (see Chapters 11 and 14).

Absorption and Activation.   Vitamin B_{12} has a unique and highly specialized mechanism of intestinal absorption which requires both gastric and ileal components. The gastric substance is "intrinsic factor," a glycoprotein which binds B_{12} in the intestinal lumen by forming an intrinsic factor-B_{12} (IF—B_{12}) complex (Castle, 1970). This complex interacts with specific receptor sites in the ileum. During this process, the IF—B_{12} complex dissociates and free B_{12} is transported across the ileal wall into the portal blood. Once in the bloodstream, free B_{12} is tightly bound to two different globulin proteins called transcobalamins I and II (Hall and Finkler, 1965). Transcobalamin I (TC I) is an α-globulin which carries the majority of B_{12} found in plasma. TC II, a β-globulin, carries less total B_{12} but is almost certainly the transport protein for B_{12} newly absorbed from the intestinal tract (Hom, 1967). TC II also facilitates uptake of B_{12} by mammalian tissues, presumably via a mediated, endocytotic process (Finkler and Hall, 1967; Rosenberg et al., 1973). The mechanisms by which B_{12} is transported intracellularly are unclear, but movement through lysosomes to mitochondria has been suggested (Pletsch and Coffey, 1972).

Once in the cell, vitamin B_{12} is converted to its coenzyme forms by a series of enzymatic reactions which have been examined in microbial and mammalian systems (Vitols et al., 1966; Walker et al., 1969; Kerwar et al., 1970; Mahoney et al., 1971). As shown in Figure 22–4, hydroxocobalamin (also called B_{12a}) is the precursor vitamin and exists with its cobalt atom oxidized to a trivalent state (CO^{+++}). B_{12a} is reduced successively to B_{12r} (Co^{++}) and B_{12s} (Co^+) by reductase enzymes which are flavoproteins requiring NAD as a cofactor. B_{12} is then converted enzymatically to Ad—B_{12} by a third enzyme called ATP:B_{12s} 5'-deoxyadenosyl transferase. The precise chemical reactions involved in CH_3—B_{12} synthesis have not been defined but are presumed to follow those shown for Ad—B_{12} during the reductase steps. Finally, the coenzymes attach to specific apoenzymes: Ad—B_{12} to methylmalonyl-CoA mutase, and CH_3—B_{12} to N^5-methyltetrahydrofolate methyltransferase.

Inherited Deficiency and Dependency.   Regardless of etiology, acquired vitamin B_{12} deficiency leads to a characteristic set of clinical and chemical hallmarks which include megaloblastic changes in the bone marrow and elsewhere; macrocytic anemia; spinocerebellar neurologic dysfunction; reduced content of B_{12} in serum and tissues; and increased urinary excretion of methylmalonate and homocystine. As noted in Table 22–4, some or all of these manifestations have been observed in a variety of different inborn errors of vitamin B_{12} me-

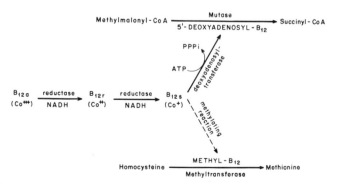

Figure 22–4 Pathway of intracellular formation of B_{12} coenzymes and the enzymatic reactions which the two B_{12} coenzymes (5'-deoxyadenosyl-B_{12} and methyl-B_{12}) cocatalyze. The methyltransferase reaction also requires N^5-methyltetrahydrofolate and S-adenosylmethionine. The broken line reflects uncertainty concerning the sequence of reactions leading to methyl-B_{12} synthesis. See text for additional details.

Table 22–4 Inborn Errors of Vitamin B_{12} Metabolism*

Phase of Metabolism Affected	Nature of Defect	Manifestation of Defect				
		Serum B_{12} Concentration	Megaloblastic Anemia	Methylmalonic-aciduria	Homo-cystinuria	In Vivo B_{12} Requirement
Intestinal absorption	IF deficiency	low	yes	yes	yes	normal
	Inactive IF	low	yes	NR	NR	normal
	Defective ileal transport	low	yes	NR	NR	normal
Plasma transport	TC I deficiency	low	no	NR	NR	normal
	TC II deficiency	normal	yes	no	no	increased
Tissue utilization	Defective Ad—B_{12} synthesis	normal	no	yes	no	increased
	Defective Ad—B_{12} and CH$_3$—B_{12} synthesis	normal	variable	yes	yes	increased

*The following symbols are used: IF = gastric intrinsic factor; TC = plasma transcobalamin; Ad—B_{12} = 5'-deoxyadenosylcobalamin; CH_3—B_{12} = methylcobalamin; NR = not reported tabolism. Children with typical "juvenile pernicious anemia" have been described with three different inherited disorders of intestinal absorption: complete lack of IF (Spurling et al., 1964); synthesis of a functionally defective IF (Katz et al., 1972); and defective ileal transport (Grasbeck et al., 1960). Each of these conditions responds dramatically to physiologic amounts of B_{12} (1 to 5 μg/day) administered *parenterally but not orally*. Infantile megaloblastic anemia was also the presenting finding in several siblings with an almost complete deficiency of the plasma B_{12} binding protein, TC II (Hakami et al., 1971). Hematologic remission again followed parenteral B_{12} administration but, in this instance, only after administration of 500 μg every second day and only so long as these huge doses of B_{12} were continued. In contrast, congenital absence of TC I produced no hematologic abnormalities, thereby indicating that only TC II-bound B_{12} modulates normal hematopoiesis (Carmel and Herbert, 1969).

At least two other mutations lead to B_{12}-responsive disorders — not because B_{12} absorption or transport are impaired but rather because coenzyme synthesis in tissue cells is blocked. The first of these disorders, described in a one-year-old boy by Rosenberg and his colleagues (1968) has already been discussed in detail in the section on methylmalonicaciduria in Chapter 14. This child had none of the hallmarks of B_{12} deficiency, yet excreted huge amounts of methylmalonate (MMA) in the urine. Physiologic B_{12} replacement was of no value, but parenteral supplementation with 1000 μg of B_{12} daily resulted in sustained biochemical and clinical improvement (Hsia et al., 1970). Although serum B_{12} was normal, cultured fibroblasts from this child contained less than 10 per cent of normal Ad—B_{12} concentration, suggesting a defect in Ad—B_{12} synthesis from the precursor vitamin. This thesis was confirmed as shown in Figure 22–5. Fibroblasts from this child took up ^{57}Co-hydroxocobalamin normally and synthesized CH_3—B_{12} as well as control cells did, but his cells were almost completely unable to make Ad—B_{12} (Mahoney et al., 1971). Since this boy's urine contained excess MMA but not homocystine, the culture studies are in good agreement with the clinical observations and suggest that he suffers from a specific defect

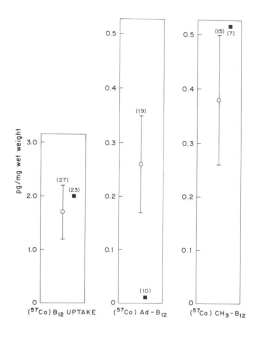

Figure 22–5   Vitamin B_{12} metabolism by intact cultured fibroblasts from controls (open circles) and child with B_{12}-responsive methylmalonicaciduria (closed squares). Fibroblasts were propagated in medium containing ^{57}Co-hydroxocobalamin (140 to 200 pg/ml). At confluence, the cells were harvested, and the cobalamins were extracted and separated by thin-layer chromatography. Control data are presented as the mean ±1 SD. Number of observations for the control and mutant lines is shown in parentheses. (Drawn from data of Mahoney et al., 1971.)

in Ad—B_{12} synthesis which impairs methylmalonyl mutase activity secondarily. The exact site of this defect, however, has not thus far yielded to studies with fibroblast extracts. It does not appear to be in the terminal adenosylation reaction (Fig. 22–4), since fibroblast extracts from this patient convert B_{12s} to Ad—B_{12} in a normal fashion (Rosenberg and Mahoney, 1973). A defect in B_{12} reduction or intracellular compartmentation remain to be investigated.

Let us now contrast the above findings with those in three patients described by Mudd (1969), Goodman (1970) and their coworkers. The first patient was an infant male who had failed to thrive from the time of birth and died at 7 weeks of age. He was not anemic and his serum B_{12} concentration was normal, but hepatic Ad—B_{12} content was much reduced and he excreted large amounts of MMA and homocystine in his urine. In addition, he had a low plasma methionine and increased urinary cystathionine. His cultured cells amplified these in vivo findings. Methylmalonyl-CoA mutase activity and N^5-methyltetrahydrofolate methyltransferase activity were markedly impaired, both reactions responding in vitro to addition of their respective B_{12} coenzymes (Mudd et al., 1970a). Further evidence for defective methionine formation was provided by growth experiments which showed that normal cells could be propagated in media containing either methionine or homocysteine as a sulfur source, whereas this patient's cells grew only in a methionine-containing medium. These findings indicated that this patient had blocks in both B_{12}-dependent reactions, presumably because neither B_{12} coenzyme was being synthesized in sufficient amounts. This thesis was corroborated by the kind of data shown in Figure 22–5: ^{57}Co-hydroxocobalamin was neither taken up nor converted to either coenzyme in anything like a normal fashion (Mahoney et al., 1971).

Subsequently, two male siblings of a consanguineous mating were described with similar but clinically less severe findings (Goodman et al., 1970). Both boys had homocystinuria and methylmalonicaciduria. Their fibroblasts showed defects in both B_{12}-dependent reactions and defective synthesis of both B_{12} coenzymes (Mahoney, 1973). One of these brothers showed marked chemical improvement on 1000 μg of B_{12} daily, indicating that this kind of defect in B_{12} metabolism is responsive in vivo as well as in vitro (Goodman, 1973). Again, the exact biochemical nature of this mutation remains to be defined.

To recapitulate, seven distinct inherited defects of B_{12} metabolism are now known: three of intestinal absorption; two of plasma transport; and two of coenzyme synthesis. Each of the intestinal defects responds to *physiologic* amounts of B_{12} given *parenterally*. The defects in TC II synthesis and coenzyme formation, however, respond only to pharmacologic (>100 times normal) doses of B_{12}.

Folic Acid

Clinicians have often considered B_{12} and folic acid in tandem because megaloblastic anemia is the hallmark of deficiency of both vitamins. These two vitamins have other prominent similarities pertinent to this discussion: both have complex systems of intestinal absorption and coenzyme synthesis; and both demonstrate a panorama of vitamin-response mutations in these transport and synthetic processes.

Like B_{12}, folic acid has a complex chemical structure (Fig. 22–6). It is composed of three moieties—a pterin ring, p-aminobenzoic acid and glutamic acid. Humans require about 50 μg of folate daily, and can satisfy this requirement by ingesting a large number of vegetables, fruits and meats rich in folic acid. There are no fewer than five coenzyme forms of folate, all of which participate in the transfer of 1-carbon units vital for the synthesis of DNA, RNA, methionine, glutamate and serine.

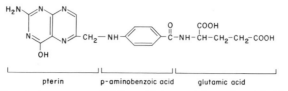

Figure 22–6 Chemical structure of folic acid (pteroylglutamic acid). Note that molecule is composed (from left to right) of a pterin ring, *p*-aminobenzoic acid and glutamic acid. In foods, the most common form of folate is the polyglutamate in which several glutamate residues are joined in γ-glutamyl linkage. The active folate coenzymes are formed by reduction of the nitrogen atoms of the pterin nucleus.

Absorption and Coenzyme Synthesis. The principal dietary form of folate is not the monoglutamate form shown in Figure 22–6 but rather folic acid polyglutamate in which one to six glutamic acid residues are linked to the parent molecule by gamma-peptide formation. The polyglutamyl form of folate cannot be absorbed intact but must be converted in the intestinal tract to its monoglutamate form (Bernstein et al., 1970). This conversion is catalyzed by a conjugase enzyme found in intestinal mucosa, stomach and pancreas. Once folic acid monoglutamate is formed, it is absorbed by active transport processes in the duodenum and jejunum. Free folate is then carried to the tissues, where a series of complex reactions convert the inactive vitamin to its active coenzyme forms (Lehninger, 1970). First, the pterin ring of folate must be reduced to its dihydro- and then tetrahydrofolate forms. Tetrahydrofolate (THF) has two principal fates. It serves as the acceptor of the β-carbon of serine when the latter is cleaved to glycine (Fig. 22–7). This carbon atom forms a methylene bridge between nitrogen atoms 5 and 10 of THF to yield N^5,N^{10}-methyleneTHF which, in turn, is reduced to N^5-methylTHF. Alternatively, THF may be converted to N^5,N^{10}-methenylTHF, the precursor of the formyl coenzyme forms of THF. These formyl- or methylTHF coenzymes are required for a number of 1-carbon transfer reactions principally concerned with purine and pyrimidine synthesis, methionine synthesis and cyclic interconversion of the folate compounds themselves. It should be emphasized that several other coenzymes participate in these "folate cycles:" pyridoxal phosphate in the decarboxylation of serine; CH_3—B_{12} in the methylation of homocystine to methionine; and NAD and ascorbic acid in the several oxidation-reduction steps.

Folate Deficiency and Dependency. Natural and experimental folic acid deficiency have been produced by dietary restriction and intestinal malabsorp-

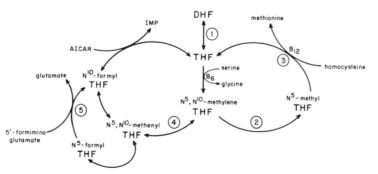

Figure 22–7 Some principal interconversions of folate coenzymes. Numbered reactions refer to enzyme systems discussed in the text: ① dihydrofolate (DHF) reductase; ② N^5,N^{10}-methylene tetrahydrofolate (THF) reductase; ③ N^5-methyl THF methyltransferase; ④ cyclohydrolase; ⑤ formiminotransferase. Other abbreviations: AICAR = 5'-aminoimidazole-4-carboxamide ribonucleotide; IMP = inosinic acid.

doxine (May, 1954). Other causes of deficiency include gastrointestinal malabsorption and the use of drugs such as isoniazid and penicillamine, which act, respectively, by competitive inhibition of PLP kinase (Vilter, 1964) and by the formation of a stable thiazolidine complex (Jaffee et al., 1964).

The diagnosis of B_6 deficiency rests on the demonstration of reduced cellular or extracellular concentrations of the vitamin, its active coenzyme or its catabolite. It is now possible to measure serum and tissue concentrations of pyridoxine and PLP by microbiologic or chemical means, and quantitation of urinary 4-pyridoxic acid also provides a useful measure of B_6 stores (Scriver and Cullen, 1965). Alternatively, indirect means have been used to estimate the adequacy of tissue B_6 content. Assay of PLP-requiring enzymes in serum or tissue has been proposed as a measure of B_6 deficiency, but the usefulness of this approach has been compromised by variability in either the affinity of specific apoenzymes for PLP or in the rate of turnover of particular apoprotein species. Until recently an even more indirect approach has depended on the metabolic response to tryptophan loading (see Chapter 21). B_6-deficient patients excrete increased amounts of kynurenine, hydroxykynurenine and xanthurenic acid because the B_6-requiring steps which catalyze the further breakdown of these tryptophan metabolites are partially blocked. We shall point out subsequently that this test can no longer be considered at all specific for B_6 deficiency.

The clinical manifestations of B_6 deficiency vary considerably with age. In infants, a potentially lethal convulsive disorder dominates the clinical scene. The precise mechanism of such cerebral dysfunction is not clear, but it may be related to reduced activity of glutamic acid decarboxylase, a PLP-cocatalyzed reaction which converts glutamic acid to the inhibitory neurotransmitter, γ-aminobutyric acid (GABA). A deficiency of GABA is then proposed to predispose the brain to hyperirritability and seizures. Adults with confirmed B_6 deficiency may present a vague symptom complex of lassitude, weakness and anorexia along with an iron-resistant microcytic, hypochromic anemia. The basis for these different clinical manifestations of B_6 deficiency in adults and infants has not been determined.

Vitamin B_6 Dependency. The six inherited disorders known to demonstrate B_6 dependency are listed in Table 22-6. None have been associated with any suggestion of B_6 deficiency, and all require 5 to 50 times the usual physiologic dose of B_6 for biochemical and/or clinical improvement. The mutant apoenzyme responsible for these disorders has been defined with the single

Table 22-6 Inherited Aminoacidopathies Demonstrating B_6 Dependency

Disorder	Clinical Hallmarks	Apoenzyme Affected
Infantile convulsions	Seizures	Glutamic acid decarboxylase
Pyridoxine-responsive anemia	Microcytic hypochromic anemia	Undefined
Cystathioninuria	Probably none	Cystathionase
Xanthurenicaciduria	Mental retardation (?)	Kynureninase
Homocystinuria	Ectopia lentis; thrombotic vascular disease; CNS dysfunction	Cystathionine synthase
Hyperoxaluria	Calcium oxalate nephrolithiasis; renal insufficiency	Glyoxylate:α-ketoglutarate carboligase

exception of those patients with pyridoxine-responsive anemia. However, the biochemical basis for the beneficial role of B₆ has been explored in only four of the five conditions where a specific apoenzyme defect is known.

In 1954, Hunt and his associates first described two infant sibs with seizures uncontrolled by anticonvulsants or physiologic doses of B_6. These children responded dramatically to parenteral administration of 5 to 25 mg of pyridoxine, as have more than 40 similar patients described subsequently. Ten years later it was proposed that this classic form of B_6 dependency was caused by a mutation in glutamate decarboxylase such that its interaction with PLP was impaired (Scriver, 1964). Following the demonstration that this enzyme existed in kidney tissue as well as brain (Scriver and Whelan, 1969), a defect in glutamate decarboxylase was confirmed by Yoshida et al. (1971). Of great importance, addition of PLP in vitro led to full correction of decarboxylase activity in the tissue of the affected patient.

Completely analogous results have been reported in two other B_6-responsive disorders: cystathioninuria (see Chapter 11) and xanthurenic aciduria (see Chapter 21). Frimpter (1965) demonstrated that liver homogenates from two patients with cystathioninuria had distinctly reduced cystathionase activity and that addition of pyridoxal phosphate to the incubation medium enhanced enzyme activity significantly (Fig. 22–10). Similarly, Tada et al. (1967, 1968) showed that the defective kynureninase activity found in liver of patients with B_6-responsive xanthurenic aciduria was restored to nearly normal values with in vitro addition of saturating amounts of vitamin B_6 (Fig. 22–10). In these three disorders, then, it seems certain that the mutant enzyme has a much reduced affinity for its coenzyme, PLP, and that holoenzyme activity can be almost totally restored by increasing the amount of PLP available for binding by the apoenzyme.

Such a mutation in apoenzyme affinity for coenzyme does not explain the B_6 responsiveness observed in many patients with homocystinuria due to cystathionine synthase deficiency (Barber and Spaeth, 1967; Yoshida et al., 1968). Several groups have reported that synthase activity in liver or cultured fibroblasts from such patients increases only slightly when PLP is added in vitro (Mudd et al., 1970, Seashore et al., 1972). Mudd (1971) argues convincingly that this small increase in activity (from <1 per cent of normal without PLP to 3 to 4 per cent with PLP) may be sufficient to restore sulfur amino acid metabolism in vivo to an extent compatible with the observed normalization of plasma and urinary concentrations of methionine, homocystine and cystine.

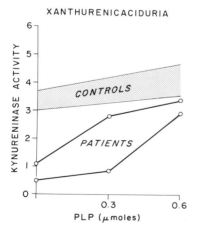

Figure 22–10 Stimulation of hepatic enzyme activity by pyridoxal-5'-phosphate (PLP) in patients with cystathioninuria (left) and xanthurenicaciduria (right). (After Frimpter, G. W.: Science *149*:1095–1096, 1965, copyright 1965, American Association for the Advancement of Science; and Tada, 1968.)

He suggests, furthermore, that in this instance B_6 may be acting to stabilize a mutant synthase apoenzyme rather than to enhance its ability to bind coenzyme. Thus, holoenzyme activity increases because there is more holoenzyme present and not, as in cystathioninuria or B_6-dependent seizures, because the specific activity of each holoenzyme molecule is increased. This intriguing notion can only be tested by purifying and quantitating the amount of synthase present — a task which appears formidable, considering the minute amount of enzyme present in available tissues.

To complete this perusal of B_6-responsive disorders, we must mention a unique infant described in 1963 by Scriver and Hutchison. On a normal B_6 intake, this child grew slowly, had repeated convulsions, was cystathioninuric and responded to an oral tryptophan load with an exaggerated increase in xanthurenic acid output. Activity of glutamic-oxalacetic and glutamic-pyruvic transaminases in serum was normal. The child responded impressively when his diet was supplemented with 2.25 to 2.5 mg pyridoxine per day — only four to five times the normal infant dose. Since several B_6-requiring enzymes were defective in this child, it is possible that he suffered from a derangement in B_6 absorption or coenzyme formation analogous to that discussed previously for B_{12} and folic acid. Studies of serum and tissue B_6 content would be of great interest in such children.

Vitamin-Responsive Disorders of Uncertain Mechanism

Table 22–7 lists all of the known vitamin-responsive disorders which may be related to amino acid metabolism. For several of these conditions, we currently lack information concerning the mechanism of the beneficial vitamin effect. Thus, no enzymatic assays have been done to explore the basis by which large doses of pyridoxine lower urinary oxalate excretion in some patients with primary hyperoxaluria (Smith and Williams, 1967). Similarly, we may assume that biotin-responsive propionicacidemia (Barnes et al., 1970) reflects some enhanced activity of the biotin-requiring enzyme, propionyl-CoA carboxylase, which is defective in this disorder, and that thiamine-responsive branched chain ketoaciduria (Scriver et al., 1971) mirrors a similar enhancement of branched-chain keto acid decarboxylase activity, but these assumptions require confirmation in vitro. Even less information exists for a peculiar X-linked form of anemia which responds to pyridoxine (Horrigan and Harris, 1964). In this instance, we have information concerning neither the biochemical basis for the disease nor the mode of action of B_6.

Finally, we must mention thiamine-responsive lactic acidosis because it may provide an example of still another mechanism of vitamin responsiveness — namely, stimulation of an alternate pathway. Brunette et al. (1972) described a patient with lacticacidosis and hyperalaninemia due to a defect in pyruvate carboxylase, the enzyme which converts pyruvate to oxalacetate. When this girl was given 5 to 20 mg of thiamine daily, accumulation of lactate, pyruvate and alanine was prevented. Importantly, thiamine is *not* the coenzyme for pyruvate carboxylase, but it is one of the cofactors needed in the pyruvate dehydrogenase complex which decarboxylates pyruvate to acetyl-CoA. Since pyruvate dehydrogenase activity was normal in the patient, it was proposed that thiamine may have prevented accumulation of lactate and pyruvate by increasing the rate of pyruvate removal via this alternate dehydrogenase pathway. A similar explanation has been proposed for those patients with the B_6-responsive form of homocystinuria in whom no increase in cystathionine synthase activity has been observed (Seashore et al., 1972), but thus far, no direct evidence supporting disposal of sulfur-containing amino acids by an alternate route has been presented.

Table 22–7 The Vitamin-Responsive Disorders of Amino Acid Metabolism

Vitamin	Disorder	Therapeutic Dose	Biochemical Basis	References
Thiamine (B₁)	Lacticacidosis	5–20 mg	Pyruvate carboxylase deficiency	Brunette et al., 1972
	Branched-chain aminoacidopathy (MSUD variant)	5–20 mg	Branched-chain ketoacid decarboxylase deficiency	Scriver et al., 1971
Pyridoxine (B₆)	Infantile convulsions	10–50 mg	Glutamic acid decarboxylase deficiency	Hunt et al., 1954; Scriver and Whelan, 1969; Yoshida et al., 1971
	Hypochromic anemia	>10 mg	Unknown	Horrigan and Harris, 1964
	Cystathioninuria	100–500 mg	Cystathionase deficiency	Frimpter et al., 1963; Frimpter, 1965
	Xanthurenicaciduria	5–10 mg	Kynureninase deficiency	Knapp, 1960; Tada et al., 1968
	Homocystinuria	25–500 mg	Cystathionine synthase deficiency	Barber and Spaeth, 1967; Mudd et al., 1970; Seashore et al., 1972
	Hyperoxaluria	100–500 mg	Glyoxylate:α-ketoglutarate carboligase deficiency	Smith and Williams, 1967
Cobalamin (B₁₂)	Juvenile pernicious anemia	<5 μg	IF deficiency or defective ileal transport	Mohamed et al., 1965; Katz et al., 1972
	Transcobalamin II deficiency	>100 μg	Deficiency of transcobalamin II	Hakami et al., 1971
	Methylmalonicaciduria	>250 μg	Defective synthesis of Ad—B₁₂ coenzyme	Rosenberg et al., 1968, 1969; Mahoney et al., 1971
	Methylmalonicaciduria, homocystinuria and hypomethininemia	>500 μg	Defective synthesis of Ad—B₁₂ and CH₃—B₁₂ coenzymes	Mudd et al., 1969, 1970; Goodman et al., 1970; Mahoney et al., 1971

Table 22-7 *Continued*

Vitamin	Disorder	Therapeutic Dose	Biochemical Basis	References
Folic acid	Megaloblastic anemia	<0.05 mg	Defective intestinal absorption of folate	Luhby et al., 1961; Lanzkowsky, 1970
	Forminotransferase deficiency	>5 mg	Forminotransferase deficiency	Arakawa et al., 1963; Arakawa, 1970
	Homocystinuria and hypomethioninemia	>10 mg	N^5,N^{10}-methylenetetrahydrofolate reductase deficiency	Mudd et al., 1972; Shih et al., 1972; Freeman et al., 1972
	Congenital megaloblastic anemia	>0.1 mg	Dihydrofolate reductase deficiency	Walters, 1967
Biotin	Propionicacidemia	10 mg	Propionyl-CoA carboxylase deficiency	Barnes et al., 1970
Niacin	Hartnup disease	40–200 mg	Defective intestinal and renal transport of tryptophan and other "neutral" amino acids	Jepson, 1972

GENETIC HETEROGENEITY

It has become almost axiomatic that any abnormal human phenotype has more than a single genotypic basis—or, in other words, that genetic heterogeneity abounds. Using vitamin responsiveness as a probe, such genetic heterogeneity is clearly apparent among the disorders we have been discussing. This genetic diversity is noteworthy because it has very real clinical implications in addition to the obvious chemical and genetic ones. For instance, the fact that some patients with methylmalonicaciduria respond to B_{12} while others do not was of crucial importance in the management of affected children, while at the same time it provided the clue to contrasting mutations affecting mutase apoenzyme structure, on the one hand, and B_{12} coenzyme synthesis, on the other (Mahoney and Rosenberg, 1970). Identical situations exist for nearly all of the vitamin-responsive aminoacidopathies. Thus, the existence of *vitamin-resistant* forms of maple syrup urine disease, cystathioninuria, homocystinuria or propionicacidemia means both that more than a single mutant gene produces the biochemical abnormalities observed and that a therapeutic trial of vitamin supplementation will be necessary to distinguish such patients from their vitamin-responsive fellows.

The genetic heterogeneity extant among these vitamin-responsive disorders takes another form—namely, that a single mutant phenotype may respond to several different vitamins, depending on the nature of the biochemical aberrations. This situation is currently typified by the different vitamin-responsive "homocystinurias." As shown in Figure 22–11, B_6-responsive homocystinuria is observed in patients with cystathionine synthase deficiency; B_{12}-responsive homocystinuria reflects a primary abnormality in CH_3—B_{12} synthesis which secondarily impairs the enzymatic methylation of homocysteine to methionine; and folate-responsive homocystinuria depends on a secondary block in methionine synthesis produced by a primary defect in N^5-methylTHF formation. To the clinician this heterogeneity is important, for he or she must not only know that patients with homocystinuria deserve a trial of vitamin therapy: Now, the alert physician must also know which biochemical constellation calls for which vitamin.

COMMENT

Individually and collectively, the vitamin-responsive inborn errors of metabolism are probably no more or no less rare than the other "Garrodian" hereditary metabolic diseases. With an increased level of awareness among physicians, and greater interest in the potential significance of the hereditary

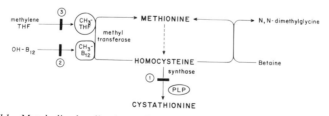

Figure 22–11 Metabolic localization of the three vitamin-responsive "homocystinurias": ① B_6-responsive cystathionine synthase deficiency; ② B_{12}-responsive defect in methyl-B_{12} synthesis; ③ folic acid-responsive N^5,N^{10}-methylenetetrahydrofolate reductase deficiency. See text for further details.

forms of vitamin dependency, it is inevitable that new patients and new vitamin dependencies will be discovered and reported more frequently in the future.

Vitamin-responsive hereditary traits have an appeal that many other genetic diseases do not share because, in theory and in practice, they are eminently treatable. Not every inherited vitamin dependency is a *disease*: for example, it is very likely that cystathioninuria and xanthurenicaciduria are benign traits which initially gained opprobrium because of a bias in the ascertainment of propositi. Nor will every late-diagnosed patient benefit clinically from treatment even though a biochemical response occurs. However, *early* diagnosis, *appropriate* treatment and *careful* supervision combined with genetic counseling could, in theory, eliminate disease resulting from the effect of mutant genes which perturb the normal participation of vitamins in cellular metabolism. We can also anticipate that synthetic forms of vitamin derivatives incorporating the specific molecular features which determine coenzyme activity will become available for therapeutic use.

At least one hazard in the vitamin-dependency success story should be anticipated. We know that too many people take supplementary vitamins for little reason other than the recommendation of an advertisement or upon the advice of physicians who like to prescribe them. Vitamins in excess can be toxic: vitamin D toxicity can cause permanent renal damage (Stickler et al., 1971); vitamin A poisoning causes serious neurological disease (Yaffe and Filer, 1971); nicotinic acid in large doses can provoke tachycardia in about a third of subjects (Ban and Lehmann, 1970). A little vitamin intake is good for us; in fact, it is essential. Does this imply that to take more of a vitamin would be better? Some people believe so, and consequently some of us are being harmed by indiscriminant vitamin intakes. We have the proof that for *some* persons in *particular* circumstances, pharmacologic doses of vitamins are essential. But should we generalize from the specific data in a few special circumstances? We believe that such generalizations *are* being made but without the benefit of evidence equivalent to that obtained in the vitamin-responsive inborn errors of metabolism.

For many diseases, we are still in search of a cause. Psychoses such as schizophrenia, behavioral aberrations and learning disorders, for examples, incapacitate many people and cause immense distress to their families. It is human nature to grasp at straws, and in such circumstances, the publication of promising perspectives which appear to bridge the gap between hope and despair (Pauling, 1968) can be seized and willingly parlayed from hypothesis to dogma. It is more likely than not that *some* patients with "schizophrenia" require vitamins in pharmacological doses (for example, see Freeman et al., 1972), but it is not likely that all patients with this multifactorial disease will respond to vitamins. Similarly, some but not all patients with upper respiratory infections will probably benefit from vitamin C, and some but not all with learning disorders may require vitamin treatment. We hope that the lessons learned from the hereditary vitamin dependencies will help us to recognize the patients with psychosis and behavioral problems who *specifically* need vitamin therapy. When we do this, we will improve the quality of medical practice while observing the dictum *primum non nocere*.

REFERENCES

Arakawa, T.: Congenital defects in folate utilization. Amer. J. Med. *48*:594–598, 1970.

Arakawa, T., Ohara, K., Kudo, Z., Tada, K., Hayashi, T., and Mizuno, T.: Hyperfolicacidemia with formiminoglutamic aciduria following histidine loading. Tohoku J. Exp. Med. *80*:370–382, 1963.

Ban, T. A., and Lehmann, H. E.: Nicotinic acid in the treatment of schizophrenias. Canadian Mental Health Association Collaborated Study. Progress Report I. Canadian Mental Health Association, Toronto, 1970.

Barber, G. W., and Spaeth, G. L.: Pyridoxine therapy in homocystinuria. Lancet (i), 337, 1967.

Barber, K. L., Lee, K. L., and Kenney, F. T.: Turnover of tyrosine transaminase in cultured hepatoma cells after inhibition of protein synthesis. Biochem. Biophys. Res. Commun. *43*: 1132–1138, 1971.

Barnes, N. D., Hull, D., Balgobin, L., and Gompertz, D.: Biotin-responsive propionicacidaemia. Lancet (ii), 244–245, 1970.

Bernstein, L. H., Gutstein, S., Weiner, S., and Efron, G.: The absorption and malabsorption of folic acid and its polyglutamates. Amer. J. Med. *48*:570–579, 1970.

Brunette, M.-G., Delvin, E., Hazel, B., and Scriver, C. R.: Thiamine-responsive lactic acidosis in a patient with deficient low-Km pyruvate carboxylase activity in liver. Pediatrics *50*:702–711, 1972.

Carmel, R., and Herbert, V.: Deficiency of vitamin B_{12}-binding alpha globulin in two brothers. Blood *33*:1–12, 1969.

Cartier, J.: Brief recit et succincte narration de la navigation faicte as ysles de Canada, Hochelage et Saguenay et autres, avec particuliers mews, langaige, et cerimonies des habitans dicelles; fort delectable a veoir (Section sub-tilled d'une grosse maladie . . .) 1545, from facsimile copy of original in British Museum. Ronald Printing Co., Montreal, 1953.

Castle, W. B.: Current concepts of pernicious anemia. Amer. J. Med. *48*:541–548, 1970.

Cazzulo, J. J., Sundaram, T. K., and Kornberg, H. L.: Mechanism of pyruvate carboxylase formation from the apo-enzyme and biotin in a thermophilic bacillus. Nature (London) *227*:1103–1105, 1970.

Federal Register, Washington, D.C., 31FR 15746, December, 1966.

Finkler, A. E., and Hall, C. A.: Nature of the relationship between vitamin B_{12} binding and cell uptake. Arch. Biochem. *120*:79–85, 1967.

Freeman, J. M., Finkelstein, J. D., Mudd, S. H., and Uhlendorf, B. W.: Homocystinuria presenting as reversible "schizophrenia"—a new defect in methionine metabolism with reduced methylene-tetrahydrofolate-reductase activity. (Abstract.) Pediat. Res. *6*:163, 1972.

Frimpter, G. W.: Cystathioninuria; nature of the defect. Science *149*:1095–1096, 1965.

Frimpter, G., Haymovitz, A., and Horwith, M.: Cystathioninuria. New Eng. J. Med. *268*:333, 1963.

Funk, C.: The Vitamins. Williams and Wilkins, Baltimore, 1922.

Garrod, A. E.: Inborn errors of metabolism (Croonian Lectures). Lancet (ii), 1–7, 73–79, 142–148, 214–220, 1908.

Goodman, S. I.: Personal communication, 1973.

Goodman, S. I., Moe, P. G., Hammond, K. B., Mudd, S. H., and Uhlendorf, B. W.: Homocystinuria with methylmalonic aciduria: Two cases in a sibship. Biochem. Med. *4*:500–515, 1970.

Grasbeck, R., Gordin, R., and Kantero, I.: Selective vitamin B_{12} malabsorption and proteinuria in young people: A syndrome. Acta Med. Scand. *167*:289–296, 1960.

Greengard, O.: The role of coenzymes, cortisone and RNA in the control of liver enzyme levels. Advances Enzyme Regulat. *1*:61–76, 1963.

Gyorgy, P.: Vitamin B_2 and pellagra-like dermatitis in rats. Nature (London) *133*:498, 1934.

Hakami, N., Neiman, P. E., Canellos, G. P., and Lazerson, J.: Neonatal megaloblastic anemia due to inherited transcobalamin II deficiency in two siblings. New Eng. J. Med. *285*:1163–1170, 1971.

Hall, C. A.: Transport of vitamin B_{12} in man. Brit. J. Haemat. *16*:429–433, 1969.

Hall, C. A., and Finkler, A. E.: The dynamics of transcobalamin II. A vitamin B_{12} binding substance in plasma. J. Lab. Clin. Med. *65*:459–468, 1965.

Hodgkin, D. C., Pickworth, J., Robertson, J. H., Trueblood, K. N., Prosen, R. J., White, J. G., Bonnett, R., Cannon, J. R., Johnson, A. W., Sutherland, I., Todd, A. R., and Smith, E. L.: The crystal structure of the hexacarboxylic acid derived from B_{12} and the molecular structure of the vitamin. Nature (London) *176*:325–328, 1955.

Hom, B. L.: Plasma turnover of [57]cobalt-vitamin B_{12} bound to transcobalamin I and II. Scand. J. Haemat. *4*:321–332, 1967.

Horrigan, D. L., and Harris, J. W.: Pyridoxine-responsive anemia: Analysis of sixty-one cases. Advances Intern. Med. *12*:103–174, 1964.

Hsia, Y. E., Lilljeqvist, A.-Ch., and Rosenberg, L. E.: Vitamin B_{12}-dependent methylmalonicaciduria: Amino acid toxicity, long chain ketonuria, and protective effect of vitamin B_{12}. Pediatrics *46*:497–507, 1970.

Hunt, A. D., Jr., Stokes, J., Jr., McCrory, W. W., and Stroud, H. H.: Pyridoxine dependency: Report of a case of intractable convulsions in an infant controlled by pyridoxine. Pediatrics *13*:140–145, 1954.

Jaffe, I., Altman, K., and Merryman, P.: Antipyridoxine effect of penicillamine in man. J. Clin. Invest. *43*:1869–1873, 1964.

Jepson, J. B.: Hartnup disease. *In* Stanbury, J. B., Wyngaarden, J. B., and Fredrickson, D. S., eds.,

The Metabolic Basis of Inherited Disease, 3rd edition. McGraw-Hill, New York, pp. 1486–1503, 1972.

Katz, M., Lee, S. K., and Cooper, B. A.: Vitamin B_{12} malabsorption due to a biologically inert intrinsic factor. New Eng. J. Med. *287*:425–429, 1972.

Kerwar, S. S., Spears, C., McAuslan, B., and Weissbach, H.: Studies on vitamin B_{12} metabolism in HeLa cells. Arch. Biochem. *142*:231–237, 1971.

Knapp, A.: Über eine neue Hereditäre von Vitamin-B_6 abhängige Störung im Tryptophan-stoffwechsel. Clin. Chim. Acta 5:6–13, 1960.

Lanzkowsky, P.: Congenital malabsorption of folate. Amer. J. Med. *48*:580–583, 1970.

Lehninger, A.: Biochemistry. Worth Publishers, Inc., New York, 1970.

Lin, E. C. C., Civen, M., and Knox, W. E.: Effect of vitamin B_6 deficiency on the basal and adapted levels of rat liver tyrosine and tryptophan transaminases. J. Biol. Chem. *233*:1183–1185, 1958.

Luhby, A. L., Engle, F. J., Roth, E., and Cooperman, J. M.: Relapsing megaloblastic anemia in an infant due to a specific defect in gastrointestinal absorption of folic acid. Amer. J. Dis. Child. *102*:482–483, 1961.

Mahoney, M. J.: Personal communication, 1973.

Mahoney, M. J., and Rosenberg, L. E.: Inherited defects of B_{12} metabolism. Amer. J. Med. *48*:584–593, 1970.

Mahoney, M. J., Rosenberg, L. E., Mudd, S. H., and Uhlendorf, B. W.: Defective metabolism of vitamin B_{12} in fibroblasts from children with methylmalonicaciduria. Biochem. Biophys. Res. Commun. *44*:375–381, 1971.

May, C. D.: Vitamin B_6 in human nutrition: A critique and an object lesson. Pediatrics *14*:269, 1954.

Minot, G. R., and Murphy, L. P.: Treatment of pernicious anemia by special diet. J.A.M.A. *87*:470–476, 1926.

Mohamed, S. D., McKay, E., and Galloway, W. H.: Juvenile familial megaloblastic anemia due to selective malabsorption of vitamin B_{12}. Quart. J. Med. *35*:433–453, 1966.

Mudd, S. H.: Pyridoxine-responsive genetic disease. Fed. Proc. *30*:970–976, 1971.

Mudd, S. H., Edwards, W. A., Loeb, P. M., Brown, M. S., and Laster, L.: Homocystinuria due to cystathionine synthase deficiency: The effect of pyridoxine. J. Clin. Invest. *49*:1762–1773, 1970.

Mudd, S. H., Levy, H. L., and Abeles, R. H.: A derangement in B_{12} metabolism leading to homocystinuria, cystathioninemia and methylmalonicaciduria. Biochem. Biophys. Res. Commun. *35*:121–126, 1969.

Mudd, S. H., Uhlendorf, B. W., Freeman, J. M., Finkelstein, J. D., and Shih, V. E.: Homocystinuria associated with decreased methylenetetrahydrofolate reductase activity. Biochem. Biophys. Res. Commun. *46*:905–912, 1972.

Mudd, S. H., Uhlendorf, B. W., Hinds, K. R., and Levy, H. L.: Deranged B_{12} metabolism: Studies of fibroblasts grown in tissue culture. Biochem. Med. *4*:215–239, 1970b.

National Academy of Sciences, National Research Council, Food and Nutrition Board: Recommended Dietary Allowances, 7th edition. National Academy of Sciences Printing and Publishing Office, Washington, D.C., Publ. 1146, 1968.

Needham, J.: Frederick Gowland Hopkins, Perspect. Biol. Med. *6*:2–46, 1962. (Note Fig. 1–18.)

Northrop, D. B.: Transcarboxylase VI kinetic analysis of the reaction mechanism. J. Biol. Chem. *244*:5808–5819, 1969.

Pauling, L.: Orthomolecular psychiatry. Science *160*:265–271, 1968.

Pletsch, Q. A., and Coffey, J. W.: Intracellular distribution of radioactive vitamin B_{12} in rat liver. J. Biol. Chem. *246*:4619–4629, 1971.

Pletsch, Q. A., and Coffey, J. W.: Properties of the proteins that bind vitamin B_{12} in subcellular fractions of rat liver. Arch. Biochem. *151*:157–167, 1972.

Rickes, F. L., Brink, N. G., Koniuszy, F. R., Wood, T. R., and Folkers, K.: Crystalline vitamin B_{12}. Science *107*:396–397, 1948.

Rosenberg, L. E.: Vitamin dependent genetic disease. Hosp. Prac. 1970. 5:59–67.

Rosenberg, L. E., Lilljeqvist, A.-Ch., and Allen, R. H.: Transcobalamin II-facilitated uptake of vitamin B_{12} by cultured fibroblasts: Studies in methylmalonicaciduria. J. Clin. Invest., *52*:69a–70a (abstract), 1973.

Rosenberg, L. E., Lilljeqvist, A.-Ch., and Hsia, Y. E.: Methylmalonic aciduria: Metabolic block localization and vitamin B_{12} dependency. Science *162*:805–807, 1968.

Rosenberg, L. E., Lilljeqvist, A.-Ch., Hsia, Y. E., and Rosenbloom, F. M.: Vitamin B_{12} dependent methylmalonicaciduria: Defective B_{12} metabolism in cultured fibroblasts. Biochem. Biophys. Res. Commun. *4*:607–614, 1969.

Rosenberg, L. E., and Mahoney, M. J.: Inherited disorders of methylmalonate and vitamin B_{12} metabolism: A progress report. *In* Hommes, F. A., and van der Berg, C. J., eds., Symposium on Developmental Biochemistry—Inborn Errors of Metabolism. Elsevier, Amsterdam, 1973. (In press.)

Scriver, C. R.: Comment on vitamin B$_6$ deficiency and dependency syndromes. *In* Gellis, S., ed., Year Book of Pediatrics, 1963–64 series. Year Book Publishers, Chicago, 1964.

Scriver, C. R.: Vitamin B$_6$ deficiency and dependency in man. Amer. J. Dis. Child *113*:109–114, 1967.

Scriver, C. R., and Cullen, A. M.: Urinary vitamin B$_6$ and 4-pyridoxic acid in health and in vitamin B$_6$ dependency. Pediatrics *36*:14–20, 1965.

Scriver, C. R., and Hutchison, J. H.: The vitamin B$_6$ deficiency syndrome in human infancy, biochemical and clinical observations. Pediatrics *31*:240–250, 1963.

Scriver, C. R., Mackenzie, S., Clow, C. L., and Delvin, E.: Thiamine-responsive maple-syrup urine disease. Lancet (i), 310–312, 1971.

Scriver, C. R., and Whelan, D. T.: Glutamic acid decarboxylase (GAD) in mammalian tissue outside the central nervous system, and its possible relevance to hereditary vitamin B$_6$ dependency with seizures. Ann. N.Y. Acad. Sci. *166*:83–96, 1969.

Seashore, M. R., Durant, J. L., and Rosenberg, L. E.: Studies of the mechanism of pyridoxine-responsive homocystinuria. Pediat. Res. *6*:187–196, 1972.

Shih, V. E., Salam, M. Z., Mudd, S. H., Uhlendorf, B. W., and Adams, R. D.: A new form of homocystinuria due to N^{5,10}-methylene tetrahydrofolate reductase deficiency. (Abstract.) Pediat. Res. *6*:135, 1972.

Smith, E. L., and Parker, L. F. J.: Purification of anti-pernicious anemia factor. Biochem. J. *43*: VIII, 1948.

Smith, L. H., Jr., and Williams, H. E.: Treatment of primary hyperoxaluria. Mod. Treatm. *4*:522–530, 1967.

Snell, E. E.: Chemical structures in relation to biological activity of vitamin B$_6$. Vitamins Hormones (N.Y.) *16*:77–125, 1958.

Snell, E. E., and Hashell, B. E.: Metabolism of water-soluble vitamins. The metabolism of vitamin B$_6$. *In* Florkin, M., and Stotz, E. N., eds., Comprehensive Biochemistry. Elsevier, New York, *21*:47–71, 1971.

Spurling, C. L., Sacks, M. S., and Jiji, R. M.: Juvenile pernicious anemia. New Eng. J. Med. *271*: 995–1003, 1964.

Stickler, G. B., Jowsey, J., and Bianco, A. J.: Possible detrimental effect of large doses of vitamin D in familial hypophosphatemic vitamin D resistant rickets. J. Pediat. *79*:68–71, 1971.

Tada, K., Yokoyama, Y., Nakagawa, H., and Arakawa, T.: Vitamin B$_6$ dependent xanthurenic aciduria (the second report). Tohoku J. Exp. Med. *95*:107–114, 1968.

Tada, K., Yokoyama, Y., Nakagawa, H., Yoshida, T., and Arakawa, T.: Vitamin B$_6$ dependent xanthurenic aciduria. Tohoku J. Exp. Med. *93*:115–124, 1967.

Vilter, R. W.: Vitamin B$_6$-hydrazide relationship. Vitamins Hormones (N.Y.) *22*:797–805, 1964.

Vitols, E., Walker, G. A., and Huennekens, F. M.: Enzymatic conversion of vitamin B$_{12s}$ to a cobamide coenzyme, α-(5,6-dimethylbenzimidazolyl) deoxyadenosylcobamide (adenosyl-B$_{12}$). J. Biol. Chem. *241*:1455–1461, 1966.

Walker, G. A., Murphy, S., and Huennekens, F. M.: Enzymatic conversion of vitamin B$_{12}$ to adenosyl-B$_{12}$: Evidence for the existence of two separate reducing systems. Arch. Biochem. *134*:95–102, 1969.

Walters, T. R.: Congenital megaloblastic anemia responsive to N^5-formyltetrahydrofolic acid administration. J. Pediat. *70*:686–687, 1967.

World Health Organization Technical Report: Series 1967, No. 362. Requirements of vitamin A, thiamine, riboflavin, and niacin. Report of a Joint FAO/WHO Expert. Group, Geneva, 1967.

World Health Organization Technical Report: Series 1970, No. 452. Requirements of ascorbic acid, vitamin D, vitamin B$_{12}$, folate and iron. Report of a Joint FAO/WHO Expert. Group, Geneva, 1970.

Wyngaarden, J. B.: Genetic control of enzyme activity in higher organisms. Biochem. Genet. *4*: 105–125, 1970.

Yaffe, S. J., and Filer, L. E., et al. (Joint Committee Statement—Committees on Drugs and Nutrition, American Academy of Pediatrics): The use and abuse of vitamin A. Pediatrics *48*:655–656, 1971.

Yoshida, T., Tada, K., and Arakawa, T.: Vitamin B$_6$ dependency of glutamic acid decarboxylase in the kidney from a patient with vitamin B$_6$ dependent convulsion. Tohoku J. Exp. Med. *104*:195–198, 1971.

Yoshida, T., Tada, K., Yokoyama, Y., and Arakawa, T.: Homocystinuria and vitamin B$_6$ dependent type. Tohoku J. Exp. Med. *96*:235–242, 1968.

Index

Note: Numbers in *italic* refer to illustrations; numbers followed by (t) refer to tables.

479